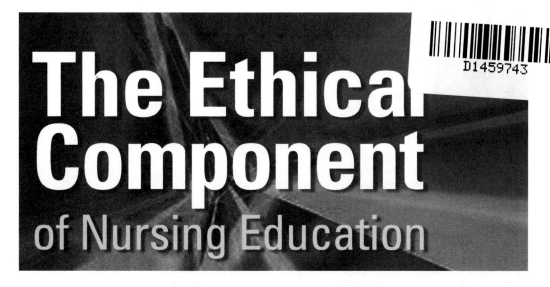

The Ethical Component
of Nursing Education

Integrating Ethics Into Clinical Experience

Marcia Sue DeWolf Bosek, DNSc, RN
Associate Professor
Department of Adult Health Nursing
Rush University College of Nursing
Program in Ethics, Department of Religion, Health & Human Values
Rush University College of Health Sciences
Chicago, Illinois

Teresa A. Savage, PhD, RN
Assistant Professor–Research
Maternal–Child Nursing, College of Nursing
University of Illinois at Chicago
Associate Director
Donnelley Family Disability Ethics Program
Rehabilitation Institute of Chicago
Chicago, Illinois

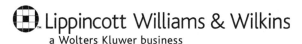
Lippincott Williams & Wilkins
a Wolters Kluwer business
Philadelphia · Baltimore · New York · London
Buenos Aires · Hong Kong · Sydney · Tokyo

Senior Acquisitions Editor: Elizabeth Nieginski
Managing Editor: Michelle Clarke
Editorial Assistant: Delema Caldwell-Jackson
Production Project Manager: Cynthia Rudy
Director of Nursing Production: Helen Ewan
Senior Managing Editor / Production: Erika Kors
Art Director: Joan Wendt
Manufacturing Coordinator: Karin Duffield
Production Services / Compositor: TechBooks
Printer: R.R. Donnelley–Crawfordsville

9 8 7 6 5 4 3 2 1

Library of Congress Cataloging-in-Publication Data

Bosek, Marcia Sue DeWolf.
  The ethical component of nursing education : integrating ethics into
clinical experience / Marcia Sue DeWolf Bosek, Teresa A. Savage.
     p. ; cm.
  Includes bibliographical references and index.
  ISBN 0-7817-4877-1 (alk. paper)
  1. Nursing ethics—Study and teaching. 2. Medical ethics—Study and
teaching. I. Savage, Teresa A. II. Title.
  [DNLM: 1. Ethics, Nursing—education. 2. Education, Nursing.
3. Ethics, Clinical—education.   RT85.B67 2006]
RT85.B67 2006
174.207—dc22

                                              2005032588

Care has been taken to confirm the accuracy of the information presented and to describe generally accepted practices. However, the authors, editors, and publisher are not responsible for errors or omissions or for any consequences from application of the information in this book and make no warranty, express or implied, with respect to the content of the publication.

The authors, editors, and publisher have exerted every effort to ensure that drug selection and dosage set forth in this text are in accordance with the current recommendations and practice at the time of publication. However, in view of ongoing research, changes in government regulations, and the constant flow of information relating to drug therapy and drug reactions, the reader is urged to check the package insert for each drug for any change in indications and dosage and for added warnings and precautions. This is particularly important when the recommended agent is a new or infrequently employed drug.

Some drugs and medical devices presented in this publication have Food and Drug Administration (FDA) clearance for limited use in restricted research settings. It is the responsibility of the health care provider to ascertain the FDA status of each drug or device planned for use in his or her clinical practice.

LWW.com

To Jim and Art
For believing that this book was a reality even before it was written

In Honor of Our Mothers
Elnere K. DeWolf and Jeanne M. Jacobs
who taught us about living and dying

and Our Fathers
Thaddeus N. DeWolf and William F. Jacobs
who are showing us how to persevere

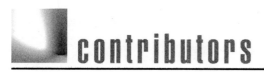# contributors

Kristin Nelson, MA
Assistant Professor
Program in Ethics, Department of Religion, Health, & Human Values
Rush University College of Health Sciences
Chicago, Illinois

Deborah Jezuit, DNSc, RN
Director of Nursing Education
College of Lake County
Grayslake, Illinois

reviewers

Pamela Altman, RN, MN, BC
Instructor
Nell Hodgson Woodruff School of Nursing
Emory University
Atlanta, Georgia

Catherine Batscha, RN, MAAPRN, ANCC
Clinical Instructor
University of Illinois at Chicago, College of Nursing
Chicago, Illinois

Cheryl Crisp, MSN, RN, APRN, BC, CDDN, CRRN
Pediatric Clinical Nurse Specialist/Research Associate
Indiana University School of Nursing
Indianapolis, Indiana

Elizabeth Gabzdyl, CNM, MSN
Clinical Instructor
University of Illinois at Chicago, College of Nursing
Chicago, Illinois

Carrie Gordy, MSN, RN, ARNP
Assistant Professor
University of Kentucky, College of Nursing
Lexington, Kentucky

Kathleen Heneghan, RN, MSN
Assistant Professor/Clinical Nurse Specialist
Department of Women's & Children's Health Nursing
Rush University College of Nursing
Assistant Director of Patient Education
American College of Surgeons
Chicago, Illinois

Andrea M. Kline, RN, MS, PCCNP, PNP-AC, CCRN
Pediatric Critical Care Nurse Practitioner
Children's Memorial Hospital
Chicago, Illinois

Olimpia Paun, PhD, APRN, BC
Assistant Professor
Department of Community & Mental Health Nursing
Rush University College of Nursing
Chicago, Illinois

Elaine Scorza, MS, RN, APRN, BC
Instructor
Department of Community & Mental Health Nursing
Rush University College of Nursing
Clinical Nurse Coordinator
Psychiatric Services
Rush University Medical Center
Chicago, Illinois

Rebekah Shepard, MS, APRN
Assistant Professor
Department of Adult Health Nursing
Department of Community & Mental Health Nursing
Rush University College of Nursing
Chicago, Illinois

Linda Spencer, PhD, RN
Director of Public Health Nursing Leadership Program
Nell Hodgson Woodruff School of Nursing
Emory University
Atlanta, Georgia

preface

The Ethical Component of Nursing Education: Integrating Ethics Into Clinical Experiences is different from other ethics textbooks on two accounts—it is based on the philosophy that ethics is embedded in relationships and interactions between nurses and patients, and that ethics education should be integrated into clinical nursing education. On the first account, ethics is often relegated to "crisis" situations involving life-and-death decisions. Ethics in nursing practice is much more than that. On a daily basis, nurses are faced with situations that raise questions about ethical commitments as well as challenge the traditional definition of "what is right and ought to be done." Additionally, changes in the healthcare system and society are creating new ethical situations never experienced before by nurses. We hope to have captured this wide diversity of ethics in this textbook.

On the second account, most nursing programs do not have a dedicated required ethics course for nursing students; rather, ethics is integrated into all nursing courses, especially clinical practica. Didactic and clinical instructors should find this textbook invaluable in guiding their instruction to capitalize on teachable moments. A teachable moment is one in which the instructor and student are (often serendipitously) provided a situation that highlights or challenges an ethical commitment. The challenge of capitalizing on teachable moments is that these moments are often unplanned and intermingled with other teaching content (such as pathophysiology or therapeutic communication), which can divert the student's/instructor's attention away from the ethical content. In addition, many clinical instructors, while skilled clinicians themselves, may never have taken an ethics course or had the opportunity to engage in ethical reflection about clinical situations in which they have been involved. Thus, many teachable moments might be missed because of lack of awareness.

Several teaching methods can be used to create teachable moments. First, a teachable moment can be created by the clinical instructor during pre- and/or post-conferences and/or guided student reflection via journaling or online discussions. Second, a teachable moment can be created by providing a guided activity that a student could engage in during clinical "down time," when assigned nursing interventions are completed and a student might find him/herself looking for something to do. Therefore, in each chapter we have included a variety of activities a student could complete in the clinical setting to maximize clinical opportunities; we have also posed a variety of discussion questions. When assigning clinical activities and discussion questions, clinical instructors should note that these activities and questions are presented with varying levels of complexity. We hope that by presenting different levels of complexity, this text will be useful to students throughout their academic program of study, regardless of the degree (associate's, bachelor's, or BSN completion) being sought. Finally, each chapter suggests printed and electronic resources that students and clinical instructors can consult for further information and guidance.

Unit 1 is composed of five chapters that are fundamental to clinical ethics. The language that is necessary to understand and communicate ethical issues is introduced in

Chapter 1. Chapter 2, History of Clinical Ethics, gives a rich background for understanding current ethical thinking and approaches. Chapter 3 helps put in context how ethics is integrated into clinical nursing practice through development of and adherence to standards of practice. The focus of Chapter 4 is on nursing students and the potential ethical situations they may face during their academic careers. Not only do we wish to prepare students for their roles as registered professional nurses, we also hope to offer meaningful exercises to help them address these unique ethical situations. Chapter 5 brings the conceptual issues and ideas into practical application. What is ethical decision making and how does one do it, or facilitate it in others? The ethical decision-making format may appear linear, but we encourage instructors and students to employ a linear approach only as an instructional format. Ethical issues are often complex and require a "peeling of the onion" process to find and sort out the medical, nursing, and contextual issues involved in an ethical situation.

Unit 2 offers an in-depth discussion of research ethics and ethical themes that recur in nursing practice. The themes are derivative of ethical principles, but we believe this language makes the concepts more accessible to students. Chapters 6, 7, and 8—Confidentiality, Truthtelling, and Advocacy—are derivative of autonomy, beneficence, and non-maleficence. Chapter 9, Allocation of Resources, is derivative of justice. Chapter 10 covers research ethics, providing an historical perspective as well as a tutorial on what nurses need to know about the topic. Whether recruiting, consenting, collecting data, or acting as principal investigator, nurses need to appreciate the differences between, and intersection of, clinical ethics and research ethics. Chapter 10 also illustrates how the common ethical themes apply to a non-clinical nursing context.

Unit 3 takes each traditional clinical rotation that nursing students experience and discusses the usual, and sometimes unusual, ethical issues that may occur in those specific settings. Although much of clinical practica occur in acute care hospitals, each chapter addresses various practice settings, for example, intensive care, the emergency department, an outpatient clinic, school, or home. Associate degree programs might not have a public health rotation, but they may incorporate home health nursing in the nursing of children or adult health practica. Some nursing programs may offer electives for students who are interested in a critical care area, such as neonatal intensive care or surgical intensive care. Chapter 11, Nursing of Children and Adolescents, discusses neonatal cases, and Chapter 12, Nursing of the Adult, includes critical care cases. Not all venues for nursing practice have been included, but it is likely that the concepts discussed in these chapters will translate to other practice areas. Given that the sequence of clinical rotations varies after the nursing fundamentals clinical experience, the clinical chapters can be used out of sequence. Our intention in these chapters was to reexamine the common ethical themes in more breadth and depth, as well as to highlight specific ethical issues that a student or practicing nurse might frequently encounter or need to be cognizant of when practicing in a specific clinical arena. This in-depth presentation could be applicable for graduate students (since there is a dearth of graduate nursing ethics curricula), but we believe that the clinical issues discussed are appropriate for the beginning nurse.

Unit 4 wraps up the book with two chapters focusing on ethical issues impacting the professional nurse's individual and professional values that cross practice settings. The work environment, workplace issues such as shift work and 24/7 coverage, scope of responsibilities, and other issues relevant to the profession of nursing are introduced.

In Units 3 and 4, the individual chapter format changes. Each chapter is divided into four sections. Section One is always Ethical Themes: Building from the Basic to the

Complex. In this section, the four common themes originally presented in Unit 2 are expanded upon and simultaneously focused to the specific clinical setting. The rationale for this teaching strategy is that students have the tendency to label content as redundant if the concept or term has been presented in a previous course or context. However, many ethical concepts and situations occur across practice settings; thus, redundancy can be an effective teaching tool. For example, a student may understand the principle of confidentiality with an adult, but may not understand the importance of confidentiality while working with an adolescent or a person with a mental illness. We believe it is useful to compare and contrast ethical concepts as the student's clinical education progresses through different patient groups and settings. Thus, our hope is that the inclusion of Ethical Themes: Building from the Basic to the Complex in each chapter is not redundant, but rather an effective teaching strategy that deepens and broadens a student's understanding. The remaining three sections of each chapter in Units 3 and 4 focus on ethical issues that frequently occur in the designated practice setting. Each section includes clinical activities and discussion questions, with resources presented collectively at the end of each chapter.

The impetus for this book was the frequent comments we and other nursing instructors have made about needing a book for teaching ethics in the clinical context. There are many wonderful books on ethics in nursing, and even more articles, and an ethics "junkie" could spend years reading them. We wanted a single reference that had enough depth so as not to treat issues superficially, but not so huge as to be prohibitively expensive or heavy. Additionally, we recognized that for any textbook to effectively integrate ethics into the clinical experience, the content had to be presented in a fashion that students could realistically read before or during the clinical experience. We hope students will indeed find this book useful not only throughout their clinical nursing program, but also into their first years of practice.

A word about the authors: We both pursued graduate degrees with an interest in ethics. We have worked as staff nurses, rotated shifts, and have been charge nurses. We have worked in various practice settings: neonatal intensive care, pediatric neurology, medical/surgical, cardiac, HIV/AIDS, and geriatric extended care. Both of us have taught at two or more baccalaureate nursing programs and have precepted master's and doctoral students pursuing degrees with a concentration in ethics. One of us (TAS) worked as a clinical nurse specialist in pediatric neurology/developmental disabilities for many years. Both of us conduct research in ethics and serve as ethics consultants at major medical centers. We often find we are polar opposites in our views, yet our differences serve to inform and educate us. Because we have differing views, we hope that our individual biases have been balanced by our collaborative effort in writing this text. We hope that our book reflects our passion for nursing ethics. Finally, we hope that students and clinical instructors find this textbook to be pragmatic, yet idealistic and inspiring.

Marcia Bosek
Teresa Savage

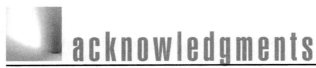

acknowledgments

The creation of this book has been impacted by many individuals. In particular, we want to thank Margaret Zuccarini for mentoring us through proposal development; Dr. Deborah Jezuit and Kristin Nelson for sharing their professional expertise; the many editors who were assigned to our book; the numerous reviewers who critically read our drafts; and Michelle Clarke for shepherding the manuscript to production. Finally, we would be remiss not to acknowledge the countless patients, families, healthcare professionals, nurse educators, and nursing students who have contributed to our understanding of nursing ethics and the realities associated with integrating ethics into nursing education.

contents

Unit 3

Clinical Ethics Issues   *181*

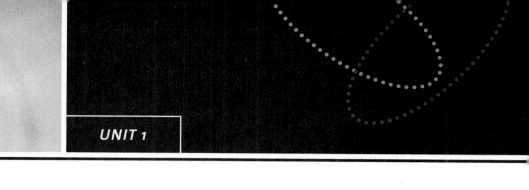

Components of
Clinical Ethics

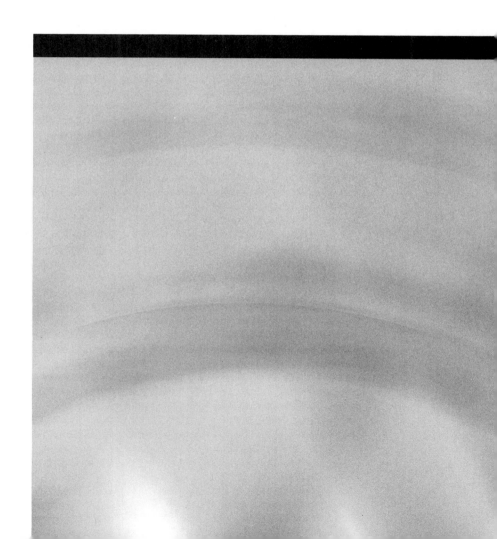

CHAPTER 1

Ethical Theories and Principles

Objectives

At the end of this chapter, the student should be able to:

1. Explain the basic premise of each major theory of ethics.
2. Identify appeals to each of these theories when they are presented in a discussion about patient care.
3. Discuss the strengths and failings of each theory as they apply to particular situations.
4. Explain the basic premise of each principle.
5. Apply each of these principles to specific patient care cases.
6. Identify conflicts among principles when applied to a case.
7. Weigh conflicting principles against one another and determine which is most compelling in a given case.

KEY WORDS

- *Advocacy*
- *Autonomy*
- *Beneficence*
- *Communitarianism*
- *Compassion*
- *Confidentiality*
- *Consequentialism*
- *Decisional capacity*
- *Deontology*
- *Due diligence*
- *Double effect*
- *Ethics of care*

- *Fidelity*
- *Informed consent*
- *Justice*
- *Nonmaleficence*
- *Paternalism*
- *Privacy*
- *Proportionality*
- *Respect*
- *Supererogation*
- *Utilitarianism*
- *Veracity*

ETHICAL THEORIES

The test of a useful theory of ethics is its ability to make sense of the world and provide guidance about how to act in it. Theories of ethics abound, and no single ethical theory has managed to capture and explain all the important elements of the moral world to the satisfaction of all or even most people. The four ethical theories discussed in this section have endured over time as ones that capture a fundamental truth about the world and the way we ought to act.

Utilitarianism

What do we mean when we talk about "doing the right thing?" Some people think that to do the right thing means to act with the intention of doing good. Thus, a person is doing the right thing (acting ethically) when he or she does something from the right intention, such as helping another person or preventing harm to another. Others claim that having a good intention is not enough. It also matters what people do and what the outcomes of their actions are.

Utilitarianism is a form of ethical theory that is concerned with the outcomes of actions. Utilitarians claim that it is the action itself that is right or wrong, not the person performing the action. As such, it is a form of a more general theory called "consequentialism." Simply put, consequentialist theories are concerned with the consequences of actions and judge whether an action is right by whether it has good consequences. All consequentialist theories share this basic foundation. Where they differ is in defining what a "good" consequence is.

A type of consequentialist theory that has become powerful in bioethics is utilitarianism. Utilitarianism as we know it began with Jeremy Bentham (1748–1832) and was refined by John Stuart Mill (1806–1873). Bentham introduced both the name "utilitarianism" and the most-recognized statement of its central thesis: The greatest happiness of the greatest number is the measure of right and wrong. This statement comes from a work Bentham published in 1776 (Bentham, 1776/1988), and it is common to hear people today use the phrase "the greatest good for the greatest number" as a rationale for social policies and practice. Though the phrase is used liberally, most people do not give much thought to what it really means. If pressed, most of us could come up with some definition for what we mean by "good" when using that phrase. For Bentham, the "good" is defined very simply as "happiness." He claimed that happiness was something that could be calculated by measuring and adding up pleasure and subtracting pain. Thus any action that brings about greater happiness for more people is a right action under Bentham's brand of utilitarianism. Mill refined this idea and strengthened the notion that pleasure and freedom from pain are the only two things desirable as ends in themselves. Mill defined utilitarianism in the second chapter of his work *Utilitarianism:*

The creed which accepts as the foundations of morals, Utility, or the Greatest Happiness Principle, holds that actions are right in proportion as they tend to promote happiness, wrong as they tend to produce the reverse of happiness. By happiness is intended pleasure, and the absence of pain; by unhappiness, pain, and the privation of pleasure. (Mill, 1863/1998, p. 14)

According to Mill, everything else we desire is desired because, ultimately, it brings us pleasure or freedom from pain.

Originally, utilitarian theories were designed for and applied to legislative matters. Most of the thought that went into utilitarian theory came from social and legal perspectives about the best ways to conduct a state and govern people. It is easy to see how this theory can be applied to other realms of moral life and why it has become particularly attractive in the realm of bioethics. First, many of the ethical problems we face in medicine are directly about people's happiness:

- The very term "quality of life" acknowledges that pleasure and pain are variables in life and need to be assessed as other life conditions change.
- It is in the forefront of decisions about withdrawing or withholding treatment as a means to end suffering.
- One reason to respect autonomy is the idea that only the patient can make an accurate determination about what course of action will bring him or her the greatest happiness, and we should therefore accept that determination as reflective of the greatest good.

Second, in medical ethics we are inevitably concerned with the distribution of medical resources. Although we do not generally have to make these decisions at the patient's bedside, we do need to be prepared to address these issues in a larger context and understand their implications for patient care. Distributing resources so that the greatest number of people can get the most benefit from them is a direct application of utilitarian theory.

Utilitarianism has been criticized as being too simplistic and unable to adequately cope with the complexities of real-life situations. We will examine three of these claims.

Utilitarianism requires us to do whatever act will bring about the greatest good, even if that means doing something we would otherwise consider immoral.

If we can bring about a good, then, according to utilitarian theory, we are required to do that action. However, there are some goods that can be achieved only through means that most of us would consider wrong. For instance, there may be times when a patient asks that her family not be informed of her diagnosis or prognosis because the patient does not want to worry them and fears the disruption in their lives that such information would bring. Yet it may seem that the family could provide valuable support for the patient. In fact you may know this particular family well enough to know that telling them about the patient's illness would bring more support and hence greater well-being to the patient than not telling. By utilitarian reasoning, it would be not just acceptable, but required, that you disclose this information to the family. However, respecting patient confidentiality is an important element of patient care. Even if you were right in your assessment of the situation, most clinicians would agree that it is absolutely wrong to disclose patient information without the patient's consent. Thus, following utilitarian reasoning could put one in a situation in which breaking ethical standards is required. This is a strong indictment of utilitarianism.

One way that utilitarians have addressed this problem is to adopt a rule-utilitarian stance. In this formulation of utilitarianism, instead of deciding what action will bring about the greatest good in each situation, rule-utilitarians advocate following a set of rules that are designed so that in most situations following them will produce the greatest amount of good overall. In the foregoing example, a rule-utilitarian would reply that, in general, disclosing confidential patient information would bring about more harm than good and therefore one should always follow the general rule of maintaining confidentiality.

True calculations of happiness are impossible.

Another criticism of utilitarianism is that in practice it is impossible for an individual or even a group to accurately calculate all the pleasure and freedom from pain that any specific act will entail. For one thing, we can never be completely sure that our actions will produce their intended results. Second, even if they do produce the desired outcome, how can we foresee all the implications of these actions and assess the effects they will have on all people, however remotely connected to the act or its outcome? In considering the total calculation of pleasure and pain, it is imperative to account for all people who will be affected by the action both now and in the future. Some acts will have implications for large groups of people over great spans of time. Then, too, there is the cumulative effect to consider. Actions do not happen in a vacuum. The social context needs to be considered. Critics argue that these are not all within the ability of the utilitarian theorist to foresee when determining what consequences a particular action will have.

Supporters of utilitarianism generally reply to this criticism by pointing out that even though not all consequences are foreseeable, the major ones are. For most situations, most of the time, a reasonable enough calculation can be made.

Utilitarianism does not consider issues of distributive justice.

Utilitarianism only requires that happiness be maximized, not that there be any sense of fairness regarding who gets to be happy. In the general formulation of utilitarianism, it is equally as legitimate to make rich people happy by buying them yachts as it is to make poor people happy by buying them homes. In health care this would mean there is no rationale for distributing resources other than to make sure that the resources do some good. Most people feel that there should be some consideration given to benefiting the least well off in society before adding resources for those who already have access to a basic minimum of health care.

There have been suggestions for changes to basic utilitarian theory to address this concern, but there is no agreement about them, and for someone who is really committed to utilitarianism, this issue may not be a concern. The only good in utilitarian theory is the maximization of pleasure and freedom from pain. Fairness is not a basic good, but may be considered a lower-level good if, in general, promoting fairness also promotes pleasure and freedom from pain. So a utilitarian would argue that if this is the case, if fairness or justice is generally a method of increasing happiness, then this is a suitable goal and can be made a criterion for distributing health care resources, not because justice or fairness is good in and of itself, but because promoting it will promote happiness in general.

Deontology

The major contender to consequentialist theory is deontological theory. "Deontology" is derived from the Greek word *deon* meaning "duty" (*Webster's College Dictionary*, 1991, p. 387). The defining difference between consequentialism and deontology is that deontologists believe that actions are right or wrong insofar as they satisfy a moral obligation or duty, regardless of whether that maximizes the good. It may happen that the same action both satisfies a moral obligation and maximizes the good, but deontologists would see the maximizing of the good as a side benefit only. There are many forms of deontological theory, but what they have in common is the determination that the action is morally right if and only if it conforms to one's moral duties and obligations. The way in which deontological theories vary is in establishing what these moral duties and obligations are.

One of the earliest and most prevalent forms of deontology is known as "divine command" theory. In this theory, the duties and obligations that are to be followed are those that have been given to people by God. Most adherents to this theory do not realize that they are practicing "divine command deontology." Rather, they are upholding and following the dictates of their religion. Almost everyone, whether they subscribe to this philosophy or not, will have some sense of duty and obligation that emanates from their acceptance of or exposure to religious mandates. However, exactly what each person believes God has commanded differs from religion to religion, if not from person to person. Examples of this theory in action, as well as its drawbacks, are profuse in the health care setting:

- Decisions about foregoing life-sustaining treatment will often involve considerations of one's obligation toward preserving life, with Orthodox Jewish patients often taking a more stringent interpretation of God's command to respect and preserve life.
- Jehovah's Witnesses, although agreeing with the duty to respect and preserve life, claim that there is a higher duty, given by divine command, not to ingest blood, and therefore refuse blood transfusions even if the consequence is that they will lose their lives or the lives of their children.
- Even people who do not identify with a particular religious tradition may have their own sense of what God requires of them. An example of this is a decision to not pursue aggressive treatment, waiting instead to see what outcome God desires, or trusting that conservative treatment will work if God so intends. This may be a reflection of a duty to trust in God and yield to the path that God has ordained.

Although the ultimate authority in divine command deontology is God, other versions of deontology do not reference a particular authority. These deontologists believe that actions are intrinsically right or wrong and that this can be discerned either through reason or intuition. No real discussion of deontology can occur without reflecting on the work of Immanuel Kant (1724–1804). Kant (1785/1959) believed that all moral duties and obligations could be determined through the application of practical reason. In Kant's view, it is incumbent on us to apply our powers of reason to ascertain which rules of obligation we should act on. Whereas the language of Kantian ethics revolves around rules, it is important to understand that these rules are about what duties and obligations we have toward others and ourselves. Ultimately, according to Kant, we must act in accordance with our obligations, which are governed by these rules.

Because obligations and duties are not self-evident, nor are they given to us from an outside authority, as other deontologists would claim, the heart of Kant's moral philosophy involves how we determine which rules to follow. Kant provides us with a formula for determining which rules (or maxims, as he calls them) are a valid reflection of our duties and obligations. This formula, or test, is called the "categorical imperative." It is also known as the universalizability criterion: "Act only on that maxim by which you can at the same time will that it should become a universal law." In more colloquial terminology, this means that we should act only if we can desire that all others act in the same way. We can test the effectiveness of this formula by examining a situation common to many medical settings: A friend of your patient approaches you and says, "I know my friend is getting the results of his biopsy today. Can you tell me what they are so I can be ready to support him?" The categorical imperative requires us to test this action to see whether, in doing so, we would be appropriately discharging our obligation to the patient. In other words, can we make "release medical information to friends of the patient" a rule that we would want everyone to follow? In general, this seems like a bad idea. Most patients would resent having a friend know private test results before they do. Many may not want the friend to know the results at all. Therefore, because we cannot generalize this action into a universal rule, we cannot release the test results to the friend.

It is quite possible that rules formulated under the categorical imperative will become very specific and that we may have to modify them as exceptions occur to us. In the foregoing example, if the patient had been a minor and the "friend" was the father of the patient needing to know the results because he had to make medical decisions for the patient, then we could formulate a rule such as, "I should release medical information to a minor patient's parent(s) so that he (they) can make informed decisions." This rule is one that we can be comfortable universalizing.

The second criterion of the categorical imperative is that no person should be treated merely as a means but, rather, as an end. Essentially what this means is that one cannot treat others as tools or use them merely to achieve an objective. People must be treated with respect. Their interests and well being must be taken into account and our interactions with them should reflect an appreciation of those and further them whenever possible. That does not mean that we cannot profit from our interactions with others. It simply means that profiting from those interactions should not be our sole aim. There is a clear and simple example of this at the heart of health care. Without patients no health care professional could earn a living. However, caring for patients merely as a means to a paycheck would not fulfill deontological requirements. In caring for them, we seek to promote their well being and do things that we might not do if our only aim was to clock in hours. In doing so we explicitly intend to receive remuneration and, according to the categorical imperative, that is acceptable as long as we are also treating patients as ends in themselves.

Kantian ethics has become almost synonymous with deontology. This is evidence of the strong impact that it has had on ethical theory in general and medical ethics in particular. It is very common to find this sort of reasoning in articles about medical ethics and even in the way health care providers talk about their obligations toward patients. Whenever terminology such as "the duty to treat," "the obligation to disclose," or "the duty to respect" appears, we can be sure that behind that language is some notion of how these rules apply generally to all patients and cannot be broken without serious grounds.

Kant rejected the idea of intuition and based his theory entirely on the idea that we can use reason to determine right action. However, others have posited that there is a very real role for a moral sense in capturing which moral duties and obligations are simply self-evident. They do not require any other rationale for adopting these duties as action guides. This is sometimes referred to as the "common sense" approach. It is attractive because many people can relate to the idea of feeling that there are some things that are just right or wrong for no other reason than that they *feel* right or wrong. A prohibition against killing is one of the obligations that many people will cite as self-evident. There are obvious problems with this approach. On the one hand, there is often wide agreement among people regarding a short list of duties that seem self-evident. On the other hand, the list is very short and is certainly not robust enough to address the full range of issues life presents. Second, although people may be in general agreement about basic obligations, such as "do not kill," the extent to which these obligations should be followed and the range of situations to which they apply will differ greatly among people. Most, but not all, will allow that the obligation does not extend to situations of self-defense. But there is much greater division among people when it comes to applying this obligation to fetuses or death row inmates.

Finally, there is another group of deontologists who believe that there is no such thing as actions that are right in and of themselves and instead look to a contractarian model of ethics to discern what duties and obligations ought to be upheld by a particular group of people in a given place and time. The driving theme behind contractarian models of deontology is that the only valid duties and obligations that exist are those that we have entered into a social contract over. However, we do not get a chance to enter into these contracts individually. Theorists of contractarian models arrive at their version of the social contract either through imagining what the ideal society would be and what duties would hold in it or by describing what they see as the model that has already come to evolve in a given society. Thus, we are born into a society and its correlated social contract. In most contractarian conceptions, goods such as basic health care are obligations that society has to the individual, and the individual then has a duty to contribute to society so that it can continue to meet its obligations to others. One of the founding ideas in these models is that we, as humans, need each other and the benefits that arise from forming communities. Whether we want to or not, we have to find a way to get along, and that means we form contracts, either implicitly or explicitly. The problem with applying the contractarian model to the field of medical ethics is that one must first know and accept the rest of the social contract.

Feminist Ethics

Feminist ethics, like any other feminist theory or politics, is not a single view or position. In general, feminists raise issues that challenge traditional assumptions about the way the world works, particularly hierarchical structures usually associated with male dominance and any systemic or organized practice that results in the oppression of any group of people. To that end, feminist philosophers often question the value of rules or formulas like those that play a central role in utilitarianism and deontology. Their concern is that that these rules reflect hierarchical thinking that values ways of being and acting that place the greatest importance on efficiency, objectiveness, obedience, and other concepts that mostly reflect the values and further the aims of the most privileged members of our society. Adhering to these rules means perpetuating the power of these values to dominate contemporary moral discourse.

For the most part, feminists do not propose the complete rejection of traditional moral theories (Donchin & Purdy, 1999). Rather, they believe that there needs to be a corrective influence on them. They note that most moral theory developed by men tends to be based on rights and obligations and it is no coincidence that this language is consistent with the legal model of property and contracts. However, this only reflects part of the moral world we live in. Feminists point out that much of the work of daily living revolves around people and relationships, and because morality is about how we understand the world and how we should act in it, we need to look to these relationships and associated values to understand morality. What do we learn when we are open to examining relationships for insights into ethics?

The first observation that we may make is that when one is in a relationship with another it is expected that each party will give special consideration to the needs of the other over the needs of people in general. This is not just part of the role of being in a relationship, it is a necessary part of the emotional commitment that naturally develops. In other words, it is not a choice but a feature of relationships that the parties will be inclined to advocate and help one another to a greater extent than, and in preference to, other people with whom they do not share a special relationship. The ethical traditions we have discussed so far, and many others, are committed to the notion of impartiality and objectiveness. Feminists will admit that there is a place for these ideas, particularly in situations in which all the players come from a fairly even playing field, but they question whether this should be our primary disposition toward others. They note that the requirement to be impartial or objective completely denies the feelings of attachment and obligations that exist within relationships. They further point out that our lives are full of relationships, which can range from the very intimate, personal relationship to very loose, general associations that nonetheless capture our allegiance. To ignore these natural ties when it comes to discharging our ethical duties seems suspect to most feminist philosophers.

A second, important observation from the feminist perspective is that there rarely exist relationships between two people or groups with absolutely identical strengths and weaknesses. Sometimes this results in a power differential between the people in the relationship. This is obvious in relationships such as parent–child, employer–employee, and government–citizen. It is essential to understand this dynamic in the health care provider–patient relationship. In relationships with a significant power differential, the party with less power is going to be greatly influenced by both the stated and perceived values that are evidenced by the party with greater power. This confers a responsibility on the party with greater power to make sure that the relationship does not become one of coercion and that he or she does not shut out the voice of the less powerful party. An ethics of impartiality/objectiveness may not be flexible enough to recognize, let alone accommodate, the needs of the weaker party. Being open to and responsive to the needs of others with whom we have a relationship has been termed an "ethics of care" even though it is not a full-fledged ethical theory. However, the underlying message, that ethics should pay attention to the content of relationships and respond to the specific and individual needs of people in a caring way instead of treating all people the same, has become such a force in ethical theory that it has been given its own name.

Another implication of the observation that people bring different strengths and weaknesses to a relationship is the fact that relationships generally develop a degree of mutual interdependence. This is not a bad thing; it is merely an acknowledgement that we seek out relationships for a reason and we can and do become significantly attached to one another. This is true for all relationships at all levels. Even pragmatically, we can see that this is a basic truth about relationships: Health care providers need patients in order to have a career, and patients need the knowledge and skill providers bring to address their health care problems. However, most provider–patient relationships develop into more than this superficial connection. Patients come to trust and respect providers, and providers learn to care about and respect patients. This makes it that much harder and unnatural for providers to step back and take an impartial view of their patients' needs. Feminist thinkers claim that they should not try to take that step back, that responding to the special needs of the patient and affirming the caring relationship are part of ethical conduct.

The role of emotions in ethics is also viewed differently in feminist theories than in the male-centered, traditional ethical theories we have studied to this point. Note that both Kant and Mill stressed the need for reason, or rational thought, as the primary means for determining moral action. Feminist theorists have suggested that another way of being moved to moral action is through the emotions. It is one thing to reason about who may be suffering and what our obligations are to them. It is another, more profound experience to empathize with those who suffer and be called to act on their behalf through that experience. Thus, our emotions may help us to recognize what people and situations are in need of moral consideration. Whether and how we act in these situations still fall under the domain of reason, but are informed by our emotional perception. The idea of paying serious attention to what our emotions can tell us also calls another assumption of many ethical theories into question. Instead of being concerned just with ethical actions, feminist thinkers tell us we should be at least as concerned with the motives from which people act (Donchin & Purdy, 1999). As an example, when the parents of a very sick child inquire about the latest rounds of tests or how the child is responding to treatment, it is important that the information be relayed in a way that is responsive to the family's needs. In the hospital setting this may mean finding a quiet corner in which the family will not have to strain to hear over all the other noises of the unit; being gentle but firm in relaying bad news, so that the family does not feel assaulted, but at the same time does not misunderstand the news; and taking time to answer questions and provide comfort so that the family feels supported. Here the nurse's motive is not just to impart news, but to be caring in so doing. This is an example of one of the main contributions of feminist thought in ethics. When considering ethical conduct, it is not just the actions that persons perform that count, but also how they perform them, what their motives are, and whether they promote positive relationships.

A final word of caution needs to be added about these examples of feminist contributions to ethical thought. Not all feminists agree that these are helpful in furthering ethical theory. In fact, some claim that to legitimize an "ethics of care" is to perpetuate the subordination of woman as caretakers. As long as women are the ones being identified with this form of ethics, or we attribute women's supposed refined or increased capacity for empathy and caring to this approach, it risks becoming a higher ethical norm to which women must aspire. Prominent bioethicists Beauchamp and Childress (2001), in their classic textbook, *Principles of Biomedical Ethics*, worried that acceptance of an ethics of care may serve to reinforce the stereotypical image of women as caretakers. They noted that nursing has been one of the first medical fields to embrace an ethic of care and that there is a danger that if it is limited to this field, it will continue to bind women to a caretaking role while discouraging men from entering a field that could become even more associated with "women's work."

Communitarianism

Most of the focus in bioethics in the United States has been on theories that promote and protect the rights of individuals. As we will see later in this chapter, an overriding concern has been placed on individual autonomy. Most ethical discussions center on the needs and rights of the patient or even the conflicting needs and rights of the patient and the health care team or other party. These are generally presented as competing claims and are settled by weighing one set of rights against another. There is another approach based in ethical theory that does not currently have much representation in the medical ethics literature. With the continued problems surrounding issues of resource allocation and the emerging awareness that there are limits to individual autonomy, we may see more ethical thought developed around the lines of *communitarian theory*. Communitarian ethical theory is based on the idea that all people and principles owe their existence to and are partly constituted by a community or group of communities. Their identity cannot be understood outside of this context.

Take any person as an example. Who is this person? Any answer will invariably lead back to a community within which that person is situated. Communities can be understood in a variety of ways—as geographical groups, nationalities, institutions, social units, and so on. Without making reference to any group, it is almost impossible to answer the question, "Who is this person?" Any other answer is likely to be unsatisfying because we understand people as being embedded in a social context. To say that someone is a "father" gives us a world of information about that person. To be a father means that one plays a particular role in a community. There is plenty of individual variation in how this role is played, but the role itself is partly constitutive of the person. In other words, the person would not be the same if we removed this role from his life. So, too, do other roles affect our lives. A communitarian would claim that it is largely these roles that combine to make us the people we are. And who we are will evolve over time depending on how we take on, discard, and alter roles. Thus a community, or nested set of communities, is integral to the identity of all people. In the same way that the individual is the moral unit in utilitarian and deontological thinking, the community is the primary moral unit in communitarian thinking. This is not to say that individuals cannot have rights or interests. Rather, it emphasizes that the good of all is best served by first considering the interests of the community. Thus, when considering what the proper moral action is, one must take into account the effect the action will have on all communities involved. In the case of any given patient this includes at least the patient, the family of the patient, the community of people directly involved with the patient's care, the health care institution, and the society in which the patient lives. There are probably many more as well. Any one of these communities could be further broken down into other communities, which will be more or less affected depending on what question is at stake and how connected the patient and issue are to those groups. One of the few examples of the clinical application of communitarian ethical thought can be found in neonatal units. There are tough decisions to be made for babies who are born with severe anomalies. If they live, many of these children will face surgery after surgery, requiring intensive hospital and home care, and may be physically, emotionally, and financially dependent on their parents for the rest of their lives. Parents have to decide whether they are capable of meeting the demands presented by such children. One of the things they have to take into account is how the presence and care of this child will affect other children living in the home. Will there be enough time and resources to adequately care for all the children in the family? Will the family be able to function as a social unit, or will it break apart in resentment and dysfunction? Although the presenting issue is whether to treat the baby, vital considerations involve the well-being of others in the home. This is an example of taking seriously the notion that the good of the community is a primary concern.

Families, neighborhoods, religions, nationalities, occupations, institutions, and others may all constitute a community. It is important to take into consideration the effect on each community when making decisions about moral action. In medical ethics, communitarians emphasize the importance of taking seriously the community that we sometimes refer to as the "institution of medicine." There are roles, norms, and expectations derived from this community that have serious implications for how health care providers should conduct themselves in the practice of medicine. Professional associations play an important part in disseminating this information and conducting public discourse on the evolution of standards and practices.

Having said that the primary unit of moral consideration is the community, we are still left with the question of how to determine the good for the community. Communitarians claim that, just like everything else, moral principles, rules, and customs are derived from the community itself. Some good may become evident because they are necessary to keep the community together or help it to function. Others may arise from the needs of the members and be consciously formed as guiding principles. The conception of good or at least the principles that reflect this are likely to change as the community evolves. Different communities may have different formulations of the good. We can easily see examples of this by looking at the differences among different national, ethnic, and religious cultures. We also see how values differ from family to family. This is one of the criticisms of communitarian ethics. How do we determine which community is the most important one, and what do we do when expectations from communities conflict? At the moment, there is no leading communitarian theory we can look to for the answer. Instead, we may approach this question in a few different ways. One way would be to give the most consideration to those communities that are most vested in the individual or issue. Another would be to weigh equally the interests of all communities. Finally, we could resist the notion of multiple communities and define the community of all human beings as the one and only relevant community. It will be interesting to see how this issue is resolved as communitarian thought gains a voice in ethical debate.

Another criticism of communitarianism is that because principles are derived from within the communities instead of having a broader or more objective justification, they are susceptible to having all the biases and deficiencies of the community from which they arise. How then can guiding principles or rules ever be anything other than flawed? How can they be critiqued at all? Communitarians answer that although the norms and values may start from within the community, they can still be guided and reformed through reason and reflective deliberation by the individuals within that community. We see this all the time in the political arena. As a national community we are constantly rethinking and revising the rules that govern our society in a quest to develop the perfect set of rules that will bring about the greatest good for our community as a whole. Thus, our principles are only as biased and limited as our best thinkers are.

Summary

There are many more ethical theories than the four types reviewed in this chapter. However, these are the ones that have had the most impact in shaping western medical ethics and which are likely to continue to do so in the future. While no one theory has been successful at providing a complete and coherent view of the world of medical ethics, each has made important contributions which shape the way we think about our professional conduct and actions.

CLINICAL EXERCISES

1. Join a nurse or interdisciplinary team as they discuss the plan of care for a patient. Listen carefully when they talk about the goals of treatment, or

even ask about these if you can. These will reveal what the clinicians consider to be "good" for the patient. What are the goods that are identified? Are these goods consistent with any particular moral theory identified in this section? Are there goods that the team has not addressed that you think ought to be addressed from an ethical standpoint?

2. Watch interactions between health care providers and patients and family. Do you notice any interactions that are improved by the attention the providers give to the way in which they carry out their duties? Can you discern motives along the lines of those emphasized in an ethics of care behind the way these duties are carried out? If appropriate, you may want to ask the provider what thoughts went into his or her decision to carry out his or her duties in that way.

3. Identify examples of moral reasoning, such as utilitarianism, deontology, ethics of care, and communitarianism, in materials published by professional nursing organizations. You might find these in codes of ethics, position papers, or articles on nursing practice.

4. Identify examples of "right" and "wrong" in the nursing literature (articles, position papers, codes, etc). How do the authors indicate that they know these are right or wrong actions?

Discussion Questions

1. Are there times when you just "know" that something is right or wrong? How do you determine where this feeling is coming from? For instance, is it based on your religious beliefs, cultural conditioning, or an intuitive moral sense? Does it matter which of these things it is based on?

2. What are the desired features of a relationship between a patient and a nurse? Between a physician and a nurse? How do issues of power affect these relationships? How do issues of interdependence affect these relationships?

3. Should the following rule be universalized? "I should lie to my patients about what modifications are necessary for them to make in their lifestyles so that they will follow more healthy lifestyles in general and not just make the changes that are necessary to address the health concern currently being treated."

4. What does it mean to you to say that society has a duty to provide basic health care to all people? What would this claim mean coming from a Kantian? From a contractarian? From a utilitarian? From a communitarian?

5. Are there any principles or goods identified by the community of nursing professionals (either a local community such as those working in your institution or a professional group at a regional or national level) that are particularly hard to realize in practice? In ethical terms, to what do you attribute this?

ETHICAL PRINCIPLES

Many people have found it much more helpful to appeal to a set of guiding principles to help make determinations of what is and is not ethical in the world of medicine rather than adopt full-fledged ethical theories about the way the world is constituted, how we know that, and what we are to do. The advantage to this is that we can avoid arguments about theoretical assumptions and move right to the business of applying moral conceptions of the good to real-life situations. We are able to do this because there is widespread agreement on the primacy and enduring value of four basic principles. However, these principles do not exist in harmony. The demands of each principle may conflict in any given case, and there is no generally accepted ranking system for appeal. These four fundamental principles are best used as tools for moral reflection and aids to decision-making rather than formulas for determining the right or best action.

Nonmaleficence

The principle of nonmaleficence is a fundamental consideration in every conception of moral and ethical life. This principle asserts an obligation to not inflict harm on others and is the basis for the injunction in many medical ethics codes to "do no harm." Intuitively, it seems appropriate that in a quest to determine the good, one should start by identifying and prohibiting harms. However, the question of what constitutes a harm is not a simple one, nor is it clear exactly what the requirements of not doing harm are. Furthermore, this principle presents a special challenge in medicine because it is not always possible to avoid doing harm while trying to restore health or achieve other goals.

Some harms are easily identifiable. From an objective standpoint, anything that reduces an individual's chances of survival or compromises his or her abilities would seem to be a harm. Some people claim that the ultimate harm is anything that results in a patient's death. However, the most important determination of harm is what the patient himself or herself considers a harm. We make a presumption that competent patients are the best judges of what procedures and outcomes will have negative consequences in their lives. An impairment of mobility might be considered a minor harm in the eyes of a patient who has sufficient social support and does not require physical dexterity or agility in his or her employment. Another patient may find the same impairment greatly affects the ability to conduct his or her life, continue employment, or pursue activities he or she enjoys. In this example, both people might consider the impairment a harm, but one deems it significantly more harmful than the other.

In some cases, something that one considers a harm may not be to another. For example, some radiation treatments involve the risk of infertility. For a woman who does not want children, already has all the children she wants, or is past the ability to reproduce this may not be considered a harm at all. A person of either gender who had looked forward to some day producing offspring might consider this radiation treatment side effect to be a great harm. Finally, what might objectively seem like a harm may actually be perceived of as a good to an individual. The best example of this is the "ultimate harm" mentioned earlier. For a person who has a terminal prognosis and is unable to get any enjoyment or satisfaction from life because of pain caused by disease and medical interventions, death may be a welcome end to his or her suffering. For many people at the end of life, more harm is caused by maintaining them on life support than by letting the natural progression of the disease end their lives. Again, this is completely dependent on the perception of the patient.

Other harms are subtler and can only be recognized by paying close attention to the needs and preferences of patients. Psychological harms, threats to independence, and anything that constrains one's ability to exercise free choice are all examples of harms that are very real to a patient but can be overlooked if we are not sensitive to the situation and the possibility of harm. Examples of these include patients who are pressured by family to make choices that go against their true wishes, clinicians who overrule a patient's priorities or values, and families who cannot make good decisions for incapacitated patients because of their own issues and needs. Vigilance, resources, and sometimes courage are needed to counter these threats of harm to patients.

The principle of nonmaleficence requires us to not inflict harm on others, but what specifically does that entail? Some have suggested that this is a passive requirement. In other words, as long as we do not actively inflict harm on someone, we cannot violate the principle of nonmaleficence. This is a very narrow reading of the principle. Consider the following example. A nurse notes that the wrong intravenous (IV) medication is hanging for a particular patient. She has to make a choice of either correcting the mistake (or causing it to be corrected) or ignoring it. If she ignores it, some amount of harm will come to the patient. At the very least, the patient will not be getting the intended benefit from the medication that was originally ordered. By the narrow definition of nonmaleficence, the nurse is not required to do anything about the mistake because the nurse did not create the harm. However, everyone would argue that the nurse has an obligation to correct the mistake. Those who uphold the narrow definition of nonmaleficence claim that preventing harm or removing harm really falls under the domain of the principle of beneficence, which is discussed later in this chapter. These sorts of distinctions, based on linguistic constructs, are not particularly instructive in helping us to determine what our obligations are toward patients. Rather than sorting out the distinct requirements of each principle, some theorists, particularly those concerned with applied rather than theoretical ethics, have moved toward combining the principles of nonmaleficence and beneficence into a single principle.

Finally, we have to recognize that medicine often requires tradeoffs. To produce a good, harm may be a necessary consequence. By almost anyone's criterion, the loss of a limb or an appendage is a harm. Yet for many persons with diabetes amputation is a necessary procedure to stop infection from spreading throughout their bodies and killing them. Most people are willing to accept this harm to achieve the greater benefit of continued life. However, just because there is a greater benefit to be realized does not mean that the patient has not incurred a harm. Measures need to be taken to help the patient to cope with this harm on the physical, psychological, and social levels. Then, too, there may be patients who do not accept the tradeoff. For them, the loss of a limb or an appendage may have more meaning than mere loss of bodily function. For instance, when pressed about reasons for refusing lifesaving amputations, some patients identify religious beliefs about being buried whole, with their body intact, as a justification for refusing the procedure. For them, the harm involved in the loss of the body part goes far behind any physical impairment and has spiritual implications. Creative solutions, such as saving the amputated body part to be buried with the patient when he or she dies, have often been successful in these cases, but the bottom line is that the patient is the one who bears the burden of any procedure, and he or she needs to be the one who determines what harms are acceptable. Such dramatic examples are not necessary to demonstrate that harms often coincide with benefits in medicine. Many medical interventions, from taking aspirin to undergoing a heart transplant, involve risks and side effects that inflict harm on a patient. Only the patient can decide whether these harms are worth the expected benefits of the intervention.

Derivative Principles of Nonmaleficence
Due Diligence

The principle of due diligence refers to the care that a reasonable person exercises in a given situation to ensure that he or she does not harm another person. In medical situations this refers to following the appropriate standards and practices of good medical care. Examples include washing one's hands before and after patient contact to prevent the spread of disease and infection, properly documenting medications given to patients to avoid duplication errors, and participating in required continuing education to stay current on the latest advances in practice and knowledge. Clearly, there could be thousands of acts that are required by the principle of due diligence depending on the setting in which one practices. Breaches of due diligence are termed negligence. Gross negligence is grounds for medical malpractice.

Double Effect

The principle of double effect is derived from Catholic moral theory regarding the permissibility of acts that will have both a harmful and a beneficial outcome. As noted earlier in this chapter, many beneficial medical interventions entail harm to the patient. Yet harm is something one is ethically required to avoid. In an attempt to resolve this dilemma, the principle of double effect establishes rules for the ethical acceptability of acts that result in both a harm and a benefit. To be justified, an act that has both a harmful and a beneficial outcome must meet the following guidelines:

1. The act itself must be either good or morally neutral.
2. The good effects must be intended and the harmful ones unintended, though they may be foreseen.
3. The harmful effects may not be a means to the beneficial or good effects.

Some sources add as a fourth criterion that the benefits of the act must outweigh the harms. In the medical context it is usually taken as a given that any treatment option a patient chooses is one in which the benefits outweigh the harms in the eyes of that patient.

A medical example that meets the foregoing criteria is that of a pregnant woman in the first trimester who is discovered to have ovarian cancer. Immediate and aggressive radiation therapy may be necessary if there is to be any chance of recovery. Although the radiation treatment may produce the morally good effect of saving the woman's life, it also entails killing the fetus. By the standards of double effect, this is a permissible act because:

1. Radiation therapy is itself a morally neutral act.
2. The intention of the therapy is to eradicate the cancer, and though it is clear that the therapy will also kill the fetus, it is not the intention to do so.
3. Killing the fetus is not what kills the cancer.

The principle of double effect has been criticized as being a rationalizing measure that can justify any decision that a patient or clinician makes. However, there are very real limitations to the use of this principle. The current state of technology in obstetrics allows for the identification of defects early in fetal development. Some defects, such as renal agenesis, the absence of kidneys, are incompatible with life. Babies with this defect will not survive long after birth. Many people who discover such a problem opt to abort the fetus instead of carrying it to term and allowing it to die. This may be a more compassionate choice for the mother because it cuts down on the time and anguish associated with carrying a baby to term who will not live and having to watch her baby die after delivery. It may or may not be a more compassionate choice for the baby depending on his or her capacity for suffering both in utero and after birth. However, by the standards of double effect, terminating a pregnancy under these conditions is not a morally valid choice. Even if our intention is good, prevention of suffering for the mother, the procedure is not justified because (1) according to Catholic moral thought, the act of terminating a pregnancy, that is, abortion, is morally bad, (2) the harmful effect of killing the fetus is intended, not merely a side effect of alleviating the mother's suffering, and (3) the abortion is the means to doing the good. This example violates all three conditions of double effect and cannot be justified by this principle.

Beneficence

Most people who work in the healing professions cite the opportunity to help others as a primary reason for entering the field. Beneficence, the principle that requires that we seek to do or produce good for others, is integral to the practice of nursing. Nursing, in all its various forms, is, at root, an attempt to do good for others. Regardless of whether the practice involves one-on-one care of patients or seemingly more removed endeavors such as research and public health, the ultimate aim is to make the lives of individuals better.

To do the good, we must first know what the good is. In the same way that we depend on patients to tell us what constitutes harm for them, it is imperative that we listen to patients' conceptions of the good. Just like notions of harm, conceptions of the good vary from patient to patient, and what one individual values may be meaningless to another. Medicine, either in the guise of research, public health, or direct patient care, fell under criticism in the past for presuming the good for others and acting on these judgments. Sterilization of individuals with mental illness or retardation was a pervasive practice until advocates for these groups finally brought the practice into the light and challenged the assumptions being made and the authority to make such decisions for others. Although most will agree that sterilization without consent is outrageous, those who participated in the practice were doing so at least partly out of the concern for the well-being of the patients and any children who might be produced by them. That this concern was misplaced and inappropriate only serves to underscore the importance of grounding the good in the actual preferences and values of patients. Much harm has been done in the name of doing good.

Even though a fundamental goal of medicine is to do good for others, it is not clear what, specifically, this principle requires of nurses. We can always identify more good that could be done, but it seems absurd to claim that anyone has an obligation to do good just because the opportunity exists. Certainly anyone is welcome to do good whenever he or she pleases, but having an actual obligation means that if one does not pursue the good or attempt to do good for another, then he or she is in violation of a moral duty and should be censured as such. The American Nurses Association (2001) described the role of nurses as "promoting, advocating for and striving to protect the health, safety and rights of the patient (Provision 3)." Thus, seeking and producing the good as it pertains to the health, safety, and rights of patients can be viewed as obligatory on the part of nurses. Further acts that produce good for others are relegated to the nice, but not obligatory, category. These are also known as acts of supererogation. Taking time to read get-well cards to a patient is a kind act that produces good for the patient, but it is not an obligation for a nurse and should not take time away from tending to the health, safety, or advocacy needs of other patients.

Derivative Principles of Beneficence
Compassion

The principle of compassion, or caring, is directly derived from beneficence. Often the good done through an act is not limited to the causal effects of the action, but depends on the way in which the action is done. Having one's dressings changed in a caring manner and a noncaring manner can be two very different experiences. Even if the amount of pain or discomfort is equivalent, the nurse who acts in a compassionate manner is likely to do far more good for the spirit of the patient than is one who does not act compassionately. Furthermore, being compassionate opens one's eyes to further psychological or spiritual suffering of the patient that can be overlooked or even purposely hidden from care providers who do not approach patients in compassionate ways.

Veracity

Veracity, sometimes referred to as honesty or truth-telling, is another ethical principle derived in large part from beneficence. The rationale for this is that patients cannot act in their own interest unless they are fully informed of their medical condition. Thus, a patient's pursuit of the good life is hampered by not knowing all relevant facts about his or her health. Even bad news, which one might be tempted to withhold out of considerations of nonmaleficence, informs patients about their life choices and helps them to pursue the best path available. In the past, it was customary not to tell people they had a fatal prognosis, based on the belief that this would spare suffering on their part. It has since become clear that there is a lot of work to be done by dying people, and to spare them this suffering is also to deny them the chance to get their affairs in order, say their goodbyes, and make peace with others, themselves, and their God. Even if it is not obvious that being truthful is to the benefit of the patient, we must respect the fact that only the patient can determine what is and is not good for himself or herself.

Note that veracity is not an absolute obligation. There are at least two instances in which truth-telling may be morally prohibited. The first is in the case of minor patients. Depending on the age and maturity of the minor, it may not be appropriate to tell the patient all the details or implications of a medical condition. Children should not be kept in the dark about their illnesses or injuries because this also causes worry and stress, but in coordination with the parents one must determine an appropriate level of detail and information to give to the child. This does not have to involve giving false information, but it may mean holding back some information in a way that would be unacceptable if the patient were an adult. The second type of case in which obligations of veracity do not hold is that in which a patient decides that he or she does not want to be informed of certain information or details. The patient may decide to appoint another person to make decisions for him or her, in which case the obligation of veracity is transferred to the decision-maker.

Patients also have the right to determine how much information they want. In these cases, the duty of veracity still holds, but needs to be expanded to include not imparting more information than the patient wants to know. A patient may decide that too many details about his or her medical condition are overwhelming and stressful and may ask only for a qualitative summary of his or her progress. Patients undergoing fertility therapy spend a great deal of time during the first part of each cycle taking medication and undergoing frequent, sometimes daily, monitoring. Some patients want to know every detail of the daily findings regarding hormone levels and egg development. Others find that they obsess about the numbers and just need to know that they are making progress and what dose of medication to take next. A simpler example of this principle can be demonstrated in another obstetric scenario. Some parents do not want to know the gender of their child when an ultrasound or amniocentesis is performed. They simply want to know whether the fetus is healthy.

Duties of veracity, although based on beneficence, are also partly derived from respect for autonomy. This comes from the notion that patients have a right to information about their bodies and to honest answers to their questions about their care. But even autonomy concerns are sensitive to the idea that part of the reason individuals need the right to information about their bodies is that it allows them to act on this information and make decisions in their best interest.

Fidelity

The principle of fidelity requires one to be faithful in relationships and matters of trust. This can be construed very narrowly as an obligation to keep promises, or more broadly as a requirement to actively uphold one's end of the patient–clinician relationship and all that that involves. At a minimum, the principle of fidelity requires that health care providers keep the promises implicit in any patient–provider relationship. On the part of the provider these expectations include acting in the best interest of the patient, maintaining confidentiality, obtaining informed consent, being honest, educating the patient, and being responsive to his or her needs. A broader interpretation entails upholding these trusts and additional ones, which might include advocacy, a deeper level of respect, and other commitments that arise as the relationship develops. The principle of fidelity may also be referred to as the principle of trust or obligation of covenant.

Paternalism

The principle of paternalism entails overriding a patient's expressed wishes, or not consulting a patient at all in his or her health care decisions, in an effort to achieve the best outcome for the patient. This practice was once common in U.S. medicine and was considered as much an obligation as any of the other principles in this chapter. Now there is great debate about whether paternalism can ever be justified toward a competent adult. It is a particularly hard case to make in our culture, which seems to value autonomy over everything else. Later chapters of this book take a deeper look at the issue of paternalism. For now, it is enough to say that the force behind paternalism is a strong and sincere recognition of the obligations of beneficence. This basic tension between autonomy and beneficence is highly characteristic of bioethics in the twenty-first century.

Proportionality

The principle of proportionality requires us to choose those actions or options that confer a greater good than harm or produce a greater benefit than burden. The higher the ratio of benefit to burden, the more ethically compelling is the act. This is similar to the utilitarian criterion, but has been specifically formulated for use in the clinical environment and is most often referenced in terms of choosing medical options. Thus it may be ethically mandatory for a clinician to offer an antibiotic for the treatment of a sexually transmitted disease because the benefit is great and the burden, both in terms of cost and side effects, is relatively low, whereas it may not be ethically required at all to offer a patient an expensive experimental drug for a disease that can be managed in other ways. It is preferable that the patient make the assessment of what treatment he or she would like to pursue, but clinicians often need to determine what treatment options should be offered to patients.

Autonomy

Concerns about breaches of autonomy were the impetus behind the bioethics movement of the 1970s in the United States. Two things happened about the same time. First, a number of medical practices came to light that were clear violations of individual autonomy. One such violation was the Tuskegee study, in which poor African-American men enrolled in a study of syphilis were never informed of an effective and inexpensive treatment that had become available for the disease and were allowed to remain sick for years and even die while being observed by medical investigators. At the same time, medical technology had developed to the point that people could be kept alive much longer than they might want. Paternalistic attitudes of clinicians, which leaned heavily toward treating at all costs, were challenged by patients and families who saw harm in keeping people alive who were either never going to regain consciousness (Karen Ann Quinlan and Nancy Cruzan) (Pence, 1995) or in treating people who were suffering so horribly that they wanted to stop all treatment and be allowed to die (Dax Cowart) (Englehardt, 1989; Wicker, 1989).

It was in this context that the field of medical ethics established itself, moving from the domain of academia to clinical settings. Whereas the medical culture around these situations has changed significantly, the focus of medical ethics has not. Autonomy remains a central concern of clinical ethics activity, and respect for autonomy is the principle most often invoked in patient care, tempered only by considerations of justice or the avoidance of harm to others.

In medicine, respect for autonomy requires us to accept the free and informed choices of competent patients or their designated decision-makers. In essence, this means that we must abide by the choices made by patients, regardless of whether they coincide with our personal values or assessments. Unlike nonmaleficence and beneficence, it is not so obvious why respect for autonomy is a fundamental principle. There are a number of opinions on this topic:

- Ultimately the only thing that truly belongs to each of us is our set of beliefs and values. They are highly personal and highly valued. Respecting decisions of others based on their beliefs and values is appropriate because it gives them their proper due as the valuable concerns that they are.
- Respecting the autonomy of others is a reciprocal arrangement. That is, we respect the right of others to make decisions that reflect their own values and beliefs because we want others to respect the decisions that we make for ourselves.
- By respecting the autonomy of another we are acknowledging that he or she is the most appropriate person to make decisions in his or her own best interest. This may have two rationales: First, the person making the decision is the one who will have to live with the consequences, and second, an individual has the best insight into what he or she values and what he or she considers good.

Whatever the reason, there is overwhelming support in our culture for the acceptance of a high level of respect for autonomy. However, our responsibility to accept the choices and preferences of others is limited to those that are authentic to a person. This is especially true in health care. We can best determine which choices are authentic by examining the criteria mentioned previously: free choice, informed choice, and competency.

Authentic choices are those that are not coerced. Both subtle and explicit coercion of patients can come from the health care providers, the patient's family and friends, the socioeconomic situation of the patient, and society in general. A truly free choice will reflect the patient's values, not those forced on him or her by others. This is not to say that patients cannot consider the effect their decisions will have on their family, fiscal situation, or society, but these considerations must be made by choice. Health care providers, family, and friends will often try to influence a patient to do what they believe is in the patient's best interest. This is a natural tendency and is done in the name of beneficence. Trying to influence a patient's decision does not need to be considered harmful as long as the patient is ultimately free to make his or her own decision and that decision is respected. However, we must be aware of influences and be ready to check them if they become a burden to the patient or get in the way of his or her making an authentic decision. Coercion can be subtle and can wear away at a patient. A patient with a terminal, though curable, disease may find his or her decision to enter hospice is never rejected, just continuously postponed while one more test or one more trial of something is done. Family and providers may be hoping that the patient will reconsider his or her decision for hospice if given a little more time. Patients may express ambivalence about some decisions or change their minds frequently about a big decision. It is important to ascertain whether that ambivalence is from internal conflict or from external influence.

Choices cannot be authentic unless they are informed. That is, a person cannot know what choice is consistent with his or her values and preferences unless he or she has access to all pertinent information. For instance, many seriously ill patients are asked to make decisions about whether they want to be resuscitated in the event of a cardiac arrest. To make this decision, they need to know what resuscitation entails and what their chances for recovery are. In our culture, most people form their impressions of cardiopulmonary resuscitation (CPR) from television shows. Depictions of resuscitative efforts are generally limited to CPR and defibrillation. They are usually shown to take a short period of time, and the people experiencing the resuscitation either die or completely recover. In reality, people who arrest may be worked on for long periods of time during which the brain receives a limited supply of oxygen, causing permanent brain damage. Other undesirable side effects can include broken or cracked ribs, a need for ventilator support, and a generally compromised level of functioning. People whose health is already compromised are far less likely to survive a resuscitation attempt or to ever leave the hospital even if they do survive it. Patients need to know this information before they can make informed decisions.

For a choice to be authentic, it must be made by a medically competent individual. The term for medical competency is decisional capacity. Legal competency and medical decisional capacity are not the same thing. A patient can be legally competent and still not meet the criteria for decisional capacity. A patient is said to have decisional capacity if he or she can:

- Express a preference (this is a minimal requirement that entails only that the patient be able to communicate by some means).
- Understand the relevant features of his or her medical condition and treatment options.
- Make a reasoned determination or show that the decision is in line with enduring values and previous decisions.

Psychiatric consultation may be helpful but is not required to make an assessment of decisional capacity. In fact, a clinician who has worked closely with a patient is more likely to be able to determine whether he or she meets these criteria than a consultant who has never worked with the patient. It is also possible for a patient to have decisional capacity at some times and not at others or to meet a high enough level of decisional capacity to make some types of medical decisions but not others. Further discussion on this topic can be found later in this book.

Respect for autonomy does not end when the patient is no longer able to communicate or make decisions for himself or herself. As long as we have some way of knowing what decisions the patient would make, we are obligated to follow his or her wishes. There are two general ways in which we can determine what a patient who is unable to communicate would want. The first way is through the use of surrogates. Surrogate decision-makers are people who are named by the patient, often a family member, who knows the patient and his or her values and preferences. They can inform the health care team of the decisions that the patient would make if he or she were able to communicate. The second way is through the use of written or verbal advance directives. This means that the patient has explicitly told another person or has written down preferences about his or her medical care in the event that he or she is no longer able to communicate them. Much more detail about surrogates and advance directives can be found later in this book. The important thing to remember for now is that decisions made by surrogates and those written in advance directives have every bit as much moral force as those expressed directly by the patient.

There is no principle of ethics that is absolute. Like other moral considerations, there are limits to clinicians' obligations of respect for autonomy. In any relationship there has to be some give and take. Whereas a patient may express a preference that certain things happen, it is still incumbent on the clinician to see that care remains within the standards of good practice. A patient cannot demand that clinicians do something that would compromise their integrity or violate their standards, nor can patients demand inappropriate treatment. A patient may refuse any treatment, including lifesaving treatment, but he or she may not demand treatment that he or she does not need or is not feasible. Limitations of autonomy may also occur out of considerations of justice or may be overridden when they cause harm to others. A classic example of limiting respect for autonomy due to justice and harm issues is the policy in the United States of notifying a patient's sexual partners when he or she has been diagnosed with a sexually transmitted disease.

Derivative Principles of Autonomy
Privacy and Confidentiality

Two related derivative principles of autonomy are privacy and confidentiality. Respect for privacy requires us to avoid intruding on the personal space and business of a patient. In health care settings, patients lose a great deal of privacy and highly value that which is left to them. Small considerations, such as knocking before entering a room or requesting permission before touching someone, can go a long way toward protecting the little privacy that patients have left. Confidentiality confers an obligation on health care providers to protect the personal information they collect on patients from being seen or used by people who do not need to know the information. This means being vigilant about holding conversations that include references to specific patients and the health care information away from the ears of people who do not have a need to know as well as keeping patient records in secure and protected places.

Advocacy

Because patients often have a hard time making their voices heard in a medical setting, *advocacy* on the part of providers is required to ensure that patients needs and values are heard and respected. Although there is a movement toward accepting the patient as a fully contributing member of the health care team, this is clearly not yet part of health care culture. Patients usually have the least powerful position, and therefore the least recognized opinions, in any health care setting. There are numerous reasons for this, which range from established attitudes about patients and how they should act to the patient's incapacitation, which limits his or her abilities to press for his or her views and needs. Someone must help these voices to be heard. Because the nurse is usually the health care provider most intimately connected to the patient, they bear a special obligation to act as advocates for their patients. This obligation is based in respect for patient autonomy. Much more will be said about advocacy throughout this book.

Informed Consent

The principle of informed consent is justified mainly by respect for autonomy. Informed consent requires that patients receive all pertinent information about their health condition and the options for treatment and that they explicitly choose their own treatments. Whereas being informed is a prerequisite to being able to exercise one's autonomy, the principle of informed consent stands on its own as an essential consideration in the ethical practice of medicine. This principle ensures that it is the patient's will, not the provider's, that is being carried out.

Justice

Justice is the primary principle that allows us to step back from the patient's perspective and take a more encompassing view of a situation. The principle of justice is also the most difficult of the four principles to apply. In part this is because there are multiple formulations of justice, none of which exactly fits the needs of all situations or the views of all people. Second, the legitimacy of applying considerations of justice differs depending on the situation. Medical ethics dilemmas and decision-making can generally be divided into two arenas: the public level and the individual level. Public-level activities refer to ethics endeavors that will affect a group or groups of people. These include policy initiatives ranging from the development of institutional procedures and regulations to national laws. Individual-level ethics activities refer to situations in which the focus is on the care of a single patient even though there may be indirect effects on others. These are the situations in which clinicians will participate on a daily basis. Considerations of justice differ greatly depending on the level of activity in which one is engaged.

The arena of ethics in which we focus on the care of individual patients requires us to consider what is owed (or due) to each person based on their being a member of the human community. Concerns about fairness or equitable distribution can only be addressed at the public level in which the needs of many can be impartially considered. To make a judgment about fairness or distribution at the individual level would mean pitting the immediate, identifiable needs of one person against the ambiguous, unknown needs of the many. For instance, there are many more people in the United States who need organ transplants than there are organs available. Organ procurement organizations have developed a set of guidelines to help to determine who should be listed for transplant and then further criteria to determine where an individual should be placed on the waiting list. Without this system clinicians would be left to decide on their own whether a particular patient deserved to have a transplant and thus leave open or deny the opportunity to some other, unknown patient. This would force clinicians to split their loyalties between their individual patients and the group of patients needing transplants as a whole and would compromise their ability to maintain roles of trust and advocacy. It would also be completely ineffectual to ask members of a health care team to determine on a case by case basis which resources each of their patients deserved. For these reasons and others, it is inappropriate to consider distributive justice issues in individual cases. Another way of saying this is that distribution decisions should not be made at the bedside.

But there is still a role for justice on the individual level. The role of justice on this level is to ensure that all people have the same rights and that these rights are respected. There are many moral theories that attempt to identify and justify what rights individuals have simply because they live in a given society. Some claim that these rights originate as part of a contractarian model. That is, individuals have a certain set of rights because as a society they have agreed that they each have these rights and will act in accordance with them. Other moral theories take a less relativistic approach to rights. For these theorists, being a member of the human race is sufficient to claim certain rights. Such theories propose various sets of rights. The Universal Declaration of Human Rights of the United Nations (1948) includes, among others, the right to freedom, liberty, and security; the right to own property; the right to enter into marriage and found a family; the right to freedom of expression; and the right of everyone "to a standard of living adequate for the health and well-being of himself and of his family, including food, clothing, housing and medical care and necessary social services." The challenge in applying these theories is to determine what a "right to medical care" entails. There have been various attempts to define a basic level or a decent minimum of health care. None of these attempts has resulted in acceptance of a general right to health care in the United States. Currently there are programs that provide for health care for the poorest children, and all health care facilities are required to provide emergency care for anyone who needs it, but this is far from establishing health care as a basic right.

Regardless of whether health care is a right, there is still work to be done in the administration of health care to ensure that the rights that patients do have are respected. Seeing that all patients are treated equally, that patients have a method for resolving their grievances, and that they are treated in a respectful manner is part of ensuring the rights of individuals. Most health care organizations and services have a patient's bill of rights that mandates the ethical treatment of patients.

Another consideration of justice on the individual level is the difference principle. This requires that like cases be treated alike and cases that are different in relevant ways be treated differently. A problem that occurs frequently in health care is the issue of patients with similar needs who have different insurance coverage. Do all patients with the same health problem have a right to be offered the same treatment or is insurance coverage a morally relevant difference such that those who have plans that do not cover more expensive treatments should not be offered those treatments? Formulary drugs are a good example of this. Most health insurance companies have a list of medications they will cover and either do not cover others or require a higher co-payment from the patient. It is usually the newer and more expensive drugs that are not covered. Physicians may prefer to prescribe these drugs when they have fewer side effects than their predecessors or when a patient experiences problems with the older drugs. However, they may not be able to treat similar patients similarly if they have different health insurance coverage. Treating patients with relevant differences differently is just as important as treating like patients alike. Some patients may require longer hospital stays or more home nursing visits or home therapy than others with the same diagnosis because they do not have adequate support at home to aid in their recovery. This is a social difference that has a direct effect on the health of the patient, and is a significant enough difference that the patients should be treated differently.

Public-level ethics activities usually revolve around questions of fairness in distributing health care resources. The requirement that we treat all people as moral equals obliges us to recognize that although people may be morally equal, they are not identical. That is, we each bring a different set of abilities and needs to the table. Treating two people with differing abilities and needs in an identical way is not necessarily the same thing as treating them fairly. Therefore, defining justice simply as fairness does not tell us much about what justice requires. There are many different ways to be fair, but each seems to leave out some important aspect of evenhandedness. The following principles of justice are representative of the most common conceptions of distributive equity in ethical theory:

To each person an equal share.

This is a simple, straightforward approach to dividing up the pie. It also only works in the most simple and straightforward situations. What it does not address is the fundamental problem stated earlier, that whereas people may be equal, their needs are not. We can see how this conception fails by using a slightly silly example. Suppose there is a very large, but nonetheless limited supply of bandages in the world. By this conception of fairness, the right thing to do is to divide the number of bandages by the number of people in the world and distribute them accordingly. So each person may get 100 bandages. This is fine for the lucky, graceful, or unadventurous folks who do not tend to scrape their knees often. But for those who do, 100 bandages over the course of their lives may be grossly inadequate. But this example is not so silly when we replace the idea of bandages with health care dollars or other limited medical resources.

To each person according to need.

This seems like an attractive proposition until it comes down to the details. One problem is defining a need. Does a short child who comes from a short family have a need for growth hormones, or is that simply a want? Another problem is comparing needs. In a world with limited resources, how do we decide which needs are the most important? Does one person's need for a heart transplant rank higher than another's need for drug detoxification? What about needs that can never be fully met? Should unlimited resources be offered to a person with AIDS even though the underlying problem will never be cured and the patient will eventually die? Does the same answer hold for a person with adult-onset diabetes or for a severely impaired newborn? The needs of some patient populations are so great that it is conceivable that the vast majority of resources would be spent on a small proportion of the general population. This is already the case in the current health care system. A significant percentage of health care dollars is spent on the last months and weeks of life. Critics of the current system claim that these health care dollars would be better spent meeting the basic health care needs of all people.

To each person according to effort, contribution, or merit.

These schemes for the redistribution of goods essentially ask us to consider social criteria as a guideline for allocating health care resources. That in itself is problematic. However, the fatal flaw with such criteria is that there is no good way to make judgments about the effort, contribution, or merit of an individual. How does the effort and contribution of a truck driver compare to that of a legislator? Some of the most important contributions in philosophy, science, and art have come from people who were not accepted in their time and even punished for their ways of thinking. Yet the fundamental flaws in this type of distributive system have not stopped people from trying to implement them. Tying medical benefits to employment is common practice. Most people get their medical insurance through their employer, and if they lose their jobs, they also lose their medical benefits. Highly paid executives often enjoy generous and comprehensive health coverage, whereas those employed in the service industry are often lucky if they have access to any sort of health plan, even one with high premiums and deductibles. Welfare programs have begun to require that people demonstrate effort, either through employment or by attending classes, to obtain benefits. This approach places an artificially high value on one's employment status, thereby undervaluing work done by parents who stay home to raise their children or by individuals who prefer unconventional work such as artists, volunteers, and entrepreneurs.

To each person according to free-market exchanges.

This is essentially the system currently in place in the United States. Individuals can either pay out of pocket for health care or invest in insurance plans to cover their needs. The rationale behind considering this a fair system is that people will pay for what they value. If they sufficiently value health care, they will spend their money on it or on insurance premiums. If they do not value health care, then they are free to spend their money on what they do value. Proponents claim that this freedom of choice is the ultimate in fairness. What this overlooks is the disproportionate burden of health care needs that some people face as well as the extremely high cost of health care. For most people it is not a matter of choosing whether they will purchase health care, but of literally not having the money to do so if they should so want to. With some hospital bills reaching the dollar value of a house, and long-term care far exceeding that, it seems overly simplistic to claim that market forces can genuinely reflect priorities.

Because none of these conceptions of fairness is perfect, in reality we try to make a system or set of rules that is as fair as possible, balancing all the considerations of fairness as well as we can. How we do this will depend on the group of people and issues involved as well as the resources at hand. In some cases it may be most important to give everyone an equal chance, in others it may be more important to see that everyone has an equal outcome. Still other health care needs, particularly those that could be designated as wants, may be better addressed through free-market practices. Rawls (1971) in *A Theory of Justice* described one way in which we, as a society, might determine how to distribute scarce resources. His model requires that the decisions-makers be blinded to their own particular situations in life (veil of ignorance). Then, with the realization that they could each find themselves in the worst-off situation, they decide what the most equitable distribution of goods is, given the particular resources and general needs of society. This happens through a process termed "reflective equilibrium" in which the participants try to determine the most effective way to use the resources at hand to address all needs with the realization that because resources are limited, not all needs will be fully met. The requirement that each person is blinded to his or her position in life is meant to ensure that the needs of the least-well-off will not be overlooked because each decision-maker knows that there is a chance that he or she will inhabit that position. Rawls also stipulated that once resources have been distributed, any further redistribution must be such that it first addresses the needs of the least-well-off and no change should ever work to the detriment of that group. Rawls acknowledged that this hypothetical model can never be duplicated in real life because the policy-makers, such as legislators, corporate leaders, and so on, can never be blinded to their actual circumstances and fortunate positions. Nonetheless, this sort of process can work if decision-makers are open to hearing and caring about the needs of all citizens.

We could also implement Rawls' notion that the ethical acceptability of a distribution plan depends on its ability to improve the lot of the least fortunate. Note that this method does not endorse any particular version of fairness. It counts on the perception and intuition of the decision-makers to determine what constitutes fairness and, in the end, to produce the most equitable distribution of goods. For Rawls, what is important is that each person realize that his or her position in life is due largely to chance rather than to any credit or fault of his or her own. This is intended to produce empathy rather than disdain for those who are sick, disabled, indigent, or face other challenges. When we each have an equal chance of finding ourselves in a less than desirable situation, we are more likely to ensure that every person has the resources to improve his or her lot in life.

Derivative Principle of Justice
Respect
Respect for persons is the primary derivative principle of justice. Respect may manifest itself as a general consideration, as efforts to help patients to maintain or preserve dignity or protect them from anything that threatens to impinge on their rights. Ultimately, respect means treating people in such a way as to recognize and value their status as fellow human beings.

SUMMARY

Nonmaleficence, beneficence, autonomy, and justice are four cornerstone principles of bioethics from which many other principles can be derived. All major ethical issues in health care will feature a concern involving one or more of these principles. Resolving ethical issues in which two or more of these foundational principles conflict requires careful weighing of all the evidence, details, and viewpoints.

CLINICAL EXERCISES

1. Review the America Nurses Association (2001) Code of Ethics for Nurses With Interpretive Statements, which is available at http://nursingworld.org/ethics/code/protected_nwcoe303.htm

   a. Note how many times references to each of the primary principles of ethics are made.
   b. What other principles, ideas, or values are stated that relate to each of these main principles?
   c. Identify potential conflicts between the principles (and/or duties) named. These may be situations that are explicitly named in the code or that you recognize as sources of conflict.
   d. How does the code recommend resolving conflicts between principles (and/or duties)?

2. Review your organization's patient's bill of rights. If one does not exist, review The Patient Care Partnership: Understanding Expectations, Rights and Responsibilities adopted by the American Hospital Association (2004), available at http://www.aha.org/aha/ptcommunication/partnership/index.html

   a. Is there a reference in this document to how the patient's rights are protected or secured? What resource is available if a patient feels his or her rights have been neglected?
   b. Having a right means that someone else has a duty. What duties are created by this bill of rights and for whom?

3. Look for instances of resource allocation in practice. Ask how these decisions are made and note whether they are left to the discretion of an individual clinician, decided by a supervisor, or made at a departmental or other institutional level.

Discussion Questions

1. Name as many desirable qualities or characteristics of a nurse as you can and how those qualities are put into action. Identify which principle or principles of ethics support that quality or action. *Example*: A good nurse is sensitive to the emotional state of the patient. Beneficence supports this quality because assessing emotional health is part of addressing the overall needs of the patient, and being responsive to the patient's mood underscores caring in the relationship.
2. Give examples not mentioned in the text of actions that are ethically required of nurses for each of the four fundamental principles.
3. How would you rank the four fundamental ethics principles in order of priority? Can you think of any instances in which you would want to change your rank order?
4. How should conflicts between principles derived from the same fundamental principle be resolved? For example, how might one resolve a conflict between confidentiality and advocacy in a situation in which advocating for a patient also entails revealing private information?

Resources

Beauchamp, T. (2000). *Philosophical ethics: An introduction to moral philosophy* (3rd ed.). New York: McGraw-Hill.

Daniels, N. (1985). *Just health care*. New York: Cambridge University Press.

Daniels, N., & Sabin, J. (2002). *Setting limits fairly: Can we learn to share medical resources?* New York: Oxford University Press.

Ethics Updates. (2003). Kant and Kantian ethics. Retrieved May 28, 2005, from http://ethics.acusd.edu/theories/kant/

The Internet Encyclopedia of Philosophy. (2005). Retrieved May 28, 2005, from http://www.utm.edu/research/iep/

International Association for Hospice and Palliative Care. (1998). The double effect of pain medication: Separating myth from reality. Retrieved May 28, 2005, from http://www.hospicecare.com/Ethics/fohrdoc.htm

Jonsen, A., Seigler, M., & Winslade, W. (2002). *Clinical Ethics* (5th ed.). New York: McGraw-Hill.

Utilitarianism Resources. (2005).Utilitarianism. Retrieved May 28, 2005, from http://www.utilitarianism.com

References

American Hospital Association. (2004). The patient care partnership: Understanding expectations, rights and responsibilities. Retrieved May 28, 2005, from http://www.aha.org/aha/ptcommunication/partnership/index.html

American Nurses Association. (2001). Code of ethics for nurses with interpretive statements. Retrieved May 28, 2005, from http://nursingworld.org/ethics/code/protected_nwcoe303.htm

Beauchamp, T., & Childress, J. (2001). *Principles of biomedical ethics* (5th ed.). New York: Oxford University Press.

Bentham, J. (1988). *A fragment on government* (R. Harrison, Ed.). New York: Cambridge University Press. (Original work published 1776)

Donchin, A., & Purdy, L. (Eds.). (1999). *Embodying bioethics: Recent feminist advances*. Lanham, MD: Rowman and Littlefield.

Engelhardt, H. T. (1989). Freedom vs. best interest: A conflict at the roots of health care. In L. D. Kliever (Ed.), *Dax's case: Essays in medical ethics and human meaning* (pp. 79–96). Dallas, TX: Southern Methodist University Press.

Kant, I. (1959). *Foundations of the metaphysics metaphysics of morals* (L. W. Beck, Trans.). New York: Macmillan. (Original work published 1785)

Mill, J. S. (1998). *Utilitarianism* (R. Crisp, Ed.). New York: Oxford University Press. (Original work published 1863)

Pence, G. E. (1995). *Classic cases in medical ethics* (2nd ed.). New York: McGraw-Hill.

Rawls, J. (1971). *A theory of justice*. Cambridge, MA: Belknap Press of Harvard University Press.

United Nations. (1948). Universal declaration of human rights. Retrieved May 28, 2005, from http://www.un.org/Overview/rights.html

Webster's college dictionary. (1991). New York: Random House.

Wicker, C. (1989). Sentenced to life. In L. J. Kliever (Ed.). *Dax's case: Essays in medical ethics and human meaning* (pp. 15–23). Dallas, TX: Southern Methodist University Press.

CHAPTER 2

History of Clinical Ethics

Objectives

At the end of this chapter, the student should be able to:

1. Describe the evolution of ethics as related to nursing practice.
2. Understand the difference between medical ethics and nursing ethics.
3. Recognize current issues in the field of nursing ethics.
4. Trace the foundation of clinical ethics.
5. Describe the current state of thinking about nursing ethics.

KEY WORDS

- *Baby Doe*
- *Bioethics*
- *Ethics committees*
- *Eugenics*
- *Medical ethics*
- *Nursing ethics*

Clinical ethics pertains to the actions and decisions clinicians, including nurses, make or facilitate in their professional practice. Some issues are related to patient care, whereas others are related to professional behaviors. Clinical ethics differs from "ordinary" ethics because it applies to a certain context, the decisions and actions in a health care setting, and to professional behaviors in the clinical context. By virtue of the professional–patient relationship, health care providers have ethical obligations and duties to patients. There is a duty to prevent harm, so that health care providers must remain competent in their skills and specialty areas. There is an obligation to tell the truth, so patients, in most cases, should be told their diagnosis and prognosis and given complete information so they can make informed health care decisions. In rare cases, the patient may not be told the diagnosis and/or prognosis if there is a strong likelihood that he or she would become suicidal or lacks the capacity to make health care decisions. Each profession has a code of ethics; nursing's code of ethics has been revised nine times since 1893, when it was first drafted as the Nightingale Pledge. This chapter describes the history of clinical ethics, especially how the field of ethics related to nursing practice has evolved.

HISTORY OF ETHICS

Ethics has been part of medicine since its inception. *Primum non nocere* is Latin for "first do no harm." Thus, doing no harm is a physician's first ethical obligation to a patient. In early medicine, this obligation was significant because a physician's ability to cure was often limited.

Nursing in the Nightingale tradition manipulated the environment to promote natural healing. Nurses did this in the home or hospital and under the supervision of physicians. Before examining the evolution of clinical ethics in nursing practice, it is instructive to first look at the evolution of ethics in medicine.

The first mention of ethics in medical publications was in 1803 when Thomas Percival referred to the public trust in medicine (Jonsen, 2000). His writings became the foundation for the code of medical ethics introduced in 1847 at the second national convention of the American Medical Association. This code, however, had more to do with protecting the profession of medicine than protecting the public trust. Practitioners of approaches now referred to as alternative therapies, such as homeopathy and naturopathy, were excluded from the profession of medicine. Through revisions in 1912, 1957, and 1966, the medical code evolved into discussions of patients' rights, competence, policing the profession, and maintaining confidentialities. There was still attention to the profession of medicine, and aspirational elements, such as caring for the poor, no longer appeared in the code.

According to Jonsen (2000), the introduction of new technologies after World War II marked the birth of "bioethics." Between 1946 and 1976, there was an exponential growth of medical advances: antibiotics, chemotherapy, vaccines and other medications for hypertension and psychiatric disorders, cardiac surgeries, cardiopulmonary resuscitation, and hemodialysis, to highlight a few. The physician needed to be more technically proficient and thus to focus on a medical specialty, which contributed to the decrease in the choice of general medicine as a family doctor. Health care costs soared, and so the government intervened with Medicare and Medicaid. To answer questions about benefit, harm, and equitable and efficacious access to and allocation of new technologies, as well as to identify who should be making those allocation decisions, the government held interdisciplinary conferences. Philosophers and theologians, as well as social scientists and physicians, were invited. At a conference in 1952, Pope Pius XII declared that the use of the new machine the ventilator was obligatory if its use was considered "ordinary means" versus extraordinary, a distinction that can be traced back to Catholic theology in the Renaissance period (Jonsen, 2000). Another topic under discussion at these conferences was the increasing ability to prolong the life of people who were old, sick, and/or disabled, including newborns with genetic conditions. New reproductive technologies, eugenics (manipulation of the gene pool through laws regarding marriage and sterilization in an effort to eliminate undesirable hereditary traits), and environmental concerns about pollution of air, water, and food were also emerging concerns for medicine. After World War II and the revelations about war crimes, including human experimentation, there was increased attention to research ethics (Chapter 10). In the struggle to "do good" there was great possibility for also doing harm. There was one major medical advance in particular that attracted the attention of a generation of philosophers and ushered in modern medical ethics, and that was organ transplantation.

First Human Heart Transplant

In 1967, Dr. Christiaan Barnard performed the world's first human heart transplant, in Capetown, South Africa. An international panel was assembled in Houston to address the ethical issues in transplantation and other medical advances, and it provided the genesis for today's major ethics think tanks and associations, for example, the Hastings Center, the Kennedy Institute of Ethics, and the Society for Health and Human Values (now the American Society of Bioethics and Humanities) (Jonsen, 1998). In the 1970s and 1980s, presidential commissions were convened, and their published proceedings have served as the foundation for ethical guidelines in the United States (Appendix A). There was a need to translate the philosophical analyses from conferences and commissions into clinically relevant information. Attention focused on the teaching of medical ethics in medical school curricula and the manner in which ethical analysis occurs in the clinical setting.

Clinical medical decision-making was becoming more complicated because there was usually more than one physician consulting on a case, patients were being included in clinical research trials, and the consumer movement was pushing for patient rights, including the right to enough information to make informed decisions. The paternalism of past eras gave way to the era of patients' rights. Facilitated by lawsuits, informed consent (a practice requiring that patients receive all pertinent information about their health condition, treatment, risks, benefits, and alternatives so they can make informed decisions) became the norm.

For today's nurses, it may seem quite strange that a physician would withhold the diagnosis and prognosis from the patient, but in the recent past (into the 1960s), physicians were considered the experts who knew best, and it was within their clinical judgment whether to divulge the diagnosis. For some conditions, treatment was not available, so patients did not have a decision to make regarding treatment. Although the legal concept of informed consent in medical treatment had been around since 1914 (*Schloendorff v. Society of New York Hospitals*) (Jonsen, 1998, p. 355), the case that catapulted informed consent into prominence involved a patient who sued his surgeon for failing to disclose the risk of paralysis with laminectomy (spine) surgery. There were a number of cases around this time, in the early 1970s, in various parts of the United States that affirmed the same principle: Patients must be fully informed prior to giving consent. Jonsen (1998) pointed out that at this time presidential commissions were discussing informed consent in human experimentation and the Tuskegee syphilis experiment was exposed. In the Tuskegee syphilis experiment, conducted from 1932 to 1972, 400 African-American sharecroppers in Tuskegee, Alabama, were followed by the Public Health Service to document the natural course of syphilis. They were not informed that they were subjects in a research study; they were deceived into thinking they were receiving free health care and were promised $50 burial money on their death. Even after penicillin was discovered as an effective treatment for syphilis, they were deliberately kept from receiving treatment. All these forces converged to emphasize the importance of the autonomy of the patient. As a result, the ethical and legal mandates to obtain informed consent prior to treatment or inclusion in research were codified, that is, translated into law.

The First Clinical Ethics Education Program

In the late 1970s, an innovative training program began at the University of Chicago. A clinical ethics fellowship program provided clinical ethics training for physicians. Fashioned after other medical training programs, ethics fellows (all physicians) attended seminars, did consultations in much the same way that medical residents performed consultations during specialty rotations, and completed a research project during the 1-year fellowship. The program emphasized the relationship between clinical decision-making and ethical decision-making. One of the founders of the program, Mark Siegler, MD, believed that one must be a physician to do ethics consultation. In 1982, one of the authors (T.A.S.) made an inquiry regarding admission into the program and was informed to call back after she completed medical school! Since that time, Dr. Siegler has admitted lawyers, nurses, psychologists, anthropologists, and other health care professionals into the program. One of the classic clinical ethics texts came out of the University of Chicago program, *Clinical Ethics*, and is in its fifth edition (Jonsen, Siegler, & Winslade, 2002).

Since that time, numerous ethics educational programs have flourished in the United States and Canada. Although nurses have been able to attend programs like that at the University of Chicago, there have been no programs exclusively devoted to preparing nurses for ethics consultation. The evolution into nursing ethics has been grounded in patient care, but not without its start as loyalty to the physician.

Evolution of Ethics in Nursing Practice

At the beginning of the nursing profession, nurses worked in hospitals or patient's homes under the direction of physicians. Nurses' training instilled the importance of loyalty to the physician. Even if the physician made an obvious error, the nurse could not challenge the physician. The nursing profession followed the discipline of both a religious community, with expectations of total devotion and self-sacrifice, and the military, with unquestioning obedience and adherence to orders. The early codes stressed the importance of maintaining the patient's confidence in the physician. Modeled after Victorian society, the nurse-as-mother was another image that was fostered. The nurse-as-mother was subservient to the physician as the head of the "family." Self-sacrifice as a mother sacrifices for her children was expected. Because physicians controlled nurses' work opportunities in homes and in institutions, it was unwise for a nurse to displease a physician. Although the patients paid the nurse directly, the nurse was unlikely to get future employment if she was no longer recommended by a physician. With the code stressing loyalty to the physician as primary, nurses often felt torn between loyalty to the physician and prevention of harm to the patient. As early as 1910, nurses wrote letters to the editor of the *American Journal of Nursing* describing situations of conflicting loyalties (Winslow, 1984). Nurses developed a number of strategies for dealing with the conflicting loyalties. The first option was to remain silent and follow orders without question. The physician, as the nurse's superior, was ultimately responsible for the outcome. The nurse's defense would be that she was following orders. This strategy failed to offer legal protection for nurses.

Another strategy was to clarify, but not question, orders. This strategy provided no protection for Nurse Somera in the Phillipines in 1929. Somera assisted a physician in a tonsillectomy. The physician ordered an injection of cocaine to be prepared. Somera asked for clarification that he had said "cocaine" and he confirmed that he did, she prepared it, the physician administered it, and the patient died. The drug he meant to ask for was procaine. Both physician and nurse were tried for manslaughter; the physician was acquitted, and the nurse was found guilty and sentenced to 1 year in prison and fined 1000 pesos. The Supreme Court of the Philippines upheld the judgment. There was an international response of outrage from nurses. It was not clear why the nurse was held responsible and the physician was not. Nursing associations in the Philippines mounted a campaign to have Somera pardoned because she had performed her duties as she was taught. They were successful; she was pardoned, and the profession of nursing was forever changed. The following statement was prepared at the International Council of Nurses Congress in 1930:

While we do not know the workings of their minds [the courts] in relation to the case, we would say that if their decisions were influenced by the thought that human life is precious and must be guarded at any cost, and that it can better be guarded by two responsible persons, a doctor and a nurse, rather than by one, a doctor and a less responsible person, we agree with them entirely. We not only agree with them but thank them for these decisions which lift nursing from a subservient place to one of equality in responsibility and dignity with that of the doctor. (Pence & Cantrall, 1990, p. 190)

The Somera case changed nursing practice, and nurses are now taught that they are responsible for the actions they implement, so they must question orders as well as clarify them.

The Somera case began the shift in nursing ethics from loyalty to advocacy (Winslow, 1984). Loyalty to the physician was present, but was waning as the primary ethical obligation of nurses. The first official code of ethics was adopted by the American Nurses Association in 1950 (see Chapter 3); it spells out that the nurse must verify orders and report unethical or incompetent behavior to proper authorities only. Nurses were still expected to show great deference to physicians. One of the authors (T.A.S.) can recall being taught in 1970 to stand up when a physician entered the nurses' station and offer her chair to the physician. She was taught that she could not give patients any information, such as telling them their blood pressure, what medication they were being given, or what their diagnosis was. She was to direct patients to speak to their physician. The idea of patient advocacy, especially if it involved conflict or confrontation, was foreign to nursing in a small midwestern medical center. In fact, the term advocacy is not found in Miller and Keane's (1972) *Encyclopedia and Dictionary of Medicine and Nursing*, which one of the authors (M.S.D.B.) used while in nursing school in the 1970s. Such was the climate when the Tuma case occurred.

The Tuma Case

Jolene Tuma was a nursing instructor in Idaho. As she and a student prepared to administer chemotherapy to a patient, the crying patient told Tuma and the student that she had controlled her leukemia for 12 years with "natural foods" and was reluctant to accept chemotherapy (Tuma, 1977, p. 546). Tuma wrote that she discussed alternative treatments, acknowledging that they were not embraced by the medical community. The patient invited her to return to explain the other treatments to her family. The patient's son told the physician, and the physician filed a complaint with the state board of nursing. Tuma was fired from her teaching position, and her nursing license was suspended. The nursing board concluded that her behavior interfered with the physician–patient relationship and was therefore unethical. Tuma argued that she had a right to inform the patient, on the patient's request, of alternative treatments. Citing the American Nurses Association (ANA) Code for Nurses, she believed she was within her scope of practice and was fulfilling her professional obligation. To her amazement, she was informed that the Idaho State Board of Nursing did not recognize the ANA Code for Nurses (Tuma, 1977). Tuma submitted a letter to *Nursing Outlook* describing the circumstances and invited nurses to comment.

Letters varied in their support. Some concluded that Tuma was acting as a patient advocate, others thought she had crossed the line into medical management. The national association, ANA, had their ethics committee review the case, but because it was under litigation, they would only issue general comments. They seemed to support Tuma in her role as patient advocate, but implied that she violated the code. Stanley (1983) criticized the ANA for not challenging the Idaho State Board of Nursing's failure to adopt the profession's code of ethics. In 1979, the Idaho Supreme Court ruled in Tuma's favor because the state practice act was too vague to be used to determine whether Tuma's behavior was unprofessional. However, there was lack of consensus within the nursing profession and health care community about whether Tuma's actions were ethical. Despite the encouragement to be patient advocates, nurses were not adequately prepared for the advocacy role. Henderson (1983) noted a dearth of literature about risk-taking and risk-takers in nursing. She called for assertive and accountable decision-makers to enter the profession. During the 1970s, two social movements that influenced nursing gained momentum: the consumer movement and the women's movement.

THE CONSUMER MOVEMENT AND THE WOMEN'S MOVEMENT

The consumer movement challenged the physician's authority and position in society. There was a resentment of the physician's arrogance and power (Winslow, 1984). Patients exerted their right to information, options, and the right to refuse treatment. Informed consent was increasingly important and, based on the Tuma case, somewhat controversial in terms of who could inform the patient. The label "patient" seemed patronizing and condescending, so terms like "client" or "consumer" became fashionable. Annas (1974) believed that patients' rights needed to be championed, and with additional training, it would be most appropriate for nurses to assume this advocacy role. He commented that nursing programs discouraged the development of independent judgment in their students, so nurse educators would need to specifically choose to teach advocacy.

The women's movement helped and hurt the nursing profession. In some ways, it empowered women to view themselves as equal to men and to expect equal pay for equal work. During World War II, women assumed many of the jobs traditionally held by men when the men entered the armed forces. However, when the veterans returned, a woman often lost her job for no other reason than a man needed it. (There were not a large number of men in nursing, so female nurses were not replaced with male nurses.) The next generation, the Baby Boomers, questioned the disparity in women's position in society, and the women's movement demanded social change, such as equality in pay, reproductive freedom, and opportunities for advancement in their careers. Nurses benefited from the collective action of women's groups, especially in the elevation of the status of women in society. However, some feminists rejected nursing as viable career and disparaged it as a menial, servant-like occupation meant for people who could not get into medical school (Muff, 1982). The media portrayal of nurses did not help, as with Nurse Ratchett of *One Flew Over the Cuckoo's Nest*. The nurse's ethical obligation to advocate for patients was dependent on society's view of nurses and nursing. The task before the profession was to educate nurses to be patient advocates, which meant they needed to acquire skills of assertiveness and risk-taking. Nurses in practice developed a communication style that allowed them to advocate for their patients without direct confrontation with physicians. For example, Nurse Anderson reports to Dr. Boone, "Infant Morris is jaundiced appearing; do you think his bilirubin level is elevated?" Dr. Boone replies, "Yes, why do not we get a bili on him in the morning." Nurse Anderson responds, "Thank you, doctor. Do you want both conjugated and unconjugated?" Dr. Boone replies, "Yes, of course." Stein (1967) documented this type of interaction and called it the "doctor–nurse game." He suggested that if a nurse like Nurse Anderson approached Dr. Boone and said, "I am ordering a bilirubin panel on the Morris baby because he's more jaundiced today," the physician would remind her that she is the nurse, he is the doctor, and he will do the ordering. Stein, Watts, and Howell revisited the doctor–nurse game in 1990 and said although gains had been made, the game persists. Savage (1995), in her doctoral dissertation, recalled interviewing a nurse who gave direct patient care half of the time and was a nurse administrator the other half. She described being unaware of the communication style she used with physicians until a social worker observed her interaction with a physician and drew it to her attention. At first she was surprised and a little embarrassed that she was "playing the game," yet she said the style was effective and less stressful than direct confrontation.

DIFFERENCE BETWEEN MEDICAL ETHICS AND NURSING ETHICS

Ethical analysis is a way of thinking and a way to break down concepts and examine them in a context and from various perspectives. Curtin and Flaherty described ethical analysis as a way "to add order and structure to ethical deliberations" (1982, p. 59). The difference between medical ethics and nursing ethics is based on the difference between the practice of medicine and the practice of nursing. Medicine focuses on the diagnosis, management, and treatment of disease and injuries, whereas nursing focuses on the "protection, promotion, and optimization of health and abilities, prevention of illness and injury, alleviation of suffering through the diagnosis and treatment of human response, and advocacy in the care of individuals, families, communities, and population" (American Nurses Association, 2003, p. 6). Often medical and nursing ethics converge when the focus is on the patient and informed decision-making. Nurses have different obligations to patients apart from the obligations physicians have to patients, and therein lies another difference between medical ethics and nursing ethics. The general term "bioethics" is sometimes used to describe the ethical issues in health and the delivery of health care, and it may broadly encompass the ethics of medical, nursing, and other health care professionals. Nursing ethics is embedded in how nurses practice nursing and how they address the ethical issues they encounter in their practice. "Ethics in nursing" and "nursing ethics" are interchangeable.

TEACHING ETHICS IN NURSING

The clinical decisions nurses make for patient care are based on respect for the patient's self-determination as well as on the teaching of self-care, disease prevention, and health maintenance. Nurses' awareness of ethics and ethical issues is useful in giving them a language to articulate the issues, but ethics should not be separated from clinical decision-making. Nursing is a morally complex activity; Levine (1989) observed that every patient interaction is a moral interaction. Ethics is much more than discussions about abortion, resuscitation, and end of life. In the 1980s, there was attention to ethics in nursing in terms of nurses' moral development, ethical decision-making models, and nurses' role on ethics committees. Numerous doctoral dissertations were devoted to measuring nurses' moral development, moral reasoning, and responses to ethical dilemmas. Ethical decision-making models, such as the one developed by Thompson and Thompson (1981), were used in nursing education. Nursing students were taught about decision-making models, but in practice, it was still not clear what the nurse's role was in the decision-making process. Were the models to be used by the nurses in making their own decisions in practice issues or were they to be used to facilitate decision-making by patients? As advocates, were nurses obligated to assist patients in their decision-making? Murphy (1993) described nurses feeling stuck "in the middle" and torn between their obligations to their patients and their desires to be loyal to the physician, their colleagues, and their employers. The drawback of being in the middle, she observed, is the powerlessness of being constrained, or the inability to view and articulate the problem in ethical terms. However, the positive aspect of being in the middle can be the opportunity to take the role of interpreter of the medical information provided by physicians or the role of mediator for conflicted families (or between physicians and patients and families) by helping them to identify values and value conflicts. Nurses can also be "in the middle" by serving as members of ethics committees, on which they can present the patient's view as they know it and also present the nursing perspective. They can also champion certain positions that empower patients and families. To fulfill this role, Murphy (1993) believed nurses need "(1) a robust conception of what it means to be a nurse, (2) some specialized knowledge, and (3) at least some professional support" (p. 4).

For example, Mr. Tron had an adverse reaction to a medication and had a cardiac arrest. He was resuscitated and transferred to the intensive care unit (ICU). Arriving at the ICU, the patient's wife asks the ICU nurse to tell her what happened. The ICU nurse is aware that the ordering physician and the previous nurse made a medication error because neither of them checked Mr. Tron's history form for drug allergies/sensitivities. The ICU nurse is unsure whether she should tell the wife about the medication error, yet she believes the patient (or in this case, his surrogate) has a right to know. The decision-making models would provide the nurse with the tools needed to follow the steps in the decision-making process, that is, identifying the ethical problem, identifying the key players, identifying the options and potential consequences, and then identifying the ramifications of each consequence. The nurse may recognize that there is an obligation to tell the truth to the patient, yet she may believe that it is the responsibility of the health care providers who made the error to divulge the incident to the patient's wife. What actions should she take if she believes the patient's wife should know about the medication error? Given that medication errors are often "system" errors, as well as errors in clinical performance, the clinical ethical issue for the ICU nurse is that the patient's wife is asking for information that the ICU nurse has and believes the wife should know, but it is information the ICU nurse is not comfortable being the one to share. Is it ethical for her to refer Mrs. Tron back to the physician and nurse from the floor? Because she was not present when the patient arrested, is it correct for her to act as though she knows what exactly happened? Or is she "copping out" by not telling Mrs. Tron what she has been told regarding the arrest? Ethical decision-making models may present a format of steps for nurses to follow, but if there is more than one course that could be followed, how does the nurse know which is the "ethical" or "more ethical" course to follow? Clinical ethics is the recognition that ethics is embedded in many of the decisions that are made in clinical care. Nurses need to be prepared to face clinical ethics decisions. This is discussed further in Chapter 5.

Nurses interested in ethics in the late 1970s recognized that nurses needed skills for managing the ethical issues that present in nursing practice. A number of books written by nurse educators, some written with nonnurses, came on the market (Bandman & Bandman, 1985; Benjamin & Curtis, 1981; Curtin & Flaherty, 1982; Davis & Aroskar, 1978; Fowler & Levine-Ariff, 1987; Jameton, 1984; Thompson & Thompson, 1981; Veatch & Fry, 1987). These authors came to ethics from various backgrounds, but they all recognized the need for nurses to be prepared to face clinical ethical issues. Many of these books have gone into their fourth editions, demonstrating the continuing need for ethics education in nursing.

The accrediting bodies for nursing education programs require ethics education, but they allow each program to decide how that education is provided (American Association of Colleges of Nursing, 1998; Commission on Collegiate Nursing Education, 2003). With the ever-increasing amount of content to be incorporated in nursing courses, ethics sometimes gets short shrift. The current expectation is that classroom instructors incorporate ethics into their lectures and readings, and the clinical instructors incorporate ethics into their pre- and postclinical conferences. Many nursing programs do not have separate ethics courses taught by nurses, although most universities have ethics courses taught in philosophy or medical humanities departments that nursing students may take as elective courses. The impetus for this textbook was to provide a resource for nursing instructors whose area of expertise is not nursing ethics.

Nursing ethics is moving into a second generation of leaders who are doing research in ethics, addressing ethical issues on an international scale, and contributing to the field of nursing ethics and the broader field of bioethics. They are at the forefront of movements toward improving palliative care, evaluating the ethical issues in genetic advances, and advocating for health care reform that improves access, resource allocation, and quality of care.

PROLIFERATION OF ETHICS COMMITTEES

Many hospitals with religious affiliations, especially Catholic hospitals, had ethics committees, but most hospitals did not. That changed after 1982 and the Baby Doe case. Baby Doe was born with a duodenal atresia (the duodenum ending in a blind pouch instead of opening into the small intestine), a tracheoesophageal fistula (an opening from the esophagus into the trachea that allows fluids to enter the lungs), and Down syndrome (an additional chromosome on the twenty-first pair, resulting in certain physical characteristics and cognitive disability). Lyon (1985) poignantly and meticulously described the events of the Baby Doe case. Two pediatricians recommended the infant be immediately transferred to a regional medical center, but the obstetrician suggested the parents do nothing and let the infant die, probably as a result of aspiration pneumonia, in a few days. After careful soul searching, the parents, who were public school teachers in Indiana, opted to forgo treatment. The expected course of events was that the infant would aspirate his stomach contents and then develop aspiration pneumonia, which, if left untreated, would lead to his death. The obstetrician wrote orders prohibiting the use of intravenous fluids. The nurses were permitted to feed the infant, but they realized that introducing liquid formula into Baby Doe's system would likely cause aspiration and death, so the infant went unfed because none of the nurses wanted to be responsible for such an outcome. Baby Doe's parents transferred him to a private room with private-duty nurses when the hospital's nurses threatened to walk out on the job if the infant was not transferred out of the nursery. Because hospital policy prevented private-duty nurses from administering medications, the hospital's nursery nurses still had to give Baby Doe his injections of morphine and phenobarbital, for sedation. One nurse described the experience as "inhumane" and "devastating" (Lyon, 1985, p. 33).

The hospital administration was concerned about their liability if an infant with a treatable condition were to die from the withholding of treatment, so they pursued legal avenues. They lost at every level, with the courts supporting the parents' right to decide for their children when given opposing medical recommendations by professionals. As a county deputy prosecutor who served as the infant's guardian *ad litem* was traveling to Washington, D.C., Baby Doe died from aspiration pneumonia at the age of 6 days. The media learned of the case when it was argued before the Indiana Supreme Court, and disability-rights groups and right-to-life organizations demanded the Reagan administration take action. As a result, a memo was sent to all hospitals that received federal funds stating that hospitals that withheld treatment in future similar cases would be viewed as discriminating against handicapped infants and would be penalized by the withholding of federal funds. Hospitals were required to hang posters stating, "Discriminatory failure to feed and care for handicapped infants in this facility is prohibited by federal law" (Lyon, 1985, p. 41). A toll-free number for reporting discriminatory actions was listed on the sign.

The American Academy of Pediatrics, the National Association of Children's Hospitals, and the Children's National Medical Center in Washington, D.C., raised a legal challenge against the Baby Doe regulations, as they were then known, and the guidelines set forth by the Reagan administration were struck down by the courts as being "arbitrary and capricious" (Lyon, 1985, p. 44). Through negotiations among federal officials, medical groups, disability groups, and right-to-life groups, the revised regulations came to stipulate that hospital ethics committees should review all such cases, and ethics committees should *always* advise physicians when the withdrawal of treatment from infants was being considered by the infants' physicians and/or parents. The guidelines recommended the composition of the committee should include "a pediatrician, a hospital administrator, an ethicist, a clergyman, a lawyer, a representative of a disability-rights organization or the parent of a disabled child, a member of the community, and a nurse" (Lyon, 1985, p. 211). This "committee approach" was also endorsed by the President's Commission for the Study of Ethical Problems in Medicine and Biomedical and Behavioral Research (1983). The nurse's role on ethics committees was not clarified, though. Some saw it as the nurse's opportunity to advocate for the patient; others saw it as a way for the profession's voice to be heard because nurses often felt disenfranchised from the decision-making process.

The nurse's role on ethics committees varied. The nurse who was directly involved with the patient might be invited to attend the ethics committee meeting to give information or ask questions, but then the nurse would have to leave when the committee began its deliberations. In other cases, some ethics committees asked one or more nurses to serve as regular committee members who always participated in the committee's deliberations. Nurses, as with all professionals on the ethics committee, bring their unique professional perspective. They can address nursing issues, help to identify options, advocate for the wishes of the patient (and family), and participate in the ethical analysis of the issues in a particular case. They can also participate in reviewing a policy for its ethical implications, and they can identify areas where ethical education is needed for nurses and other employees of the institution or agency.

Although ethics committees proliferated, nurses were not always included as members, and nursing access was often thwarted by the requirement that the attending physician must approve their referral to the committee. In cases where the physician was viewed as the possible source of the ethical distress, nurses had no avenue for obtaining an ethics consultation.

At one time the Joint Commission on Accreditation for Healthcare Organizations required that each institution have a mechanism for employees for resolving ethical problems, but the requirement has since disappeared from their regulations. Now the emphasis is on patient's rights, and the institution no longer has to provide a clearly articulated process for the resolution of ethical problems (Joint Commission on Accreditation for Healthcare Organizations, 2004).

Nursing Ethics Now and in the Future

The current state of nursing practice challenges us to operationalize nursing ethics. Advocacy and patient rights are the priorities, yet nurses find themselves again "in the middle." Constrained by health care costs and third-party payers, nursing is the largest expense in health care facilities, so facilities' management tries to structure nursing care delivery to flex up and down in response to revenues—not in response to patient needs. Prospective payment schemes, in which insurance companies pay a fixed amount for a hospitalization according to the patient's diagnosis regardless of the actual costs, brings about a perverse incentive to reduce services and limit utilization. If patients' stays are shorter than anticipated, then, through prospective payment plans, the facility "makes" money from the shortened stays. That money can then compensate for times when other patients' lengths of stay exceed what is anticipated but their additional days in the facility are not covered by insurance. Nurses who want to implement a plan of care based on patient needs are restricted to "what is covered by insurance" versus "what is needed." This approach demands that interventions are justified and supported by evidence, and it can lead to a stunted creativity in how nurses approach patient care. It fosters a "cookie-cutter" approach in applying a prepaid formula based on diagnosis and not based on individual needs and responses. Nurses are challenged to meet their ethical obligations to patients while also serving as stewards of resources, and they are challenged to be satisfied with the quality of care that they deliver under these limiting circumstances.

The nursing shortage reflects an aging workforce, more attractive career options outside of nursing to people who would have previously considered the profession of nursing, the decimation of nursing staffs in the 1990s during managed care's heyday, and people's disenchantment and frustration with the way nursing is currently being practiced (Nevidjon & Erickson, 2001; Weinberg, 2003). Nursing ethics, centered on patient care, is the means by which nurses justify their plans of care and their use of resources in implementing these plans. It is the weapon nurses use to combat the ultimate commodification (making a commodity) of health care.

SUMMARY

Nursing ethics permeates all aspects of nursing practice and professional relationships. Nursing no longer has loyalty to the physician as its primary ethical obligation. Collegiality and collaboration, based on mutual respect, is the basis for the nurse–physician relationship. Provided they are followed in response to an individual patient's needs, the use of clinical pathways (plans of care for certain conditions, based on expected outcomes, that can be individualized and used to guide care) and standing orders (prewritten unit-based physician's orders that can be implemented under specific circumstances) allows for nursing decisions that increase responsibility and accountability in nursing practice. In managing their units and departments, nurse managers are expected to apply business principles, which can ethically fall short when utilitarianism is embraced. Nurses are often instrumental in writing hospital policies, yet those policies may not reflect nursing ethics. For example, there is literature to support family presence at resuscitations of loved ones (Eichhorn et al. 2001; MacLean et al. 2003; Meyers et al. 2000; York, 2004), yet most institutions either prohibit family presence or do not have a policy explicitly permitting it (Kleinpell, 2003). Nurses who appreciate the value of family presence can work toward establishing these policies at their institutions.

Nurses need the education and language to identify ethical issues, analyze ethical situations, and articulate ethical reasoning, especially in light of the nursing shortage and its resulting threat to safe nursing practice. Efficiency and patient and family responsibility cannot replace expert nursing care in health care settings, such as the ICU, nursing home, ambulatory care center, or the patient's home. Nursing ethics will assist nurses to shape their practice and health care delivery in society.

CLINICAL EXERCISES

1. Identify the mechanism in your institution or agency for resolving ethical problems. When was it started, who started it, and how has it changed?

2. Identify what ethics content is presented in your institution or agency's orientation for newly employed nurses.
3. Ask an experienced staff nurse on your unit or in your agency how nursing ethics has changed since he or she began practicing.
4. Identify professional associations or societies that include nurses and whose focus is ethics.

Discussion Questions

Give rationales for each of your decisions.

1. In the example of Mr. Tron and the medication error, discuss whether you, as the ICU nurse, would tell Mrs. Tron about the medication error.
2. Should nurses be required to obtain the permission of the attending physician before requesting an ethics consultation through the ethics committee? Give the rationale for your answer, and then give the rationale for the opposing argument.
3. If the communication style as described in the "doctor–nurse game" is efficient and less stressful than confrontation, should it be fostered?
4. Identify actions and decisions that are challenging current ethical norms. For example, whereas Western medicine agrees that a patient has the right to know his or her medical diagnosis, family members for a patient of Asian descent may request that the physician not disclose a terminal diagnosis to the patient based on respect for the patient's culture. Discuss how you, as a nurse, would handle those situations.

References

American Association of Colleges of Nursing. (1998). *The essentials of baccalaureate education for professional nursing practice*. Washington, DC: Author.

American Nurses Association. (2003). *Nursing's social policy statement* (2nd ed.). Washington, DC: Author.

Annas, G. J. (1974). The patient rights advocate; can nurses effectively fill the role? *Supervisor Nurse, 5*(7), 20–25.

Bandman, E L., & Bandman, B. (1985). *Nursing ethics in the lifespan*. Norwalk, CT: Appleton-Century-Crofts.

Benjamin, M., & Curtis, J. (1981). *Ethics in nursing*. New York: Oxford University Press.

Commission on Collegiate Nursing Education. (2003). *Standards for accreditation of baccalaureate and graduate nursing programs*. Washington, DC: Author.

Curtin, L., & Flaherty, M. J. (1982). *Nursing ethics—Theories and pragmatics*. Bowie, MD: Brady.

Davis, A. J., & Aroskar, M. A. (1978). *Ethical dilemmas and nursing practice*. New York: Appleton-Century-Crofts.

Eichhorn, D. J., Meyers, T. A., Guzzetta, C. E., Clark, A. P., Klein, J. D., Taliaferro, E., et al. (2001). Family presence during invasive procedures and resuscitation: Hearing the voice of the patient. *American Journal of Nursing, 101*(5), 48–55.

Fowler, M. D. M., & Levine-Ariff, J. (1987). *Ethics at the bedside: A source book for the critical care nurse*. Philadelphia: Lippincott.

Henderson, G. (1983). Nurses as risk-takers. In J. C. McCloskey & H. K. Grace (Eds.). *Current issues in nursing* (pp. 593–597). Boston: Blackwell Scientific.

Jameton, A. (1984). *Nursing practice—The ethical issues*. Englewood Cliffs, NJ: Prentice-Hall.

Joint Commission on Accreditation for Healthcare Organizations. (2004). *2004 Critical access hospital standards: Ethics, rights, and responsibilities*. Oak Brook, IL: Author.

Jonsen, A. R. (1998). *The birth of bioethics*. New York: Oxford University Press.

Jonsen, A. R. (2000). *A short history of medical ethics*. New York: Oxford University Press.

Jonsen, A. R., Siegler, M., & Winslade, W. J. (2002). *Clinical ethics: A practical approach to ethical decisions in clinical medicine* (5th ed.). New York: McGraw-Hill.

Kleinpell, R. M. (2003). Advanced practice. RNs support family presence with codes, but policies lacking. *Nursing Spectrum (Florida Edition), 13*(15), 6.

Levine, M. E. (1989). Beyond dilemma. . . The crucial issues of nursing ethics: the day-by-day, one-on-one relationship between the nurse and the patient. *Seminars in Oncology Nursing, 5*(2), 124–128.

Lyon, J. (1985). *Playing God in the nursery*. New York: WW Norton.

MacLean, S. L., Guzzetta, C. E., White, C., Fontaine, D., Eichhorn, D. J., Meyers, T. A., et al. (2003). Family presence during cardiopulmonary resuscitation and invasive procedures: Practices of critical care and emergency nurses. *American Journal of Critical Care, 12*(3), 246–257.

Meyers, T. A., Eichhorn, D. J., Guzzetta, C. E., Clark, A. P., Klein, J. D., Taliaferro, E., et al. (2000). Family presence during invasive procedures and resuscitation: the experience of family members, nurses, and physicians. *American Journal of Nursing, 100*(2), 32–43.

Miller, B. F., & Keane, C. B. (1972). *Encyclopedia and dictionary of medicine and nursing*. Philadelphia: WB Saunders.

Muff, J. (Ed.). (1982). *Women's issues in nursing: Socialization, sexism, and stereotyping*. Prospect Heights, IL: Waveland Press.

Murphy, P. (1993). Clinical ethics: Must nurses be forever in the middle? *Bioethics Forum, 9*(4), 3–4.

Nevidjon, G., & Erickson, J. I. (2001). The nursing shortage: Solutions for the short and long term. *Online Journal of Issues in Nursing, 6*(1), manuscript 4. Retrieved January 2, 2005, from http://nursingworld.org/ojin/topic14/tpc14_4.htm

Pence, T., & Cantrall, J. (1990). *Ethics in nursing: An anthology*. New York: National League for Nursing.

President's Commission for the Study of Ethical Problems in Medicine and Biomedical and Behavioral Research. (1983). *Deciding to forego life-sustaining treatment: Ethical, medical, and legal issues in treatment decisions*. Washington, D. C.: U. S. Government Printing Office.

Savage, T. A. (1995). *Nurses' negotiation processes in facilitating ethical decision-making in patient care*. Unpublished doctoral dissertation, University of Illinois at Chicago, Health Science Center.

Stanley, T. (1983). Ethical reflection on the Tuma case: Is it part of the nurse's role to advise on alternative forms of therapy or treatment? In J. C. McCloskey & H. K. Grace (Eds.). *Current issues in nursing* (pp. 715–726). Boston: Blackwell Scientific.

Stein, L. I. (1967). The doctor–nurse game. *Archives of General Psychiatry, 16*, 699–703.

Stein, L. I., Watts, D. T., & Howell, T. (1990). The doctor–nurse game, revisited. *New England Journal of Medicine, 322*(8), 546–549.

Thompson, J. B., & Thompson, H. O. (1981). *Ethics in nursing*. New York: Macmillan.

Tuma, J. L. (1977). Professional misconduct. *Nursing Outlook, 25*, 546.

Veatch, R. M., & Fry, S. T. (1987). *Case studies in nursing ethics*. Philadelphia: Lippincott.

Weinberg, D. B. (2003). *Code green: Money-driven hospitals and the dismantling of nursing*. Ithaca, NY: Cornell University Press.

Winslow, G. R. (1984). From loyalty to advocacy: A new metaphor for nursing. *Hastings Center Report, 14*(3), 32–40.

York, N. L. (2004). Implementing a family presence protocol option. *DCCN: Dimensions of Critical Care Nursing, 23*(2), 84–88.

CHAPTER 3

Ethical Standard of Practice

Objectives

At the end of this chapter, the student should be able to:

1. Analyze the 2001 American Nurses Association's Code of Ethics for Nurses.
2. Identify moral values.
3. Describe his or her code of ethics as a professional nurse.
4. Discriminate between non-maleficence and beneficence.
5. Define standards and scope of practice for registered nurses.
6. Discriminate among differences in standards for the general, specialty, and advanced practice nurse.
7. Strategize on the challenges of abiding by the 2001 American Nurses Association's Code of Ethics for Nurses.
8. Locate policy and position statements relevant to nursing issues.

KEY WORDS

- *Codes of ethics*
- *Scope of practice*
- *Standards*

To understand the ethical standards of practice, it is necessary to understand "standards and scopes of practice," codes of ethics, policy statements, position statements, and other guidelines for nursing practice. The general public, even those who receive nursing care, may not be able to describe what a nurse does. The "standards and scope of practice" describe nursing responsibilities in general, yet measurable, terms. The standards may also be used in specialty nursing practice. One commonly accepted ethical standard for nurses is the American Nurses Association's Code of Ethics for Nurses. Students will have the opportunity to critique the usefulness of this new code for guiding clinical practice, particularly with regard to the ethical concepts of nonmaleficence and beneficence. This chapter describes "standards and scope of practice" and the use of policy and position statements and illustrates the applicability of the Code of Ethics for Nurses.

CODE OF ETHICS

Barnett (2001) claimed that "the development of a code of ethics for a profession is a fundamental attribute that defines a vocation as a profession" (p. 6). Whereas a code of ethics defines a profession's ethical standards and expectations, codes of ethics are not stagnant. Codes of ethics should be modified and revised as the profession is faced with new situations.

The Florence Nightingale Pledge, which was written by Lystra Gretter in 1893, is believed to be the original nursing code of ethics (Box 3-1). Gretter used the Hippocratic Oath, taken by physicians, as an example. In this original pledge, the nurse's dependence on the physician is very noticeable.

After the Nurse's Associated Alumnae of the United States and Canada aborted their effort to draft a code in 1896, the *American Journal of Nursing* published a code in 1926 (Box 3-2). However, the American Nurses Association (ANA) never ratified this code. In fact, there was no "official nursing code of ethics" until the 1950 House of Delegates of the ANA adopted a Code for Professional Nurses (Pinch, 2000) (Box 3-3).

BOX 3-1

The Florence Nightingale Pledge

I solemnly pledge myself before God and presence of this assembly, to pass my life in purity and to practice my profession faithfully.

I will abstain from whatever is deleterious and mischievous, and will not take or knowingly administer any harmful drug.

I will do all in my power to maintain and elevate the standard of my profession, and will hold in confidence all personal matters committed to my keeping and family affairs coming to my knowledge in the practice of my calling.

With loyalty will I endeavor to aid the physician in his work, and devote myself to the welfare of those committed to my care.

Available at http://carenurse.com/creeds/nightengale.html

BOX 3-2

A Suggested Code: A Code of Ethics Presented for the Consideration of the American Nurses' Association[1] in 1926

This suggested Code is under consideration by the American Nurses' Association. It is in no sense final. It is published in order that the Association may have the benefit of the suggestions or criticisms of all its members. Individual nurses and nursing organizations should make a thoughtful study of it during the coming year. Suggestions from other groups also, such as medical, hospital, public health, or social work are invited.

Heir throughout the ages of those who have nurtured the young, the weak and the sick, the mother, the kindly neighbor, the knight on the battlefield, the nun and the deaconess within or without enclosing walls—nursing emerges as a profession from its historic setting in an attempt to meet the present demands of society. The most precious possession of this profession is the ideal of service extending even to the sacrifice of life itself, its incessant effort is to meet the need of the world for skilled and tender care in illness and for wise guidance in attaining and maintaining health, the constant obligation of the profession is to keep abreast of all scientific advancement relating to health.

In common with the other professions, nursing faces the necessity for crystallizing into language those ethical principles which shall be a guide to conduct commonly called a code of ethics. The purpose of such a code is not to provide rules of conduct covering specific types of situations arising in the practice of a profession but rather to create a sensitiveness to ethical situations and to formulate general principles which, rooted in conviction and supported with enthusiasm, create the individual habit of forming conscious and critical judgment resulting in action in specific situations.

The American Nurses' Association, aware of the continuing growth and development of the profession and the necessity for constant adaptation to present social need, has accepted the responsibility imposed upon it by its position of leadership and has formulated the following Code of Ethics. It proposes to subject the Code to the thoughtful scrutiny of its members at each Biennial meeting of the Association in order that it shall be supported as a dynamic force in the life of the profession.

The nurse is primarily a citizen. The fundamental basis of ethics is the same for every profession. The obligation of each individual is to serve society as well as possible by contributing that for which he is best fitted. The obligation of society is to see that the individual has opportunity to develop and to realize the fullest health and happiness possible without interfering with others. This statement is in harmony with the highest ideals of nursing as a profession of service. Nursing beyond peradventure meets a basic human need; the nurse who fails to safeguard her health except in occasional situations of extreme need or in war or other catastrophe becomes an economic liability. Economic independence is admittedly one of the first duties of every citizen, while the nurse who fails to find happiness in her work is not truly a nurse. Self realization and the most complete development of individual capacities are the ideals of present-day society for all of its members. There is no ground for expecting the nurse to be an exception to this rule nor its corollary

(Continued)

BOX 3-2 (CONTINUED)

that self-development can best be nurtured in the soil of economic self-respect. That woman can best fulfill her obligation to state and nation who has a decent margin of time and energy for recreation and with which to keep in touch with current events.

The use of the term "professional" implies exalted purpose, sound preparation and conformance to requirements imposed by the state which evidence such preparation. No worker is welcome to the ranks of nursing who does not put the ideal of service above that of remuneration. The nurse to be considered professional must be willing to subscribe to the purpose of licensure by registering in at least one state, and, if possible, in the state in which she practises. Professional growth and development are promoted by membership in professional organizations, both national, state and local, by attendance at meetings and conventions and by constant reading on professional subjects. Yet further growth may be assured by attendance on institutes and postgraduate courses.

The nurse as a professional worker is a public servant and has many-sided relationships.

The Relation of the Nurse to the Patient

The nurse should bring to the care of the patient all of the knowledge, skill and devotion which she may possess. To do this, she must appreciate the relationship of the patient to his family and to his community. Therefore the nurse must broaden her thoughtful consideration of the patient so that it will include his whole family and his friends, for only in surroundings harmonious and peaceful for the patient can the nurse give her utmost of skill, devotion and knowledge, which shall include the safeguarding of the health of those about the patient and the protection of property.

The Relation of the Nurse to the Medical Profession

The term "medicine" should be understood to refer to *scientific* medicine and the desirable relationship between the two should be one of mutual respect. The nurse should be fully Informed on the provisions of the medical practice act of her own state in order that she may not unconsciously support quackery and actual infringements of the law. The key to the situation lies in the mutuality of aim of medicine and nursing; the aims, to cure and prevent disease and promote positive health, are identical, the technics of the two are different and neither profession can secure complete results without the other. The nurse should respect the physician as the person legally and professionally responsible for the medical and surgical treatment of the sick. She should endeavor to give such intelligent and skilled nursing service that she will be looked upon as a co-worker of the doctor in the whole field of health.

Under no circumstances, except in emergency, is the nurse justified in instituting treatment.

The Relation of the Nurse to the Allied Professions

The health of the public has come to demand many services other than nursing. Without the closest interrelation of workers and appreciation of the ethical standards of all groups and a clear understanding of the limitations of her own group, the best results in building positive health in the community cannot be obtained.

BOX 3-2   (CONTINUED)

Relation of Nurse to Nurse

The "Golden Rule" embodies all that could be written in many pages on the relation of nurse to nurse. This should be one of fine loyalty, of appreciation for work conscientiously done, and of respect for positions of authority. On the other hand, loyalty to the motive which inspires nursing should make the nurse fearless to bring to light any serious violation of the ideals herein expressed; the larger loyalty is that to the community, for loyalty to an ideal is higher than any personal loyalty.

Relation of the Nurse to Her Profession

The nurse has a definite responsibility to her profession as a whole. The contribution of individual service is not enough. She should, in addition, give a reasonable portion of her time to the furtherance of such advancements of the profession as are only possible through action of the group as a whole. This involves attendance at meetings and the acquisition of information at least sufficient for intelligent participation in such matters as organization and legislation.

The supreme responsibility of the nurse in relation to her profession is to keep alight that spiritual flame which has illumined the work of the great nurses of all time.

¹Read before and discussed by the Association at Atlantic City, May 1926, and referred back to the Committee on Ethical Standards for further study and final report at the Biennial in 1928.

Source: Originally published in the *American Journal of Nursing 26*(8), 599–601 (1926). Reprinted with permission from American Nurses Association, *Code of ethics for nurses with interpretive statements,* © 2001 nursesbooks.org, American Nurses Association, Washington, D.C.

Some minor changes were made to the code in 1956, but a major revision was completed in 1960. Another revision occurred in 1968, and the Interpretive Statements were a prominent addition to the 1976 version. Although the basic provisions of the Code remained the same, the Interpretive Statements underwent a serious revision in 1985. (Pinch, 2000, p. 35)

One reason for the 1968 revision was to "eliminate any reference to 'private ethics'" and instead to focus on "personal ethics which reflect credit upon the profession" (Pinch, 2000, p. 35). In addition, the language of the code became more generic, using the term "health professions" rather than referring specifically to physicians. The 1976 revision included nonsexist language and used the broader term "client" rather than "patient" (Pinch, 2000). The 1976 Code for Nurses is given in Box 3-4.

The conflict of interests experienced by many nurses who worked for health maintenance organizations (HMOs) and managed care was one major impetus for the 2001 revision of the code. This latest revision took 5 years to accomplish. The ANA presented nine drafts, which members debated before the 2000 ANA House of Delegates finally adopted the latest revision. One key change was the title of the document, which was changed from Code for Nurses to Code of Ethics for Nurses.

BOX 3-3

1950 American Nurses Association Code for Professional Nurses

Professional nurses minister to the sick, assume responsibility for creating a physical, social, and spiritual environment which will be conducive to recovery, and stress the prevention of illness and promotion of health by teaching and example. They render health service to the individual, the family, and the community and co-ordinate their services with members of other health professions involved in specific situations.

Service to mankind is the primary function of nurses and the reason for the existence of the nursing profession. Need for nursing service is universal. Professional nursing service is therefore unrestricted by considerations of nationality, race, creed, or color.

Inherent in the code is the fundamental concept that the nurse subscribes to the democratic values to which our country is committed.

With reference to the following statements, the profession recognizes that a professional code cannot cover in detail all the activities and relationships of nurses, some of which are conditioned by personal philosophies and beliefs.

1. The fundamental responsibility of the nurse is to conserve life and to promote health.

2. The professional nurse must not only be adequately prepared to practice, but can maintain professional status only by continued reading, study, observation, and investigation.

3. When a patient requires continuous nursing service, the nurse must remain with the patient until assured that adequate relief is available.

4. The religious beliefs of a patient must be respected.

5. Professional nurses hold in confidence all personal information entrusted to them.

6. A nurse recommends or gives medical treatment without medical orders only in emergencies and reports such action to a physician at the earliest possible moment.

7. The nurse is obligated to carry out the physician's orders intelligently, to avoid misunderstanding or inaccuracies by verifying orders and to refuse to participate in unethical procedures.

8. The nurse sustains confidence in the physician and other members of the health team; incompetency or unethical conduct of associates in the health professions should be exposed, but only to the proper authority.

9. The nurse has an obligation to give conscientious service and in return is entitled to just remuneration.

10. A nurse accepts only such compensation as the contract, actual or implied, provides. A professional worker does not accept tips or bribes.

11. Professional nurses do not permit their names to be used in connection with testimonials in the advertisement of products.

(Continued)

> ## BOX 3-3   (CONTINUED)
>
> **12.** The Golden Rule should guide the nurse in relationships with members of other professions and with nursing associates.
>
> **13.** The nurse in private life adheres to standards of personal ethics which reflect credit upon the profession.
>
> **14.** In personal conduct nurses should not knowingly disregard the accepted patterns of behavior of the community in which they live and work.
>
> **15.** The nurse as a citizen understands and upholds the laws and as a professional worker is especially concerned with those laws which affect the practice of medicine and nursing.
>
> **16.** A nurse should participate and share responsibility with other citizens and health professions in promoting efforts to meet the health needs of the public—local, state, national, and international.
>
> **17.** A nurse recognizes and performs the duties of citizenship, such as voting and holding office when eligible; these duties include an appreciation of the social, economic, and political factors which develop a desirable pattern of living together in a community.
>
> *Source:* Originally published in the *American Journal of Nursing* (1950). Reprinted with permission from American Nurses Association, *Code of ethics for nurses with interpretive statements,* © 2001 nursesbooks.org, American Nurses Association, Washington, D.C.

As you read the 2001 Code of Ethics for Nurses with Interpretive Statements (American Nurses Association [ANA], 2001) (see Box 3-5 on page 58), consider what moral values are represented in this code. A value

---

represents a way of life. The development of values relates to one's self-identity. Value development derives from life experience; therefore, each person discovers what his/her values are as life is experienced. . . . This notion of self-discovery negates the notion that values are rigidly prescribed and taught as a set of "ought to's." Rather, values develop from association with other people, the environment, and with self. . . . A value is something that is chosen from alternatives, is acted on, and contributes to the person's creative integration and personality development. A value is a stance taken and is expressed through behaviors, feelings, imagination, knowledge, and actions. (Steele, 1983, p. 1)

STANDARDS AND SCOPE OF PRACTICE

Despite movies and television shows depicting nurses, the general public does not have a clear notion of what nurses do and what guides their practice. There is

---

BOX 3-4

1976 American Nurses Association Code for Nurses

1. The nurse provides services with respect for human dignity and the uniqueness of the client, unrestricted by considerations of social or economic status, personal attributes, or the nature of health problems.

2. The nurse safeguards the client's right to privacy by judiciously protecting information of a confidential nature.

3. The nurse acts to safeguard the client and the public when health care and safety are affected by the incompetent, unethical, or illegal practice of any person.

4. The nurse assumes responsibility and accountability for individual nursing judgments and actions.

5. The nurse maintains competence in nursing.

6. The nurse exercises informed judgment and uses individual competence and qualifications as criteria in seeking consultation, accepting responsibilities, and delegating nursing activities to others.

7. The nurse participates in activities that contribute to the ongoing development of the profession's body of knowledge.

8. The nurse participates in the profession's efforts to implement and improve standards of nursing.

9. The nurse participates in the profession's efforts to establish and maintain conditions of employment conducive to high-quality nursing care.

10. The nurse participates in the profession's effort to protect the public from misinformation and misrepresentation and to maintain the integrity of nursing.

11. The nurse collaborates with members of the health professions and other citizens in promoting community and national efforts to meet the health needs of the public.

Source: Originally published by the American Nurses Association (1976, 1985). Kansas City, MO: Author. Reprinted with permission from American Nurses Association, Code of Ethics with Interpretive Statements, © 1976, 1985 nursesbooks.org, American Nurses Association, Washington, DC.

---

often the misconception that physicians direct nursing care and that nurses "serve" physicians as their assistants. Even during a hospitalization, patients may not be aware of all that nurses do in the course of delivering patient care. Nurses are accountable to the public for their practice, and to that end, the ANA has articulated standards and scope for nursing practice. Over time, the standards and scope have been revised, and each state has a Nurse Practice Act that describes the scope of practice for nurses in that state. "Standards are authoritative statements by which the nursing profession describes the responsibilities for which its practitioners are accountable" (ANA, 2004, p. 1). The scope of practice describes "the *who, what, where, when, why,* and *how* of nursing practice" (ANA, 2004, p. 1).

For example, Nurse Brian Starr, who works in a neonatal intensive care unit, is licensed by his state's Board of Nursing as a Registered Professional Nurse. Under that license, he can deliver nursing care in any setting, but he chooses to specialize in neonatal intensive care nursing. To practice ethically, he adheres to the standards of practice in neonatal nursing, and he maintains his competency of the evolving knowledge within this specialty. His psychomotor skills remain current. He has a greater depth of knowledge in this specialty than someone in adult health nursing. The "scope of nursing" allows the neonatal nurse and, for example, the adult health nurse to practice nursing, but to work in different specialties.

The standards for practice follow the nursing process and have broad categories of assessment, diagnosis, outcomes identification, planning, implementation, and evaluation (ANA, 2004, p. 3). There are also standards for the nurse to follow as a member of the profession of nursing. These additional standards focus on quality, education, evaluation of professional practice, collaboration, ethics, research, resource utilization, and leadership (ANA, 2004, p. 3).

Nurse Starr is expected to conduct patient assessments, develop for each patient a nursing care plan that is individualized and consistent with the current state of knowledge in neonatal nursing, implement the plan of care, and effectively communicate the plan to all other appropriate health care providers. He is also expected to participate in activities at his institution that monitor and improve the quality of nursing practice, to keep his knowledge base and skills current, and to keep current with the guidelines, statutes, rules, and regulations governing his practice.

Nurse Starr should contribute to the professional development of his colleagues through the sharing of his knowledge. His nursing care should be done in collaboration with other members on the health care team. He should practice judicious stewardship with resources; should integrate research findings in his practice; and provide leadership in his institution, his practice area, and the nursing profession.

It may sound overwhelming that a nurse can work 40+ hours a week in a physically and emotionally demanding profession while also caring for his or her family, participating in community activities, meeting the expectations of the standards of practice, and finding time to rejuvenate his or her energies. The work environment must be conducive to safe nursing practice and must facilitate nurses' ability to adhere to the standards of practice. Each nurse, as a professional, must commit to adhering to the standards of practice, and each nurse must work within his or her place of employment and with the state nurses' association to structure a work environment that is conducive to adherence to the standards of practice.

POLICY AND POSITION STATEMENTS

Health care is dynamic, and it changes with new discoveries and changing attitudes. To be current with new knowledge and the changing health care delivery system, standards of practice change. Interested groups often issue policy or position statements that reflect their current thinking on various topics. It can be helpful for nurses to be familiar with statements that are relevant to the nurses' practice areas. Nurses can determine individually or as a group how relevant and useful the statements are in their practice. One case that has been in the news recently illustrates the need for nurses to examine the positions of various groups.

Terri Schiavo was a 40-year-old woman who experienced anoxic brain damage in 1990. She became the focus of national attention when her husband, as surrogate decision-maker, sought to have her feeding tube removed. Her parents opposed removing the feeding tube and sought to have the husband removed as surrogate. The issues that were disputed were the husband's ability to represent his wife's interests, the allegations that he had not provided the rehabilitative treatments he promised to provide when he won a malpractice settlement, and whether she was in a persistent vegetative state for which further rehabilitation would be futile. Terri Schiavo lived in a hospice in anticipation of her death after the removal of the feeding tube. She had been moved back and forth between the hospice and a nursing home when the feeding tube was removed. When a court ruled that the tube could be removed, it was removed for 6 days. In an unprecedented action, the Florida legislature passed Terri's Law, which gave Florida Governor Jeb Bush the power to reverse the courts' decision and order the feeding tube reinserted. This law was overturned by the Florida Supreme Court, which stated that the law violated separation of powers between executive and legislative branches. The U.S. Supreme Court refused to hear the case, which meant that the ruling of the lower court stood. Although there are many issues in this case that merit detailed discussion, the purpose of presenting it in this section is to identify where policy or position statements might assist nurses in analyzing similar situations. In this case, two issues under dispute were whether Terri Schiavo was in a persistent vegetative state and whether the feeding tube could ethically be removed. Nurses can refer to policies in their institutions and position statements of national or local professional organizations regarding the persistent vegetative state and minimally conscious states, their diagnosis and prognosis, and considerations regarding forgoing nutrition and hydration.

The Florida courts decided, based on the evidence presented, that Terri Schiavo was in a persistent vegetative state. Her parents contended that she could focus and follow visual stimuli and that she responded to her parents by smiling and making sounds. Against a court order, they released a videotape supposedly demonstrating these abilities. A speech pathologist swore an affidavit that she believed, based on examining records and videotapes, that Schiavo was not in a persistent vegetative state but was in a minimally conscious state.

Because both conditions reflect significant brain damage and limitations in functioning, this difference may seem like splitting hairs. However, some people, especially Terri Schiavo's family, believed she would improve with rehabilitation. For example, the American Academy of Neurology (AAN) (1995) has practice parameters on the assessment and management of the persistent vegetative state (PVS). In the statement, the AAN described how the clinical diagnosis of PVS is made and that, in the case of nontraumatic injuries (such as Schiavo's injury), the diagnosis of *permanent* can be made after 3 months. It also stated that the physician and the patient's surrogate must determine the appropriate continuation or withdrawal of artificial nutrition and hydration. Nurses can refer to this statement to see the AAN's recommendations on how the diagnosis of PVS should be made. The AAN statement, however, does not advise how to resolve conflict when the clinical diagnosis of PVS is in dispute. In cases where the patient's family members disagree about the best course of action for the patient, health care professionals can refer to policy and procedures that are already in place to determine how to proceed.

The practice of withdrawing nutrition and hydration from people in "permanent" vegetative states (vegetative states persisting longer than 1 year) is common, according to Dr. Ronald Cranford, bioethicist and neurologist at the University of Minnesota

Bioethics Center. Cranford (2003) maintained that there are approximately 25,000 to 35,000 people in the United States in a permanent vegetative state, and "tens or hundreds of times every week … hundreds of thousands of times a year" nutrition and hydration are withdrawn. If the family does not agree that the patient is "hopeless" or if there is conflict among the family, then, in his practice, nutrition and hydration are not discontinued.

Seven years earlier, Cranford was asked whether the adjective "permanent" should be dropped from the AAN practice parameters in light of the case of a woman recovering from a vegetative state after being in it for 3 years. Because recoveries were infrequent, he disagreed with dropping the label of "permanent," and he dismissed the woman's recovery as not being a "meaningful recovery" because she still required the use of a wheelchair and had an attention span of 15 minutes (Cranford, 1996). One might conclude that whereas the AAN finds it permissible to withdraw nutrition and hydration from a person in a persistent or permanent vegetative state, not all neurologists will use its practice parameters to make such a diagnosis or to medically manage such conditions. As in the example just cited, some neurologists find it ethically permissible to remove nutrition and hydration, when the family requests it, from patients who have severe brain damage but who are not actually in vegetative states.

Another guide that could be pertinent in cases of people with PVS is the statement that Pope John Paul II made in March 2004 at an international congress entitled "Life-Sustaining Treatments and Vegetative State: Scientific Advances and Ethical Dilemmas." Such statements by the pope are interpreted as Church policy. The pertinent passages in the Pope's statement are as follows:

I should like particularly to underline how the administration of water and food, even when provided by artificial means, always represents a natural means *of preserving life, not a* medical act. *Its use, furthermore, should be considered, in principle,* ordinary and proportionate, *and, as such, morally obligatory insofar as and until it is seen to have attained its proper finality, which, in the present case, consists in providing nourishment to the patient, and alleviation of his suffering. . . . The evaluation of probabilities founded on waning hopes for recovery when the vegetative state is prolonged beyond a year cannot ethically justify the cessation or interruption of* minimal care *for the patient, including nutrition and hydration. Death by starvation or dehydration is, in fact, the only possible outcome as result of their withdrawal. In this sense it ends up becoming, if done knowingly and willingly, true and proper euthanasia by omission . . . such an act is always* a serious violation of the law of God, *since it is the deliberate and morally unacceptable killing of a human person.* [Emphasis as in original text] *(John Paul II, 2004)*

The Pope's statement indicates the unacceptability, according to Church policy, of removing a feeding tube and discontinuing nutrition and hydration for someone in a persistent vegetative state. What does this policy mean for a Catholic patient (e.g., Terri Schiavo)? What does this policy mean for a Catholic health care provider? What does it mean for a Catholic institution? The World Federation of Catholic Medical Associations (WFCMA) issued a public statement that discourages the use of the adjective "permanent" and reinforces the pope's statement. Regarding nutrition and hydration, the WFCMA (2004) says,

---

The possible decision of withdrawing nutrition and hydration, necessarily administered to VS patients in an assisted way, is followed inevitably by the patients' death, as a direct consequence. Therefore, it has to be considered a genuine act of euthanasia by omission, which is morally unacceptable.

In other religions, such as Judaism, there is no single authority, such as the Pope is in Roman Catholicism. Followers of Judaism use the writings of preeminent halakhic (Jewish law) scholars and ethicists for guidance in informed decision-making. One such scholar, Dr. David Bleich (1998), stated "that the life of a mentally incompetent person, and even of a patient in a permanent vegetative state, must be prolonged to the extent possible so long as the patient does not suffer extreme pain" (p. 88). Another scholar, Rabbi Feinstein (as cited in Resnicoff, 1998), agreed that the "life of a mentally incompetent, or a person in a permanent vegetative state, must be prolonged as much as possible so long as the person is not experiencing pain."

Nurses who provide care for patients who are in a persistent vegetative state should be aware of the policies, practice parameters, and guidelines that relate to this issue. By helping families to gather pertinent information on forgoing nutrition and hydration, nurses can facilitate decision-making by families when patients' wishes are unknown (for more on ethical decision-making see Chapter 5). For some nurses, if treatment decisions (and hence their nursing care) become inconsistent with positions held by the groups to which these nurses belong and the groups whose values they embrace, their ability to continue to remain involved in patients' care may be affected. A nurse may conscientiously object to participating in the removal of nutrition and hydration, even if that was the patient's wishes (for more on conscientious objection see Chapter 16). Shannon and Walter (2004) suggested that the papal allocution will affect Catholic health care institutions, health care providers, and patients if it is interpreted by Catholic bishops to mandate tube feedings in cases of PVS. Repenshek and Slosar (2004) disagreed and believed that the pope's statement allows for consideration of the specifics of any individual case, so that tube feedings are not obligatory and can be discontinued for patients in PVS.

Terri Schiavo's feeding tube was removed March 18, 2005, by court order, and she died March 31, 2005, 13 days after its removal. Her case polarized the ethics community and the nation, who saw the removal of the tube as either respecting her right to refuse medical treatment or the murder of a vulnerable, disabled woman. [For more details about the Schiavo case, see the Terri Schiavo Information Page (2005).]

CODES OF ETHICS

Codes of ethics are created to benefit the public. Codes of ethics "Must be constructed carefully, with the understanding that behavior not explicitly deemed unethical will, by default, be accepted as ethical" (Barnett, 2001, p. 8). However, just having a code of ethics is not sufficient. Professional organizations must also investigate allegations of behavior that is contrary to the organization's code and must enforce it. In all likelihood, the majority of allegations of behavior contrary to the Code of Ethics for Nurses are related to the ethical principles of non-maleficence and beneficence. Usually, enforcement of an organization's code of ethics (such as the ANA's code) results only in loss of membership within the professional organization. Codes of ethics are not usually legally binding, but they may be used by individual state licensing boards to establish practice expectations and standards.

THE 2001 ANA CODE OF ETHICS FOR NURSES: ASPIRATIONS AND CHALLENGES

The 2001 ANA Code of Ethics for Nurses represents the highest aspirations for the ethical practice of professional nurses in the United States (Box 3-5). These aspirations represent the ideal action a nurse should, and therefore ought to, achieve in his or her daily practice. Most of the time, these aspirations will be realistic challenges that a professional nurse will agree with and be able to achieve. However, the possibility exists that a professional nurse will find himself or herself in a dilemma when situational variables or other ethical commitments are in conflict with the ideals set forth in the 2001 Code of Ethics for Nurses. The section presents an exemplar (illustrating the provision in action) and a challenging situation (illustrating the difficulty a nurse might experience when attempting to meet the expectation) for each provision of the code.

(Each provision listed below is reprinted with permission from American Nurses Association, *Code of ethics for nurses with interpretive statements*, © 2001 nursesbooks.org, American Nurses Association, Washington, D.C.)

Provision 1

The nurse, in all professional relationships, practices with compassion and respect for the inherent dignity, worth, and uniqueness of every individual unrestricted by considerations of social or economic status, personal attributes, or the nature of health problems.

Exemplar
An obese patient with necrotizing fasciitis was unable to see the large surgical wound that was created when necrotic abdominal tissue was removed. The wound was draining into a drainage bag. After the student nurse provided morning care, the patient complemented the nursing student's care with, "Thank you so much for not gawking at me the first time you saw my wound, and for always closing the door." The patient went on to explain how some medical students would barge in, leaving the door open, and gawk at her wound while exclaiming, "Awesome!" Provision 1.1 reminds nurses that all nursing encounters should promote the dignity of each patient.

Challenges
1. You are working in the post-anesthesia recovery (PAR) unit and are assigned to care for a patient who just underwent an appendectomy. When the patient is admitted to the PAR, a guard accompanies him. The anesthesiologist explains that the patient is currently incarcerated for child abuse. For the last 3 years, you have been a "big sibling" to a child who was

BOX 3-5

2001 American Nursing Association Code of Ethics for Nurses

1. The nurse, in all professional relationships, practices with compassion and respect for the inherent dignity, worth, and uniqueness of every individual, unrestricted by considerations of social or economic status, personal attributes, or the nature of health problems.

2. The nurse's primary commitment is to the patient, whether an individual, family, group, or community.

3. The nurse promotes, advocates for, and strives to protect the health, safety, and rights of the patient.

4. The nurse is responsible and accountable for individual nursing practice and determines the appropriate delegation of tasks consistent with the nurse's obligation to provide optimum patient care.

5. The nurse owes the same duties to self as to others, including the responsibility to preserve integrity and safety, to maintain competence, and to continue personal and professional growth.

6. The nurse participates in establishing, maintaining, and improving health care environments and conditions of employment conductive to the provision of quality health care and consistent with the values of the profession through individual and collective action.

7. The nurse participates in the advancement of the profession through contributions to practice, education, administration, and knowledge development.

8. The nurse collaborates with other health professionals and the public in promoting community, national, and international efforts to meet health needs.

9. The profession of nursing, as represented by associations and their members, is responsible for articulating nursing values, for maintaining the integrity of the profession and its practice, and for shaping social policy.

Source: Reprinted with permission from American Nurses Association, *Code of ethics for nurses with interpretive statements,* © 2001 nursesbooks.org, American Nurses Association, Washington, D.C.

physically abused by an uncle and, as a result, you have strong opinions about people who abuse children.

2. Last year, you were the first one on the scene of a motor vehicle accident with fatalities that were caused by a drunk driver. Since that time, you have been involved in a variety of social causes advocating for tougher penalties for people who cause traffic fatalities while driving drunk. You are working in the PAR unit and are assigned to care for a patient who suffered chest and abdominal injuries during an automobile accident. When the patient was admitted to the PAR, you learned that he was driving with a blood alcohol level of 1.6 when he ran a red light and hit a minivan. Two children and the driver of the other vehicle were pronounced dead at the scene of the accident.

Situations like these create tension between the nurse's ability to have respect for persons even when the nurse has little or no respect for the person's actions.

Provision 2

The nurse's primary commitment is to the patient, whether an individual, family, group, or community.

Exemplar

Mr. Keith, an 89-year-old man with an internal cardiac defibrillator, asks that the device be removed even though he is at risk for a fatal arrhythmia. He is a widower, and his adult children do not want him to remove the device. He tells them that he experiences significant pain and discomfort when the defibrillator shocks him, which is occurring more frequently, and that he would prefer to die from his failing heart than to live this way. All the other medical options available to treat his arrhythmia have been exhausted. His children oppose his decision, but Mr. Keith has decisional capacity, therefore, his request will be honored.

Challenge

You are the discharge-planning nurse for a neurosurgical unit. Mr. Post is a 30-year-old who experienced a spinal cord injury when he lost control of and was thrown from his motorcycle. He sustained a C4 ASIA A injury, rendering him tetraplegic. It is likely he will require around-the-clock assistance. He has refused to consider a long-term care facility, stating that, "Nobody with an active mind lives at those places." He has asked to live with his parents; however, his parents have not agreed to this request. As you talk with the parents, you find out that both of them have several chronic illnesses that affect their physical strength and stamina. In fact, 2 days before their son's injury, the parents listed their house for sale, and they were planning to buy a condominium in a retirement community. They would be unable to care for their son in their condominium. How should the nurse proceed because Provision 2 requires that her primary commitment is to be an advocate for Mr. Post and not for his parents?

Provision 3

The nurse promotes, advocates for, and strives to protect the health, safety, and rights of the patient.

Exemplar

Provision 3.2 states that "A nurse has a duty to maintain confidentiality of all patient information." One nursing student illustrated his commitment to confidentiality by explaining that "All nursing students write only initials on the paperwork we submit to our instructors. While on the unit, we keep all papers turned over, so no patient information is ever visible to other persons walking down the hallway. I have never heard a nursing student mention a patient's name in conversation off the clinical unit."

Challenge

You are working the night shift on a surgical unit. At 4 A.M., you realize that your patient's bag of intravenous (IV) fluids is running out. When you check the physician's orders (1 liter of lactated Ringer's over 10 hours × 1 bag), you notice that there is no order for any additional IV fluids. At 3:30 A.M., the surgical resident on call told you, "I am exhausted. I am going to try to get a couple hours of sleep before I have to operate again this morning. Please do not call me unless it's really urgent." Based on your experience with the resident and your knowledge of your patient's medical condition, you conclude that the resident would reorder the patient's current IV fluids if you were to notify her. However, knowing that the resident's skills can be impaired by lack of sleep, you are reluctant to interrupt the resident's sleep. Because no additional IV fluid orders exist, is it more ethical to saline-lock the patient's IV access, to anticipate the resident's orders by hanging another bag of the same solution for which you do not have an order, or to wake the resident and get her to write the order?

Provision 4

The nurse is responsible and accountable for individual nursing practice and determines the appropriate delegation of tasks consistent with the nurse's obligation to provide optimum patient care.

Exemplar

Provision 4.3 states, "Individual nurses are responsible for assessing their own competence. When the needs of the patient are beyond the qualifications and competencies of the nurse, consultation and collaboration must be sought from qualified nurses, other health professionals or other appropriate sources." A nursing student was assigned to care for a patient who was scheduled to have hemodialysis at 10 A.M. in the patient's room. The student realized that hemodialysis could possibly alter the effectiveness of some of the medications that were scheduled to be given to the patient at 8 A.M. Recognizing her limited knowledge of pharmacokinetics, the student (after consulting with his nursing instructor) collaborated with the hospital pharmacist to determine which drugs could be safely administered during dialysis and which would have to be held until after the dialysis was complete.

Challenge

While you are in the middle of a complex dressing change, a nursing aide comes to you, stating, "Mrs. Reneau wants to go to physical therapy without her IV. Transport is already here, so I need you to disconnect her IV now." The hospital's policy states that only a registered nurse may initiate or discontinue an intravenous infusion. Because the hospital also has a policy that every peripheral IV site must have a saline-lock, can you delegate the task of disconnecting the IV to the nursing aide because you believe the potential risk to the patient is minimal? Although it is tempting to delegate a task that you believe is of minimal risk, it would violate policy and could potentially harm the patient, and so delegating to the nursing assistant is not an ethical option.

Provision 5

The nurse owes the same duties to self as to others, including the responsibility to preserve integrity and safety, to maintain competence, and to continue personal and professional growth.

Exemplar

A staff nurse on an oncology unit recognized that a patient was being significantly undermedicated for pain. After confirming with other staff nurses that there was a knowledge deficit among the staff regarding long-term pain management with oncology patients, the nurse discussed this observation with her clinical manager. As a result, the clinical manager arranged for the clinical nurse specialist from the pain management service to provide a series of in-services to the oncology staff nurses. This illustrates the oncology staff nurse's and the clinical manager's commitment to Provision 5.2's requirement that professional nurses must have "a commitment to life-long learning."

Challenge

You are working the night shift in an intensive care unit that is staffed with two registered nurses. You have been unable to take a break because your assigned patients have been unstable and have required frequent monitoring. You are now experiencing symptoms of hypoglycemia and you realize that you need to eat. However, the cafeteria closed 30 minutes ago, there are no vending machines in the unit, and the hospital has a policy that employees who eat food from the patient nutrition center will be fired. Because the other nurse is busy stabilizing a new patient and is unable to relieve you, do you continue to work, or do you drink a glass of orange juice from the patient nutrition center?

Provision 6

The nurse participates in establishing, maintaining, and improving health care environments and conditions of employment conducive to the provision of quality health care and consistent with the values of the profession through individual and collective action.

Exemplar

One morning, during change-of-shift report, a nurse commented, "We ran out of morphine again last night. I am so frustrated with always running out of medications during the night." Other nurses concurred with this observation, and together they approached their nursing supervisor with this concern. The nursing supervisor suggested that the unit's nurses should complete the hospital's "unusual occurrence" form each time the unit ran out of a routinely stocked narcotic. As a result of creating a clear paper trail that documented the continued shortage of routinely stocked medications on the unit, the pharmacy instituted a new inventory schedule and a new distribution system. The actions of these nurses represent a commitment to Provision 6.3's requirement that nurses address concerns through appropriate organizational structures.

Challenge

The unit director for a busy neonatal intensive care unit (NICU) communicates the following challenge to the nursing staff: "If the NICU does not use any agency staffing during the last 2 weeks of the year, each nurse will receive an end-of-the-year bonus!" This challenge places the nursing staff in a potential conflict of interest (for more on ethical issues related to staffing see Chapter 17). To receive the promised bonus, the nurses may be tempted to accept staffing ratios that would not be acceptable if the bonus challenge were not in place.

Provision 7

The nurse participates in the advancement of the profession through contributions to practice, education, administration, and knowledge development.

Exemplar

Nurse Angostino and Nurse Beckham, staff nurses in orthopedics, attend an annual conference on joint replacement. They instruct other staff nurses about the evidence supporting clinical pathways, pain management, and different models of nursing care delivery in orthopedic nursing. They also convert their presentation into a manuscript for a nursing journal and submit it for publication.

Challenges

1. In Interpretive Statement 7.1, the ANA states, "Nurses can also advance the profession by serving in leadership or mentorship roles." For example, Nurse Cohen has a number of unstable patients. The nursing instructor, in consultation with the charge nurse, assigns a student to one of Nurse Cohen's patients. Nurse Cohen asks the charge nurse to get the student reassigned because he believes that precepting a student will take too much time and he cannot safely manage his workload and precept a student on this particular day. Is Nurse Cohen's request unethical?
2. The nursing administration of a large academic medical center expects staff nurses who hold elected leadership positions in the staff nurse organization to attend committee meetings on their days off because they are unable to take time during their regular shifts to attend meetings. Does this provision support the administration's stance that staff nurses who hold leadership offices in the hospital nursing staff organization should fulfill these duties on personal time, without financial compensation from the hospital?

Provision 8

The nurse collaborates with other health professionals and the public in promoting community, national, and international efforts to meet health needs.

Exemplar

Nurses from across the United States rallied to support the health care needs in New York City that followed the September 11 attack on the World Trade Center. Individual nurses, nursing groups, and nursing organizations collaborated with the American Red Cross and other governmental and health agencies to provide not only professional nursing services, but also financial, material, and emotional support.

Challenge

Nurse Zoloff, a nurse working in a medical office, has been told that he cannot give appointments to patients who have outstanding balances on their bills unless they make a $10 co-payment. He realizes that some patients have to choose among paying their rent, buying groceries, and paying their medical bills. However, he has been reprimanded for violating this policy and giving appointments to patients who have not paid their co-pays. There is a patient who is requesting an appointment, who owes a balance, and who cannot make the co-pay. What should Nurse Zoloff do?

Provision 9

The profession of nursing, as represented by associations and their members, is responsible for articulating nursing values, maintaining the integrity of the profession and its practice, and shaping social policy.

Exemplar

A group of nurses in the state nurses association drafted a position statement on the use of genetic technologies and forwarded it to their board of directors for review and adoption. The process of drafting the position statement involved numerous meetings, trips to the library, and hours of writing and editing the draft. The nurses donated their time to their nursing organization to accomplish this task.

Challenge

Because "the profession of nursing is represented by associations," do nurses have an ethical obligation to be active members in national and/or specialty nursing organizations? If so, what level of involvement is ethically mandatory? For example, some nurses will state, "Even though I do not attend any meetings, my dues help to support the political lobbying that promotes the interests of nurses." Are financial contributions enough? A local district of a national nursing organization that has a membership of 700 nurses. However, during a recent election of officers, the slate of officers was uncontested, and there was no candidate identified for president. When the ballots were counted, it was found that fewer than 25 members had voted. Thus, one must question how this local district will be able to carry out its mandate to articulate nursing values and shape social policy with such a limited involvement by its members.

SUMMARY

Codes, policy, standards, and position statements are used by professions to communicate not only minimal expectations, but also the ideals the profession is aspiring to achieve. Individual nurses, the nursing profession, and the public need to realize that achieving these ethical aspirations may not be easy at times. In fact, if achieving these ethical ideals were easy, then there would be no need to create ethical codes, policies, standards, and position statements, and nurses would not experience conflict and indecision while attempting to do what is right or what ought to be done.

CLINICAL EXERCISES

1. Talk with a nurse about:

   - The nursing organizations in which he or she holds a professional membership.

- Whether his or her organization has a code of ethics.
- Whether the nurse find the 2001 ANA Code of Ethics for Nurses or other codes or position statements to be helpful resources. Why or why not?

Discussion Questions

1. What moral values are expressed through the 2001 ANA Code of Ethics for Nurses?
2. Briefly describe an action that you took or witnessed professionally that illustrates a commitment to do good/what is right. What guidance (if any) does the 2001 ANA Code of Ethics for Nurses provide in relation to your example of a commitment to do good/what is right?
3. Briefly describe an action that you took or witnessed professionally that illustrates a lack of commitment to do good/what is right. What guidance (if any) does the 2001 ANA Code of Ethics for Nurses provide in relation to your example of a lack of commitment to do good/what is right?
4. Compare the nine provisions of the 2001 ANA Code of Ethics for Nurses with the 11 points of the 1975 Code for Nurses. Discuss at least one difference.
5. Create a position statement that communicates your clinical group's stance on the practice of having nursing students rotate among all three shifts (and weekends) during their leadership/management and community health clinical rotations.
6. Compare and contrast the standards, policies, and position papers written by various nursing and health care organizations and by special-interest groups and religious organizations regarding:

- Informed consent.
- Palliative care and pain control.
- Forgoing nutrition and hydration.

Resources

American Academy of Neurology. (1995). Practice parameters: Assessment and management of patients in the persistent vegetative state. Retrieved March 5, 2005, from http://www.aan.com/professionals/practice/pdfs/pdf_1995_thru_1998/1995.45.1015.pdf

American Association of Managed Care Nurses. (2004). *Managed care nursing practice standards*. Glen Allen, VA: Author.

Association of Rehabilitation Nurses. Position statements are available at http://www.rehabnurse.org/profresources/index.html

International Society of Nurses in Genetics (ISONG). Position statements are available at http://www.isong.org/about/position_statements/index.html and http://www.isong.org/practice/standards/index.htm (retrieved May 15, 2005).

John Paul II. (2004). Address of John Paul II to the participants in the International Congress on "Life-Sustaining Treatments and Vegetative State: Scientific Advances and Ethical Dilemmas." Retrieved May 15, 2005, from www.vatican.va/holy_father/john_paul_ii/speeches/2004/march/documents/hf_jp-ii_spe_20040320_congress-fiamc_en.html

National Mental Health Association. (2005). Standards for responsible management of consumer information. Retrieved May 15, 2005, from http://www.nmha.org/position/ps34.cfm

National Association of the Deaf. (2003). Position statement on mental health services for people who are deaf and hard of hearing. Retrieved May 15, 2005, from http://www.nad.org/infocenter/newsroom/positions/mentalhealth.html

National Black Nurses Association. Position papers and briefing papers are available at http://www.nbna.org/papers.htm

References

American Academy of Neurology. (1995). Practice parameters: Assessment and management of patients in the persistent vegetative state. *Neurology, 45*, 1015–1018.

American Nurses' Association. (1926). A suggested code: A code of ethics presented for consideration of the American Nurses' Association. *American Journal of Nursing*, 26(8), 599–601.

American Nurses Association. (1950). A code for professional nurses. *American Journal of Nursing, 50*(7), 392.

American Nurses Association. (1976, 1985). *Code for nurses with interpretive statements*. Kansas City, MO: Author.

American Nurses Association (2001). *The code of ethics for nurses with interpretive statements*. Washington, D.C.: Author.

American Nurses Association. (2004). *Nursing: Scope & standards of practice*. Washington, DC: nursesbooks.org

Barnett, P. D. (2001). *Ethics in forensic science: Professional standards for the practice of criminalistics*. Boca Raton, FL: CRC Press.

Bleich, J. D. (1998). *Bioethical dilemmas: A Jewish perspective*. Hoboken, NJ: KTAV Publishing House.

Cranford, R. (1996). Vegetative recovery. NPR All Things Considered, January 3, 1996. Retrieved May 15, 2005, from http://www.npr.org/templates/story/story.php?storyId=1041888

Cranford, R. (2003). Families struggle with life support issues. NPR Morning Edition, October 23, 2003. Retrieved March 5, 2005, from www.npr.org/features/feature.php?wfId=1476123

John Paul II. (2004). Address of John Paul II to the participants in the International Congress on "Life-Sustaining Treatments and Vegetative State: Scientific Advances and Ethical Dilemmas." Retrieved May 15, 2005, from www.vatican.va/holy_father/john_paul_ii/speeches/2004/march/documents/hf_jp-ii_spe_20040320_congress-fiamc_en.html

Nightingale Pledge. (1983). Retrieved November 9, 2005, from http://carenurse.com/creeds/nightengale.html

Pinch, W. J. E. (2000). Revisions to ANA Code of Ethics are in the works: A look at the process. *Nebraska Nurse, 33*(1), 35.

Repenshek, M., & Slosar, J. P. (2004). Medically assisted nutrition and hydration: A contribution to the dialogue. *Hastings Center Report, 34*(6), 13–16.

Resnicoff, S. H. (1998). Physician-assisted suicide under Jewish law. Retrieved May 15, 2005, from www.jlaw.com/Articles/phys-suicide.html

Shannon, T. A., & Walter, J. J. (2004). Implications of the papal allocution on feeding tubes. *Hastings Center Report, 34*(4), 18–20.

Steele, S. M. (1983). Values and values clarification. In S. M. Steele & V. M. Harmon (Eds.). *Values clarification in nursing* (2nd ed.) (pp. 1–37). Norwalk, CT: Appleton-Century-Crofts.

Terri Schiavo Information Page (2005). Retrieved May 15, 2005, from http://abstractappeal.com/schiavo/infopage.html

World Federation of Catholic Medical Associations. (2004). Considerations on the scientific and ethical problems related to vegetative state. Retrieved May 15, 2005, from http://www.vegetativestate.org/documento_FIAMC.htm

CHAPTER 4

The Student Role

Objectives

At the end of this chapter, the student should be able to:

1. Differentiate between examples of academic honesty and dishonesty, and between errors and violations.
2. Identify boundaries used to maintain professional relationships.
3. Propose strategies for minimizing the occurrence of academic dishonesty.
4. Consider personal and professional values when proposing strategies to maintain professional relationships with patients, students, and other health care professionals.

KEY WORDS

- *Academic dishonesty*
- *Error*
- *Fabrication*
- *Violations*

Ethical expectations for nursing students are not limited to clinical practice, but also extend into other aspects of the professional role, such as academics and interprofessional relationships. These ethical expectations have been set by the nursing profession, as well as by society. Thus, nursing students may experience ethical conflicts when their personal moral compasses or values do not coincide with the expectations of the profession and society.

Nursing in the United States is perceived by the public to be one of the most ethical and honest professions (Gallup Poll News Service, 2003). However, at the same time, academic dishonesty among college students is becoming more prevalent (Bailey, 2001). These two conflicting perceptions may create a potential dilemma for the nursing profession. How can nursing maintain its ranking as an ethical and honest profession if nursing students are not committed to the same ethical standards in their academic careers as practicing nurses?

ACADEMIC HONESTY

Academic honesty is a fundamental value held by universities and colleges. When students act honestly in their academic endeavors, the students' knowledge and skills can be accurately evaluated and they will be more likely to successfully begin their new careers, ultimately benefiting their patients. Thus, academic honesty not only benefits the students' professional future, but also creates good for society while maintaining the university's or college's reputation (Purdue University, Office of the Dean, 2003).

ACADEMIC DISHONESTY

Academic dishonesty is defined as "dishonesty in connection with any University activity. Cheating, plagiarism or knowingly furnishing false information to the University. . . . Moreover, knowingly to aid and abet, directly or indirectly, other parties in committing dishonest acts is in itself dishonest" (Purdue University, Office of the Dean 2003). Box 4-1 lists behaviors that illustrate academic dishonesty. A variety of reasons have been suggested for the increased incidence of academic dishonesty including the "publish or perish" philosophy, dilution of academic standards, competition for scholarships and academic recognition, limited or stagnant moral development among students, and easy access to copious amounts of information on the Internet (Bowman, 2002; Brown, 2002).

When a student engages in academic dishonesty, the student's potential to be successful in the future is weakened. For example, Sally pays Joan to take the pharmacology final exam in her place, explaining "the college requires a 75% average on all exams to continue in the program, and I know I can not do it on my own." Thus, if this deception is not noticed and Sally is allowed to matriculate into a clinical course, her future success as a nurse and the safety of her future patients may be threatened by her substandard pharmacology knowledge base.

Academic dishonesty involves acts of deception and illustrates a lack of commitment to veracity (truth-telling). Veracity is one of the common themes discussed in depth in Chapter 7 and is further explored in the various clinical chapters. In addition, Chapter 10 discusses research misconduct. Therefore, this chapter does not include further discussion of the concept of deception, but instead discusses examples

BOX 4-1

Behaviors Illustrating Academic Dishonesty

"Substituting" on an exam for another student

"Substituting" in a course for another student

Paying someone else to write a paper but submitting it as one's own work

Giving or receiving answers by the use of signals during an exam

Copying, with or without the other person's knowledge, during an exam

Doing class assignments for someone else

Plagiarizing published material, class assignments, or lab reports

Turning in a paper that has been purchased from a commercial research firm or has been obtained from the Internet

Padding items of a bibliography

Obtaining an unauthorized copy of a test in advance of its scheduled administration

Using unauthorized notes during an exam

Collaborating with other students on assignments when collaboration is not allowed

Obtaining a test from the exam site but completing/submitting it later

Altering answers on a scored test and then submitting it to be regraded

Accessing and altering grade records

Stealing class assignments from other students and submitting them as one's own work

Fabricating data

Destroying or stealing the work of other students

Source: Purdue University, Office of the Dean. (2003). Academic integrity: A guide for students. Retrieved September 29, 2005, from http://purduekellely.iupui.edu/academic/integrity.aspx Reprinted with permission.

of academic and professional misconduct and presents suggestions for avoiding these academic and professional pitfalls.

Cheating

Although acts of cheating have undoubtedly been around since the beginning of objective evaluation of student work, acts of cheating are escalating and becoming more accepted by high school and college students (Brown, 2002). Even if a student does not initially set out to cheat—for example, "While I was stretching, I noticed that the person next to me had written down '14' as the answer"— the commission of an act of cheating is always intentional (Brown, 2002). Despite the initial intent of the student in this example, if the student made a conscious choice to record the other student's answer of '14' on his or her test, the student was cheating. There are a variety of traditional means for cheating: writing information on one's hand, on a pencil, or on a gum wrapper; hiding answers within the graffiti on the student's desk (The Blur of Sanity, 2005); copying from another student's test; obtaining copies of previous exams; using hand signals (Brown, 2002); turning in a paper purchased from the Internet; and destroying or altering grade records (Purdue University, Office of the Dean, 2003).

However, the increased availability and capabilities of technology have created new and more insidious ways to cheat. Personal digital assistants (PDAs) are used widely by health care professionals for rapid retrieval of data and statistics. In addition, cell phones with text messaging capabilities are becoming common. PDAs and text messaging provide students with a quiet, accurate, and speedy mechanism for accessing information during an exam. For example, a PDA can be used to quickly access information about a specific drug during a pharmacology exam. Text messaging not only allows students to communicate with one another during an exam, but it also allows them to communicate with individuals outside of the examination room. For example, a student in the exam could text message someone not in the exam for answers to specific questions.

When recognized incidents of cheating do not result in negative consequences, students who do not engage in cheating may become disadvantaged. For example, if grades are assigned based on the statistical distribution of an exam, the possibility exists that a noncheater might be assigned a lower letter grade than would have been assigned if the cheating had not occurred. Thus, acts of cheating may create questions of fairness in which noncheating students may be put at a disadvantage when competing for awards and scholarships based on grade point averages. Although individual disciplinary actions regarding acts of cheating need to be dealt with privately, mechanisms need to be put in place to notify other students and constituents that individuals who engage in academic dishonesty are disciplined according to the university or college policy (Smith, 2000).

Plagiarism

Plagiarism is intellectual theft (Kralik, 2003).

Plagiarism occurs when a writer presents another person's intellectual property as his or her own. While some students may deliberately and knowingly lift portions of a document (or even an entire document), most students inadvertently plagiarize by neglecting to properly cite the sources that they use when writing their research papers. (Bowman, 2002, p.12)

Plagiarism represents a lack of commitment to honesty. It is the intentional or unintentional theft of someone else's words and thoughts. Plagiarism is disrespectful to the person whose work is plagiarized, as well as disrespectful to the reader. When an author (whether a student or professional writer) plagiarizes, the author is pretending that his or her work is unique when in fact this is not true. Thus, the reader's time,

BOX 4-2

University of Kentucky Department of Chemistry Plagiarism Certification

Please read the following statement. If you accept this statement, please sign and date it in the space provided and give your signed statement to your instructor. NOTE: This statement may not be required by your instructor, but if it is, then you MUST complete and return this form before turning in any assignments in the class.

I certify that ALL of the following are true:

1. I have read and fully understand the consequences of plagiarism as discussed in the Student Rights and Responsibilities handbook and the Chemistry Department web page on plagiarism.

2. I fully understand the definition of plagiarism and recognize specifically that it includes copying of assignments, paraphrasing, reusing old lab reports, and related acts.

3. I recognize that the **minimum** penalty for plagiarism is an **E in the course.**

4. If I am unsure about whether something constitutes plagiarism, I will consult my instructor **before** I turn in the assignment.

5. I have given correct information on this form.

Name (Print): _____   Date: _____

Source: University of Kentucky, Department of Chemistry (1998). Plagiarism certification. Retrieved April 23, 2004, from http://www.chem.uky.edu/courses/common/plagcert.html
Used with permission.

and perhaps money (if the document was purchased), may be wasted when he or she reads a plagiarized document. Therefore, academic institutions and publishers may require persons to communicate their understanding of plagiarism (Box 4-2).

During my academic career, I have uncovered many instances of plagiarism simply because the documents submitted by the students did not "sound like" them. For example, a junior nursing student who was struggling to maintain a C average submitted a term paper about a specific respiratory disease. In this paper, she succinctly and in clear detail explained complex pathophysiological concepts. At the end of the paragraph, she included an end-note citation listing the author and publication date of a pathophysiology book that was not required in the student's class. I had a copy of this text on my office bookshelf and used the index to find the section in the book that pertained to the paper topic. It was clear that the student had presented the words from the book exactly as they were printed, but she had failed to give complete credit to the original author. For some paragraphs the student used, she did not attribute credit at all. Complete credit would have required the student not only to indicate the author and year of publication, but also to use quotation marks (or blocking for longer quotations) and to indicate page numbers for any direct quotations.

Prior to discussing these findings, I obtained all the references the student listed in her paper from the college library. Because this scenario preceded current confidentiality requirements, I was able to see that no one else had checked out each book cited on the reference list since the student's sister, who was also a nursing student, had the year before. Although the faculty reviewing this case could not be sure, we concluded that, in all likelihood, this paper was originally written (and plagiarized) by the student's sister the year before, and the current student engaged in an act of plagiarism by submitting her sister's work as her own.

Another example of plagiarism occurred when a student submitted a paper to me that used ethical terms that were not used in the class readings or during the class discussions. In addition, the logic of the student's argument was difficult to follow, so in an effort to better understand the points the student was attempting to make, I obtained the student's cited references from the library. When I was reviewing the references in the student's paper, I noticed that the student had taken an entire paragraph from reference 1 but had attributed reference 2 as the source. Throughout the paper, the student repeatedly copied a section verbatim from one source while citing another reference as the source. I concluded that the student had intentionally acted to hide acts of plagiarism by attributing the plagiarized thoughts to a different reference in an attempt to confuse anyone who tried to confirm the references.

Although most instances of plagiarism are intentional, the possibility exists for plagiarism to occur unintentionally. A student e-mailed a paper to the professor. The professor "ran the paper" through a plagiarism computer program, and the program indicated that a paragraph in the paper was a verbatim quotation from a published article. When the faculty member confronted the student with the program's findings, the student acknowledged having read the reference and claimed to have correctly attributed credit by the use of direct quotations and a complete reference. The student produced a hard copy of the paper supporting this claim. To settle this disagreement, the faculty person went back to the student's original e-mailed file and noted that the student did, in fact, use quotation marks as claimed. After further investigation, the faculty person realized that the electronic file lost formatting when it was run through the plagiarism software, and the student had not engaged in plagiarism.

Students and other authors need to be aware of the possibility that whenever a file is converted from one computer program to another computer program, the file's formatting may be altered; therefore authors should review the accuracy of all reformatted computer documents prior to submitting them for review or publication. In addition, reviewers (professors, peer reviewers, and/or editors) must also be aware of the possibility that a document may lose important formatting features if read or opened using a different computer program. It is important to remember that formatting issues related to computer program conversion do not meet the definition of plagiarism because they are honest errors, and thus students and authors should not be penalized in these cases.

Self-plagiarism is a form of plagiarism in which the author reuses his or her previous written work but presents it as new. Students do this when, for example, they submit a paper on assisted suicide originally written for a nursing ethics class for additional credit in the nursing professional issues course the next term.

Self-plagiarism (or what is sometimes referred to as duplicate publications or "salami slicing") is an example of scientific misconduct that occurs when an author or researcher reuses previously published text in a new manuscript without giving appropriate credit, which violates the original publisher's copyright. When writing two articles (one for a research journal and one for a clinical journal) based on the same research study, the only way to prevent self-plagiarism is to rewrite the duplicate sections and cite the first article in the reference list of the second article (self-citation) (Lowe, 2003).

"Cyberplagiarism" is a term that has recently been coined. It refers to authors plagiarizing content they found on Internet sites. Cyberplagiarism is a growing phenomenon that is complicated by writers' misbelief that Internet information is part of the public domain, and thus its use does not require documentation. The Internet's easy access is a double-edged sword for plagiarizers. Although information can easily be cut and pasted into a new document, a variety of plagiarism programs are being developed to assist professors and editors to identify incidents of cyberplagiarism (Eysenbach, 2000), such as www.turnitin.com

There are many actions and strategies a student could implement to minimize the likelihood of engaging in academic misconduct. First, the student should establish a moral compass for his or her academic and professional life by setting high, but achievable, standards. For example, a student could decide, "I will always be honest in my academic and professional careers," or, "I will take advantage of each learning experience as it occurs." Second, students need to be organized so they have sufficient time to study and complete assignments. Plagiarism and cheating are often the result of being unprepared or of not having the time needed to complete a project independently. Third, students need to develop a consistent note-taking system when researching a topic, and they need to keep working copies of their papers and assignments. These strategies may support a student's efforts in defending himself or herself against accusations of academic misconduct. Fourth, when submitting work electronically, one should always send a copy to oneself so that one can verify the electronic formatting of the document. Fifth, one should pay attention to the referencing details required by the style of referencing (depending on the appropriate style guide, e.g., that of the American Psychological Association or the American Medical Association) one is using to format the document. Finally, one should proofread the paper!

The following are suggestions for preventing academic dishonesty:

- Increase student awareness that academic dishonesty is not tolerated and has severe consequences (Bailey, 2001).
- Develop a computer function that integrates an "attribute" (gives credit to source) (Eysenbach, 2000, p. 6) to the "copy and paste" function.
- Use multiple versions of the same test, increase the use of proctors who move around the examination room, and do not allow students to keep any personal effects besides one pencil (Brown, 2002).
- Use a completely different examination if giving a make-up exam (Brown, 2002).
- Protect computer passwords and files to prevent theft of data on computers (Purdue University, Office of the Dean, 2003).
- Require students to participate in an academic exercise that explains academic honesty and reference citation practices and expectations (Bailey, 2001).
- Provide orientation sessions where students can discuss the expectations for professional honesty, especially those related to documentation in the patient record (Bailey, 2001).

- Attach a Charge of Academic Dishonesty Form in the student's permanent academic record after an act of academic dishonesty has been proven (Lang, 2002).

CLINICAL DISHONESTY

Fabrication

Fabrication occurs when the writer presents data or information that has no factual basis. In other words, the writer makes up the data. During academic exercises, a student may fabricate or "fudge" statistics or incident rates for a specific disease when the data are unknown to the student.

In the clinical practice, students may also be tempted to fabricate patient information. Fabrication may occur when the student forgets to complete an action. For example, a student fails to check the patient's pulse rate prior to giving the patient a dose of Lanoxin, but falsely records an apical pulse of 78 "because that is what the pulse has been for 3 days, and I do not want my clinical instructor to write me up." As another example, information may be fabricated when the practitioner forgot what the objective measurement was. For example, "I weighed Mr. Jones, but I do not remember what he weighed. Yesterday, he weighed 168 pounds. His edema is less today, so I'll record 165."

Fabrication of data in the clinical setting violates the principles of nonmaleficence and beneficence. When data are fabricated, clinical decisions could end up being made using inaccurate data or observations, which could cause harm to the patient. When nurses fabricate patient data, the nurse is acting out of self-interest and not out of a commitment to promoting good for the patient. When objective data are missing, because the nurse either did not collect them or forgot them, actions to fabricate the data serve only to create a picture of competence related to the nurse's performance. They do not prevent harm or do good for the patient.

ERRORS

Errors are not a form of dishonesty. The Institute of Medicine (2000) defined an error as "The failure of a planned action to be completed as intended (i.e., error of execution) or the use of a wrong plan to achieve an aim (i.e., error of planning)" (p. 28). An error is not an intentional act, but a deviation from the standard accepted way of acting. The determination of an error should not be decided solely by the consequences of the action. Rather, an error occurs any time the standard has not been followed. An error can be classified as being active, such as a medication or documentation error, or latent, such as lack of prevention (Hall, 2002). Table 4-1 describes the eight types of errors that can occur.

Nursing students, from the first day of class, are taught the importance of knowing and following the standards of care. One of the first standards a nursing student is taught notes the "Five Rights of Medication Administration": the right patient, drug, route, time, and dose. Whereas the American Nurses Association (ANA) (2001) Code of Ethics for Nurses with Interpretive Statements does not discuss errors directly, this code does discuss competency:

Table 4-1	**Types of Nursing Errors**
Type of Error	Illustration
Lack of attentiveness	Inability to monitor patient needs and progress due to inadequate staffing ratios.
Lack of agency/fiduciary concern	Failure to act as a patient advocate, such as not questioning an order or reporting significant changes in the patient's condition.
Inappropriate judgment	Making a wrong clinical judgment because of not collecting the right data or faulty reasoning about the data collected.
Medication errors	Missed medications, wrong dosages, or inaccurate intravenous rates.
Lack of intervention on the patient's behalf	Because of lack of attentiveness, the nurse does not notice that the patient is unresponsive due to being in a hypoglycemic state.
Lack of prevention	Not cleaning up spilled water on the floor in a patient's room, which the patient subsequently slips on while walking to the bathroom.
Missed or mistaken physician or other health care provider's orders	Misunderstanding that the physician's order is to add 40 mEq of KCl to the current IV bag and giving the KCl IV push instead.
Documentation errors	Recording nursing actions prior to implementation or failing to document changes in the patient's condition.

Source: Benner, P. et al. (2002). Individual, practice, and system causes of errors in nursing: A taxonomy. *Journal of Nursing Administration,* 32(10), 509–523.

Only those individuals who have demonstrated the knowledge, skill, practice experiences, commitment, and integrity essential to professional practice are allowed to enter into and continue to practice within the profession. Nurse educators have a responsibility to ensure that basic competencies are achieved, and to promote a commitment to professional practice prior to entry of an individual into practice. Nurse administrators are responsible for assuring that the knowledge and skills of each nurse in the workplace are assessed prior to the assignment of responsibilities requiring preparation beyond basic academic programs. (ANA; 2001, Provision 3.4. Reprinted with permission from the American Nurses Association, *Code of ethics for nurses with interpretive statements,* © 2001 nursesbooks.org, American Nurses Association, Washington, DC.)

This code also stipulates that "the nurse retains accountability and responsibility for the quality of practice and for conformity with standards" (Provision 4.1). It is important to note that an intentional violation of the standard of care is not an error. A violation is "a deliberate—but not necessarily reprehensible—deviation from those practices appreciated by the individual as being required by regulation, or necessary or advisable to achieve an appropriate objective while maintaining safety and the ongoing operation of a devise or system" [Merry & McCall Smith (2001), as cited in Runciman, Merry, & Tito, 2003, electronic p. 3].

Examples of a violation include a hospital administrator forcing a health care professional to work despite mandatory overtime regulations and an employee not wearing personal protective equipment as directed by the Occupational Safety and Health Administration (OSHA). Thus, any discussion of errors and violations should focus on the person's intentions and actions and not on the direct consequences (Runciman et al., 2003).

There is a need to change the current culture of silence surrounding the occurrence of errors to a culture in which health care professionals feel safe to identify errors and to work to minimize their causes. Adopting a policy of disclosing an error to a patient and/or significant other would be a major paradigm shift for many health care workers. In the past, errors were not disclosed because of fears of legal retaliation. However, after implementing full disclosure policies, hospitals have found that full disclosure actually decreases the occurrence of law suits (Watson, 2003). This position is further supported by the National Patient Safety Foundation (2000):

When a health care injury occurs, the patient and the family (or representative) are entitled to a prompt explanation of how the injury occurred, and its short and long-term effects. When an error contributed to the injury, the patient and the family or representative should receive a truthful and compassionate explanation about the error and the remedies available to the patient. They should be informed that the factors involved in the injury will be investigated so that steps can be taken to reduce the likelihood of similar injury to other patients. (Reprinted with permission of the National Patient Safety Foundation © 2000.)

Determining how to best disclose an error requires a team approach (Watson, 2003). The nurse should notify his or her supervisor and the patient's primary care provider. In addition, the nurse may want to discuss the event with the hospital's legal counsel or risk management person. The Institute of Medicine (2000) recommends that a "nationwide mandatory reporting system should be established that provides for the collection of standardized information by state governments about adverse events that result in death or serious harm" (p. 87) as a means for promoting the public's ability to make informed, autonomous decisions. However, strategies would be needed to protect the confidentiality of individual patient data. In addition, nursing organizations, such as the Association of Perioperative Registered Nurses (AORN), are working to develop voluntary reporting systems for errors and "near misses" related to specific nursing functions (Watson et al., 2002).

Nurses have an ethical responsibility to maintain patient safety that includes minimizing and reporting the incidence of errors. As discussed previously, patients cannot make informed decisions about future health care if they are unaware that an error and its related consequences have occurred. The occurrence of negative consequences and not disclosing all the facts to the patient are acts of harm toward the patient. This inability to make future plans based on accurate data is a violation of the principle of beneficence, or the promotion of good for the patient (Kelly, 2002).

A utilitarian would suggest that the decision to disclose an error should be made after considering *the greatest good for the greatest number*. This mental exercise requires the decision-maker to consider both the short- and long-term harms and benefit to all stakeholders (i.e., patient, nurse, hospital, society). Honesty and open disclosure will create the greatest good because they promote the possibility of preventing similar errors in the future.

A deontologist's decision about whether to report an error will rest on his or her belief that health care professionals have a moral duty to be truthful (Kelly, 2002). Based on the belief that moral duties should always be followed regardless of the consequences that may result, a deontologist could also support the need for the mandatory reporting of errors in honor of the moral obligation to respect persons.

PROFESSIONAL RELATIONSHIPS AND BOUNDARIES

All therapeutic professional relationships (be they between two health care professionals, between the patient and the nurse, or between the nursing student and the faculty) are built on a foundation of trust, and therefore may also be referred to as "a fiduciary relationship." A fiduciary relationship is a "special confidence reposed in one who, in equity and good conscience, is bound to act in good faith and with due regard to the interests of one reposing the confidence" (Hall, 2001, p. 4). Thus, professional relationships require that boundaries be established between the two individuals as means for promoting trust and maintaining personal privacy. Boundaries often are constructed to preclude the sharing of information that a person considers private. Thus, the creation of boundaries is different for each person depending on his or her values and on how transparently he or she lives his or her life. For example, the elderly often maintain stronger boundaries around talking about sexual practices than might teenagers. Spirituality is a topic many health care providers are uncomfortable discussing, and thus they may create protective boundaries even when their patients are eager to incorporate spiritual practices into their plans of care (Post, Puchalski, & Larson, 2000).

When power is unequally distributed between two people, professional boundaries assist in preventing an abuse of power (Hall, 2001). For example, it is commonly accepted that health care professionals have more power than their patients, faculty members have power over their students, and physicians have more power than other health care employees. A variety of boundaries are commonly maintained during professional relationships. For example, in a nurse–patient relationship, the nurse maintains boundaries to protect his or her personal information by not discussing, for example, his or her financial status, his or her current problems with raising teenagers, or the fact that his or her spouse has an addiction problem. Boundaries can also be created by how people refer to themselves and others. For example, having students refer to faculty members by titles, such as "doctor" or "professor," rather than by their first names promotes the notion that professors and students are not equals and that a professional distance should be maintained.

When boundaries are violated during a professional relationship, the possibility exists for harm to occur, especially to the person with less power. Harm can occur when the person who violates the boundary attempts to meet personal needs at the expense of the other. Thus, the possibility exists for "physical, verbal, emotional, sexual and financial harm" (Cameron, 1997, p. 142) to occur. Boundary violations can result from poor judgment or economic problems. Examples of poor judgment could include a counselor touching a distraught patient in a manner the patient may perceive as sexual, such as stroking the hair, or a male health care provider performing an "unnecessary" breast exam on an attractive female patient. Boundary violations due to economic problems can occur when a faculty member invites a financially destitute student to live in a guestroom in the faculty member's home or when a student explains to his or her academic advisor, "I will not be able to continue in the program unless someone co-signs my loan. Do you know anyone that would do this for me?"

The Nurse–Patient Relationship

Due to their professional roles, knowledge base, interpersonal skills (sometimes referred to as charisma), and social status in the community (Hall, 2001), health care providers (including nurses) may hold power over their patients. Thus, it is the health care providers' responsibility to prevent the misuse of their power for personal reasons when interacting with patients. Although everyone would agree that it is unethical for a health care provider to engage in a sexual relationship with a current patient, there is less professional consensus about whether it is ethical to initiate personal relationships with a former patient (Hall, 2001).

Because nurses are perceived by patients as caring and knowledgeable advocates, patients will often share extremely personal information with them, such as sexual issues or psychological problems. Once this information is learned it cannot be unlearned, and therefore the nurse may have an unfair power advantage over the patient if a social relationship were to begin. For example, during the beginning stages of a personal relationship, intimate personal information, such as a history of sexual abuse, rape, or eating disorders, is typically not shared. Thus, if a nurse enters a personal relationship knowing intimate information, the ability to form a relationship as equals may not be possible (Hall, 2001).

In addition, the possibility exists that a patient will be unable to separate his or her initial professional perceptions about the nurse from his or her subsequent personal feelings. The inability to separate personal and professional feelings may limit the patient's ability to voluntarily enter a nonprofessional relationship with a health care provider. For example, a patient may state, "The night nurse saved my life when I began to bleed. There is nothing I would not do to repay him." As a means of promoting voluntary consent, the state of California legally requires that physicians maintain a 2-year period of no contact with a patient prior to initiating a nonprofessional relationship. Even though this legal statute exists, many believe that it is unethical for a physician to engage in a sexual relationship with anyone who is, or who ever has been, a patient (American Psychiatric Association, 1993; Hall, 2001; Zelas, 1997). However, little has been written about whether nurses should be held to the same ethical standard.

The Student–Faculty Relationship

Student–faculty relationships share many of the same power issues previously described in nurse–patient relationships. There is an inequity of power between students and faculty. Faculty members gain power through their academic position, as well as through their professional knowledge base. They have the ability to influence a student's academic progression through a plan of study, as well as influence over the student's ability to successfully gain employment following graduation. For example, the potential exists for a personal relationship between a faculty member and a student to occur in return for the faculty member giving the student a favorable grade or writing the student a favorable reference letter.

Similarly, students may find themselves in a position of having information about a professor that, if it were to become public, could create negative consequences for the professor. For example, Joe Kramer is a student volunteer assisting Prof. Smith in a writing project and has access to the professor's office. While checking references on one of Dr. Smith's articles, Joe accidentally discovers that Dr. Smith has been visiting child pornography Internet sites. The potential exists that Joe could use this information for personal gain, for example, saying to Dr. Smith, "I will not share this information if you make sure I get the department scholarship that pays all tuition and fees for my senior year."

Student–Student Relationships

Based on their shared desire for a nursing education, nursing students are required to spend a great deal of time together and to develop professional relationships with fellow students that, under other circumstances, they might never have chosen to develop. In student–student relationships, students are required to work together (in clinical groups and group projects) to assist each other to learn, grow professionally, and share educational resources. Throughout nursing education, there is an expectation that students will share their professional knowledge and experiences so that other students may learn vicariously through them. For example, in postconference, a clinical instructor may direct a student to explain to the other students the assessment and critical thinking steps instituted when a patient with documented deep vein thrombosis does not awaken. During this type of group interaction, the students realize that this experience of having a patient with a deep vein thrombosis could happen to any of them.

Other learning experiences in one's nursing education have the potential of placing a nursing student in a situation where his or her privacy is threatened, changing the nature of a relationship with another student. Many physical assessment courses include a laboratory experience in which students work in pairs to practice the physical assessment skills of inspection, palpation, auscultation, and percussion. Practicing these skills may require the student to expose or discuss his or her body parts in ways the student would not typically share in a peer relationship. Examples include students performing breast exams on each other and students asking each other review-of-system questions about their weight and diet histories. Thus, educational measures that require the disclosure of personal information while in professional relationships with fellow students and/or faculty instructors may be extremely stressful, and these measures have the potential to permanently affect these relationships.

A variety of rationales have been proposed to support the practice of these laboratory exercises, including the effective allocation of scarce resources and the promotion of empathy for patients. Nursing schools often defend the practicing of skills on student partners with economic reasons, saying that the use of professional actors for physical-assessment and history-taking laboratories may be economically unfeasible based on the school's tuition and laboratory fees. In addition, faculty may defend the use of student-partner laboratory experiences by saying they are a means of impressing on students how difficult many patients may find it to disrobe in front of, or answer personal questions asked by, the student as a health care professional. Although comments like this may heighten a student's empathy, they may also be perceived by students as being coercive and uncaring. When a student asks a patient sensitive questions or performs a physical examination, there is an assumption that the experience may (1) benefit the patient's plan of care, (2) benefit the student's knowledge, and, thus, (3) benefit other patients in the future. However, when the same questions or exams are conducted between student partners, there is no assumption that the examination will benefit the student being examined. Thus, there may be a difference in motivation for participation. In addition, there is also the potential that the student–faculty relationship could be threatened if private information about the student is communicated to the faculty through other students' written assignments or if a faculty person is present during the student-partner examination (Morgan, 2001).

Morgan (2001) proposed a variety of strategies for promoting discussion between faculty and students about educational practices that challenge the professional relationship between students and their professors. These strategies also allow potential students to make informed decisions about their educational options:

1. Include a statement in the college bulletin indicating that nursing students will be asked to assume the role of patients during laboratory courses.
2. Give students options in their written assignments, for example, describing how "you, a family member, or a friend" is meeting your/their developmental needs.
3. Ensure that successful completion of an assignment does not mandate the disclosure of honest personal data. For example, when creating a family pedigree chart, a student should be allowed to opt to not disclose his or her HIV status or age.
4. Avoiding overlapping relationships between faculty members and students. For example, it may not be ideal for a student's academic advisor to also be that student's clinical instructor. Furthermore, faculty members should avoid developing counseling relationships with students who they may also encounter in the academic arena.
5. Focus on long-range educational goals, such as "the student will develop accurate assessment skills," rather than on particular educational activities.

Another strategy for minimizing disclosure of student sensitive information is to allow students to hire a professional actor for all simulation activities. Although this option does protect student confidentiality, this strategy may disenfranchise students with limited financial resources.

SUMMARY

Nursing students and practicing nurses are exposed to a variety of situations in which they need to make a conscientious decision about how to proceed. Although the temptation to engage in academic dishonesty is great for some, such acts do not result in long-term benefits and do not fulfill the nurse's responsibility to act virtuously. Similarly, when equity of power does not exist, the possibility exists for the nurse to take advantage of others, or to be taken advantage of, in various relationships with patients, peers, and other health care professionals. Thus, the nurse must carefully weigh the benefits and burdens of engaging in personal relationships with present or past professional contacts prior to developing them.

CLINICAL EXERCISES

1. Ask the nurse you are working with on the clinical unit whether he or she has ever had an experience in which a patient, or a patient's significant other, did not respect the nurse's professional boundaries.
2. Investigate whether your university or college has a policy regarding personal relationships between students and faculty, students and staff, or undergraduate students and graduate students in teacher assistant positions.
3. Does your university or college have a policy on academic honesty or plagiarism? Talk to your clinical instructor, course director, or academic advisor about actions the faculty takes to promote academic honesty.

Discussion Questions

1. Identify the professional boundary issues that should be considered before entering into nonprofessional relationships in the following situations:

    a. You are a 21-year-old nursing student enrolled in the Leadership Management clinical rotation. In this clinical rotation, students are assigned to "work" five 8-hour shifts for a 10-week period. On Monday, an 84-year-old patient with congestive heart failure is admitted to the unit and is accompanied by his 25-year-old grandchild. Just before the end of the shift, the grandchild suggests having dinner together that evening.

    b. You are a 63-year-old nurse working in the health center of a retirement community. Over a period of 2 years, you have had almost daily interactions with a spouse of one of the health center's patients. Six months after the patient dies, you meet the spouse by accident at the supermarket, and the spouse suggests having dinner together on your next day off.

    c. You are a 45-year-old nurse working in a community home for adults with developmental delays. A sibling of one of the patients visits several times a week, and one day the sibling suggests going to dinner together over the weekend.

    d. The family of a patient who died after being hospitalized for several weeks invites you and another nurse to eat supper with them at a restaurant owned by family friends. They explain, "You meant so much to our Mom, and we talked a lot about how you should experience this special ethnic food."

    e. You did join the family in the previous situation for dinner at the restaurant. At the end of the meal, the family begins to plan the next family outing and says to you, "What day would work better for you? You have to come. You're part of the family now!"

2. The final exam in a nursing ethics course was a take-home ethical case analysis. While grading these exams, the professor notices similarities between two of them. Read the following test-question answers from each student and then state whether you believe these students cheated or plagiarized each other's work. Explain your answer.

Test Question—Identify what ethical issues are present in the following cases.

Student A's answers:

- The staff nurse must follow the rules (if there are any) and laws that guide nursing practice.
- Is it ethical to resuscitate a patient who has completed a Durable Power of Attorney?
- Lack of family education about what it means to be a DNR, after all it was the patient's fifth admission to the hospital

Student B's answers:

- The staff nurse should follow the rules (and there are any) that guide practice in this nursing situation.
- Is the action of resuscitating a patient ethical since he has a Durable Power of Attorney?
- No family education about what a DNR means.

3. Paraphrase and correctly reference the following quotation:

   Plagiarism occurs when a writer presents another person's intellectual property as his or her own. While some students may deliberately and knowingly lift portions of a document (or even an entire document), most students inadvertently plagiarize by neglecting to properly cite the sources that they use when writing their research papers. (Bowman, 2002, p.12)

4. During a clinical rotation in the post-anesthesia recovery unit, a nursing student is assigned to a patient who just had her pregnancy terminated. While assessing the patient, the nursing student realizes that the patient is an English major at the same faith-based college the nursing student attends. The patient says to the nursing student, "Please do not tell anyone about my operation. The college is so conservative. I do not think people will understand or accept my position."

   - Later, the patient says to the nursing student, "Would it be possible to ride back to campus with you? I could not find a car to borrow. My room-mate dropped me off on her way to student-teaching practicum. Unfortunately, there are not any taxi cabs out here in the sticks." What personal and professional boundaries should the nursing student consider before responding to the patient's request?
   - When saying goodbye to the nursing student, the patient asks, "Would you be able to check in on me this evening? I do not have anyone to talk to about what I have experienced today."
   - The nursing student decides to visit the patient in her dormitory room after supper. After thanking the student for coming, the patient states, "I feel awful. I have a temperature of 102.5 degrees. What should I do? Can you help me?" What are the professional and personal boundaries the nursing student should consider before answering?

5. An interdisciplinary group of students and faculty are planning to participate in a 2-week volunteer project in a developing country in Central

America. Due to the collegial nature of this trip, the trip may foster personal relationships between students and faculty. What actions and conversations should occur prior to (and during) this trip to avoid the blurring of student–faculty privacy boundaries?

6. If the literature is correct that being an ethical nursing student is a prerequisite for becoming an ethical practicing nurse, do you believe that nursing schools should screen applicants for honesty? Explain your answer. If you agree that applicants should be screened, how would you propose this screening occur?

Resources

Bosek, M. S. D. (2004). NCLEX results to disclose or not disclose: An ethical analysis. *JONA Healthcare Law, Ethics & Regulation, 6*(2), 39–41.

Indiana University Writing Tutorial Services. (1998). Plagiarism: What it is and how to recognize and avoid it. Retrieved February 2, 2005, from http://www.indiana.edu/~wts/pamphlets/plagiarism.shtml

Jezuit, D. L., Rosenberg, L., & Murphy, C. M. (1999). Ethics in practice. A student nurse's perception of right and wrong. *JONA's Healthcare Law, Ethics and Regulation, 1*(3), 16–19.

National Student Nurses Association. (1999). Code of professional conduct. Retrieved February 2, 2005, from http://www.nsna.org/pubs/pdf/CodeofProfessionalConduct.pdf

National Student Nurses Association. (2001). Code of academic and clinical conduct. Retrieved February 2, 2005, from http://www.nsna.org/pubs/pdf/code_of_ac.pdf

Purdue University Online Writing Lab. (2003). Avoiding plagiarism. Retrieved February 2, 2005, from http://owl.english.purdue.edu/handouts/research/r_plagiar.html

Spector, N., & Sheets, V. (2004). NCLEX results to disclose or not disclose. *JONA Healthcare Law, Ethics and Regulation, 6*(2), 38–39.

Standler, R. B. (2000). Plagiarism in colleges in USA. Retrieved February 2, 2005, from http://www.rbs2.com/plag.htm

References

American Nurses Association. (2001). *The code of ethics for nurses with interpretive statements.* Washington, DC: Author.

American Psychiatric Association. (1993). *The principles of medical ethics with annotations especially applicable to psychiatry.* Washington, DC: Author.

Bailey, P. A. (2001). Academic misconduct: Responses from deans and nurse educators. *Journal of Nursing Education, 40*(3), 124–131.

Benner, P., Sheets, V., Uris, P., Malloch, K., Schwed, K., & Jamison, D. (2002). Individual, practice, and system causes of errors in nursing: A taxonomy. *Journal of Nursing Administration, 32*(10), 509–523.

Bowman, V. (2002, March). The campaign against plagiarism: Academic initiatives. *LIRT News,* p. 12.

Brown, D. L. (2002). Spotlight on...Cheating must be okay—everybody does it! *Nurse Educator, 27*(1), 6–8.

Cameron, M. E. (1997). Legal and ethical issues: Professional boundaries in nursing. *Journal of Professional Nursing, 13*(3), 142.

Eysenbach, G. (2000). Report of a case of cyberplagiarism- and reflections on detecting and preventing academic misconduct using the internet. *Journal of Medical Internet Research, 2*(1), e4. Retrieved on December 2, 2005 from http://www.jmir.org/2000/1/e4/

Gallup Poll News Service. (2003, December 1). Public rates nursing as most honest and ethical profession. Retrieved September 29, 2005, from http://poll.gallup.com/content/default.aspx?ci= 9823&pg=1

Hall, J. K. (2002). Systems do not make mistakes—people do. *JONA's Healthcare, Law, Ethics, and Regulation, 4*(2), 23.

Hall, K. H. (2001). Sexualization of the doctor–patient relationship: Is it ever ethically permissible? *Family Practice, 18*, 511–515.

Institute of Medicine. (2000). *To err is human: Building a safer health system.* Washington, DC: National Academy Press.

Kelly, G. A. (2002). Living at the sharp end: Moral obligations of nurses in reporting and disclosing errors in health care. *Critical Care Nursing Clinics of North America, 14*, 401–405.

Kralik, D. (2003). Editor's note: Cyberplagiarism...what is it? *Journal of Advanced Nursing, 43*(6), 539.

Lang, J. M. (2002, May 14). Dealing with plagiarists. *The Chronicle of Higher Education.* Retrieved January 5, 2004, from http://chronicle.com/jobs/2002/05/2002051401c.htm

Lowe, N. K. (2003). Editorial: Publication ethics: Copyright and self-plagiarism. *Journal of Obstetric, Gynecologic, and Neonatal Nursing, 32*, 145–146.

Morgan, J. E. (2001). Confidential student information in nursing education. *Nurse Educator, 26*(6), 289–292.

National Patient Safety Foundation. (2000). Talking to patients about health care injury: Statement of principle. Retrieved May 1, 2004, from http://www.npsf.org/html/statement.html

Post, S. G., Puchalski, C. M., & Larson, D. B. (2000). Physicians and patient spirituality: Professional boundaries, competency, and ethics. *Annals of Internal Medicine, 132*(7), 578–583.

Purdue University, Office of the Dean. (2003). Academic integrity: A guide for students. Retrieved September 29, 2005, from http://purduekelley.iupui.edu/academic/integrity.aspx

Runicman, W. B., Merry, A. F., & Tito, F. (2003). Error, blame, and the law in health care-An antipodean perspective. *Annals of Internal Medicine, 138*(12), 974–979. Retrieved on November 11, 2005, from http://www.annals.org/cgi/content/full/138/12/974

Smith, R. (2000). Cheating at medical school: Justice must be done and seen to be done. *British Medical Journal, 321,* 398.

The Blur of Insanity (2005). Cheating tricks. Retrieved September 29, 2005, from http://www.blurofinsanity.com/blurhomeframes02.html

University of Kentucky, Department of Chemistry (1998). Plagiarism certification. Retrieved April 23, 2004, from http://www.chem.uky.edu/courses/common/plagcert.html

Watson, D. (2003). Creating a culture of safety. *AORN Online, 77*(2), 268, 270–271.

Watson, D., Cooper, T. A., Groah, L., Hickey, P., Killen. A. R., Sandel, D., et al. (2002). First, do no harm. *AORN Online, 76*(5), 752, 754–755.

Zelas, K. (1997). Sex and the doctor–patient relationship. *New Zealand Medical Journal, 110,* 60–62.

CHAPTER 5

Ethical Decision-Making

Objectives

At the end of this chapter, the student should be able to:

1. Use the nursing process to guide ethical decision-making.
2. Identify values that influence ethical decision-making.
3. Identify resources and barriers to ethical decision-making.
4. Discriminate between nurse values and patient values during ethical decision-making.
5. Identify strategies for promoting individualized ethical decision-making.
6. Identify multiple potential actions for resolving an ethical situation.

KEY WORDS

- *Decision-maker*
- *Ethical decision-making*
- *Ethical situation*
- *Nursing process*

Although many similarities can occur among different ethical situations that revolve around the same ethical question, there is no "one size fits all" solution for such situations. Therefore, nurses need to develop ethical decision-making skills, including the ability to identify ethical issues, the ability to discern who is an appropriate decision-maker, the ability to prioritize the values and outcomes that are being promoted, and the ability to access resources and evaluate outcomes.

ETHICAL DECISION-MAKING

Nurses experience ethical situations on a daily basis. In this book, the terms "ethical situation," "ethical issue," "ethical question," "ethical problem," and "ethical quandary" will be used interchangeably. An ethical situation occurs when an individual perceives that there is a conflict regarding the right thing to do. Many of these ethical questions come up routinely, often several times a day; for example, "Should I tell the patient I forgot I promised to bring fresh ice water?" However, other larger ethical issues, such as assisted suicide and whistle-blowing, are rare occurrences that may occur only once, if ever, during a nurse's professional career. When a nurse experiences an ethical situation, the nurse must identify what role he or she should assume related to the decision-making process that is required by the situation. Specifically, the nurse must consider whether he or she will need to make the decision or whether the patient will need to make the decision.

Depending on the specific issues and questions involved in ethical problems, nurses may take on a number of roles in ethical situations. First, may fill the role of facilitator/organizer by arranging patient-care conferences. At patient-care conferences, everyone involved in the ethical situation (the patient, the patient's significant others, and the health care team members) can simultaneously hear the same information and discuss the options. Patient-care conferences may facilitate the ethical decision-making process.

The second role nurses may fill during the ethical decision-making process is that of agitator. As an agitator, during interdisciplinary rounds, the nurse raises questions and seeks clarification from members of the health care team. For example, the nurse could ask the patient's family doctor, "What are the medical goals for this patient?"

The third role nurses can fill during the ethical decision-making process is that of clarifier/educator. Often nurses assume this role when patients and/or significant others ask, "Can you explain what the doctor just told us? He spoke so fast and we did not understand all the words he used."

Finally, nurses may serve as supportive listeners to patients and/or surrogate decision-makers as they grapple with the realities associated with the patients' prognoses.

Decision-Making by a Nurse

In ethical situations related to the actions of nurses or other health care providers, nurses are often required to assume the decision-maker role. When serving as decision-makers during ethical situations, nurses must first identify the types of ethical issues that need to be resolved. First, is the ethical issue one that affects the nurse's personal or professional values, thus requiring the nurse to decide how he or she must act? For example, in the ice-water scenario presented previously, the nurse realizes that the ethical question is related to his or her professional values. Because of the failure to keep a promise, he or she now needs to make a decision about what to tell the patient.

Next, is the ethical issue one that revolves around the patient's values? In certain situations, nurses may need to make ethical decisions for or on behalf of patients. For example, when admitted to the surgical unit from the post-anesthesia recovery unit, a 19-year-old patient asks whether her fiancé can stay at her bedside during the night. The nurse initially permits the patient's fiancé to stay in her room. An hour later, when the nurse enters the room, the patient is crying and the fiancé is saying, as he pushes the tray table away from the patient, "Do not be such a baby. I do not know why you can not reach it yourself. I am going to have to spend the night just to make sure you are not being lazy." At this point, the nurse realizes that he or she will need to make a new decision about whether allowing the fiancé to stay past the hospital's visiting hours is in the patient's best interest. Although the temptation is great to make the decision based on the nurse's values and beliefs (i.e., this guy is a jerk, she would be better off without him!), the nurse needs to make a patient-centered decision based on the patient's values. The effect of values on decision-making will be discussed in more depth later in this chapter.

Facilitating Patient Decision-Making

In many ethical situations, the nurse's role is to serve as an advocate by providing the patient (or surrogate decision-maker) with the information and skills necessary to make an informed decision. When the patient is the decision-maker, the nurse may need to assist the patient with the decision-making process by clarifying terms, educating the patient about the involved anatomy, and assisting the patient with identifying and prioritizing his or her values. For example, a 30-year-old male patient says to his nurse, "The doctor was just here and said that I have an infection of my epididymis and need immediate surgery. I do not know what to do or think. I do not even know what an epididymis is or does. All I know is that I am in severe pain, and I am having trouble thinking clearly because of the pain pills. What would happen if I did not have surgery?"

ETHICAL DECISION-MAKING GOALS

The goal of ethical decision-making is to determine the *right* solution for the issue at hand, or "what ought to be done." Initially, determining what is right (or what ought to be done) seems like it should be easy. As children, we learned rules and absolutes to help guide our sense of right or wrong and, thus, our decision-making. Some of these rules are based on social conventions such as, "A man should open a door for a woman," "Honesty is the best policy," and "Women and children first." Other rules have a religious basis, such as the Golden Rule's "Do unto others as you would have them do unto you."

When seeking assistance with ethical decision-making, nurses will often say, "Just tell me the right thing to do." This request implies a belief that there is one, and only one, *right solution* for resolving a specific ethical issue. Therefore, if the nurse can identify this one correct action, then the nurse will know how to resolve this situation, as well as how to resolve any future situations that revolve around the same ethical issue. This viewpoint is commonly referred to as "the cookie-cutter approach" to decision-making, in which every solution (like every cookie made using the same cookie cutter) is the same. For the cookie-cutter approach to work, one must believe that every time an ethical situation involving a specific issue occurs, such as whether to initiate tube feedings or when to stop aggressive treatment, the internal and external dynamics are the same and, thus, one solution fits all situations. However, this approach is unrealistic.

REALITIES IN DECISION-MAKING

Obstacles to Recognizing an Ethical Situation

A variety of factors may keep nurses (or other decision-makers) from recognizing when ethical situations are occurring. DeWolf (1989), in researching the ethical decision-making process used by medical-surgical nurses, noted that five precipitating factors must occur before nurses perceive that an ethical situation is taking place. The first factor is that the nurses experience an emotional reaction, such as anger, or report feeling emotionally uncomfortable. Second, the nurses feel a sense of urgency related to the perception that there is little or no time available to make a decision. Third, the nurses personalize the situation by considering how they would want the situation to be resolved if they were the patient. Fourth, the nurses recognize that a communication failure occurred, and that information pertinent to making the decision is lacking. Fifth, the nurses recognize that there is a disagreement among the involved health care professionals as to what the correct course of action is.

In describing the ethical decision-making process implemented by emergency department nurses, Bosek (2001) noted that nurses often perceived that an ethical situation is occurring based on their prior experiences in similar situations. They also become aware of a current ethical situation if the situation is highlighted by, or discussed with, others during conversations.

Strategies for Fostering the Recognition of Ethical Situations

Several suggestions about how to foster the recognition of ethical situations among nurses and other decision-makers are based on these research findings. First, ethical discussions and decision-making should not occur in isolation. Decision-makers need to have access to peers, significant others, and leaders for assistance in clarifying their perceptions and their labeling issues.

Second, in the majority of ethical situations (questions about whether to begin cardiopulmonary resuscitation being a prime exception), decision-makers really do have time to consider their options, and they need to be reminded that a sense of urgency is unfounded and that making good decisions requires time.

Third, personalizing the situation, as the nurses did in DeWolf's research, by using "The Granny Test" strategy (considering what you would want done if this was your grandmother), for example, is an attempt to create a "one size fits all" solution. Personalization ignores the individual features of the situation, so ethical decision-makers should not engage in it. In addition, personalization works only if the decision-maker accepts the following assumptions:

1. I love my grandmother and only want the best for her.
2. Everyone loves his or her grandmother in the same way I love mine.

Fourth, because nurses may not experience emotional reactions when faced with frequently occurring ethical situations, they need to continue to develop their theoretical knowledge bases regarding ethics and current ethical issues. This is necessary because nurses may become "immune" to the emotional dynamics associated with recurring ethical situations. It is also necessary because nurses' ability to become emotionally involved during clinical ethical situations may be limited by current staffing practices that reduce their ability to develop relationships with patients and their significant others and by staffing practices that create multiple and competing duties for them.

The continuing development of nurses' theoretical knowledge bases can occur via brown-bag lunch discussions about ethical situations described in the media or via journal club discussion about articles published in the nursing literature. In addition, nurse managers need to provide forums in which staff nurses can discuss ethical situations that recently occurred on the unit. These discussions would provide novice nurses with the opportunity to learn vicariously through the experiences of their peers.

Fifth, nurses need to continue to develop strong communication skills, as well as the moral courage, to ask pointed questions, to seek clarification, and to defend their personal and professional values. They also need to work with their institution's nursing structure to create an organizational ethical climate that is open to ethical discourse.

ETHICAL DECISION-MAKING USING THE NURSING PROCESS

Although many ethical situations involving the same ethical question may share similar features, no two ethical situations are alike. The individuals involved in each situation are different and have different beliefs, values, experiences, and life goals. Because each ethical situation is different, the possibility of creating a "rulebook" that a nurse could memorize in preparation for future ethical situations is unrealistic. Thus, it behooves the professional nurse to develop skills for using an assortment of decision-making approaches.

A variety of models and strategies have been proposed as guides for facilitating ethical decision-making. Although each model has its special focus (e.g., Curtin [1982] emphasized the consideration of rights, Shelly [1980] suggested that the decision-maker take into consideration biblical principles, and Savage [1990] proposed a facilitation model [Opacich, 1996]), all models include four steps (Bosek & Savage, 1999):

1. Identify the ethical problem.
2. Identify and consider alternatives.
3. Implement a choice.
4. Evaluate the decision-making process and its outcome (p. 78).

Because these four steps are very similar to the steps in the nursing process (assessment, diagnosis, goals, intervention and rationale, and evaluation), they should be familiar to nursing students.

Table 5-1 illustrates how the nursing process can be used to guide ethical deliberations. The situation regarding the patient advised to have surgery for his infected epididymis is used in this example.

Assessment

Subjective data include the patient's statements reflecting his lack of knowledge regarding not only the anatomical role of an epididymis, but also the possible biological, social, and psychological effects of removing the epididymis. Objective data

Table 5-1 Application of the Nursing Process to Ethical Decision-Making

Assessment	Nursing Diagnosis	Goals	Interventions	Rationale	Evaluation

Subjective
• I do not know what an epididymis is or does
• I don't know what to do or think
• Unclear what would happen if surgery not done
• Patient's sexual history
• Patient's reproductive goals
 	
Objective
• Infected epididymis
• Taking pain meds
• Difficulty thinking clearly
	Threats to informed consent related to knowledge deficit and/or impaired decisional capacity secondary to pain medications as evidenced by comments about not knowing what role an epididymis serves in the male body and not thinking clearly	• Patient will verbalize an accurate understanding of the anatomical role of an epididymis
		• Patient will verbalize values related to being the biological father of future children
		• Patient will make an informed decision about what treatment option to initiate that reflects his values
			Assessment
			• Assess patient's values and goals about fatherhood by asking open-ended questions
			• Assess the patient's understanding of the male reproductive system using an anatomical drawing
			
			Actions
			• Investigate sperm-banking procedures
			• Arrange for a representative from the fertility clinic to meet with patient and partner prior to making a decision
			• Discuss pain control with physician to identify whether alternate medications without sedation would be possible
			
			Education
			• Based on patient's knowledge deficits provide education about the male reproductive system
			• Steps required for making an informed decision:
			  1. Understands problem
			  2. Understands options
			  3. Understands pros and cons associated with each option
			  4. Able to explain choice made
				• Autonomous decisions should be made using the patient's values and goals
				• Accurate knowledge is fundamental to making an informed decision
				
				• Identifies a potential option
				• Provides resources for promoting patient's knowledge base regarding reproductive options
				• Pain medication could decrease cognitive functions
				
				• Patient-centered education is built on the patient's existing knowledge base
				
				• Information regarding informed consent may help the patient to be confident in decision-making
					Were the goals met? If not, why?

include the patient's sexual history and current medical symptoms. Further information that is currently unknown includes the patient's reproductive goals.

Diagnosis

Because how the diagnosis is framed will influence the goals and interventions generated, identification of the ethical issue at hand is a crucial step in the decision-making
process. Sometimes, identification of the ethical problem at hand may be missed due to
the nurse's lack of experience with similar issues or because the nurse is too focused on
the concurrent physiological problems. For example, based on the available data, an
inexperienced nurse might identify the nursing diagnosis as, "Potential for alterations
in coping due to fear of surgery." However, a nursing diagnosis related to the ethical
issues at hand should include, "Threats to informed consent related to knowledge
deficit and/or impaired decisional capacity secondary to pain medications."

Goals

When identifying the goals of ethical decision-making, it is important that the goals
reflect the values, beliefs, and life ambitions of the focus person. Thus, when identifying the goals for the decision-making process, the nurse must be able to discriminate
between his or her personal beliefs and values and those held by the focus person. For
example, the nurse might identify goals such as "eliminate infection" and "no further
pain." The patient may agree with these goals but also have other goals, such as "be
the biological father of two more children" and "remain physically intact (no changes
to body image)." Goals related to the ethical diagnosis should include "Patient will
make an informed decision based on accurate knowledge."

Interventions and Ethical Rationale

Interventions comprise assessments, actions, and education. During any ethical decision-making process, it is imperative that nurses identify and clarify (assess) the focus
person's values, as well as the values of the other stakeholders involved in the situation (values clarification is discussed further in Chapter 12). In the foregoing example,
the nurse could assist the patient in clarifying his goals and values related to fatherhood. How important is it to the patient and his partner that he be capable of being the
biological father of his children?

"Actions" include gathering whatever further information is needed for ethical
decision-making. For example, the nurse could investigate whether sperm banking
prior to surgery is an option. The nurse could also arrange a patient-care conference
with the surgeon, a representative from the hospital's fertility clinic, and the patient
(and his partner) for the purpose of identifying potential actions and their expected
consequences as related to the fertility goals expressed by the patient.

"Education" includes the nurse educating the patient (and his partner) about the
male reproductive system. In addition, the nurse needs to educate the patient about
the ethical requirements of an "informed decision."

Evaluation

Evaluation can be done both immediately after the decision is made and just prior to
implementation of the decision. At these points, the decision-maker can review

whether the original question has been answered and can consider whether the chosen action supports the identified goals and the goals' related values. If the answer to any of these is "no," then the decision-maker needs to review the decision-making process. Through this retrospection, the decision-maker may discover that the original goals have been revised or reprioritized. For example, the patient, after talking with his partner, may have revised his goals related to fatherhood to be broader than just the ability to inseminate.

Evaluation should also occur after the identified action has been implemented and the situation is resolved. The decision-maker should review the ethical decision-making process for problem areas, including further information that is needed but is not available, resources that would have been beneficial, and values or strategies that were not considered. Finally, the decision-maker should evaluate the consequences and intents associated with the implemented action for congruence with the decision-maker's life goals and values. Based on this evaluation, actions may be taken to change the variables that precipitated the ethical situation, thus preventing future similar ethical problems.

DECISION ANALYSIS MODEL

The decision analysis model (DAM) (Bosek, 1995; Keeney, 1982; MacLean, 1989) is one strategy that is available to assist individuals with identifying and prioritizing desired outcomes and values of potential actions that could be taken to resolve ethical problems. The DAM (Table 5-2) is a grid formatted with a horizontal and a vertical axis. On the horizontal axis, the decision-maker identifies key values or outcomes (typically three or four) to be promoted throughout the decision-making process. These values or outcomes are then prioritized, with the number 1 assigned to the lowest priority and the number 4 assigned to the most important outcome to promote. When identifying these values and outcomes, the decision-maker needs to remember that each of the identified outcomes must be able to occur simultaneously.

On the vertical axis, the decision-maker identifies all the possible actions for resolving the ethical issue. After the values or outcomes and actions have been identified, the next step is to calculate the probability that the identified action might promote each desired value or outcome. Each action has 100 points to be distributed among the various values and outcomes. After the points have been distributed, the

Table 5-2	**Decision Analysis Model**				
	Value/ Outcome	Value/ Outcome	Value/ Outcome	Value/ Outcome	Total Score
Action					
Action					
Action					
Action					
Action					

fifth step is to calculate the expected score by multiplying the value or outcome priority number by the probability. Finally, an expected total score is calculated for each proposed action by adding the expected scores generated for the action. Based on the values or outcomes identified in the DAM, the decision-maker should implement the action with the highest expected total score. However, prior to implementing the action, the decision-maker should stop to ask, "Does this action make sense?" For example, a nurse could use the DAM to determine the best way to travel to a professional convention being held thousands of miles away. The total score could suggest that hitchhiking would be the preferred action. However, to many, this action might seem ill-advised. A review of the prioritized values or outcomes might reveal that the decision-maker had identified "low cost" as the top priority and had assigned "safety" a lower priority. After the value or outcome priorities have been revised, the DAM might suggest that flying would be preferred to hitchhiking or driving.

Previously, the point was made that the goals for decision-making should reflect the focus person's values or desired outcomes rather than the values or desired outcomes of the nurse. Consider the following situation. A nurse on a cardiac surgical unit discovers that the family of a patient has just completed the ritual sacrifice of a chicken over the patient's bed. The family states, "We believe that this ritual will promote the patient's healing, and we will need to repeat the ritual every day until he is healed" (Burton & Bosek, 2000). How the nurse frames the ethical question will affect not only the values and desired outcomes, but also the possible options. For example, the nurse could frame the ethical issue as follows:

- What is the best way to keep this patient from harm (Table 5-3)?
- What is the best way to respect the family's religious values (Table 5-4)?

Resources for Facilitating Ethical Decision-Making

A variety of resources are available to help facilitate the ethical decision-making process for nurses (Bosek, 1993a). If the ethical issue that needs to be resolved involves a question of what is best for a specific patient, then the primary resource the nurse should consult is the patient and/or the patient's surrogate decision-maker. The patient and the patient's surrogate are the best sources for ascertaining what values, goals, and priorities should be used to guide the nurse's decision-making. For example, when faced with the ethical question of whether to initiate tube feedings, the nurse should engage the patient and/or surrogate in a dialogue to determine the patient's values and beliefs about whether food and hydration are basic rights that should be provided, regardless of the means.

Professional publications are another resource available to nurses to facilitate their ethical deliberations. Professional publications include "codes of ethics" and "professional position statements," which were discussed in Chapter 3. Additionally, institutional "policy and procedure" manuals outline standardized approaches for a variety of situations that are often associated with ethical questions, for example, removal of life-sustaining treatment, comfort and palliative care, informed consent and refusal of treatment, implementation of advance directives, and treatment of premature infants with extremely low birth weight.

Many nursing journals (e.g., *AJN*; *JONA's Healthcare Law, Ethics, and Regulation*; *Orthopaedic Nursing*; *Pediatric Nursing*) have ethics columns. In addition, a

Table 5-3	What Is the Best Way to Keep This Patient From Harm?			
	Value/Outcome	Value/Outcome	Value/Outcome	
	Patient Is Free From Physical Harm (#3)	Hospital Standards Are Maintained (#2)	Family's Religious Values Are Respected (#1)	Total Score
Action Prohibit future sacrifices	50% (50 × 3 = 150)	50% (50 × 2 = 100)	0% (0 × 1 = 0)	150 + 100 + 0 = 250 (Action to be implemented)
Action Allow the sacrifice to continue without any modifications	0% (0 × 3 = 0)	0% (0 × 2 = 0)	100% (100 × 1 = 100)	0 + 0 + 100 = 100
Action Allow the sacrifice to occur in the autopsy room with the patient wearing isolation gear	33% (33 × 3 = 99)	33% (33 × 2 = 66)	34% (34 × 1 = 34)	99 + 66 + 34 = 199
Action Have the family sacrifice the chicken at home and bring a video for the patient to watch	40% (40 × 3 = 120)	40% (40 × 2 = 80)	20% (20 × 1 = 20)	120 + 80 + 20 = 220

variety of nursing textbooks address specific ethical content. Finally, a variety of ethics publications are accessible to nurses via libraries and the Internet. Every nurse should become familiar with the published resources available in the nurse's station or office, in the institutional library, and on the Internet.

Most institutions have an identified ethics mechanism. All nurses should have access to it. In addition, each institution should have a policy regarding the use of the identified ethics mechanism. First, this policy should indicate how to access the ethics mechanism. For example, can any employee initiate an ethics consult? Can a patient and/or significant other contact the ethics mechanism? If so, does the patient's primary health care provider or team need to be notified or to approve? Second, is there a charge for accessing the ethics mechanism? If there is a charge, is the charge billed to the patient, to the department of the person initiating the consult, or to the institution's chief financial officer? Third, the policy should stipulate

Table 5-4	**What Is the Best Way to Respect the Family's Religious Values?**			
	Value/ Outcome	Value/ Outcome	Value/ Outcome	
	Patient Is Free From Physical Harm (#1)	Hospital Standards Are Maintained (#2)	Family's Religious Values Are Respected (#3)	Score
Action Prohibit future sacrifices	50% (50 × 1 = 50)	50% (50 × 2 = 100)	0% (0 × 3 = 0)	50 + 100 + 0 = 150
Action Allow the sacrifice to continue without any modifications	0% (0 × 1 = 0)	0% (0 × 2 = 0)	100% (100 × 3 = 300)	0 + 0 + 300 = 300 (Action to be implemented)
Action Allow the sacrifice to occur in the autopsy room with the patient wearing isolation gear	33% (33 × 1 = 33)	33% (33 × 2 = 66)	34% (34 × 3 = 102)	33 + 66 + 102 = 201
Action Have the family sacrifice the chicken at home and bring a video for the patient to watch	40% (40 × 1 = 40)	40% (40 × 2 = 80)	20% (20 × 3 = 60)	40 + 80 + 60 = 180

whether initiating the consult is optional or mandatory and whether following the ethics mechanism's recommendation is optional or mandatory. For example, a hospital may stipulate, "Any time a decision is being considered to withdraw ventilator support for the purpose of letting death occur, the ethics mechanism must be contacted, and its recommendations must be followed." This is an example of mandatory to consult and mandatory to implement recommendations. In some institutions, it may be optional to consult the ethics mechanism and optional to follow its recommendations.

Traditionally, institutions have one of two types of ethics mechanisms: institutional ethics committees (IEC) or ethics consultants. Each mechanism has strengths and limitations, and each institution must decide what type of ethics mechanism to implement based on its needs.

Institutional Ethics Committee

An institutional ethics committee is made up of a group of interdisciplinary health care professionals, such as a nurse, a physician, a dietician, a pharmacist, a chaplain, a representative from the business office or administration, an ethicist, and possibly a community representative. Depending on how the committee fits into the institution's hierarchy, the committee's membership may vary. For example, if the IEC is a committee sponsored by the department of nursing, the committee may have several nurses, be chaired by a nurse, and report to the director of nursing. However, if the IEC is part of the medical department, then the committee may have more physician members, may be convened by a physician, and may report directly to the hospital's chief operating officer.

One of the strengths of an IEC is its ability to consider an issue with input from a wide variety of perspectives. For instance, a nurse may consult the IEC about an incident in which a physician discontinued all pain medications for a patient, stating, "There is no physiological reason why this patient should require pain medications." However, during the night shift, the patient cried and reported her pain as a 10 on a 0–10 scale. In this case, the IEC's interdisciplinary membership would allow the committee to have expert input concerning the ethical, pharmacological, pathological, and psychological aspects of this issue, as well as input regarding the communication and system protocols that should be followed when initiating a change in a patient's plan of care.

Limitations associated with the use of an IEC include time limitations. Many IECs meet on a preset date (e.g., the third Tuesday of the month at 1 P.M.) because of the difficulties associated with convening a large, diverse group of individuals. Thus, many IECs provide only a retrospective review and are unable to provide input for an ongoing, current situation.

Although an interdisciplinary focus has many benefits, an interdisciplinary membership may also negatively affect the committee's deliberations. For example, if the department of medicine sponsors the committee, nonphysician members may feel constrained about expressing views that are contrary to those held by the physician members. In addition, the mechanism for identifying potential IEC members may influence the committee's deliberations. Are members identified because they have had course work in ethics or because they express an interest in ethics? The potential also exists that a health care professional (HCP) may be assigned to participate on an IEC as a form of punishment or remediation by a supervisor who believes that participating may make the HCP a more ethical practitioner. Finally, the potential exists for IEC members to provide input based on their personal values and beliefs rather than as unbiased representatives of their profession. For example, an IEC member might state, "I do not buy into this brain death criterion. If a person's heart is beating, then they are alive and I do not care what the policy claims."

Ethics Consultant

Many institutions opt for ethics consultants as their identified ethics mechanism (Bosek, 1993b). An ethics consultant has expertise in the field of ethics, often gained through academic coursework, such as a graduate degree in health care ethics or philosophy. Ethics consultants often provide immediate ethical support to the institution over the phone. They also provide an on-call service to the institution, agreeing to be at the institution within a specified time after being paged, such as within 6 hours of being contacted, and/or conduct routine rounds at the institution. Thus, the use of an ethics consultant allows an institution to have ethical assistance prospectively, as well as retrospectively.

A limitation of the ethics consultant mechanism is that an individual consultant cannot provide as broad a review of the situation as an interdisciplinary team. In addition, because an ethics consultant may have limited health care knowledge, the possibility exists that the consultant may not recognize the ethical nuances associated with various treatment options. For example, if a nurse practitioner at a primary health care center contacts an ethics consultant regarding which of four possible birth-control options is ethically preferable for a sexually active 13-year-old with limited cognitive abilities, the consultant might not know enough about the factors associated with developmental delay to give an educated answer.

> ### Case Study 5-1
>
> Two elderly sisters live in a two-flat apartment building. Both sisters are seen by the same home health nurse. Angela lives on the first floor. She has severe congestive heart failure (CHF). Belinda lives on the second floor. She requires assistance for all activities of daily living. Angela is the primary caregiver for Belinda. Both sisters have repeatedly expressed the intent to remain in their homes. Because the sisters never married and have no other siblings, they have no other family. When the home health nurse arrives, she determines that Angela's CHF is not responding to the current treatment plan and Angela needs to be hospitalized. However, Angela refuses to go to the hospital because that would leave Belinda without a caregiver. The home health nurse contacts the nursing supervisor and states, "I do not know what to do. If I advocate for Angela, I put Belinda at risk, but if I advocate for Belinda, then I put Angela at risk!"
>
> 1. Identify the ethical situation to be resolved. Then complete the decision analysis model from the perspectives of the following individuals:
>
>   - The home health nurse.
>   - Angela.
>   - Belinda.
>
> 2. Discuss how the nurse could use available resources to assist in making a decision about resolving this ethical situation.

SUMMARY

Ethical decision-making is a complex process that requires the nurse to be inquisitive, analytical, and thoughtful while also acting with moral courage. Although barriers to ethical decision-making exist, there are numerous resources available in the health care arena to facilitate individualized ethical deliberations.

CLINICAL EXERCISES

1. What type of ethics mechanism has your clinical institution adopted?

   • What department or office sponsors the ethics mechanism?
   • To what office or person does the ethics mechanism report?
   • Which of the following types of structure applies to the use of the ethics mechanism?

   Optional to consult/optional to implement recommendations?
   Mandatory to consult/optional to implement recommendations?
   Mandatory to consult/mandatory to implement recommendations?

2. Ask the nurse you are working with about the types of ethical situations he or she has encountered recently in the clinical setting.
3. Identify three resources available in your hospital or university library that a nurse might consult to assist in resolving a clinical ethical situation.

Discussion Questions

1. Describe a clinical situation you witnessed or experienced that involved an ethical issue or question.
2. For the situation you described in answer to question 1, discuss whether you or the identified decision-maker experienced any of the obstacles to recognizing an ethical situation that were discussed in this chapter.
3. Use the nursing process to analyze the case you identified in question 1.

Resources

Fry, S., & Johnstone, M. J. (2002). *Ethics in nursing practice: A guide to ethical decision making* (2nd ed.). Abingdon, Oxon, UK: Blackwell.
Narrigan, D. (2004). Examining an ethical dilemma: A case study in clinical practice. *Journal of Midwifery & Women's Health, 49*(3), 243–249.
The Josephson Institute (2002). *Making ethical decisions.* Los Angeles: Author.

References

Bosek, M. S. D. (1993a). A comparison of ethical resources. *MEDSURG Nursing, 2*(4), 332–334.
Bosek, M. S. D. (1993b). What to expect from an ethics consultation. *MEDSURG Nursing, 2*(5), 408–410.
Bosek, M.S.D. (1995). Optimizing ethical decision making: The decision analysis model. *MEDSURG Nursing, 4(6),* 486–488.
Bosek, M. S. D. (2001). Ethical decision making by emergency nurses. *Journal of Nursing Law, 7*(4), 31–41.
Bosek, M. S. D., & Savage, T. A. (1999). Ethics. In D. D. Ignatavicius, M. L. Workman, & M. A. Mishler (eds.). *Medical-surgical nursing across the health care continuum* (pp. 75–92). Philadelphia: WB Saunders.
Burton, L. A., & Bosek, M. S. D. (2000). When religion may be an ethical issue. *Journal of Religion and Health, 39*(2), 97–106.

Curtin, L. (1982). No rush to judgment. In L. Curtin & M. J. Flaherty (eds.). *Nursing ethics: Theories and pragmatics* (pp. 57–63). Bowie, MD: Robert J. Brady.

DeWolf, M. S. (1989). *Clinical ethical decision-making: A grounded theory method.* (Doctoral dissertation, Rush University, 1989.) Dissertation Abstracts International, *50*(11), 4980.

Keeney, R. L. (1982). Decision analysis: An overview. *Operations Research, 30*(5), 803–838.

MacLean, S. L. (1989). The decision-making process in critical care of the aged. *Critical Care Nursing Quarterly, 12*(1), 74–81.

Opacich, K. J. (1996). Ethical dimensions in occupational therapy (pp. 627–650). In *The occupational therapy manager* (rev. ed.). Bethesda, MD: American Occupational Therapy Association.

Savage, T. A. (1990, October). *The unrecognized role of the nurse in ethical decision-making.* Paper presented at the University of Illinois College of Medicine Symposium: "A time to live...A time to die: Medical ethics in the '90's." Rockford, IL.

Shelly, J. A. (1980). *Dilemma: A nurse's guide for making ethical decisions.* Downers Grove, IL: InterVarsity Press.

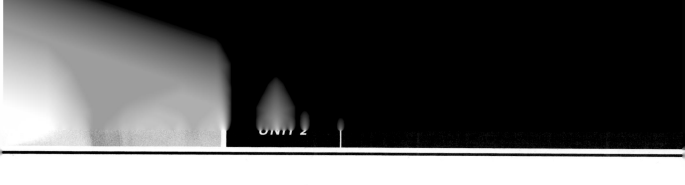

Ethical Themes
and Research Ethics

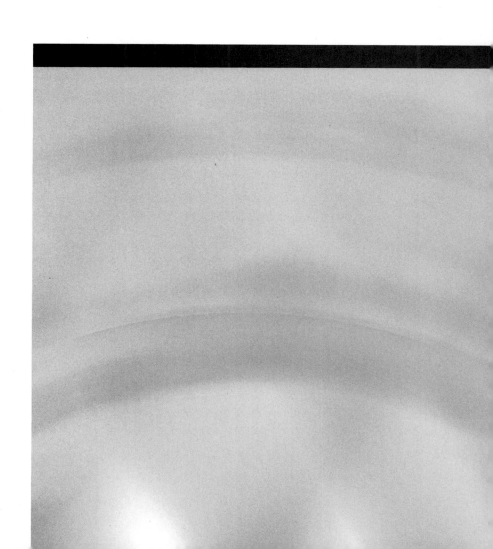

CHAPTER 6

Confidentiality

Objectives

At the end of this chapter, the student should be able to:

1. Discriminate between confidential and nonconfidential patient information.
2. Discuss basic actions every nurse must implement to protect patient confidentiality.
3. Analyze special threats to patient confidentiality from the health care environment and information services.
4. Propose solutions for protecting patient confidentiality during special circumstances.

KEY WORDS

- *Anonymity*
- *Confidentiality*
- *HIPAA*

- *Privacy*
- *Privacy Rule*

Confidentiality is a primary ethical principle that must be maintained throughout every nurse's professional practice. It is one of the four common ethical themes in nursing practice that will be expanded on in each of the chapters in Unit 3: Clinical Ethical Issues.

CONFIDENTIALITY DEFINED

"Loose Lips Sink Ships" is a famous slogan from World War II Navy publications used to warn against the accidental disclosure of military plans to the enemy through casual verbal or written communication. More recently, hospitals have had "Mum's the Word" campaigns to heighten the awareness of all health care professionals about the importance of confidentiality. Although a breach of confidentiality by nonmilitary nurses may not be a threat to national security, such a breach could result in grave harms to the patient, the nurse, the institution, and/or the nursing profession as a whole.

Confidentiality has been defined in a variety of ways:

- "Keeping the secrets of the patient" (Hall, 1996, p. 3).
- Controlling "access to sensitive personal information" (Lo, 2000, p. 42).
- Holding "in confidence all personal matters committed to [one's] keeping and all family affairs coming to [one's] knowledge in the practice of [one's] calling" [The Original Nightingale Pledge of 1893, as cited in The Nightingale Pledge for Nursing Student's Pinning Ceremony (2001)].
- Keeping something "classified, restricted, undisclosed, secret, or private" (Parsons & Parsons, 1992, p. 37).

Despite differences in focus, each definition shares the idea that patient-related information must not be disclosed. Thus, nurses must become knowledgeable about what information must not be disclosed, which information can be disclosed, and who should have access to that information.

RATIONALE FOR KEEPING INFORMATION CONFIDENTIAL

The American Nurses Association (ANA) Code of Ethics for Nurses with Interpretive Statements (American Nurses Association [ANA], 2001) states that "associated with the right to privacy, the nurse has a duty to maintain confidentiality of all patient information" (p. 12). The right to privacy was first discussed as a legal right in an article published in the *Harvard Law Review* in 1890 (*Nurse's Legal Handbook*, 1999). A person's right to privacy is supported by the ethical principle of non-maleficence because actions taken to maintain privacy are undertaken to decrease harm to the individual and his or her reputation.

Protecting patient confidentiality is necessary for establishing and maintaining a trusting relationship. When the patient knows that the nurse will keep in confidence any information provided, he or she will be willing to establish and maintain a professional nurse–patient relationship. Failure to maintain patient confidences (about information or secrets) will erode this relationship and ultimately result in harm not only to the patient, but also to the nurse and nursing. Thus, failure to maintain confidentiality will always result in some type of harm.

The Health Information Portability and Accountability Act (HIPAA)

The first federal privacy standards to protect patients' medical records and other health information provided to health plans, doctors, hospitals, and other health care providers took effect on April 14, 2003. Developed by the U.S. Department of Health and Human Services (DHHS), these new standards provide patients with access to their medical records and more control over how their personal health information is used and disclosed (U.S. Department of Health and Human Services [USDHHS], 2003, p. 1).

Privacy Rule

The Standards for Privacy of Individually Identifiable Health Information, commonly referred to as the Privacy Rule, was created in response to the 1996 Health Insurance Portability and Accountability Act (Public Law 104-91) (HIPAA). The Privacy Rule addresses how health care providers (including researchers), health plans, and health care clearinghouses convey patient information electronically. Failure to comply with the Privacy Rule can result in either civil or criminal legal charges by the Health and Human Services' Office for Civil Rights (OCR) under HIPAA (USDHHS, 2003). With all the focus on maintaining confidentiality, the "primary intent to provide better access to health insurance, limit fraud and abuse, and reduce administrative costs" (Dickey, 2002, pp. 2–3) can easily be forgotten.

These laws provide a minimum acceptable standard related to how a patient's medical records and personal health information are to be kept confidential. For example, patients are guaranteed access to their medical records and must be provided a written statement on how the agency, company, and/or health care provider will use his or her health care information. In addition, limits have been placed on the type and scope of personal information shared between health care entities or non–health care–related entities—for example, life insurance companies, banks, or marketing agencies. Finally, patients have been given the power to request special accommodations for protecting their health care information—for example, requesting that the primary care provider contact the patient at work rather than home with laboratory results (USDHHS, 2003).

The standards also require that health care entities create policies and procedures to protect patient information. Health care entities (health plans, hospitals, clinics, etc.) must provide patients with written privacy procedures and provide employee confidentiality education (USDHHS, 2003).

Maintaining confidential patient information is not limited to the United States. Comparable laws exist in other countries. In Canada, for example, there is Manitoba's (1998) Freedom of Information and Protection of Privacy Act, Alberta's (2005) Freedom of Information and Protection of Privacy, and British Columbia's (2003) Freedom of Information and Protection of Privacy Amendment Act.

Discussion Exercises 6-1

You are assigned to a cardiac unit for your clinical rotation. As you enter your patient's room, the patient yells at you, "I am going to sue this hospital and every employee! My boss called the hospital and the switchboard operator told him that I was in the cardiac unit before she forwarded the call to my room. I did not want anyone—especially my boss—to know that I have had a heart attack. I thought my diagnosis would be kept confidential!"

1. Do you believe that this patient's confidentiality was violated?
2. How should you respond to his concerns?
3. What recommendations would you suggest to the switchboard operator?

WHAT INFORMATION IS CONFIDENTIAL?

Whereas the concept of confidentiality is a well-accepted ethical commitment, little pragmatic guidance exists for knowing what specific information must be kept confidential or the actions necessary to maintain these confidences. In fact, the ANA (2001) claimed that all patient information is confidential, which sets a very high standard for nurses to meet.

In the literature, there is one common description of what confidential information is: "individually identifiable health information, including genetic information" (ANA, 1999, p. 1). This descriptor is helpful in assisting the nurse to understand that confidentiality applies to information and is not the same as anonymity.

Anonymity is generally associated with charitable giving or providing tips to the police about a crime when a person does not want his or her identity linked to an action. Unfortunately, health care organizations cannot function using an anonymity standard. Health care providers would not be able to provide organized sequential care and treatment if every patient, much less every laboratory test, was anonymous. Because of the difficulty in maintaining anonymity with test results, HIV testing centers, for example, use code numbers that are not linked with any patient identifiers (i.e., the number is placed on the blood tube and given to the person). To receive HIV results, the person being tested must initiate the call to the center and provide the code.

Nurses must learn to recognize what data meet the individually identifiable definition, which include basic demographic data, such as date of birth, social security number, mother's maiden name, and address. A variety of health-related information is identified and documented in a patient's written record including diagnosis, laboratory values, test results, physical exam findings, subjective patient comments, and insurance and/or financial information. Individually identifiable data are any information that would either provide someone access to further information (such as financial records or bank accounts) or provide information about the individual's life. For example, if a physician is overheard calling in a prescription for AZT (azidothymidine), the eavesdropper can ascertain that the person is likely to be HIV+.

The concept of identifiability is important for nursing students as well as other health care professionals to remember. Nursing students are also responsible for maintaining patient confidentiality in their written clinical work. Because the potential exists for a student's written clinical work and/or clinical worksheets to get misplaced, students should not include patient identifiers, such as name, initials, social security number, address, date of birth, or room number, on any written notes or assignments. Instead, if necessary, students can refer to the patient as "Ms. M," where the M could refer to the patient's first name or, for example, be a signifier in a code system in which the patient is referred to by the initial two letters down in the alphabet from his or her actual name. For example, Mr. Brown would be referred to as Mr. D and Ms. Lopez as Ms. N. In addition, an adult patient's age can be communicated in years or a child's age in months, which is less identifiable than a birth date.

Discussion Exercises 6-2

A well-loved and well-respected physician is hospitalized on your unit. This physician-patient requests that his chart be "locked up" because he does not want information contained in his history and physical to become widely known.

1. Should this chart receive special protection? If so, how would you propose to protect this chart?
2. Your unit conducts walking rounds at change of shift where report is given at the doorway to the patient's room to the entire nursing team. Should any modifications be made to this routine in light of the patient's request? For example, should everyone on the team be included in the report? Where should report occur? If you identified specific modifications, do these modifications meet the concept of universality (see Chapter 1)?
3. What persons do you believe should be able to access this physician-patient's chart?
4. What criteria should be considered before deciding whether a nursing student or medical student should be assigned to care for this physician-patient?

WHO CAN ACCESS CONFIDENTIAL INFORMATION?

Basically every piece of data recorded and observed by a health care professional would fit into the category of individually identifiable information; thus, the nurse must consider with whom these data may ethically and legally be shared. HIPAA and the so-called Final Rule for Privacy (Office for Civil Rights, 2002) stipulate that patients may access their medical records and "restrict disclosures of protected health information to the minimum needed for healthcare treatment and business operations" (Phoenix Health Systems, 2005, p. 4). Thus, the standard for determining whether patient information can be disclosed is commonly referred to as "disclose only on the need-to-know basis."

To apply the need-to-know standard, the nurse must consider the question, "Can this person do his or her job safely and knowledgeably without this information?" If the answer is yes, then the information should not be disclosed. For example, a housekeeper does not need to know that a patient is HIV+ because he or she should already be using standard precautions when cleaning. However, if the HIV+ patient also has tuberculosis, the housekeeper needs to be informed to follow airborne precautions, but does not need to know the actual diagnosis.

One common threat to maintaining confidentiality is the use of signs to alert employees to individualized patient needs. Frequently, nurses put up signs on the door to a patient's room or on the wall over the bed stating warnings such as the following:

- Hard of hearing.
- No blood draws or BPs in left arm.
- No lab tech draw—Nursing blood draw only.
- Fall precautions.
- Airborne precautions. Do not enter if you have not had the chickenpox.

Although the intent behind each of these signs is to prevent harm to either the patient or an employee, each sign discloses a clue to the patient's identity and condition. For example, "No blood draws or BP in the left arm" is generally related to a history of a mastectomy or shunt access for dialysis, and "Fall precautions" could imply that the patient has cognitive and/or motor deficiencies.

When signs are used in areas within public view (i.e., the patient's door), every effort must be taken to convey the warning while preventing disclosure of patient information. Some agencies have adopted the use of a colored dot system instead of using a text message. For example, a sign with a solid red circle indicates that the patient has a do-not-resuscitate status. Another strategy for protecting patient confidentiality related to warnings to protect both the employee and/or the patient is to include warning instructions directly on the laboratory; diagnostic and/or transportation requisition form, such as "Airborne precautions" or "No blood draws in left arm." Warnings designed to protect just the patient could be communicated via the patient's identification band if the warning must be followed for the entire admission or via a separate wrist band for warnings that might be time limited, such as fall precautions or NPO (nothing by mouth). There is a great need for improved mechanisms for communicating important patient information while protecting patient confidentiality.

The increasing use of computerized health care records and electronic billing and patient databases has compounded the question of who should have access to specific patient information, especially when information is shared between agencies, such as hospitals and third-party payers. In the future, health care agencies will have to create a variety of access levels by the use of passwords to protect and limit the dissemination of identifiable information. For example, the patient's financial and demographic information would be accessible to the billing office and discharge planner, but not to the nurse or dietician. In contrast, the nurse and dietician would be able to access the patient's total protein laboratory data, but the billing office and discharge planner would not be able to obtain this information. Although these types of protections are available for computerized records, the traditional written patient care record does not offer this type of protection, but rather relies on the integrity of the health care provider to seek only the information necessary to the care that he or she intends to provide.

To ensure that the coordination of the patient's care is not compromised, nurses will need to know their agency's policy and procedure about actions taken to protect the communication of confidential patient information by verbal, written, and electronic (including Internet, e-mail, and fax) means. Although the presence of these policies will streamline the majority of situations in which confidential patient information needs to be shared, the nurse will still be required to make independent judgments about whether to disclose information. In these situations, the nurse should continue to follow agency policies and consider and verify the other person's/agency's need to know the patient's status. Often there is a perception of urgency when in reality a delay of an hour or even a day may not create harm to the patient's plan of care or recovery. Whenever questions arise regarding the communication of patient information that is not covered by current policy and procedure, the nurse should contact his or her supervisor and, when appropriate, include the patient or the patient's surrogate decision-maker for guidance in how to proceed.

Although the general standard for deciding whether to disclose patient information is the need-to-know standard, the possibility exists that a nurse or other health care professional might have to violate this standard because of a competing commitment to prevent a harm to self or others. For example, if a patient discloses imminent plans for suicide or murder, the nurse or other health care professional may need to disclose this information to individuals who do not normally meet the need-to-know criterion, such as the police or security guards. This quandary is discussed in greater length in Chapter 14.

Example of HIPAA Standards Protecting Confidentiality

A well-known nursing faculty member from the local university shares a table with a staff nurse from the neurological unit in the hospital cafeteria. After noticing that the nursing faculty member is not in uniform, the nurse asks, "Is not the university on spring break this week?" The faculty member responds, "Yes, the students are on spring break. I figured you would know that my daughter is having a seizure work-up on your unit this week." The nurse replies, "Yes, I noticed the similar name, but I was unaware that she is your daughter. Because I have not been assigned to care for her, I have not heard anything about her medical problems or reasons for being hospitalized."

Example of Failure to Protect Confidentiality

During the 3 P.M. intershift report, the day nurse states,

In room 928 is Mr. S. He is a member of the Hospital Trustees. His wife is related to X family. The X family is the one that gave the one million dollar endowment for the "Closer than Home Residence" for families that need a place to stay close to the hospital. Anyway, he is here today with. . . .

Sharing the patient's and extended family's special relationship to the hospital is an example of disclosing patient information that does not directly affect his care. This disclosure also has the potential to create harm to the other patients on the unit if Mr. S. were to receive preferential treatment because of his special connections to the hospital.

Example of Failure to Protect Confidentiality

The nurse enters a postpartum patient's room. The patient's husband is in the room and notices on her chart the term "multipara." He asks what the term means. The nurse explains that "multipara" indicates a woman who has carried two or more viable pregnancies to term. He states that there must be some mistake because this is his wife's first pregnancy.

This case illustrates how a nurse can inadvertently disclose private information that may appear to be common knowledge because the medical record clearly states that this is the woman's second pregnancy. However, the woman's decision to not disclose her previous pregnancy to her spouse illustrates her decision that he did not need to know this, even though her health care providers did.

To prevent situations like this from happening, nurses need to be vigilant in protecting patient information kept at the patient's bedside. These actions might include keeping the chart closed when not documenting and asking the patient's permission to have visitors present during any interaction between the patient and the health care staff. In addition, patient orientation information should describe the patient's and/or family's responsibility for maintaining confidentiality. In addition, some agencies require the patient's permission to have the information kept at the bedside.

When a breach of confidentiality does occur, the nurse should follow the agency's policy and procedure for addressing such situations, which may include contacting the risk management representative and completing an unusual-occurrence form. In this case, the nurse should acknowledge the husband's confusion and follow up with the patient privately to determine how the patient desires to respond to this incident. Although the nurse is obligated to act to protect the patient's confidentiality, he or she is not obligated to lie to protect the patient's reproductive history from her husband.

SUMMARY

Maintaining confidentiality is a fundamental obligation for every nurse during every patient encounter. Patient information should be shared only on a need-to-know basis. Confidentiality is necessary to establishing and maintaining a trusting nurse–patient relationship and ultimately to prevent harm to the patient. The nurse's ability to maintain the confidentiality of patient information is complicated by the use of multiple communication methods (intershift report, patient charts, computer records, and location of telephones) in addition to the complexity of the health care delivery system and interdependence with third-party payers. HIPAA (1996) is an attempt to establish clear guidelines and expectations for every health care provider and health care agency.

CLINICAL EXERCISES

1. Identify whether your clinical agency has a policy on confidentiality.

   - How does your clinical agency define confidentiality?
   - What safeguards are included to protect the confidentiality of information?
   - Are any consequences listed for intentional or unintentional breaches of confidentiality?

2. Examine your state law(s) regarding confidentiality.
3. Talk with a staff nurse about what actions he or she takes to maintain confidentiality in the clinical setting.
4. Spend 10 to 15 minutes in a public area (hallway, elevator, lounge, cafeteria) of your clinical site, college of nursing, or other public building.

   - Are you able to hear or see any information that you believe is confidential that you should not be able to see or hear?

- Was this confidential information potentially accessible to others? If so, to whom?
- What recommendations would you make to decrease the type of breaches to confidentiality you observed?
- Based on your observations, what recommendations do you believe should be made to improve a policy on confidentiality?

5. Ask the staff nurse you are working with about the notes he or she takes during report.

- What type of information is included?
- How does the nurse discard these notes when they are no longer needed?
- Has the nurse ever lost his or her notes? What actions should be taken by the nurse if this does occur?

Discussion Questions

1. While doing your preparation for your next clinical day (e.g., care plan, reading about the disease), your roommate/significant other says, "Tell me about your patient."

- What information can you share and still maintain confidentiality?
- Does the fact that your roommate is a nursing student in the same class but different clinical group influence what information you can share?

2. Based on the HIPAA regulations, what precautions should a nursing student take with written assignments? What information should not be included in a student's clinical preparation notes, care plans, or written assignments?
3. If a nursing student repeatedly breaches patient confidentiality in his or her academic paperwork, what should the penalties be?
4. If a nursing student is found to be discussing confidential patient information in a public space, such as the cafeteria, what should the penalties be?

Resources

American Nurses Association. (1995). Position statements: On access to patient data. Retrieved November 16, 2005, from http://www.nursingworld.org/readroom/position/joint/jtdata.htm

Buppert, C. (2002). Complying with patient privacy requirements. *Nurse Practitioner, 27*(5), 12–32.

Canadian Nurses Association. (2001). *Position statement: Privacy of personal health information*. Ottawa: Author.

Gostin, L. O., Lazzarini, Z., & Flaherty, K. M. (n.d.). Legislative survey of state confidentiality laws, with specific emphasis on HIV and immunization. Retrieved November 16, 2005, from http://www.epic.org/privacy/medical/cdc_survey.html

Jones, R. L. (1995). Client confidentiality: A lawyer's duties with regard to Internet e-mail. Retrieved November 16, 2005, from http://www.kuesterlaw.com/netethics/bjones.htm

Manning, W. L. (1997). Medical records, privacy & confidentiality. Retrieved November 16, 2005, from http://www.netreach.net/~wmanning/privacy.htm

Office of the Information and Privacy Commissioner of Alberta. (2005). 10 years overseeing access and privacy: 1995–2005. Retrieved November 16, 2005, from http://www.oipc.ab.ca/home/

Salladay, S.A. (2002). Confidentiality: Stop the gossip. *Nursing, 32*(4), 78.

Wysoker, A. (2001). Legal and ethical considerations. Confidentiality. *Journal of the American Psychiatric Nurses Association, 7*(2), 57–58.

References

Alberta. (2005). Freedom of information and protection of privacy guidelines and practices. Retrieved November 16, 2005, from http://www3.gov.ab.ca/foip/guidelines_practices/2005/index.cfm

American Nurses Association. (1999). Position statements: Privacy and confidentiality. Retrieved November 16, 2005, from http://nursingworld.org/readroom/position/ethics/Etprivcy.htm

American Nurses Association. (2001). *Code of ethics for nurses with interpretive statements.* Washington, DC: Author.

British Columbia (2003). Freedom of Information and Protection of Privacy Amendment Act. Retrieved on November 16, 2005, from http://www.legis.gov.bc.ca/37th4th/3rd_read/gov13-3.htm

Dickey, S. B. (2002). Silence is not enough: Maintaining confidentiality in an electronic world. *American Nurses Association Ethics & Human Rights Issues Update, 1*(3), 1–6. Available at http://www.nursingworld.org/ethics/update/vol1no3b.htm

Hall, J. K. (1996). *Nursing: Ethics and law.* Philadelphia: WB Saunders.

Lo, B. (2000). Resolving ethical dilemmas: *A guide for clinicians* (2nd ed.). Philadelphia: Lippincott, Williams & Wilkens.

Manitoba (1998). Freedom of Information and Protection of Privacy Act. Retrieved November 16, 2005, from http://www.gov.mb.ca/chc/fippa/introduction/whatis.html

Nurse's legal handbook (4th ed.) (1999). Springhouse, PA: Springhouse Corp.

Office for Civil Rights. (2002). HHS...Standards for privacy of individually identifiable health information. Final rule. *Federal Register, 67*(157), 53181–53723. Retrieved on November 16, 2005, from http://www.hipaadvisory.com/regs/regs_in_PDF/finalprivmod.pdf

Parsons, A. H., & Parsons, P. H. (1992). *Health care ethics.* Toronto: Wall & Emerson.

Phoenix Health Systems (2005). *HIPAA primer.* Retrieved November 16, 2005, from http://www.hipaadvisory.com/regs/HIPAAprimer.htm

The Nightingale Pledge for Nursing Student's Pinning Ceremony. (2001). Retrieved November 16, 2005, from http://www.accd.edu/sac/nursing/honors.html

U.S. Department of Health and Human Services. (2003). Protecting the privacy of patients' health information. Retrieved November 16, 2005, from http://www.hhs.gov/news/facts/privacy.html

CHAPTER 7

Truth-Telling

Objectives

At the end of this chapter, the student should be able to:

1. Understand the moral differences between truth-telling and lying.
2. Provide examples of rationales supporting truth-telling and lying.
3. Discuss the nurse's moral obligation to be truthful.
4. Outline actions a nurse could take after deception has occurred.
5. Discuss strategies for a nurse to employ when another health care professional is not being truthful.
6. Discuss mechanisms for promoting truthfulness in the clinical setting.

KEY WORDS

- *Deception*
- *Excuses*
- *Lying*
- *Promises*
- *Trust*
- *Truth*
- *Truth-telling*
- *Veracity*

This chapter reviews the foundational concepts, obligations, and criticisms related to the ethical principle of veracity (referred to in this book as truth-telling). Truth-telling is one of four common ethical themes occurring in nursing practice that will be expanded on in each of the chapters of Unit 3: Clinical Ethical Issues.

The Importance of Truth-Telling

The importance of telling the truth is taught to children in multiple ways. Parents and teachers are quick to point out that "honesty is the best policy." Children read about Pinocchio, who becomes embarrassed when his nose grows after he tells a lie. In nearly every TV courtroom show we see the bailiff direct the witness, "Repeat after me. I promise to tell the truth, the whole truth and nothing but the truth. So help me God." These examples imply that one should tell the truth rather than a lie to avoid bad consequences. Negative consequences associated with not telling the truth include the loss of respect between the two parties and the subsequent harm to their relationship. Thus, a foundational ethical premise behind the need to tell the truth is trust.

Trust

For the health care system to work accurately and efficiently, trust must exist among all persons and agencies involved. "Trust simplifies human life by endowing some expectations with assurance" (Whitbeck, 1995, p. 2502). Thus, trust is the unrestricted certainty that another (person, agency, or even inanimate object) will perform as expected.

Patients should be able to trust that their health care providers are competent and will act to promote the patients' best interest. For example, a patient who is a "tough stick" must trust that the nurse assigned to restart an intravenous access has the requisite skills necessary to accomplish the task. Additionally, trust rests on the belief that the nurse has the requisite problem-solving skills and compassion for determining when to protect the patient's limited veins rather than attempting "one more stick." Thus, patients must be able to trust that nurses and other health care professionals will fulfill their responsibilities by always placing the patients' interest first (Whitbeck, 1995).

Nurses must also trust that the patient will be truthful and fulfill his or her responsibilities. The nurse's ability to remove harm and promote good for a patient rests on the nurse's ability to trust in the data provided by the patient in addition to the patient's ability to keep promises and fulfill responsibilities. Ethical issues involving the perception of noncompliance can occur when patients are unable to maintain or implement their portion of the health care plan. Additionally, the patient could experience harm from unnecessary or omitted interventions if the information he or she disclosed is inaccurate or incomplete (Whitbeck, 1995).

Trust relationships are also forged between health care agencies and their employees. When hiring nurses, the health care agency trusts that the nurse will come to work as scheduled and will carry out the responsibilities of the assigned role. Employees trust that the health care agency will in fact provide an orientation and the resources necessary to carry out the assigned responsibilities (e.g., supplies, support staff, policies and procedures) and financial compensation for the hours worked. Similar examples exist for agencies with trusting relationships. Accreditation bodies trust that conditions noted at a health care agency during an inspection will be maintained between inspections. Health care agencies trust that third-party payers, such as insurance companies, will reimburse them for care that has been contracted for and provided.

Finally, persons and agencies must trust in the actions of inanimate objects. On a daily basis, nurses trust that intravenous devices will deliver fluids and medications at the correct rate and that labeled bottles contain the identified substance. Patients trust that an internal defibrillator will work when needed and that emergency call lights are functional. Thus, "trust involves both confidence and reliance" (Whitbeck, 1995, p. 2501).

THE OBLIGATION TO TELL THE TRUTH

The obligation for truth-telling by health care professionals is based on other foundational commitments to respect people, prevent harm, do good, and honor autonomy. Arguments can be made based on these principles that both support and oppose truth-telling. For example, truth-telling is supported by a deontological approach to ethics because truth-telling is a morally praiseworthy action in and of itself. A deontologist would explain that one has a duty to tell the truth, and, like every other duty, the truth should always be upheld regardless of the outcomes that occur from the act of truth-telling. Thus, a deontologist would suggest that telling the truth fulfills the categorical imperative for universality, which requires that we act in the same fashion as we wish others would act if they were in a similar situation.

Utilitarians, however, evaluate the moral appropriateness of an action by weighing the anticipated harms and benefits that are expected from the action. Actions that promote the most good or happiness for the most persons are considered morally justifiable. Based on this theory, the obligation to be truthful is not always shared by utilitarians because truthfulness may not be the action that would create the most happiness for the most people. Box 7-1 discusses ethical codes and the obligation for truth-telling.

DISCRIMINATING BETWEEN TRUTH AND NONTRUTH

Truth

Truth is a "statement or belief which corresponds to the reality" (*Funk & Wagnalls New International Dictionary*, 1996, p. 1350). The determination of an idea's truthfulness depends first on the speaker's intentions. When attempting to communicate a truthful statement, the speaker's intention is to communicate the reality that he or she understands. When telling the truth, the speaker is not communicating through words or action ideas meant to deceive the other person. For example, a lost visitor stops a nursing student in the hallway and asks, "Which is the medical records department?" The nursing student, believing that the medical records department is part of the business office, directs the visitor to the second floor. This

> **BOX 7-1**
>
> ## Obligation for Truth-Telling
>
> Although the obligation for truth-telling has deep historical roots socially, it is interesting to note that early ethical codes, such as the Nightingale Pledge or Hippocratic Oath, did not require truthfulness (Bok, 1999; Lo, 2000).
>
> In the earlier ANA (1976, 1985) codes, Provision 10 required nurses to "participate in the profession's efforts to protect the public from misinformation and misrepresentation and to maintain the integrity of nursing" (p. 15). The associated interpretive statement (Provision 10.1) did not specifically address a nurse's day-to-day obligation to be truthful, but rather emphasized his or her role in protecting the client from nontruthful statements from commercial companies.
>
> This omission is not corrected in the ANA (2001) code; instead, Provision 1.4 stipulates that "patients have the moral and legal right . . . to be given accurate, complete and understandable information in a manner that facilitates an informed judgement" (p.8). Although Interpretive Provision 1.4 includes all the criteria for truth, the ANA authors, for unknown reasons, avoided using the terms truth, truth-telling, truthfulness, and veracity. Refer to Discussion Question 4.

nursing student is attempting to provide a truthful answer based on his or her current experiences and beliefs. Thus, this nursing student is conveying a truthful answer even if he or she is conveying incorrect information because the criterion of intention is fulfilled.

In contrast, after being asked, "Is this your first shot?" the nursing student replies, "No, I have done it several times." However, the student fails to include the fact that the several times were all done on a mannequin. Because the nursing student intentionally left out key information with the intention of creating an image of experience, the student's comment does not meet the standard for truthfulness. Thus, another criterion for creating truth is full disclosure. Without full disclosure, the patient could make decisions, such as letting the nursing student perform the injection, based on incomplete or inaccurate information, which would be a violation of the patient's right to self-determination.

Rationale in Support of Truth-Telling

Lo (2000) identified several rationales supporting the need for truth-telling and against the use of lies. First, there is an ethical presumption that lying is wrong. According to the Judeo-Christian tradition, "you shall not bear false witness against your neighbor" (Exodus 20:16). According to the Islamic tradition, "cover not the truth with falsehood, nor conceal the truth you know" (Quran 2:42; Ali, 1989). Thus, lying should be avoided because it diminishes the social trust within a community, group, or relationship. Second, people desire to be autonomous in their decision-making, and complete, accurate information is needed before an informed decision can be made. Third, the communication of truthful information creates greater long-term benefits than harms (Lo, 2000). Fourth, lies and deception can require a lot of emotional energy to maintain. Once a lie is told, the liar must remember not only the truth, but also the details of the lie so as not to get caught in it later. Finally, the risk of having the lie accidentally exposed increases with the number of people involved and the complexity of the situation. Thus when faced with temptations to deceive, health care professionals need to reframe the question from "What should the patient be told" to "What is the best way to communicate this information to this patient?" (Lo, 2000). Thus, the old adage, "Oh, what a wicked web we weave when we practice to deceive" remains a useful slogan for nurses.

Nontruth: Lies and Lying

The opposite of truth is nontruth. However, Western society rarely uses this term; instead, we commonly speak of a lie or lying. Each of us has lied at one time or another and will undoubtedly lie again sometime in the future. In fact, it is estimated (based on parental feedback) that 19.4% of children lie (Stouthamer-Loeber, 1986). Young children frequently exhibit mild deception through "simple denial, bragging and exaggeration, tales of fantasy or 'white lies'." However, "chronic lying, deliberate feigning of physical or emotional distress, cheating others out of money, or making false allegations" (Lu & Boone, 2002, p. 90) are serious actions designed to intentionally deceive another person. Examples of false verbal comments that are not lies or attempts at deception include spontaneous confabulations and memory failures displayed by patients with brain injuries (Schnider, 2001).

Lies can occur through the deliberate omitting of information, the providing of incomplete information, or the providing of false information. In addition, the manner in which the information is conveyed can also create a false impression, for example, tone of voice, nonverbal mannerisms, and choice of wording.

White Lies

White lies are falsehoods of trivial importance that are not intended to create harm for any person. White lies are offered most frequently during daily social interactions as a form of accepted and often expected acts of etiquette. Patients may tell white lies to minimize distress to family and health care providers. For example, a nauseated patient might reply "I am OK" while simultaneously experiencing dry heaves over an emesis basin. White lies help us out of touchy situations without hurting someone else's feelings. For example, when your grandmother asks, "Did I knit your birthday sweater too big?" most of us might reply, "Oh, I love my sweaters roomy. This way I can wear a turtleneck underneath," regardless of our real opinion of how the sweater fits (Bok, 1999).

Similarly, white lies are often told to brighten people's spirits during a dismal situation, as flattery, or even to express appreciation for undesired gifts (Bok, 1999). Undoubtedly, each of us has at some point in our lives said white lies similar to the following:

- "Look at the bright side: Dislodging your IV access gave me the opportunity to practice my IV insertion skills."
- "That new uniform style makes you look slimmer."
- "Thanks, but no thanks, I am on a diet" (when offered a piece of candy from a patient in isolation).

Thus, white lies seem to have an established function in Western society because of their ability to minimize seemingly insignificant issues or events that, if blown out of proportion, could create greater harms or obligations for others (Bok, 1999). For example, if, instead of a telling a white lie covering up how he or she actually feels, a person replied, "I am so depressed. Everything is going wrong," the person initiating the question might perceive an obligation to provide assistance or at least offer a sympathetic response when no such intention was present at the beginning of the verbal exchange.

Rationale to Justify Lying

If, in justifying lying or telling the truth, a person refers to the potential consequences that he or she is attempting to maximize or minimize, the person is implementing a utilitarian approach. Because utilitarians evaluate the moral appropriateness of an action by weighing the anticipated harms and benefits that are expected from the action, it follows that actions that promote the most good or happiness for the most persons would be considered morally justifiable. Bok (1999) pointed out that this simplistic view "appears to imply that lies, apart from their resultant harm and benefits, are in themselves neutral" (p. 50). However, most persons in Western society would disagree and consider that "we should allow an initial presumption against lies" (p. 50). A variety of consequences have been used to support the use of lies.

Preventing Harm

One of the most common reasons given for not telling the truth is to protect others from harm. Nurses may use this strategy when contacting a family member by phone after a patient has died. A nurse might say, "Ms. Phon, your father has taken a turn for the worse. Would you like to come to the hospital?" Although the nurse's comment is not an outright lie (dying is definitely a turn for the worse), the nurse is not completely forthcoming because the comment does not provide an accurate representation of the reality of the situation. The euphemism "taken a turn for the worse" is an attempt to motivate the daughter to come to the hospital, but also limit the daughter's emotional trauma so she can drive safely to the hospital. If the daughter does not agree to come to the hospital, the nurse will need to augment the previous comments by disclosing that the patient is in fact dead, thus acknowledging that the nurse's initial comments were not completely truthful. Nurses often justify this type of deception based on the belief that when a person learns about a loved one's death, support systems should be available to assist with grieving.

Similarly, prevention of harm has been used by health care professionals to justify not telling patients the truth about their test results or diagnosis. This perception of harm might include loss of hope, ineffective coping, or refusal to continue with therapy (Lo, 2000). However, this rationale is shortsighted because it does not consider the potential long-term harm to the patient–health care provider relationship if on learning the truth, the patient does not agree that the health care provider's deception was appropriate.

Promoting Good

When claiming that a lie created good, this good is often associated with the liar and not others. For example, an employee might lie about not swiping in at the beginning of the shift, an attempt to hide the fact that he was actually late to work, stating, "Oh, I forgot to swipe in." Similarly, a biotech company might lie about use of embryonic tissues based on a belief that if the experiment works, society will greatly benefit (Bok, 1999).

Moral Qualities of the Person Being Told the Lie

Many claim that it is morally appropriate to return a lie with a lie. This rationale could gain some support from the principle of universality. As mentioned earlier, universality claims that if an action is correct in this situation, the same action would be appropriate to use in every similar situation. Thus, a liar could not complain about being lied to without undermining the appropriateness of his or her lie (Bok, 1999). For example, a nursing unit honors requests to be off on a holiday based on seniority. After being denied the shift off, a new employee calls in *sick* on New Year's Eve. In response to this apparent lie, the nursing supervisor replies, "You will need to provide a written statement from your primary health care provider to qualify for sick pay and prior to being able to return to work (even though no policy exists)".

During times of war, the military and public justify lying to the enemy, which may create a necessary diversion so that strategies can be instituted to win a battle (Bok, 1999). Taken at face value, this idea of lying to the enemy does not seem applicable to most nurses, except perhaps those in the military. However, the enemy concept may apply to competing hospitals and agencies vying to recruit nurses during a nursing shortage. For example, Hospital A's nursing administrator may lie by omission to Hospital B's nursing administrator about Hospital A's anticipated revised salary and benefits package as a means to gain an edge in recruiting newly graduated nurses. Similar comparisons might be made regarding research endeavors, an institution's financial status, or interactions between applicants for the same position or scholarship. However, Carr (2004) argued that "bluffing is nothing more than a form of lying. . . . Bluffing in business might be regarded simply as game strategy—much like bluffing in poker, which does not reflect on the morality of the bluffer" (p. 443).

The Truth Is Not Desired or Welcomed

There are times when a person may decide that he or she does not want to know the truth. This decision may be based on fatigue, depression, severe illness, cultural norms, or competing priorities. For example, a critically and/or terminally ill patient may elect not to know the most current diagnosis or lab result due to lack of energy or limited cognitive or emotional resources to adequately deal with new information. Immigrants from other cultures, such as Japan or Korea, may not value autonomy as strongly as Americans do, and thus health care professionals might be directed to limit the information disclosed to such patients. Other times, people may desire not to learn the truth until after a special or major event, such as a wedding or certifying exam. This rationale shares many similarities with the first rationale related to preventing harm. However, the major difference is related to the fact that the lie may be out of respect for another's preference not to be told rather than being based on paternalism (the liar's beliefs about what is right or wrong).

Using Truth to Build a Therapeutic Nurse–Patient Relationship

A high quality therapeutic nurse–patient relationship requires that mutual trust be present. Without honesty, a person cannot establish a pattern of positive trusting experiences. Clear communication is another factor that contributes to trust. A trusting person exhibits the following characteristics:

A feeling of comfort with growth in self-awareness and an ability to share this awareness with others; acceptance of others as they are without needing to change them; openness to new experiences; long-term consistency between words and actions; and the ability to delay gratification. (Sundeen, Stuart, Rankin, & Cohen, 1998, p. 152)

Thus, it is easy to recognize that truthfulness is a key component for developing these trusting characteristics. When a nurse conveys a truthful message and his or her actions match the message, the patient develops trust in the nurse, and the start of a therapeutic relationship is formed. For example, a nurse states, "I want to know how that pain shot helps your pain. I'll be back to check on you in 15 minutes." The patient is able to recognize not only the truth of the nurse's message, but also the nurse's caring when the nurse does in fact return to verify the effectiveness of the pain medication.

Discussion Exercises 7-1

During change of shift report you learn the following information: "This 36-year old female was admitted for multiple fractured ribs and liver contusion secondary to a motor vehicle accident (MVA). She developed a large blood clot that was treated with IV heparin (and 2 days ago was started on Coumadin (warfarin). Yesterday, the laboratory notified the attending physician that this woman is pregnant, however, the patient has not yet been informed about the pregnancy. Since she has received Coumadin (warfarin) in addition to the various scans and X-rays, the physician wants to meet with the perinatologist prior to disclosing this information to the patient." Until the patient is notified, the treatment regimen continues as ordered.

1. Do you believe there are any issues with truth-telling or deception in this case? Explain.
2. What should you do or say if the patient comments, "I am a little worried. I just realized that I missed my period. Do you think it is just because of my being so sick?"
3. Should the nurse refuse to participate in this patient's care, continuing the Coumadin and/or to sending the patient for any scans/X-rays?
4. If the decision is made to hold today's Coumadin dose, what explanation will you give the patient if she asks why she has not received her routine daily Coumadin dose?

Communicating Bad News

As discussed previously, the temptation to use nontruth during times of crisis or disappointment is great. Sometimes, a nontruthful statement is used to ease an emotional response, for example, telling a family member their loved one "slipped away peacefully" even if this was not the case.

The temptation also exists to use nontruthful statements to *soften* the perception of the news for either the message sender (health care professional) and/or the message receiver (patient), for example, "Your cancer is not responding as well as we hoped to the chemotherapy," when in fact there has been no beneficial change in status. The use of nontruthful statements during these difficult discussions creates added stress because the message sender must decide either to continue on the nontruthful path or acknowledge the deception to subsequently convey the truth about the situation. Once the message receiver is aware of the deception, he or she may then be unable to believe future messages based on the inability to trust the truthfulness of the message or the message sender's intentions.

Even though nurses usually are not responsible for initially disclosing bad news related to a diagnosis ("The second blood test confirms that you are HIV+"; "The transplanted heart is being rejected"), they are often responsible for clarifying the information given by the primary health care provider. In addition, the nurse is often responsible for conveying undesirable news about delayed or canceled tests or procedures, critical changes in a loved one's physical status, and medication errors. Thus, nurses need to develop strong communication skills as well as the self-confidence necessary to discuss topics that may prove to be emotional or embarrassing to the patient, the family, or the nurse.

When preparing to impart bad news, the nurse should collect and understand the facts that need to be presented and be able to discuss the news in terms the other person can understand. When possible, bad news should be given in person in a private setting (Farber, 2002). The patient's current knowledge about the topic and how much information the patient desires should be verified: "And if they ask us to 'tell it to me straight' ... no matter how difficult, we must use our humanity to tell them, and we must never question whether it was the right thing to do" (Neff, Lyckholm, & Smith, 2002). Gallagher, Waterman, Ebers, Fraser, and Levinson (2003) suggested that a patient's distress might be less when the bad news is given in a factual, compassionate, and sympathetic fashion, which may include an apology if appropriate.

Often nurses worry about showing their emotions and "not looking professional." However, sharing one's tears with a family when a patient dies may assist the family to recognize that your concern is genuine while at the same time providing the family permission to grieve. The nurse needs to make sure that he or she has sufficient uninterrupted time for these tough conversations. This may mean negotiating with another nurse to answer one's pages, phone calls, and/or call lights. Finally, the nurse needs to summarize the conversation and identify what the next step(s) will be (Farber et al., 2002).

Following the Disclosure of Nontruth

Despite having a commitment to promoting truthful communications, a nurse might find himself or herself in a position of following a deceptive communication between a patient and another health care professional. In the ideal world, the nurse will discover this occurrence and have ample opportunity to decide how to proceed; however, this is not always the case, especially when one is confronted directly by a patient about the deception. There are no hard and fast rules for determining how to proceed. If asked directly, "Why did Dr. X lie to me?" the nurse can honestly state "I do not know" and assist the patient to determine how he or she would like the incident handled. Ideally, the nurse should attempt not to be caught in the middle between the patient and a physician or other person with higher authority. An obligation to be a patient advocate may require the nurse to be part of future conversations, thus forcing him or her into a potentially adversarial confrontation. The nurse should involve the nursing supervisor for assistance, refer to relevant policy and procedures, and remember risk management principles when documenting the incident. In many cases, bringing the topic into the open will be incentive enough to promote open and honest dialogue and, thus, defuse the situation.

If the deceptive comment was made by an unlicensed assistive personnel (UAP) under the supervision of the nurse, then the nurse must take primary responsibility in correcting the patient's knowledge and clarifying the plan of care. In addition, the nurse has the obligation to educate the UAP on the ethical obligation for honest communication, investigate (and rectify when possible) the reason for the deception, and work to create an environment of trust between the patient and the entire health care team.

SUMMARY

For nurses, truth-telling is an expected action based on a professional commitment to respect persons and their autonomy. Telling the truth requires an intention to communicate information that conforms to reality. Persons can engage in telling nontruths via lies and white lies. A variety of rationales can be used to defend the use of both truthful and nontruthful statements. When making decisions about telling the truth, nurses need to consider not only their intentions and the expected outcomes, but also other coexisting moral commitments and obligations. Telling the truth should be a primary commitment for the professional nurse.

CLINICAL EXERCISES

Before posing any questions, be sure to explain to the other person that your clinical assignment is about truth-telling. This explanation should provide the person with a pragmatic understanding for why you are asking questions that might appear at face value to be "politically incorrect."

1. Check your agency's policy and procedure manual to see whether a policy on disclosure of information or truth-telling exists.
2. Talk with the nursing staff (including ancillary personnel) about "white lies" health care professionals might say to a patient and/or their significant others. Are there particular situations or events that may be more likely for the use of white lies?

Discussion Questions

1. Ask a family member or friend if he or she has ever lied to another family member or friend.

   a. If so, what reasons did he or she provide to justify the lie?
   b. If not, what reasons did he or she provide for not lying?

2. Ask a family member or friend if he or she has ever not told his or her physician the truth about symptoms or treatment.

a. If so, what reasons did he or she provide to justify the lie?
b. If not, what reasons did he or she provide for not lying?

3. Bok (1999) proposed that there should be

   at least one immediate limitation on lying: in any situation where a lie is a possible choice, one must first seek truthful alternatives. . . . And only where a lie is a last resort can one even begin to consider whether or not it is morally justified. (p. 31)

   a. Do you agree that lying should only be done as last resort?
   b. Can you think of a lie that has no truthful alternatives?

4. The ANA (2001) Code of Ethics for Nurses With Interpretive Statements does not include the word "veracity" or "truthfulness." Does this mean that the professional nurse does not have an obligation to be truthful?

5. Bok (1999) claimed that "lying requires a *reason*, while truth-telling does not" (p. 22). What is your assessment of this assertion? Provide an example to illustrate your position.

Resources

Aitken, S. (2000). Deception and lies. *Nursing Standard, 14*(32), 22–23.

American Nurses Association. (1994). Position statement: Polygraph testing of health care workers. Retrieved November 14, 2005, from http://www.nursingworld.org/readroom/position/workplac/wkpolygr.htm

American Nurses Association, & Computer-Based Patient Record Institute, Inc. (1995). Position statement: Position paper on authentication in a computer-based patient record. Retrieved November 14, 2005, from http://www.nursingworld.org/readroom/position/joint/jtcpri2.htm

Crow, K., Matheson, L., & Steed, A. (2000). Informed consent and truth-telling: Cultural directions for healthcare providers. *Journal of Nursing Administration, 30*(3), 148–152.

Kant, I. (1898). On a supposed right to tell lies from benevolent motives. In I. Kant (T. K Abbott, Trans.) *Kant's critique of practical reason and other works* (5th ed.). London: Longmans, Green, and Co. Retrieved on November 14, 2005, from http://oll.libertyfund.org/Intros/Kant.php

Kinsella, L. (2001). Truthtelling in patient care: Resolving ethical issues. *Nursing, 31*(12), 52.

Quek, T. (n.d.). The truth about a child's compulsive lying. Retrieved November 14, 2005, from http://webhome.idirect.com/~readon/lies.html

References

Ali, A. Y. (Ed.). (1989). *The holy Quran: Text, translation and commentary* (New rev. ed.). Brentwood, MD: Amana Corp.

American Nurses Association (1976, 1985). *Code for nurses with interpretive statements*. Kansas City, MO: Author.

American Nurses Association. (2001). *Code of ethics for nurses with interpretive statements*. Washington DC: Author.

Bok, S. (1999). *Lying: Moral choice in public and private life*. New York: Vintage Books.

Carr, A. Z. (2004). Is business bluffing ethical? In T. L. Beauchamp & M. E. Bowie (Eds.). *Ethical theory and business* (7th ed.) (pp. 443–447). Englewood Cliffs, NJ: Prentice-Hall.

Farber, N. J., Urban, S. Y., Collier, V. U., Weiner, J., Polite, R. G., Davis, E., et al. (2002). The good news about giving bad news to patients. *Journal of General Internal Medicine, 17*(2), 914–922.

Funk & Wagnalls New International Dictionary (Comprehensive ed.). (1996). Chicago: World Publishers.

Gallagher, T. H., Waterman, A. D., Ebers, A. G., Fraser, V. J., & Levinson, W. (2003). Patients' and physicians' attitudes regarding the disclosure of medical errors. *JAMA, 289*(8), 1001–1007.

Lo, B. (2000). *Resolving ethical dilemmas: A guide for clinicians* (2nd ed.). Philadelphia: Lippincott, Williams & Wilkens.

Lu, P. H., & Boone, K. B. (2002). Suspect cognitive symptoms in a 9-year old child: Malingering by proxy? *Clinical Neuropsychologist, 16*(1), 90–96.

Neff, P., Lyckholm, L., & Smith, T. (2002). Truth or consequences: What to do when the patient does not want to know. *Journal of Clinical Oncology, 20*(1), 3035–3037.

Schnider, A. (2001). Spontaneous confabulations, reality monitoring, and the limbic system—a review. *Brain Research Reviews, 36*, 150–160.

Stouthamer-Loeber, M. (1986). Lying as a problem behavior in children: A review. *Clinical Psychology Review, 6,* 267–289.

Sundeen, S. J., Stuart, G. W., Rankin, E. A. D., & Cohen, S. A. (1998). *Nurse–client interaction: Implementing the nursing process* (6th ed.). St. Louis: Mosby.

Whitbeck, C. (1995). Trust. In W. Reich (Ed.). *Encyclopedia of bioethics* (pp. 2499–2504). New York: Simon & Schuster Macmillan.

CHAPTER 8

Advocacy

Objectives

At the end of this chapter, the student should be able to:

1. Define patient advocacy, workplace advocacy, and professional advocacy.
2. Identify opportunities to advocate for patients.
3. Understand the nursing profession's obligation to advocate.
4. Describe actions the nurse could take in advocating for patients.
5. Give an example of how the nursing profession advocates for patients.
6. Give examples of how the nursing profession advocates for its workplace environment.

KEY WORDS

- *Advocacy for patients*
- *Advocacy for the profession*
- *Autonomy*
- *Code of ethics*
- *Competency*
- *Decision-making capacity*

- *Empowerment*
- *Incompetent*
- *Moral courage*
- *Moral distress*
- *Therapeutic relationships*

Members of every health care profession believe they have a responsibility to act as a patient advocate. No single profession "owns" the role as advocate, but nursing has promoted this role as integral to good nursing care. What does it mean to be a patient advocate? This chapter focuses on the nurse's role as patient advocate, as well as the broader concept of advocacy in nursing. Advocacy is one of the four common ethical themes in nursing practice that will be expanded on in each of the chapters of Unit 3: Clinical Ethical Issues.

What Is Advocacy?

Imagine that you travel to a foreign land where you do not know the culture or language. How do you get your needs met? You can attempt to communicate through gestures or using pictures, but you cannot be sure that you are being understood. It would certainly help if you had an advocate, someone who knows the country's culture, language, and the system in which you are attempting to interact. The health care system is analogous to a foreign land for many patients. This language is full of jargon, abbreviations, and colloquialisms. Most health care institutions have a hierarchy, policies, procedures, standards, routines, and rituals that seem mysterious to patients, families, visitors, and students learning to be health care professionals. As nursing students become familiar with health systems, they become insiders. As insiders, health care professionals have an obligation to assist patients to navigate the health care system to get their needs met. However, the nursing student first needs to learn the role of the professional nurse, how the nursing process is enacted, and how nursing care is delivered in the specific health care setting.

Along with understanding the disease process, diagnostic procedures, treatments, symptom management, and psychosocial implications of health promotion, maintenance, and restoration, nurses need to learn the system in which patient care occurs. In some systems, such as the ambulatory setting, healthy individuals seek preventative activities like screening tests. Patients with symptoms seek diagnostic tests, and diagnosed patients seek treatment. As part of the nursing process, the nurse learns the reason for and the patient's expectations of the visit. Nursing assessment begins at the first interaction with the patient and continues through the entire patient contact period. Patient education, clarification, and reinforcement of information occur, along with an assessment of the patient's understanding. A patient may be prepared for an examination or educated on medication administration. The nurse may help a patient to understand information given by another professional. In this setting, the nurse acts an advocate by helping meet the patient's expectations of this outpatient visit. The word advocacy comes from Latin *advocare*, meaning "to call to one's aid." To advocate on behalf of a patient is to come to his or her aid or to give voice to his or her concerns. Providing information to the patient and keeping him or her informed aids the patient in the encounter with the health care system.

There are numerous mentions of advocacy in the American Nurses Association (ANA) (2001) Code of Ethics for Nurses With Interpretive Statements. In the Canadian Nurses Association (CNA) (2002) Code of Ethics for Registered Nurses, eight values are described that are key to nursing practice. To effectuate many of those values, the nurse must advocate for the patient. In both codes, the nurse is expected to advocate for the rights of patients for safe, humane, and culturally competent nursing care. Advocacy in this example might mean that the nurse should contact a medical translator for a patient whose first language is not English. The ANA code also uses the term "advocates" in discussing the nurse's duty to protect the patient's privacy, ensure that the patient and important others have a voice in decision-making, and protect the patient from incompetent, unethical, illegal, or impaired practice of any health care provider.

Advocating for institutional change on behalf of all patients is also included in the ANA code. The Canadian code beckons nurses to "advocate for practice environments that have the organizational structures and resources necessary to ensure safety, support and respect for all persons in the work setting" (CNA, 2002, p. 8).

THE CALL TO ADVOCACY

Myra Levine (1989), one of the earliest nurse ethicists, described every interaction between a nurse and patient as a moral interaction. Meeting a patient, taking a history, being present during the examination, and performing an examination are profoundly moral interactions and need to be conducted with respect and competency. Patients often are vulnerable and depend on health care providers to instruct them on what to expect, explain findings, explain options, and give advice, when appropriate. Although there is a hierarchy of professionals in terms of power and authority in the health care setting, the nurse has power over the patient in many encounters because of the special knowledge the nurse has. The nurse is usually in control of the situation, with patients being told where to go and what to do. The nurse often has information that the patient does not have, such as how to navigate the health care system. Even the most sophisticated patients may not know the particular nuances of the health care setting that can affect their care. The nurse can "run interference" for the patient by educating him or her and removing barriers so the patient can achieve the desired goals.

Whose Goals to Promote?

The goals might be negotiated between the patient and health care provider or might be articulated by the patient but not endorsed by the health care team. Conflict can occur if the goals of the patient and the professionals are not the same and are even incompatible. Does the nurse advocate for what the patient wants against the nurse's better judgment? For example, a patient with breast cancer wants to use only homeopathy and diet to combat the cancer. Her oncologist recommends a lumpectomy, radiation treatments, and oral chemotherapy. Does the nurse advocate for the patient by supporting her decision to forgo traditional treatment or does he or she try to educate the patient to accept the traditional treatment? If the patient has not discussed her preferences with the oncologist, the nurse can facilitate a discussion between them. In addition, the nurse can assist the patient to obtain information about the pros and cons of the various types of treatment the patient is considering. While respecting the patient's right to make a decision consistent with her values, the health care team is also expected to offer their recommendations based on their experiences and knowledge of the state-of-the-art techniques relating to the particular condition. Ultimately the decision is the patient's.

THE STRENGTH TO ADVOCATE

Nurses with less experience may hesitate to assume an advocacy role. Working in health care requires humility in light of the growing amount of medical information.

A nurse may feel that he or she does not know enough to question a physician or fellow nurse. It is very appropriate for the nurse to ask for information about a decision or course of action. The nurse may also do some research through the library, Internet, or personal contacts. Knowing standards of care, policies and procedures, and professional position or policy statements are helpful in advocating. Knowing the patient's wishes and communicating with the patient, family (if appropriate), and the health care team are also very helpful in advocating. A nurse can advocate for the patient by providing the patient with necessary information or facilitating decision-making by talking with the patient. Allowing the patient to speculate, think out loud, and use the nurse as a sounding board is part of the therapeutic relationship. As nurses experience more opportunities to advocate, they will become more comfortable with the role.

At a minimum, nurses advocate for patients by avoiding preventable harms. The nurse can do this in several ways: maintaining competence in the area of nursing in which he or she practices, applying critical thinking skills when implementing the treatment plan, and acting to promote the health and safety of patients while they are in his or her care. Individual acts of the nurse, as well as participation in groups designed to avert iatrogenic illnesses and injuries (those caused by the medical treatment or health care staff) for the patient population, are acts of advocacy. For example, as a nurse is reviewing newly written physician orders, she notices that the new medication may interact with a current medication the patient is receiving. Instead of assuming that the physician was aware of all the medications taken by the patient or that the pharmacy will identify the potential drug interaction as the order is filled, the nurse contacts the physician to discuss the order. Doing so prevents a potential harm to the patient. In another example, the nurses on a particular unit observe that there has been an increase in patient falls. The nurses on that unit come together to examine the root cause for the falls and devise a plan to reduce their incidence. Advocacy, based on the ethical principles of autonomy of the patient, beneficence, and nonmaleficence, is an ethical obligation of the nurse.

Case Study 8-1

Nurse Anchor is assigned to a 73-year-old woman with a wound on her foot. Dressing changes have been very uncomfortable, and Nurse Anchor suggests that he give the patient pain medication prior to changing the dressing. The surgeon, Dr. Carney, arrives on the unit earlier than expected and begins to change the dressing. Nurse Anchor comes into the room and asks Dr. Carney to wait until he can medicate the patient. The surgeon says to the patient, "You do not mind if I get this over with, do you? I'll hurry so it will not hurt as much." The patient hesitates for a moment, and says, "I suppose so." How can the nurse advocate for this patient?

Possible response. Nurse Anchor says to his patient, "If you want, I can give you your pain medication now like we discussed and we can ask Dr. Carney to return in 15 minutes. Would you prefer that?" Nurse Anchor realizes that many patients, especially elderly patients, do not question physician authority, and the nurse believes the patient would prefer not to experience pain during the dressing change. The nurse said what he thought the patient wanted to say; he "gave her a voice."

Case Study 8-2

During her pediatric rotation, Student Nurse Baker is with a 3-year-old boy in the playroom. The policy on the pediatric unit is that all procedures are performed in the procedure room and not in the playroom because the playroom is considered a safe place. A medical student comes in and says to the child, "There you are, I have been looking for you. I need to take a quick look at you," and begins to examine the child.

Possible response. Student Nurse Baker informs the medical student that the playroom is an "exam-free zone" and she will bring the child to the procedure room so that the medical student can complete her examination. The medical student agrees and stops examining the child until they have all moved to the procedure room.

Suppose the medical student insists on completing her exam in the playroom and says she will not do anything to hurt the child. The student nurse responds with, "He needs to know that this is a safe place and he can come here to play. If you need to do the exam now, I will bring him to the procedure room for you." The student nurse has advocated for the child, who cannot speak for himself. The medical student was prioritizing her need to complete the exam over the child's need to feel safe in the playroom.

Now suppose that the child experienced acute respiratory distress while in the playroom. The student nurse would act immediately to save the child's life, prioritizing his need to breathe over his need to feel safe in the playroom. Advocacy requires analyzing the situation and deciding what actions will give the patient a voice and will advance his or her interests.

RELATIONSHIPS BETWEEN HEALTH CARE PROFESSIONALS

The Doctor–Nurse Game

Much has been written about the "doctor–nurse game" since the phrase was coined by Stein (1967). The communication style signified by this "game" represents deference on behalf of the nurse to the authority of the physician. In this sort of relationship, the nurse identifies the patient's needs or problems and makes recommendations to the physician, but in a passive way so that it appears the physician is arriving at the recommendations on his own. The use of the male pronoun is intentional because most physicians were men and nurses women in 1967. Savage (1995) found that this type of communication style persisted because nurses found it was effective when they advocated for their patients. For example, an experienced nurse on a bone marrow transplant unit notices a patient may be having beginning signs of graft-versus-host disease. She contacts the physician, a first-year resident, and describes the patient's signs and symptoms. The physician thanks her for telling him and starts to hang up. She adds, "Is there anything you want me to do . . . any medication to order or blood to have drawn?" She is expecting him to proceed in the usual way that graft-versus-host disease is managed, and because he did not, she attempts to elicit the expected response without openly telling him what should be done. As part of the resident's education, the nurse could be asking in a Socratic fashion what should be done next, but it is more likely that she has found that leading the resident to the expected response will result in getting the orders that she believes is best for her patient. However, the interaction seems to perpetuate the "doctor–nurse game."

The doctor–nurse game, issues involving physician–nurse relationships, and fear of physicians have been reported in the United States (Mason, 2002), the United Kingdom (Radcliffe, 2000), Mexico (Hojat et al., 2001), Australia (Ahern & McDonald, 2002), and Canada (Boychuk Duchscher, 2001). It also has been found that patient outcomes, as well as nurses' job satisfaction, are greatly affected by the quality of the nurse–physician relationship (Aiken, Havens, & Sloane, 2000; Longo, Young, Mehr, Lindbloom, & Salerno, 2002; Rosenstein, 2002). Furthermore, new graduates have described interacting with physicians as a major source of anxiety (Boychuk Duchscher, 2001). Why are these facts important in advocacy? When the nurse must challenge the status quo on behalf of the patient, moral courage is required, and the doctor–nurse game only makes this more challenging.

Handling Conflict Between Team Members

In the foregoing case examples of advocacy, the nurse (and student nurse) had to interact with a physician (and medical student) to advocate for their patients. In both cases, the nurses questioned the physicians' actions. It is quite possible that the physicians could have reacted angrily and become verbally abusive toward the nurses; fearing that outcome, the nurses might not have spoken up. It is also possible that the nurses could be concerned about their ongoing relationship with the physicians; thus they might have thought that the lesser of two evils would be to allow the physicians to continue. Speaking up on behalf of patients requires moral courage. If, in either case, the nurse did not get the outcome she desired, she would need to decide what to do next. Within a health care system, she could follow the chain of command in the nursing structure. She could notify the charge nurse. The student nurse could have contacted her instructor or the staff nurse assigned to her patient. Although these scenarios describe what seem like minor issues, they represent fundamental ethical issues for nurses. The nurses are acting to prevent harm (principle of non-maleficence) to their patients and to promote patient well-being (beneficence).

Relationships among nurses, student nurses, physicians, and medical students directly affect patient care. As with all human interactions, there are complex issues involving hierarchy, gender, personalities, and other intangible factors. Sometimes the intensity of the work of health care is used as an excuse for a lack of civility in interactions in the health care setting. Use of respectful language, professional decorum, and diplomacy when necessary should ensure effective communication and functional relationships among health care professionals.

Case Study 8-3

Nurse Ash observes an orthopedic resident going into her patient's room, so she follows him in. He removes the patient's dressing and opens the sterile dressing he intends to apply. As he is donning his sterile gloves, the tips of the fingers of the glove brush up against the patient's bedside table, but he continues. What should the nurse do if she believes the physician has contaminated his glove? Because the physician proceeds with changing the dressing, the nurse might assume that he was unaware of the contamination. It is possible, though, that the physician was aware, and was anxious to complete the dressing change even though he risks infecting his patient.

Possible response: Nurse Ash begins to open another package of sterile gloves for the physician and says, "Let me open these for you. I notice you just contaminated your right glove." The nurse is stating the observation she made and offering assistance to the physician to avoid possible harm to the patient.

Suppose the physician responds, "No, I did not contaminate my glove." What should the nurse do if she is certain the glove has been contaminated? The interaction with the physician may feel uncomfortable for the nurse, yet the duty to prevent harm to the patient is paramount. The nurse says, "Because it's possible that you did contaminate your glove, even though you do not think you did, the safest course of action to avoid possibly infecting the wound is to change your gloves. I have another pair here for you." Again, the nurse states objectively what is known, and offers an option that is in the patient's best interests.

Uncertainty, Dilemma, and Distress

Ethical issues are often embedded in the clinical context, where there are sociopolitical forces of power, institutional culture, and professional codes. The "right" course of action is often not clear, hence the frequent reference to an issue being gray rather than black and white. Jameton (1984) used the language of uncertainty, dilemma, and distress (p. 131). There can be ethical uncertainty, a question of whether the problem is an ethics problem. There are ethical dilemmas when a choice must be made between two equally unpleasant alternatives. An example of a dilemma might be the decision to amputate a gangrenous limb. The patient does not want to lose a limb, but does not want to die of septicemia.

Even if the nurse clearly identifies what he or she believes is the right course of action, there may be resistance to that course. To challenge the status quo once again requires the courage to speak up on behalf of a specific patient or a population of patients. Nurses may experience moral distress as they analyze a situation; they may not always be able to articulate the ethical components but will describe feeling that something "is not right." In advocating for patients, nurses decide what is the "right" thing to do. Here are additional examples of situations in which a nurse could advocate for a patient. Think of different courses of action the nurse could take and a rationale for those actions.

Case Study 8-4

Nurse Hunt works in home health care nursing. She visits a gentleman, Mr. Dash, who had a stroke. His son and daughter check on him and run errands for him, but he lives alone and eats frozen microwave dinners. His appearance and his home are unkempt and disheveled. When checking his medication, Nurse Hunt discovers that he has nearly full bottles of antihypertensive and anticoagulant medications. He said he sometimes forgets whether he has taken them and figures it is better to skip them than take a double dose. Despite pillboxes, schedules, and other reminders, he does not regularly take his medication. His blood pressure is 230/150. Nurse Hunt begins to call the physician to report her findings and Mr. Dash asks her not to, saying he does not want any more medication, hospitalization, or therapy. He wants to be left alone.

Possible actions. The nurse believes that she needs to act quickly. Does she comply with the patient's wishes to be left alone, or does she contact the physician and seek medical input? She considers whether she knows the patient well enough to accept his refusal of treatment, or if she has the time to assess his decision-making capacity. She is concerned that if she does not act quickly, the patient could experience another stroke. She explains to Mr. Dash that she thinks he could be in imminent danger of having another stroke, and should that happen while she is there, she would call an ambulance. She also tells him that he could be experiencing depression, which is interfering with his ability to make decisions. She would like the three of them, Mr. Dash, the physician, and herself, to make a plan on what to do about his blood pressure. He has the right to refuse treatment, but she would like to make sure he is fully capable of making the decision to forgo life-sustaining treatment.

In this scenario, Nurse Hunt does not know Mr. Dash very well, and because there is not such a relationship to draw on, she hesitates to act on his request at the cost of his health. She thinks his present condition could negatively affect his ability to make decisions. This may appear to be the antithesis of advocacy, yet it is not. The nurse respects the autonomy of the patient. For the patient to exercise autonomy, he must first be competent and have decision-making capacity. Competence is decided by a court of law, and he has not been declared incompetent, so he is presumed to be competent. Decision-making capacity, however, is not a legal condition; it is a "real-life" state and can be transient. Depending on the current situation, a patient may or may not have decision-making capacity. In light of the lack of time to assess the patient's capacity, the nurse is acting to preserve life.

Now suppose that Nurse Hunt knew Mr. Dash quite well, knew of his desire to forgo further treatment, knew of his family's agreement to honor Mr. Dash's wishes, and believed he had decision-making capacity in his decision to forgo treatment. His current request not to have his hypertension treated is consistent with their previous discussions. Nurse Hunt explains to Mr. Dash that his hypertension may precipitate another stroke, and it may be further disabling but it may not cause his death. She encourages him to complete an advance directive so a surrogate can make decisions for him if he is incapacitated. Nurse Hunt may have suggested to Mr. Dash and his physician that a "Do Not Resuscitate" order be written so that any health professional in the home at the time of an arrest will not be legally compelled to resuscitate him. Although Nurse Hunt may have strong feelings that Mr. Dash should accept treatment, she is advocating for what he, as a competent adult who has decision-making capacity, wants.

Case Study 8-5

Nurse Gorrell works on a medical unit. He is caring for an 82-year-old man who had a myocardial infarction and is experiencing left heart failure. Consistent with his advance directives, and with his family's agreement, a "Do Not Resuscitate" order was written. He is receiving palliative care. In the morning a phlebotomist prepares to draw blood. Nurse Gorrell checks the orders and discovers that the order for routine laboratory tests was not canceled. He calls the intern to get an order to cancel the blood work, but the intern says he still wants it. The intern says the attending will ask him what the patient's potassium is and he'll have to have an answer for him. Nurse Gorrell then asks what the intern intends to do if the potassium result is abnormal, and he replies, "Nothing. That's not the point. The point is, I have to have the information if I am asked."

Possible response. Nurse Gorrell is not convinced that the patient should endure the discomfort and expense of a blood test that will not alter his course of treatment. He advises the intern that he is going to ask the phlebotomist to wait until he speaks to the attending physician. Once he reaches the attending, he asks whether it is necessary to obtain the potassium level, and the attending agrees it is not necessary.

Suppose the attending said that he is curious to see whether the potassium level has changed, but that knowing the level will not persuade him to change any treatment. Nurse Gorrell then suggests that the patient be asked if he will agree to a test that is not for his benefit but for the physician's knowledge. Or the nurse may ask the physician if he believes the value of knowing the results outweighs the discomfort and cost to the patient. The nurse may not be able to prevent the blood from being drawn even if he believes there is no justifiable reason to do so; however, he should bring the issue of unnecessary tests on dying patients to the appropriate group within the institution. There may be a continuous quality improvement (CQI) committee or a committee addressing palliative or comfort care for dying patients. In the process of developing a unit or department policy, dialogue can occur between professional groups so that there will be an understanding of each group's perspective and a mutually agreeable policy can be enacted.

LEARNING HOW TO ADVOCATE

In a bibliometric analysis of articles on patient advocacy, Mallik and Rafferty (2000) concluded that advocacy by U.S. nurses has become "more contentious and militant as nurses seek to empower themselves with the advocacy role" (p. 8). Foley, Minick, and Kee (2002) found that nurses learn advocacy in a haphazard manner that is dependent on situations. They identified three ways that nurses learn advocacy. In the first, the nurse identifies how he or she learned to "stand up for others" in the past. Standing up for one's siblings against a bully is an example of how a nurse may have experienced advocacy prior to coming into the profession. Learning by watching how other nurses advocate is the second way. The third is by gaining confidence through experience, validation, and mentoring. As nurses are socialized into the profession, they should be alert for opportunities to share their inside knowledge of the health care system and advocate for patients by helping them to navigate it.

ADVOCACY FOR THE PROFESSION

The American Nurses Association in the United States, the Canadian Nurses Association in Canada, and other associations in the United States and elsewhere exist for a number of reasons. One major purpose is to advocate for the health and welfare of their citizens or special patient populations and for the advancement of the nursing profession. The 1991 ANA Code of Ethics for Nurses With Interpretative Statements (ANA, 2001) represents the profession's expectations of its members. Most of the provisions in the 2001 ANA code pertain to client–patient interests, whereas some address workplace issues. All codes provide the ethical impetus for advocacy.

Workplace Advocacy

Having a work environment that is conducive to optimal performance is a goal of nursing. Staffing and workload determinations are critical to the nurse's performance. The nurse prioritizes and delegate tasks. Having too many patients or patients who are acutely ill requires the nurse to shift time and attention to those patients. Although it may be idealistic to expect nurses to deliver the highest quality care every day, nurses do strive to achieve this. On those days that they believe they will not be able to devote the amount of time and attention to patients who need it the most, they advise their managers and negotiate for the optimal assignments. If this type of workload dilemma occurs chronically, the nurses must advocate for a change, such as increasing the number of nurses on their unit, decreasing the patient census, or referring more acute patients to better-staffed units. This type of negotiation is part of workplace advocacy. The nurses may be part of a collective bargaining unit of their professional organization, such as the UAN (United American Nurses, AFL-CIO) of the American Nurses Association, or may have a structure within their nursing division like shared governance through which they can negotiate change with the organization's administrators.

Nurses often work through their professional association to advocate for better working conditions. Staffing, workload, and delegation are key issues that immediately affect patient care. Other workplace issues include nurse safety and health. Workplace violence, such as may occur in the emergency department or on a psychiatric unit, threatens the health of nurses, patients, other employees, and visitors. Nurses advocate for security measures that provide for safe delivery of care. Other environmental workplace issues include freedom from sexual harassment and avoidance of hazardous materials or situations conducive to workplace injury.

Mandatory overtime, especially in times of nursing shortages, is a source of conflict between nurses and administrators. Fatigue can lead to errors, and nurses who want to prevent the possibility of harm to patients may resist mandatory overtime. The conundrum that occurs with the "proof" that mandatory overtime risks patient safety is that nurses will risk their own health to avoid harm to patients. Many nurses have stories of a near-miss of patient harm that occurred when they were working overtime but that they did not report for various reasons. In a nurse's estimation, for example, the fatigue from overtime contributed to the likelihood of error. The operative issue is that nurses judge whether they are capable of safely providing several hours of patient care beyond the end of their shift; with mandatory overtime, their judgment about the safety of care is irrelevant. They are ordered to remain on the unit and take care of patients until they are relieved; if they leave at the end of their shift without reporting off to another nurse, they could be accused of patient abandonment. Each institution should have a definition of patient abandonment, and the nurses should have input into the definition and procedure for safely transferring care. The principle of non-maleficence, or preventing harm, holds for the prevention of harm to the nurse and others who deliver care, as well as for prevention of harm to the patients. Identifying unsafe situations, either for patients or staff, is an ethical obligation of health care providers.

To attract people into the profession of nursing, the work life of nurses needs to be continuously evaluated. Educational preparation, entry level for practice, and socialization into the profession are important issues for discussion. Workplace issues, in addition to those described earlier, include the use of needle-less intravenous systems, latex allergy management, and work-related disability benefits, and should be addressed in every facility employing nurses. Ongoing education through in-services, formal education with tuition reimbursement, and paid release time to attend conferences also should be the focus of advocacy. On a broader societal scale, nursing, through professional organizations, advocates by disseminating position statements on important issues for patients and families and for nurses. At the end of 2005, the ANA has 84 position statements including those pertaining to blood-borne and airborne diseases; ethics and human rights issues; social causes and health care; drug and alcohol abuse; nursing education, practice, and research; consumer advocacy and workplace advocacy; and the use of unlicensed assistive personnel. They have also issued joint statements with other professional and consumer groups. Practicing nurses can aid in the efforts to improve their profession by participating in their association's advocacy activities.

SUMMARY

For nursing to thrive, nurses need to advocate for the profession. This differs somewhat from patient advocacy, but patients benefit from successful advocacy for the profession. Advocacy, based on the principles of autonomy of the patient, beneficence, and nonmaleficence, is an ethical obligation of the nurse.

CLINICAL EXERCISES

1. Identify how your patient might benefit by your advocacy today.
2. Review the ANA (2001) Code of Ethics for Nurses With Interpretive Statements for provisions related to patient advocacy. What specific assistance does the code provide for the situation you identified in Clinical Exercise 1?
3. Find policies and procedures in your current clinical setting that reflect workplace advocacy. Suppose you have a latex allergy. Is there a policy that addresses how you are to observe standard precautions in light of this?
4. Discuss with a staff nurse in your clinical setting how he or she assesses the decision-making capacity of patients.

Discussion Questions

1. Observe the consent process with one of the patients in your clinical setting.

   - How was the patient's decision-making capacity assessed?
   - Was there any information you thought should have been given to the patient but was not? What would you have done differently?
   - What was the nurse's role in the consent process? Would you do anything differently than what the nurse in this case did? If so, what would you do and why?

2. Your patient has been diagnosed with a terminal illness. His family asks that he not be told his diagnosis, and the physician agrees not to tell him at this time. During his morning care, he tells you that he thinks he is not being told everything.

- What do you say to him, and why?
- Do you believe he has a right to know?
- Do you believe his family is making decisions for him in his best interests?
- Ask a staff nurse in your clinical setting how he or she would handle a situation like this.

3. The family of your patient with a brain tumor in intensive care wishes to bring in a reflexologist—someone who attempts to heal through applying pressure to specific areas of the patient's feet and hands.

- How should you advocate for your patient and family in this case?
- What criteria would you consider to determine whether this intervention is in your patient's best interests?
- Who ultimately decides whether this intervention can be performed for your patient?
- What alternative could you propose to balance the patient's values with his medical needs?

4. You are caring for a patient who has no family. The patient recently underwent surgery for removal of a cancerous tumor of the bowel. The insurance company authorized 6 days of hospitalization, and you believe the patient will not be ready for discharge by the sixth day.

- How do you advocate for the patient?
- What resources are available to you to advocate for the patient?

Resources

American Nurses Association Commission on Workplace Advocacy. Information on ANA activities regarding appropriate staffing, health and safety issues, patient safety and advocacy, workplace rights, and other resources for nurses is available at www.nursingworld.org/wpa/infolnks.htm

Canadian Nurses Association. (2002). Code of ethics for Registered Nurses. Available at http://cna-aiic.ca/CNA/practice/ethics/code/default_e.aspx

Federal Citizen Information Center. Support group and consumer information is available at www.pueblo.gsa.gov

Library of Congress. Legislative information and links for tracking bills in Congress are available at http://thomas.loc.gov/

United American Nurses, AFL-CIO. Information is available at http://nursingworld.org/uan

References

Ahern, K., & McDonald, S. (2002). The beliefs of nurses who were involved in a whistleblowing event. *Journal of Advanced Nursing, 38*(3), 303–309.

Aiken, L. H., Havens, D. S., & Sloane, D. M. (2000). The Magnet Nursing Services Recognition Program: A comparison of two groups of Magnet hospitals. *American Journal of Nursing, 100*(3), 26–36.

American Nurses Association. (2001). *Code of ethics for nurses with interpretive statements*. Washington, DC: Author.

Boychuk Duchscher, J. (2001). Out in the real world: Newly graduated nurses in acute-care speak out. *Journal of Nursing Administration, 31*(9), 426–439.

Canadian Nurses Association. (2002). Code of ethics for Registered Nurses. Available at http://cnaaiic.ca/CNA/practice/ethics/code/default_e.aspx

Foley, B. J., Minick, M. P., & Kee, C. C. (2002). How nurses learn advocacy. *Journal of Nursing Scholarship, 34*(2), 181–186.

Hojat, M., Nasca, T. J., Cohen, M. J. M., Fields, S. K., Rattner, S. L., Griffiths, M., et al. (2001). Attitudes toward physician–nurse collaboration: A cross-cultural study of male and female physician and nurses in the United States and Mexico. *Nursing Research, 50*(2), 123–128.

Jameton, A. (1984). *Nursing practice: The ethical issues*. Englewood Cliffs, NJ: Prentice Hall.

Levine, M. E. (1989). Ethical issues in cancer care: Beyond dilemma. *Seminars in Oncology Nursing, 5*(2), 124–128.

Longo, D. R., Young, J., Mehr, D., Lindbloom, E., & Salerno, L. D. (2002). Barriers to timely care of acute infections in nursing homes: A preliminary qualitative study. *Journal of the American Medical Directors Association, 3*(6), 360–365.

Mallik, M., & Rafferty, A. M. (2000). Diffusion of the concept of patient advocacy [Electronic version]. *Journal of Nursing Scholarship, 32*(4), 399–404.

Mason, D. J. (2002). MD–RN: A tired old dance. *American Journal of Nursing, 102*(6), 7.

Radcliffe, M. (2000). Doctors and nurses: New game, same result. *BMJ, 320*(7241), 1085.

Rosenstein, A. H. (2002). Nurse–physician relationships: Impact on nurse satisfaction and retention. *American Journal of Nursing, 102*(6), 26–34.

Savage, T. A. (1995). Nurses' negotiation processes in facilitating ethical decision-making in patient care. *Dissertation Abstracts International, 56*(12), 6675B.

Stein, L. I. (1967). The doctor–nurse game. *Archives of General Psychiatry, 16*, 699–703.

CHAPTER 9

Allocation of Resources

Objectives

At the end of this chapter, the student should be able to:

1. Identify issues of macro allocation in apportioning resources.
2. Articulate the ethical theories underpinning allocation decisions.
3. Describe the issues of micro allocation that nurses may face.
4. Describe the genesis and evolution of the U.S. health care delivery system.
5. Discuss the pros and cons of the managed care movement.

KEY WORDS

- *COBRA*
- *Delegation*
- *Distributive justice*
- *EMTALA*
- *Fee-for-service*
- *Health care rationing*
- *Health maintenance organization (HMO)*
- *Hill–Burton Act*
- *Managed care*
- *Medicaid*
- *Medicare*
- *Preferred provider organization (PPO)*
- *Single-payer program*
- *Universal coverage*

Figures vary, but there are at least 40 million people in the United States who do not have health care insurance and/or have difficulty obtaining health care. There has been debate over the last 50 years on whether health care is a right or a privilege. Because there are finite resources in health care, allocation decisions have to be made. This chapter focuses on issues of macro and micro allocation with regard to the apportionment of resources. Resource allocation is one of the four common ethical themes occurring in nursing practice that will be expanded on in each of the chapters of Unit 3: Clinical Ethical Issues. This chapter discusses the issues facing all health care providers, not just nurses, and is intended to give the reader an overall picture of the environment in which he or she will be working.

JUSTICE IN HEALTH CARE

Distributive justice is the fair allocation of the benefits and burdens of society. Although there are numerous principles of justice (as discussed in Chapter 1), this chapter deals with distributive justice. How health care is delivered is a matter of justice. Who gets health care, how much they get, and at what cost are all questions of justice. In an ideal world, a person needing health care should be able to go to a health care facility and receive the appropriate level of services required to diagnose, treat, and/or manage his or her condition, without regard for ability to pay. Good health is vital to a society's survival, but in the United States there is a philosophical debate as to whether health care is a basic right or a privilege. If it is a basic right, what level of health care should be available? If it is a privilege, how does one acquire the privilege?

THE U.S. HEALTH CARE SYSTEM

In the United States, the health care system is very complex. This section provides a rather simplified overview of the health care system. Although there are extensive regulations regarding the delivery of health care in hospitals, nursing homes, ambulatory facilities, and patient homes and through emergency medical services, health care is treated as a commodity, something available for purchase. One accesses most services through a professional health care provider, such as a physician, nurse practitioner, nurse, or paramedic. Legislation such as the Hill–Burton Act of 1946 (U.S. Department of Health and Human Services, 2000) and the Emergency Medical Treatment and Active Labor Act of 1985 (Social Security Administration, 2003) ensures that patients cannot be turned away from a health care facility based on inability to pay. They must be treated or stabilized before transfer to another facility, such as a county facility for the indigent.

Since the Roosevelt administration in the 1940s, there have been changes in the health care delivery system of the United States and in the values underpinning the system. Most Americans did not have health insurance in the 1940s, and to attract and retain workers, companies offered health insurance as a job benefit when it was difficult for them to provide higher salaries (Califano, 1986). The company bore the expense and the employee and dependents were covered for hospitalizations and tests. Today, there are usually higher deductibles and often more restrictions on what is covered. As medical advances occurred, the cost of health care rose and health insurance costs consumed an increasing percentage of company expenditures. Medical research and training of the health care workforce were often subsidized by cost shifting in hospitals, that is, teaching and research hospitals charged more for tests or drugs than did community hospitals, driving costs higher still.

Because most health insurance coverage was tied to employment, products and services produced in the United States were more expensive, and companies complained of the inability to compete in a global marketplace. Efforts such as wage and price freezes failed to curb the escalating costs. Medical knowledge was increasing exponentially, and certain cultural and sociopolitical movements, such as the women's movement and the consumer movement, contributed to consumer expectations of the highest quality health care.

Employees feared that they would not be able to get health insurance if they left their current job because insurance companies had a "preexisting condition" exclusion clause. The Consolidated Omnibus Budget Reconciliation Act (COBRA) of 1986 mandated that employers had to offer continued insurance coverage for up to 18 months to employees who left or were discharged. The Health Insurance Portability and Accountability Act (HIPAA) of 1996 had provisions for extending employer insurance to employees who left their jobs, although it made it possible for an employer to raise premiums to a level that was prohibitive for the employee, thereby making insurance coverage unattainable.

Health Maintenance Organizations

One attempt at containing costs was the managed care movement. The best-known type of managed care organization is the health maintenance organization (HMO). HMOs started in California with the Kaiser Permanente Company in the 1930s (Hendricks, 1993). This type of health insurance was intended to cover the costs of hospitalizations, tests, physician bills, and durable medical equipment needs. Health check-ups, office visits, outpatient procedures, and prescriptions were less expensive, and the cost was borne by the patient. For example, in the 1970s, under a traditional health insurance plan, when a couple in their 40s wanted a thorough yearly physical examination, they would contact their physician, who arranged for a week-long hospitalization. During the hospitalization, the couple would undergo tests that would not be covered if done on an outpatient basis. The insurance would pay for the hospitalization, tests, and any physicians' bill, such as radiology for reading X-rays or anesthesiology for anesthesia during tests. This approach, the fee-for-service approach, gave the couple a choice of which physician they saw and what tests they wanted. The hospitalization was more of a convenience for them.

Fast forward to the 1990s. In an HMO, the couple would select a primary care physician from a list of physicians in the HMO. They would schedule an appointment for their yearly examination and see the physician in the office. At that appointment, if there were any medically indicated tests, the physician would authorize them, usually to be done on an outpatient basis. Hospitalization would only occur if there was an acute illness or if a test, such as a cardiac catheterization, required it. Even then, the HMO might only pay for a 23-hour admission, in which the patient would be monitored after the test and discharged in less than 24 hours. Another person in the HMO would have the responsibility of reviewing the use of health care resources and could deny authorization of payment for hospitalizations, procedures, equipment, or referrals not covered by the plan or medically necessary. This reviewer might or might not be a health care professional and would never examine the patient.

The HMO system was intended to contain costs by instituting a level for approval by another party other than the primary care provider. Instead of health care on demand, the patient must have had a medical necessity attested to by an HMO-employed physician and a utilization reviewer. However, the HMOs had many problems. Early in the HMO experiment, it was found that in some HMOs, increased physician income was tied to decreased use of HMO resources (Graig, 1999). It was also revealed that in some HMOs, physicians were prohibited from recommending services not included in the HMO coverage; this was called the "gag" clause. Other difficulties with HMOs were "drive-through" deliveries, in which women were discharged within 24 hours of giving birth, even though in some instances their infants had to remain hospitalized for 48 hours because of the need for a state-mandated newborn screening blood test. There seemed to be daily news stories of someone being denied treatment by their HMO—someone losing their leg because they were discharged from the hospital prematurely (*Wickline v. California*, 1986) or someone dying because they were denied recommended treatment (*McClellan v. Health Maintenance Organization of Pennsylvania*, 1992). The backlash against HMOs resulted in legislation outlawing gag clauses or requiring HMOs to inform patients if physician income was tied to resource utilization (Graig, 1999). However, by the mid-1980s, HMOs were becoming the primary method for health care coverage for most Americans. Patients were being asked to pay increasing portions of the monthly premium previously paid entirely by their employer, and co-pays and deductibles were increased.

Because the HMO was tied to the employee's benefits, the federal benefits law known as ERISA (Employee Retirement Income Security Act of 1974) permitted an HMO to "avoid all state law liability, including liability for medical malpractice, when engaging in actions that constitute benefits determination rather than clinical" determinations (Moskowitz, 1998, p. 373). Essentially patients could not sue their HMO for damages caused by denial of treatment. Although HMO administrators could deny authorization for treatment based on how they determined benefits, they maintained that it was the physician who was responsible for the medical decision-making. So when patients could not pay for treatment that the HMO denied, the administrators were, in effect, making a medical decision. Courts have recently allowed patients to sue HMOs (Forster, 2000).

Preferred Provider Organizations

A hybrid of the fee-for-service and HMO is the preferred provider organization (PPO). Companies negotiate with a number of hospitals, physicians, and other providers who discount their services to the companies' employees. Employees are offered a panel of providers and hospitals from which to choose. Going to a hospital or provider outside the PPO panel results in higher costs to the employee.

Medicare/Medicaid

People not getting health insurance through an employer have the option of self-pay or a government program, Medicare or Medicaid. For Medicare, one has to be older than 65, on hemodialysis, blind, or otherwise disabled. Medicaid, operated by the states, has varying eligibility requirements, but was intended for women and children and people with disabilities or chronic medical conditions. To be eligible, one has to be indigent, or to "spend down" to the level of poverty. The spend-down amount is the amount that a patient's monthly income exceeds the Medicaid allowance for living expenses. For example, let's say that a patient's medical expenses are $5000/month. If a patient's household income is $3000/month and to be eligible for Medicaid the household income for a family of four cannot be more than $1533/month, he must spend $1467/month (his spend-down amount) on medical expenses before Medicaid will pay any medical expenses.

COBRA (1986) and HIPAA (1996) have had an impact on making health care more accessible to more people, but there is still a long way to go.

ACCESS TO CARE

The issues in allocation of health care resources often revolve around payment. In most other developed countries, the government (a single-payer program), a public–private partnership, or both cover health care. Having a single-payer program reduces administrative costs. The citizens of these countries are taxed at a higher level than citizens in the United States. In World Health Organization rankings of overall health system performance, the United States is ranked 37 of 54 industrialized nations (191 nations total), yet the United States spends more for health care than any other country. The U.S. spends 1.8 times per capita more than Japan and up to 2.8 times per capita more than Germany (Le Bow, 2002, pp. 145–149). Around 40 million people, or 15% of the U.S. population, do not have health insurance, and another 50 million are underinsured or do not have adequate health care insurance coverage to meet their needs (Le Bow, 2002, pp. 17–18).

Health care financing is not the only issue. Disparities in health care also occur based on race, ethnicity, and age (American Nurses Association [ANA], 1998). Certain groups are more vulnerable than others, such as African Americans, Latinos, immigrants, children, the elderly, and people with mental illness, all of whom can face many barriers to care. People with chronic illnesses, such as AIDS, and people with disabilities where lack of transportation presents real physical barriers have difficulty accessing health care services (Friedman, 1994). Nurses can assist in reducing disparities by practicing culturally competent nursing, which will attract formerly disenfranchised patients, thereby making health care accessible, and implementing or participating in systematic interventions that include involvement of stakeholders in the community, again improving accessibility (Cooper, Hill, & Powe, 2002).

MANAGED CARE

As stated, the purpose of managed care organizations such as HMOs is to control health care costs by scrutinizing expenditures. Not only is having a medical necessity critical to obtaining services, but a review of the services by another party is also usually required. The process is intended to ensure that no unnecessary services are provided. The problem occurs when it becomes cumbersome to get the necessary services approved in a timely fashion.

Managed care involves planning for services for a specific pool of "covered lives." An employer negotiates with the managed care organization (MCO) to deliver services at an agreed-on price. The employer will pay a specific amount per employee, and the employee will also pay a monthly premium and an additional amount if dependents are also covered under the same plan. The employee is also expected to meet a yearly deductible in out-of-pocket expenditures and may have co-pays (additional out-of-pocket expenditures) when getting prescriptions filled or utilizing other services. The premiums and the investments made by the company with premium funds form the basis for paying for the following: the health care costs of the covered lives, any out-of-network referrals and treatment, administrative costs, other business expenses such as capital expenditures and advertising, and profits to shareholders.

There are various types of MCOs (a full discussion of which—not-for-profit companies, tax benefits to companies, and for-profit companies—is beyond the scope of this book). The for-profit MCOs have an obligation to make money for their shareholders; however, there is a concern that they might do this by reducing utilization, and the obligation to their shareholders might conflict with their obligation to provide health care services to their enrollees. Even in not-for-profit MCOs there is concern that there are incentives and disincentives to reduce utilization. Instead of thinking about an individual patient and his or her needs, an MCO considers the needs of the entire pool of enrollees and strives to hold utilization to a minimum.

Health Promotion/Maintenance Programs

The MCO may also promote programs that improve or maintain health, such as smoking cessation, weight reduction, stress management, seat belt use, helmet use, domestic violence screening, use of child car seats, mammography, and immunizations for flu, pneumonia, hepatitis B, and the usual childhood diseases. Although this may appear to be humanitarian in purpose, it is actually also a cost containment method. A healthier pool of enrollees decreases use of expensive medical procedures and treatments. Despite the motivation for these programs, this trend is beneficial to the enrollee.

Use of Clinical Pathways by Managed Care Organizations

The use of clinical pathways to determine hospital lengths of stay is becoming more widespread in MCOs. According to the patient's diagnosis, the MCO will pay a fixed amount for the hospitalization. (This was fashioned after the federal government program of DRGs, or diagnosis-related groups.) The patient is expected to have a predictable course, so the anticipated treatments and days of hospitalization can be reimbursed at a fixed amount. If the patient encounters problems and the hospitalization is extended, the MCO does not pay any additional amount unless the patient's diagnosis changes.

For example, if a patient is hospitalized for an appendectomy and recovers more slowly than expected, the hospital is not reimbursed by the MCO for the additional length of stay. The hospital's utilization reviewer might contact the physician to see whether the patient could be discharged home at the expected time, according to the clinical pathway for appendectomy. The ethical concern is that the patient may be discharged prematurely and the family expected to provide postoperative care in the patient's home. The principle of nonmaleficence, or preventing harm, is central. The family may be anxious and willing to have the patient home, but is it in the patient's best interests to be discharged at this point? Hospitalization is intended so that the patient can receive vigilant monitoring through nursing care. It may be possible to arrange home health nursing, even 24-hour nursing, if needed, which costs less than hospitalization. Ideally, patient needs should dictate the provision of services, but clinical judgment and fiscal responsibility are closely linked and can influence physician judgment.

Prescribing in a Managed Care Organization

Medical justification can also pose potential conflicts for physicians in their prescribing practices. One example is the use of generic medications in MCO formularies. Generic drugs are less expensive than name brands and are as effective in most cases. However, in some cases, generics are different and do not provide the desired effect. For example, some patients do not get seizure control when they take carbamazepine versus Tegretol. According to LegalMedsOnline.com, as of April 1, 2005, generic carbamazepine cost approximately 16¢ per tablet and nongeneric Tegretol cost approximately 37¢ per tablet. The primary care physician must document that generic substitution is not acceptable for the MCO to authorize payment above the generic medication cost.

Prescription drug prices have been rising more rapidly than any other health care cost. Box 9-1 explains some of the factors in the rising costs of prescriptions.

Financial Incentives/Disincentives

Another issue with HMOs is the use of financial incentives and disincentives as a method of cost containment. Some MCOs provide a bonus to their physicians at year's end if resource use is lower than expected, thereby freeing up funds. This places physicians in the position of considering their personal financial gain at the cost of underprescribing services for their patients. The conflict of interest is apparent. For physicians who resist the influence of financial incentives on their clinical decision-making, there are disincentives, such as being threatened with exclusion from the MCO or MCO network if they are seen as overutilizing resources. In for-profit MCO's, there have been reports of excessive salaries and benefits packages for top administrators at the same time their organization was denying treatment for bone marrow transplantation

---

BOX 9-1

Prescription Drug Prices

Prescription drug prices have been rising more rapidly than any other health care cost (Graig, 1999). U.S. patent laws allow pharmaceutical companies to slightly alter a medication and repatent it to prevent generic drugs from entering the market. In addition, direct marketing to the consumer via television and print ads increases demand for brand-name products even when generic or older, much less expensive medications are as effective. More of the health care dollar will be spent on medications as the world's population ages. Examination of the responsible allocation of resources is forcing U.S. politicians to address the marketplace mentality of prescription drug pricing.

or other "expensive" treatments. From a business standpoint, the MCO administrators face a conflict between obligations to stockholders and obligations to patients.

What to Do?

Possible Solutions at the Government Level

The ranks of the uninsured and underinsured are growing, and there does not seem to be a consensus endorsing any particular plan for health care reform. Many options are being explored to combat the problem. The state of Oregon, for example, developed a program for covering all its citizens through employer-based insurance and a redesigned Medicaid program (Hadorn, 1991). For the people insured through their Medicaid program, a prioritized list of treatments was developed and a cut-off point determined. Treatments falling below the cut-off point were not funded. Critics of the plan declared it to be rationing of health care (Kitzhaber, 2003). Although some authors declare the Oregon Health Plan to be a success (Floyd, 2003), others believe its success, as measured by a reduction in the percentage of uninsured individuals (17% in 1992 to 11% in 1997), can be attributed to raising revenue through a cigarette tax and moving Medicaid recipients to managed care (Oberlander, Marmor, & Jacobs, 2001, p. 6). These authors identify the true success of the plan to increasing public awareness and garnering support for raising taxes.

The present system in the United States becomes a rationing system when the uninsured or underinsured cannot get treatment. In effect, health care is rationed to those who can afford it. One of the best-known solutions being explored is universal coverage. Universal coverage would provide a basic level of health care to all and a method of deciding how other health care resources should be allocated. Many other countries, such as the United Kingdom and Canada, have universal coverage. The following are only a few of the options being explored—a whole book could easily be devoted to the topic of solutions to this growing problem.

Possible Solutions at the Personal Level

Complementary and Alternative Medicine

A popular solution to combat the rising costs of health care is to utilize complementary and alternative medicine (CAM) at the patient's cost instead of traditional medicine. With limited accessibility to traditional, or allopathic, medicine, the use of CAM therapies is increasing (Parkman, 2002). Many of these therapies are more affordable for the consumer than traditional health care and there are data—both evidence based and anecdotal—of success with CAM therapies. There is an interest in integrating allopathic medicine and CAM. Third-party payers are including coverage for treatments such as chiropractic adjustments, acupuncture, acupressure, hypnotherapy, biofeedback, reflexology, and massage therapy. The National Institute of Health has established the National Center for Complementary and Alternative Medicine to study the efficacy of such treatments.

Informal Caregiving

Another trend caused by reduced accessibility to health care is informal caregiving by family or friends. With barriers to inpatient hospitalization and decreased hospital stays, families are expected to provide care to a sick or disabled relative. Even with home health nursing, family members have to assume more direct care responsibilities. There are certain advantages to receiving care at home—the familiar environment, the "control" one has in one's own home, and the reduced possibility of medical error or nosocomial infection. However, the dynamics of the family relationships change and there is a risk of caregiver burden. In additional, the family member may learn specific caregiving tasks, but lack the depth of knowledge for assessment and interpretation of findings that the professional caregiver would have. The American Nurses Association (ANA, 1995a) position statement on informal caregiving calls for recognition of informal caregiving as a "precious health care resource" and seeks financial, emotional, and respite support for caregivers (p. 1).

NURSES' ROLE IN MACRO ALLOCATION

Political Action

There are a number of ways that nurses can influence resource allocation. On the level of macro allocation, nurses can affect policy through their involvement with their professional associations. For example, the authors of this book provided testimony to Illinois legislators regarding a proposed ban on cloning. They were instrumental in drafting the state association's position statement that rejected a ban but favored regulation (Illinois Nurses Association Council on Ethics and Human Rights, 1999). Other nurses in the association were integrally involved in decisions regarding allocation of the tobacco settlement monies that came to each state. At community levels, elected and/or appointed health officials make allocation decisions regarding support of certain programs, such as a free clinic for uninsured patients, immunization programs, injury prevention programs, and obesity prevention and body image programs aimed at teens. Nurses can influence the allocation decisions by becoming involved in the decision-making process. Presenting testimony, submitting data, and informing the decision-makers, such as board of health members and city, county, and state politicians, can affect allocation of health resources.

Nurses can also influence allocation decisions regarding hospital beds, trauma centers, specialty programs (such as transplant programs), and other health facilities. For example, if a facility requires a certificate of need to be approved by government bodies, information will be gathered and public hearings held to demonstrate the need for the proposed facility, such as an ambulatory facility or addition to a hospital. Nurses, like other concerned citizens, can influence the process by testifying, as a private citizen or as a representative of their professional organization, in support of or opposition to a proposed facility. Nursing has a long and proud history in advocacy through political activism for a just health care system. Rains and Barton-Kriese (2001) conducted a study of nursing students and political science students to identify how they acquired the skills and desire to become politically active. In their qualitative study, they interviewed 17 students (9 nursing, 8 political science) and concluded, "nursing seemed grounded in application and service, demonstrating by involvement that they could 'walk the walk'. Political science involvement originated in theory, and resulted in more articulate discourse on the subject; they could 'talk the talk'" (p. 219). The authors recommend that nurse educators and other practicing nurses mentor nursing students in political activism. Rodgers (2001) proposed service learning as an alternative to traditional nursing courses in public health. Service learning can teach the student about activism, community engagement, and allocation of resources on a first-hand basis. Students perform a needs assessment through connecting to citizens of a specific community, learning their health needs and priorities, and planning projects within the limits of the available and attainable resources.

The overarching ethical principle in allocation decisions is justice. Deciding what is just is a political process that must be informed by the public, health care professionals, and politicians. In a utilitarian model of distributive justice, there may be more emphasis on health promotion and disease prevention and less emphasis on expensive technologies with low or unknown efficacy. For example, a county may support an immunization program for children but may decide not to pay for bone marrow transplant for neuroblastoma. Utility is maximized in terms of having many children immunized and reducing the morbidity and mortality from childhood diseases. However, it could be perceived that the immunization program is being funded by denying funding for bone marrow transplants for children with neuroblastoma. In the utilitarian equation, a greater good for a greater number (maximum happiness) is achieved (through the immunization program) at the cost of sacrificing the few (children with neuroblastoma).

An egalitarian approach would be to strive to provide equal health care. However, what is "equal," will equal be adequate, and does equal mean equal access or equal amount of services? An example of an egalitarian allocation is a flu inoculation program. When the allotment of flu shots is great, people who ask for the flu shot will likely get one, and it is distributed on a first-come, first-served basis. When the allotment is low, flu shots may be reserved for those at greatest risk of complications from the flu, like the elderly or chronically ill, but again, that group would get flu shots on a first-come, first-serve basis. For this same example, the utilitarian approach might be to offer the flu shot to people whose productivity would be adversely affected by the flu (healthy employed people) or to those whose illness would require an inordinate amount of resources (people with chronic illness or disability).

NURSES' ROLE IN MICRO ALLOCATION

Nurses may not be directly involved in issues of macro allocation, except as a concerned citizen or as an activist. However, nurses are actively involved in decisions on micro allocation. The principle of justice influences how nurses allocate their time. Nurses assess the needs of their patients and prioritize their time accordingly. A number of factors can influence how they allocate their time.

Staffing

Over the last few decades, there have been periods of nursing shortage and nursing abundance. With the evolution of managed care, the major fixed cost in health care facilities has been labor. When facilities could not increase revenue, an expenditure they chose to decrease was professional nursing staff. Unlicensed assistive personnel (UAP) were hired to perform multiple tasks from mopping the floors to distributing meal trays to taking blood pressures. Nurses were expected to delegate appropriate tasks and supervise the UAP, thereby freeing the professional nurse's time to perform duties that the UAP could not. Nurses, especially those who were socialized into primary nursing versus functional or team nursing, had difficulty adjusting to the new model. Those of us educated in the 1970s viewed the change as déjà vu. Although the UAP model was reminiscent of the functional nursing model of the 1960s and 1970s, the major difference was the acuity level of patients and the increased knowledge and scope of practice of the professional nurse. The UAP model seemed like a step backward for nursing, and it seemed like patients were placed at risk of harm. Unfamiliar with the skills required for delegation, nurses accustomed to the primary care nursing model experienced the ethical distress of not being able to deliver the kind of nursing care they believed was holistic and ethically appropriate. Nurse administrators encouraged their nursing staff to "work smarter, not harder." Nevertheless, nurses who were accustomed to primary care mourned the loss of this model of nursing care delivery.

Even in well-staffed units, there are times of short staffing. Nurses miss work because of illness, or there is reduced staffing during low census or vacation times. When patient care is jeopardized, staffing is a micro allocation issue. Nurses pitch in and work overtime, or part-time employees pick up extra shifts to deal with an increase in census or acuity. When low staffing levels become chronic, either because of a shortage of nurses, unfilled nursing positions, or increased patient acuity or a combination of these, decisions have to be made to decrease the potential for harm to patients. Closing units, putting trauma centers on bypass, and transferring patients to other units are options for resolving short staffing. "Floating," having a nurse from one unit work on a different unit, has been a common solution. With the increased specialization areas of nursing, however, it may not be appropriate to float a nurse from a pediatric unit to an adult cardiac care unit. Within departments, nurses form float pools, where they intentionally rotate between various units in their departments. They remain familiar with the unit practices and patient populations and feel competent in delivering nursing care on these units. In the absence of that type of program, nurses may be reluctant to float and may conscientiously refuse an assignment on an unfamiliar unit. Before the refusal, however, the nurse negotiates with nursing management to work out an equitable arrangement that meets patients' needs and does not compromise the nurse's integrity (ANA, 1995b).

Case Study 9-1

Mrs. Lam, a staff nurse on the geriatric rehabilitation unit, comments to her nurse manager that it seems as though more patients are experiencing falls than in the past. Her nurse manager shares the observation at a staff meeting. The nurses agree with Mrs. Lam's observation about the increase in falls, but explain that their workloads are too heavy for them to monitor their patients or assist them when they are ambulating or transferring. The following day, the nurse manager asks the staff to volunteer to retrospectively review the charts of the last 6 months to determine whether there actually has been an increase in falls. The staff nurses are concerned that they cannot give patient care and do a chart review on the same shift, and because many of them have been working overtime to cover short staffing, they do not want to spend their time off in doing chart reviews. They inform the nurse manager that although they would like to have the information, they do not believe each shift is adequately staffed to allow them to review charts and they will not do chart reviews on noncompensated time. The nurse manager cannot authorize overtime pay for chart review. What should the nurse manager do? What responsibility does the staff have to investigate this clinical issue?

The nurse manager speaks with a nursing instructor who supervises students on her unit and suggests as a "management in action" project that the students could perform a chart review. The nurse manager meets with the student group to discuss the issue of falls and information from the chart that may be pertinent. In 4 weeks, the students reviewed all of the charts and presented the raw data to the nurse manager. The nurse manager returned to her staff and asked them to review the data for any connections to increased falls. Mrs. Lam observed that the falls were occurring in patients of a particular physician in a specialty program. These patients were receiving medications that in combination were likely causing orthostatic hypotension (a rapid drop in blood pressure with position change), and, in turn, were causing patients to faint upon rising. The nurse manager presented the data to the physician and pharmacist on the unit, and they developed a plan to monitor patient's responses to the medication. The nurse manager also presented the data to nursing administration as evidence that increased staffing is needed to monitor patients and assist them in ambulation and transferring.

The staff nurses faced a dilemma in wanting the data regarding increased falls, yet feeling they could not allocate any direct patient care time to the chart review. The nurse manager had limited resources to get the data, so she asked for volunteers, but the already-overworked staff would not volunteer. The students contributed to investigating and solving a clinical problem, learned continuous quality improvement techniques, and provided a valuable service to the staff as reciprocity for their preceptorship during the students' clinical rotation.

Appropriate Level of Care

Another micro allocation issue for nurses is the determination of the appropriate level of care for a patient. There are three levels of care: tertiary, or the most technologically complex and sophisticated; secondary, which may also be technologically complex but is aimed at reducing morbidity or restoring health in those with a chronic condition or disability; and primary, which is focused on prevention and health promotion.

Tertiary Level of Care

Hospitals providing tertiary care provide the most sophisticated technological medical and nursing care. Trauma centers, specialty intensive care units, transplants centers, centers of excellence for various conditions, such as women's health or Alzheimer disease, are found in tertiary care centers. The placements of these centers are macro allocation issues, but in this section, the focus will be on micro allocation issues, which occur within the unit or at the bedside and can cause ethical distress in the health care professionals involved.

Trauma Centers

In trauma centers, patients without the ability to pay must be treated or at least stabilized before they are transferred. To deny treatment based on ability to pay would violate the Emergency Medical Treatment and Active Labor Act (EMTALA), also known as the antidumping act (Social Security Administration, 2003). Emergency departments

(EDs) are not adequately reimbursed, yet they are mandated to treat. Nurses experience frustration when patients seek their primary care in the ED. The patients receive fragmented and very expensive care and the limited resources of the ED are expended for nonemergency cases. Some hospitals have responded by instituting "fast track" or "urgent care" programs in the ED so patients for whom the ED is the only portal into the health care system can receive care, patient education, and perhaps social services.

Intensive Care Units

Treatment decisions in intensive care units (ICUs) can also pose ethical conflicts for nurses. In practice, admission to an ICU is sometimes limited to patients who are expected to benefit from such care. The judgment about the potential benefit creates ethical distress in some health care providers. Studies have described differences among physician, nurse, patient, and family estimation about the benefits of ICU treatment (Skowronski, 2001; Wu et al., 2002). There is not always agreement about the benefit of ICU admission, yet physicians usually have unilateral decision-making power. Whereas nurses sometimes question the appropriateness of the admission or disagree with a resuscitation plan, their major concerns are often their ability to provide adequate staffing and their lack of input into clinical decisions (Oberle & Hughes, 2001).

Most patients who die in ICUs have a terminal condition (Hammes & Rooney, 1998). These patients who die usually are acutely ill and require a level of care they cannot receive in another setting, so they end up in the ICU. Although ICU nurses want to see their patients receive the highest quality care, they may not always believe that the ICU is the appropriate place for them. The lack of a more appropriate place, such as an inpatient hospice, or of sufficient resources in the home leaves few options. One resolution might be to have dedicated hospice beds within or near the ICU so that patients can receive intensive care and prepare for their death. This would require allocation decisions at the unit or hospital level in which nurses should be involved. Another solution would be to have an intermediate care unit with a higher nurse–patient ratio than the regular units but a lower one than the intensive care units.

Quality of Life

Another micro allocation issue surrounds quality-of-life assessment by ICU staff. Certain situations provoke ethical questions. As mentioned, patients with terminal illnesses can pose ethical dilemmas. Some health care providers may believe that other patients without terminal illnesses are more appropriate candidates for intensive care. There is a trend in some institutions to develop "futility policies" to describe certain categories of patients who will not be admitted to intensive care (*Philadelphia Inquirer*, 2002). Patients with impaired cognition, such as those with advanced dementia, intellectual disabilities, or conditions referred to as a persistent vegetative state or a minimally conscious state, raise questions of futility. The intensive care treatment may extend the lives of these patients but may not alter their cognitive status. Advocates of the futility policy suggest that finite resources are better utilized in patients who can benefit. Opponents of the futility policy believe the policy discriminates against people with disabilities and that those patients merit intensive care regardless of their cognitive status. Rubin (1998) considered the determination of futility as a process of negotiation between patient/family and health care providers. Nurses from intensive care and nurses who are knowledgeable about these patient populations should participate in the development of ICU admission policies.

Transplantation

Many tertiary medical centers have transplant programs employing surgeons, nurses, social workers, administrators, and other health care professionals. Although organ procurement organizations (OPOs) maintain waiting lists for patients needing organs, the decision to place a patient on the waiting list is made by the members of the transplant program. Nurses are involved in the assessment of the patient, the patient's social situation, and the patient's willingness and ability to follow through with the postoperative regimen.

The factors involved in organ transplantation are myriad and complex. On an individual basis, nurses in the transplant programs should be nonjudgmental about patient's cause of organ failure, such as alcohol or intravenous drug use, yet in the decision about allocation of an extremely scarce resource, should continued substance abuse be considered? Should a patient's "fame" or social status permit them to be placed higher on the list? Another ethical issue for nurses in deciding who gets on the list is that the ability to continue to operate a transplant program depends on successful cases. Putting a very ill patient on the list could result in having a higher death rate than other centers, thereby jeopardizing the center's future.

Other ethical issues in transplantation are defining brain death (New Jersey permits a family to reject the diagnosis of brain death based on their religious beliefs), organ retrieval (different protocols exist for declaration of death prior to removing organs), and live-donor donation (fully informing the donor of the high-risk nature of the surgery). Nurses are involved in caring for the patient undergoing evaluation for brain death, caring for the body after brain death has been declared prior to organ retrieval, and caring for the well patient who is donating a kidney or portion of liver. They also participate in the informed consent process with the live donors and with family members. Moreover, it is the nurses who assist in explaining brain death to the family. Health care providers in the ICU caring for the patient who is brain dead should not be involved in asking for organ donation from the family. The family might interpret that as indicating that the health care providers do not have the patient's best interests in mind, so personnel from the OPO are usually contacted to be available to meet with the family at an appropriate time to discuss organ donation.

Secondary Level of Care

Nurses often have key roles in admission decisions regarding acute rehabilitation. Rehabilitation nurses evaluate patients in the acute care facility to determine their eligibility for admission to a rehabilitation facility. The process is not completely value-neutral. Patients' potential for rehabilitation, including their family support and their attitude, may be considered. The nurse, in consultation with other team members, makes a recommendation about the appropriateness of the admission. The same process occurs in long-term care, although in both cases, financial eligibility may be the deciding factor on whether a patient gets admitted. The ethical questions of who gets services and who decides permeate these decisions.

Primary Level of Care

An example of micro allocation in primary care is the inaccessibility of routine gynecological care to women with disabilities. Women in wheelchairs or women with intellectual disabilities pose a clinical challenge to health care providers who plan to perform a routine pelvic examination and Pap smear. It is common for these women not to be offered these types of examinations. Despite the Americans with Disabilities Act

(1991), there is a lack of facilities and lack of knowledgeable health care providers, which limit the accessibility of these routine-screening exams for women with disabilities. Nurses can facilitate screening by referring women to specialty clinics or learning how their clinic can accommodate patients who have special needs.

SUMMARY

Nurses should be aware of the ethical underpinnings of resource allocation decisions. In deciding where to work, the nurse can examine the mission of the institution or agency and discuss how the mission is operationalized. A mismatch of the nurse's values with the institution's values can result in ethical distress for the nurse.

With global concerns over terrorism and war, resource allocation will not get any easier. This can be seen from recent discussions over who should be candidates for smallpox vaccination. Nurses should strive for responsible stewardship of health care resources while advocating for services that meet their patients' needs. It is likely that health care reform will occur in incremental levels, so nurses should keep up to date on the changes and voice their concerns for adopting a just health care system.

CLINICAL EXERCISES

1. Within your assigned unit, identify any policies related to allocation of resources. Are there policies related to admission to the hospital or to your specific unit? Are there policies or guidelines regarding eligibility for admission to an intensive care unit? What is the rationale for the admission/eligibility criteria? Who makes the decision?
2. Think about one of the patients you are assigned to on this particular rotation. What are the resources the patient needs? How is "need" determined? Who decides?
3. Identify three ways you believe costs could be reduced in the area in which you are assigned. Will these reductions affect patient care, and if so, how will you ensure that quality is not adversely affected?
4. Identify guidelines for determining length of stay for the types of patients on the unit where you are assigned. Do you agree with the guidelines? If not, why not?
5. What is the cost of a 1-day stay at the local hospital, a long-term care facility, an elder day care center, and a child day care center? What is included in this cost?

Discussion Questions

1. Using a prescription website, such as LegalMedsOnline.com, calculate what your patients would be paying on a monthly basis for their routine medications through this program.

   - What is the difference between generic and brand name drugs? Ask your patients if they have prescription drug benefits. If so, do they know what they pay for their prescriptions?

- With your instructor's guidance, talk with your patients about how finances and insurance coverage influence their decisions (e.g., they may skip appointments or medications because of the financial cost).

2. Again with your instructor's approval and guidance, talk with your patients, if they are willing, about their insurance coverage.

   - Do they have a PPO, an HMO, Medicaid, Medicare, or no insurance?
   - What factors influenced their insurance choices?
   - What changes would your patient like in his or her current policy?

3. Investigate your college's student health insurance policy.

   - Is it an HMO or a PPO? Does it have a ceiling on the maximum payout? For example, some policies have a $1,000,000 lifetime limit, or $50,000/year maximum payout.
   - Does your policy cover organ transplantations?
   - Does it cover treatment for substance abuse? If so, is this coverage inpatient or outpatient?

4. Discuss with the charge nurse how decisions are made to limit admissions on the unit where you are assigned. How does staffing or patient acuity influence the decision? What other factors influence the decisions to admit or limit admission of patients?

5. Divide your clinical group into two parts: utilitarians and egalitarians. Make a pie chart showing how the "Ethical Insurance Company" benefits should be allocated based on each of these theoretical approaches. Justify and explain how the pie is divided. Items to be included are, but are not limited to, preventive care, acute care, rehabilitation, substance abuse rehabilitation, psychiatric care, and research.

6. List all of your living immediate family and prioritize how you would decide who gets flu shots if there were only enough for half of them. Justify your decisions.

Special Topic: *Using Research in Resource Allocation*

Evidence-Based Practice

In addition to clinical pathways, the use of evidence-based medicine and evidence-based practice are gaining in popularity. Their appeal is based on the belief that the quality of health care and thus health care outcomes can be improved by using scientifically supported health care interventions. The effectiveness of a given intervention is reported and the evidence is evaluated. The evidence can be a double-blind, randomized clinical trial, an open-label clinical trial, a case report, or a consensus panel statement. In nursing, there may be evidence that would support continuing a particular practice or evidence to the contrary. Much of nursing practice in the past has been based on tradition and has not been rigorously evaluated (Jennings & Loan, 2001). Justice in resource allocation, in terms of stewardship, would require that, when feasible, nursing interventions are supported by evidence that they are effective for their intended purposes. Stewardship is the wise and responsible use of resources. However, in times of nursing shortages, nurses may not be able to devote energies to collecting and presenting the evidence (Turrill, 2000). In the medical literature, there are examples of evidence-based guidelines that are not followed because of lack of awareness or the inability "to overcome the inertia of previous practice" (Hesdorffer, Ghajar, & Iacono, 2002). Responsible resource allocation would require evaluation of current practices in light of persuasive evidence.

Nursing education programs, especially those preparing advance practice nurses, have incorporated courses on evidence-based practice into their curriculums. For nurses to make informed decisions about adopting practices based on available evidence, they need to have details about the study (design, recruitment, etc.) and the skills to critique both quantitative and qualitative research. Courses as well as current textbooks can facilitate their preparation in judging evidence on which to base their practice (DiCenso, Guyatt, & Ciliska, 2005; Melnyk & Fineout-Overholt, 2005).

There is a cautionary note to include about outcomes research. The instruments that are developed to evaluate outcomes are used to justify interventions through demonstrating cost effectiveness. However, the purpose of the intervention may not be to improve the patient's score on some functional measure or to reduce costs of treatment, but to improve the patient's quality of life.

Outcomes Research

Rehabilitation outcomes research offers examples of measuring outcomes with the FIM, or Functional Independence Measure. A patient with tetraplegia would not be able to demonstrate improvement on the FIM instrument, which measures physical function and the need for assistance. Failure to show improvement on this scale could mean that an extension of the patient's hospital stay may be denied. Yet it is invaluable to that patient that he or she have the skills and technology to control the environment—a longer hospital stay would enable this patient to acquire these skills and achieve a greater level of control of the environment. A third-party payer might not accept the rehabilitation physician's justification for additional hospital days when they will not improve the FIM score. The FIM is an inappropriate measure of the need for therapies in the case of a person with tetraplegia, but may be quite appropriate for someone who experienced a stroke (Kirschner, 2001).

Resources

American Health Research Institute. (2000). *Health care reform: Specifics, economics and legislative actions and philosophy of health care*. Washington, DC: Abbe Publishers Association.

American Nurses Association. Position statements are available at www.nursingworld.org

Deber, R. B. (2003). Health care reform: Lesson from Canada. *American Journal of Public Health, 93*(1), 20–24.

Geyman, J. P. (2002). Family practice in a failing health care system: New opportunities to advocate for system reform. *Journal of the American Board of Family Practice, 15*(5), 407–416.

Goodman, M. (1998). Ethical issues in health care rationing. *Nursing Management, 5*(4), 29–33.

Graig, L. A. (1999). *Health of nations: An international perspective on U. S. health care reform*. (3rd ed.). Washington, DC: Congressional Quarterly.

Holm, S. (1998). The second phase of priority setting: Goodbye to the simple solutions: The second phase of priority setting in health care. *BMJ, 317*, 1000–1002.

Mariner, W. K. (1995). Rationing health care and the need for credible scarcity: Why American can not say no. *American Journal of Public Health, 85*(10), 1439–1445.

Massachusetts Medical Society. (1989). A national health program for the United States: A physicians' proposal. *New England Journal of Medicine, 320*, 102–108 [full text available at www.pnhp.org/publications/a_national_health_program_for_the_united_states.php?].

Mok, E. (2001). Hong Kong healthcare system and its challenges. *Journal of Nursing Administration, 31*(11), 520–523.

Rodwin, V. G. (2003). The health care system under French National Health Insurance: Lessons for health reform in the United States. *American Journal of Public Health, 93(*1), 31–37 [full-text article available online].

Sarikonda-Woitas, C., & Robinson, J. H. (2002). Ethical health care policy: Nursing's voice in allocation. *Nursing Administration Quarterly, 26*(4), 72–80.

Strelioff, G. D. (2003). Canadian health care system. *Journal of the American Board of Family Practice, 16*(1), 87–88.

References

American Nurses Association. (1995a). *Position statement on informal caregiving*. Washington, DC: Author.

American Nurses Association. (1995b). *Position statement on the right to accept or reject an assignment*. Washington, DC: Author.

American Nurses Association. (1998). *Position statement on discrimination and racism in health care*. Washington, DC: Author.

Americans with Disabilities Act (1991). Retrieved November 11, 2005, from www.ada.gov

Califano, J. A. (1986). *America's health care revolution: Who lives? Who dies? Who pays?* New York: Random House.

Cooper, L. A., Hill, M. N., & Powe, N. R. (2002). Designing and evaluating interventions to eliminate racial and ethnic disparities in health care. *Journal of General Internal Medicine, 17*(6), 477–486.

DiCenso, A., Guyatt, G., & Ciliska, D. (2005). *Evidence-based nursing: A guide to clinical practice*. St. Louis, MO: Elsevier Mosby.

Emergency Medical Treatment and Active Labor Act. 42 U.S.C. 1395dd of the Consolidated Omnibus Budget Reconciliation Act of 1986.

Floyd, E. J. (2003). Healthcare reform through rationing. *Journal of Healthcare Management, 48*(4), 233–241.

Forster, H. P. (2000). Legal trends in bioethics: Managed care. *Journal of Clinical Ethics, 11*(4), 378.

Friedman, E. (1994). Money is not everything: Nonfinancial barrier to access. *Journal of the American Medical Association, 271*(19), 1535–1538.

Graig, L. A. (1999). *Health of nations* (3rd ed.). Washington, DC: Congressional Quarterly.

Hadorn, D. C. (1991). The Oregon priority-setting exercise: Quality of life and public policy. *Hastings Center Report, 21*(3), Suppl 11–16.

Hammes, B. J., & Rooney, B. L. (1998). Death and end-of-life planning in one Midwestern community. *Archives of Internal Medicine, 158*, 282–390.

Hendricks, R. (1993). *A model for national health care: The history of Kaiser Permanente*. New Brunswick, NJ: Rutgers University Press.

Hesdorffer, D. C., Ghajar, J., & Iacono, L. (2002). Predictors of compliance with the evidence-based guidelines for traumatic brain injury care: A survey of United States trauma centers. *Journal of Trauma, 52*(6), 1202–1209.

Jennings, B. M., & Loan, L. A. (2001). Misconceptions among nurses about evidence-based practice. *Journal of Nursing Scholarship, 33*(2), 121–127.

Kirschner, K. L. (2001). Ethical implications of outcomes research. *American Journal of Physical Medicine & Rehabilitation, 80*(5), 392–399.

Kitzhaber, J. (2003). The road to meaningful reform: A conversation with Oregon's John Kitzhaber. Interview by Jeff Goldsmith. *Health Affairs, 22*(1), 114–124.

Le Bow, B. (2002). *Health care meltdown: Confronting the myths and fixing our failing system*. Boise, ID: JRI Press.

*McClellan v. Health Maintenance Organization of Pennsylvania.*413 Pa. Super. 128, 604 A.2d 053 (1992).

Melnyk, B. M., & Fineout-Overholt, E. (2005). *Evidence-based practice in nursing & health care: A guide to best practice*. Philadelphia: Lippincott Williams & Wilkins.

Moskowitz, E. H. (1998). Clinical responsbility and legal liability in managed care. *Journal of the American Geriatrics Society, 46*(3), 373–377.

Oberlander, J., Marmor, T., & Jacobs, L. (2001). Rationing medical care: Rhetoric and reality in the Oregon Health Plan [Electronic version]. *Canadian Medical Association Journal, 164*(11), 1583–1587.

Oberle, K., & Hughes, D. (2001). Doctors' and nurses' perceptions of ethical problems in end-of-life decisions. *Journal of Advanced Nursing, 33*(6), 707–715.

Parkman, C. A. (2002). CAM therapies and nursing competency. *Journal for Nurses in Staff Development, 18*(2), 61–65.

Penn hospital to limit its care in futile case, severely brain-damaged patients will not get certain treatments, as a rule. (2002, November 4). Philadelphia Inquirer, p. A01.

Rains, J. W., & Barton-Kriese, P. (2001). Developing political competence: A comparative study across disciplines. *Public Health Nursing, 18*(4), 219–224.

Rodgers, M. W. (2001). Service learning: Resource allocation. *Nurse Educator, 26*(5), 244–247.

Rubin, S. B. (1998). *When doctors say no: The battleground of medical futility*. Bloomington, IN: Indiana University Press.

Skowronski, G. A. (2001). Bed rationing and allocation in the intensive care unit. *Current Opinion in Critical Care, 7*(6), 480–484.

Social Security Administration. (2003). Private examination and treatment for emergency medical conditions and women in labor. Retrieved May 15, 2005, from http://www.ssa.gov/OP_Home/ssact/title18/1867.htm

Turrill, S. (2000). A situational analysis: The potential to produce evidence-based nursing practice guidelines within a regional neonatal intensive care unit. *Journal of Nursing Management, 8*(6), 345–355.

U.S. Department of Health and Human Services, Office for Civil Rights. (2000). Your rights under the community service assurance provision of the Hill–Burton Act. Retrieved May 15, 2005, from http://www.os.dhhs.gov/ocr/hburton.html

Wickline v. California. 183 Cal App. 3d 1065, 228 Cal Rptr. 661, review granted, 231 Cal Rptr. 560, 727 P.2d 753 (1986).

Wu, A. W., Young, Y., Dawson, N. V., Brant, L., Galanos, A. N., Broste, S., et al. (2002). Estimates of future physical functioning by seriously ill hospitalized patients, their families, and their physicians. *Journal of the American Geriatrics Society, 50*(2), 230–237 (2002).

CHAPTER 10

Research Ethics

Objectives

At the end of this chapter, the student should be able to:

1. Describe the tenets of the Nuremberg Code and other applicable codes covering human subject research.
2. Identify the ethical themes of advocacy, confidentiality, truth-telling, and allocation of resources in the conduct of research.
3. Identify the ethical issues in conducting research with human subjects.
4. Describe the elements of informed consent for participation in research.
5. Determine the adequacy of protection of human subjects in proposed research studies.

KEY WORDS

- Assent
- Clinical equipoise
- Clinical trials
- Human subject research
- Informed consent
- Institutional review board (IRB)
- Nontherapeutic research
- Placebo
- Randomization
- Recruitment
- Research ethics committee (REC)
- Standard treatment
- Therapeutic misconception
- Therapeutic research

Research is the

---

class of activities designed to develop or contribute to generalizable knowledge. Generalizable knowledge consists of theories, principles, or relationships (or the accumulation of data on which they may be based) that can be corroborated by accepted scientific observation and inference. (Levine, 1986, p. 3)

In this chapter, only research with human subjects will be discussed.

Clinical trials, in which new interventions are compared to standard interventions, are common research designs and are considered the gold standard of medical research. The interventions tested in clinical trials can be devices, procedures, or pharmaceutical agents. After extensive laboratory testing and animal studies (if appropriate) have been done, the intervention is then tested on human subjects. Before the researchers conduct the study with human subjects, they must obtain approval from an oversight committee, known as an institutional review board (IRB) in the United States and a research ethics committee (REC) in Canada. The oversight committee reviews a detailed proposal in which the investigators describe the purpose of the study; the previous research; all procedures that will be done with human subjects; the potential risks and benefits; the measures that will be taken to minimize risks; any alternatives to participation; copies of the consent form, all instruments, recruitment scripts, and advertisements; and the sponsor's project booklet, if applicable. Many advances in health care have been achieved through human subject research.

Nurses participate in research on a variety of levels—as recruiters of subjects, as collectors of data, as research coordinators and data managers, and as principal investigators. Regardless of the nurse's role, the nurse, along with all other members of the research team, must conduct the study in an ethical manner. This chapter covers the ethical issues that pertain to human subject research and specifically illustrates application of the ethical themes in an activity other than clinical nursing.

ETHICAL THEMES

Advocacy

The principal investigator has a responsibility to fully inform a potential research subject about possible risks and benefits and to answer questions that enable the potential subject to decide whether to participate. In clinical research, the principal investigator may be the person's physician, or the physician may be the one who is recruiting patients from his or her practice to participate in a study. Although the patient should be told that there may be no direct benefit to him or her for participating in the study, patients often have a *therapeutic misconception* that their physician would not ask them to participate if the physician did not believe it would benefit them. For example, a study evaluating the effect of a drug to treat malignant melanoma, a frequently fatal form of skin cancer, is being conducted at a medical center. Dr. Douglas is an oncologist who is one of the investigators. After Dr. Douglas diagnoses a patient, Mr. Smith, with malignant melanoma, he describes the standard treatment and tells the patient that there is also an experimental treatment that may be better than, the same as, or worse than standard treatment in terms of curing the skin cancer. The doctor further explains what each treatment is and tells the patient that if he (the patient) decides to participate in the study, he must agree to be randomized (i.e., arbitrarily assigned) to either the standard treatment group or the experimental treatment group. A document that details all the procedures that the research subject would undergo, the possible risks and benefits, the alternatives to participation, and the costs if any is presented to the patient for him to review, discuss, and sign (if he is willing to participate). Patients sometimes interpret the physician's request that they consider participating in the study as a sign that the study has therapeutic value. This therapeutic misconception is difficult to dispel because patients are often hopeful that the experimental treatment is superior to the standard treatment, especially if the standard treatment does not offer a high rate of cure.

Advocacy for the patient ensures that he or she understands the information provided and knows whom to call for additional information. The patient who becomes a research subject should be informed that it will be determined by chance which treatment he or she will receive and that it is possible that if he or she is in the experimental group, he or she may not benefit and may, in fact, suffer harm. The principal investigator should fully explain to the patient the measures that will be taken to minimize potential harm, but it is also necessary to emphasize to the patient the possibility of unforeseen harm.

Truth-Telling

Patients who become subjects often do not understand that their involvement in research is not intended to benefit them. Clinical research, especially randomized trials, is intended to benefit future patients. There needs to be a sufficient, statistically calculated number of subjects in a clinical trial to determine the probability that one treatment is superior to another. At least one portion of the subjects in a clinical trial will not benefit, and to judge the efficacy of a treatment, it is necessary to compare the subjects who respond to treatment with those who do not. Because the investigators do not know which treatment is superior, it is ethical for them to enroll subjects in a study. *Clinical equipoise* is the state of not knowing which treatment is better. In the previous case of a malignant melanoma study, there is a standard treatment and there is an experimental treatment. It is not known by anyone which treatment is superior. When people with malignant melanoma enter the study with the hope of being helped, if clinical equipoise exists, it is still ethical to enroll those subjects as long as they understand that they will be randomized and that they may not benefit from being in the study. If the data show that one treatment is superior to the other or that one treatment causes unacceptable harm, then there is no longer clinical equipoise, and it is no longer ethical to enroll subjects in the study. The study must be designed in such a way that the fewest number of subjects are recruited to determine statistical significance and that the data are analyzed in a timely fashion so that the study is conducted only as long as is necessary to determine efficacy.

Confidentiality

All data collected in the research process should be kept confidential and, if possible, should be coded so that the risk of breaches in confidentiality is minimized. There are a number of phases of research in which confidentiality measures should be taken: recruitment, documentation of informed consent, data collection, data coding and analysis, and reporting of results.

The first phase is recruitment, the phase in which researchers attempt to enroll participants in their study. The Health Information Privacy and Accountability Act of 1996 (HIPAA) contains specific regulations regarding access of medical records for research. Researchers may post IRB-approved flyers that describe their study and the eligibility for inclusion in public areas like clinics, grocery stores, churches, and libraries. Anyone wanting further information is directed to call a phone number. The researchers may prepare a letter that physicians can mail to certain patients, but the researchers do not have the names of the patients, and they will only get them if the patients call the researchers and give them their names.

All data should be coded so that identifying information is minimized. This reduces the chance of subjects being identified if the data were to be seen by anyone else. Researchers take steps to protect their data by using codes rather than names, using passwords for computer access to protect their computer files, and by locking their records in file cabinets in locked offices.

Resource Allocation

In the early 1990s, a number of U.S. academic medical centers were temporarily barred from reviewing and approving research studies at their institutions. According to the Office for Protection from Research Risk, these institutions were not following the rules put forth and adopted by 17 federal agencies; therefore permission to perform research at a number of institutions was suspended. Following the suspension of research, each institution's IRB, the special committee charged with research review, approval, and oversight, was required to re-review every study that was active. At one institution alone, it was estimated that the cost of the second review was in the millions of dollars. The dramatic gesture of suspending active studies and mandating a second review of each study's protocol illustrated that human subject research must be conducted in an ethical manner, and that the federal agency that permitted local institutions to approve research would not tolerate sloppy record-keeping. At the institution of one of this book's authors (T.A.S.), there were more than 1300 studies to be reviewed, and three institutional review boards met 4 hours a day, 3 days a week to review and deliberate the research protocols. All the institutions whose research was suspended later invested millions of dollars in hiring and training staff and providing resources to improve research oversight.

HISTORY OF RESEARCH ETHICS

Past Abuses in Research

Abuses in research made clear the need for regulatory bodies to oversee human subject research. In 1891, a physician in Stockholm, Sweden, who wanted to test a smallpox vaccine on calves ended up using children from an orphanage because calves were too expensive to acquire and maintain. The head physician of the orphanage gave his consent for experimentation on the children (Lederer, 1995, p. 51). Eighteen years later, in a Philadelphia orphanage, more than 100 children younger than the age of

8 years were injected in their eyes with tuberculin, an extract of *Tuberculin bacillus* (Lederer, 1995). Even though the medical community had adopted certain strategies for the ethical conduct of research, such as requiring researchers to be responsible for the welfare of subjects, obtaining consent, and being willing to experiment on themselves first, abuses continued to occur. Reform finally came in response to a number of experiments done without consent.

The most egregious research abuses occurred during World War II in concentration camps. These experiments became known through the Nuremberg War Crime Trials after the war. Prisoners in concentration camps, especially Dachau in Germany and Auschwitz in Poland, were used for medical experimentation. The experiments fell into three categories: military purposes, racial hygiene purposes, and sadistic curiosity.

A number of experiments were carried out for military purposes. Hypothermia was studied by submerging prisoners in ice water and measuring their vital signs until they died. Other experiments involved exposing prisoners to conditions that simulated the high-altitude conditions that pilots would encounter if they had to eject from their planes. Potential antidotes to poisons were investigated by first having prisoners ingest the poisons, or by delivering them to prisoners via bullets or arrows. Prisoners were also forced to drink seawater. In addition, vaccines for communicable diseases were tested on prisoners, and limbs were amputated and transplanted.

Racial hygiene was promoted through a number of programs, such as the Aktion T-4 program, which was instituted to exterminate people with disabilities, especially infants and children (Burleigh, 1994). Techniques for inducing sterility in women and for castrating men as well as methods for promoting fertility in women were studied. The Nazi regime intended to expand throughout Eastern Europe and populate the conquered territory with desirable races only.

The third category of human experimentation was conducted by Joseph Mengele. He had an interest in twins research, and he often used one twin as the control for the experiment he performed on the other. One such experiment was to inject dye into one twin's eyes and observe whether the irises changed color. To conclude the experiment, both twins were killed and post-mortem examinations done.

The conduct of the physicians who performed these human experimentations was horrendous. Their total disregard for the humanity of their subjects was so shocking that one might suspect they were forced to commit these acts, but in many cases, they were not. Historians maintain that not only did these physicians willingly perform such experiments, but they enthusiastically volunteered to perform them (Annas & Grodin, 1992; Lifton, 1986; Proctor, 1988). Many people in these physicians' societies viewed these human subjects as having a "life unworthy of living" (Proctor, 1988).

One of the remaining ethical questions relating to the Nazi experiments is whether to use their data. Moe (1984) argued that if using the Nazi experiment data can benefit others, then the data should be used with the acknowledgment of the "incomprehensible horror that produced them" (p. 7). Others condemned the use of the data and declared those who used them were complicit (Gaylin, 1989; Spiro, 1985). The Doctors' Trial in 1947 culminated in seven researchers being executed and nine being given long prison sentences (Hornblum, 1998). The Nuremberg Code was developed as a guide for all medical researchers. However, despite the Nuremberg War Crime Trials and the development of the Nuremberg Code, exploitation of human subjects continued.

Beecher (1966) published an exposé of abuses in which he reviewed 50 studies and found 22 that were unethical. Among the 22 unethical studies, 2 were particularly infamous: the Jewish Chronic Disease Hospital cancer study and the Willowbrook State School hepatitis study. Elderly patients at the Jewish Chronic Disease Hospital were injected with live cancer cells to learn the rate of rejection of those cells. The patients, however, were not informed that they were part of such a study (Brody, 1998). At Willowbrook, a state school for significantly disabled children, admissions had been closed except to one isolated ward. For children to be admitted to this ward, their parents had to consent to have them be infected with hepatitis. If they declined, their child would not be admitted (Brody, 1998). These two studies occurred in the 1960s, nearly two decades after the Nuremberg Trials and the development of the Nuremberg Code.

Another study that gained a great deal of attention started in the 1930s and continued into the 1970s. This study was the Tuskegee syphilis experiment conducted by the U.S. Public Health Service (Jones, 1993). The study was intended to describe the clinical course of syphilis throughout a man's lifetime. Nearly 400 black sharecroppers with syphilis and 201 control subjects without the infection were followed from 1930 to 1972. They were required to submit to various tests, to give blood and cerebrospinal fluid samples, and to abstain from any treatment. Early treatments for syphilis produced significant toxicity, but in the 1940s, penicillin, which was not toxic, became available. A nurse who was a liaison between the U.S. Public Health Service and the men enrolled in the study prevented the infected patients from getting treatment. The subjects were told that they would be dropped from the study and would not receive the burial money (about $50) that had originally been offered to them as an incentive to recruit them into the study. The study became public when an Associated Press reporter broke it in the *Washington Star* on July 25, 1972 (Jones, 1993, p. 204). In response to the story, public outcry moved Congress to pass the National Research Act; this, in turn, resulted in the Belmont Report, issued by a committee that drafted regulations for protecting humans subjects in research.

Research on Prisoners

Another group that is vulnerable to unethical biomedical research is the prison population. Hornblum (1998) detailed years of research performed on prisoners in Holmesburg Prison in Pennsylvania and in other prisons throughout the country. For example, despite accusations of sloppy research and exploitation by one of his primary researchers, Dr. Albert M. Kligman's dermatology studies continued for 20 years. When Kligman first saw the prison, he is quoted as saying, "All I saw before me were acres of skin. It was like a farmer seeing a fertile field for the first time" (Hornblum, 1998, p. 37). Although the prison had an institutional review board, a committee responsible for research approval and oversight, it was ineffective in protecting the prisoners from such research abuses. Thick, jargon-filled research protocols were mailed to IRB members, IRB meetings were not held, and pharmaceutical companies sent checks for hundreds of dollars "in gratitude of" the IRB members' service. When Dow Chemical ended its relationship with Kligman because of the risks his research posed for prisoners and the prisoners started suing him, his research on prisoners finally came to an end (Hornblum, 1998, p. 243).

A by-product of prisoners' involvement in research came to light during congressional hearings in 1972. Prisoners who participated in biomedical research were able to earn much more money than the 15 to 25 cents/day other prisoners earned from regular prison work. Some prisoners who participated in research earned from

$10,000 to $20,000/year. This kind of money gave them extraordinary power over other inmates, and it contributed to the sexual abuse of weaker and poorer inmates. Inmates who resisted "volunteering" for research were gang-raped (Hornblum, 1998). As a result of this issue becoming public, special regulations now exist pertaining to research with prisoners.

Evolution of U.S. Regulations on Human Research Subjects

The lessons from the Nuremberg Code were lost on some U.S. researchers, who saw the code as "a good code for barbarians, but an unnecessary code for ordinary physician-scientists" (Hornblum, 1998, p. 298). This attitude symbolized an arrogance that valued career advancement over the safety of, and respect for, human subjects.

Notwithstanding the Nuremberg Code, it was not until 1974 that the United States enacted regulations protecting human subjects. The National Institutes of Health already had policies protecting human subjects who were involved in federally funded research, and those policies were raised to federal regulations in 1974 (U.S. Department of Health and Human Services, Office for Human Research Protections, 2004a, b).

The National Commission for the Protection of Human Subjects of Biomedical and Behavioral Research was established through the National Research Act. After 4 years of meetings, the commission issued its report, known as the Belmont Report, after the Belmont Conference Center at the Smithsonian Institute where the commission held its meetings. In response to this report, the Department of Health and Human Services and the Food and Drug Administration (FDA) revised their regulations and developed specific guidelines. These guidelines were codified as Title 45, Part 46, of the Code of Federal Regulations (45 CFR 46). They were adopted by 16 federal agencies over a period of years, and the FDA adopted a portion of them. One of the primary measures instituted to protect human subjects was the federal government's mandate for institutional review boards.

INSTITUTIONAL REVIEW BOARDS

The Belmont Report (1979) described the ethical conduct of human subject research and the creation and implementation of IRBs. The guiding principles for research are respect for persons, beneficence, and justice. The informed consent process demonstrates respect for persons. Potential subjects should receive information that they can understand and comprehend so that they can decide whether to volunteer. Beneficence is achieved by explaining to potential subjects the risk/benefit ratio, all possible harms, any possible benefits, and the eventual societal benefit of the research. The fair selection of subjects reflects justice. Inclusion of vulnerable groups, such as children or those who are economically disadvantaged, must be justified.

IRBs are guided by these principles. The reasoning behind having local IRBs rather than having one central IRB within the federal government is that a local committee represents the community's values. As dictated by 45 CFR 46, the IRB should be composed of people with the ability to critically review research projects and of nonscientific community members. The IRB must contain nonaffiliated members, that is, people who have no direct relationship with the IRB's institution. The members' terms should be staggered so that senior members can orient new members because there can be a steep learning curve if one has never served on an IRB before. Each member should become familiar with the Nuremberg Code.

The Belmont Report was adopted all or in part by 17 federal agencies and was published in the *Federal Register* in 1979. Known as The Common Rule, 45 CFR 46 lists all the requirements for conducting human subject research, including all the specifications for the composition and function of an institutional review board. Institutions, such as hospitals or universities, may apply for a federal-wide assurance (FWA), which means that if they follow certain procedures, their IRB is empowered by the federal government to review and approve human subject research. Agencies that do not have an FWA must apply for a single-project assurance (SPA), which means they must send every single proposal to the appropriate federal agency. Even if the research will be conducted outside of the United States, IRB approval must be obtained before the research can be started.

Most academic medical centers, hospitals, and other facilities where research is conducted either have one or more IRBs or contract with free-standing IRBs to have their proposals reviewed. The IRB should contain a mix of researchers with varied backgrounds so that it is likely that someone on the IRB has expertise relevant to any type of proposal. For example, institutions that have cancer research centers should have IRBs that contain researchers and clinicians with oncology expertise. IRBs also should include researchers with in-depth knowledge about research design, methodology, and statistics. The scientific merit of a proposal may have been evaluated prior to its coming to the IRB for disposition, but because ethical research requires good science, IRB members must be qualified to critique a study's design, as well as its actions, to protect the subjects' rights. As listed in the Nuremberg Code, the proposal should have scientific merit, and if information in the proposal is not persuasive, the proposal should be returned to the investigator for more information.

Some IRBs may invite experts to participate on an ad hoc basis to provide them with information to help them to understand a particular aspect of a proposal. Some IRBs ask the principle investigator to attend the meeting and present his or her proposal, after which he or she is excused before discussion and voting occurs.

At IRB meetings, which usually last 4 to 5 hours, members discuss and vote on a number of proposals, from 10 to 20, depending on the complexity of the proposed studies. Each member may also be assigned proposals for expedited review. Studies involving more than a minimal risk to human subjects and studies involving children, pregnant women, prisoners, or individuals who do not have decisional capacity must have full board review. The outcome of full board review is that the proposal is approved, is returned to the principal investigator with requests for modifications, or is not approved.

If a proposal poses no more than minimal risk or if it is a minor change to previously approved research within its approval period, then the proposal may not require full board review. Although the same standards are applied to research submitted for expedited review, most institutions only have 2 members review the proposal rather than having the full board of 10 to 15 people review it. In expedited reviews, IRB members can approve proposals or ask for them to be modified, but they cannot reject them. If the reviewers are inclined to reject a proposal, then the proposal is referred to the full board for review.

One other type of review can be done. If a researcher believes that his or her project is *not* human subject research, then an exemption can be requested. For example, a physician, nurse, and medical student agree to review case reports published over a 20-year period in a well-known journal. They will perform a content analysis of the case reports, looking for issues related to health disparity, and they will calculate correlations in how often they agree in identifying themes of the content of the case reports. The case reports are in the public domain, and no identifying information on any patient, living or dead, will be revealed in their review. If they have any question about whether this project could be construed as human subject research and therefore should come under IRB review, they should submit a brief proposal to the IRB asking for a determination of exemption. Sometimes this communication can occur through a phone call or e-mail.

INFORMED CONSENT

The cornerstone of human subject research is informed consent. Respect for persons is demonstrated through the consent process. There are eight elements in informed consent (Box 10-1). Getting the subject to sign the consent form, however, is not the final objective. The signature should only designate a point in the informed consent process where the subject understands and agrees to participate. Therefore, informing and clarifying should occur *throughout* the entire research process.

Because most biomedical research is done in the clinical context, it may be confusing for patients to distinguish research from treatment. For example, Mrs. Vaughn is admitted for surgery. A resident physician examines her, explains the procedure she will undergo, and asks her to sign the consent form for surgery. Later that evening, the resident returns and asks Mrs. Vaughn whether she agrees to participate in a study looking at an experimental adhesive that would be used on her skin instead of sutures. All the risks and benefits are explained, the option of not participating and

---

BOX 10-1

Elements of Informed Consent

1. The subject understands the purpose and duration of research and procedures to be done.

2. All reasonably foreseeable risks or discomforts are explained to the subject.

3. All reasonably expected benefits, if any, are explained.

4. All appropriate alternatives to participation are disclosed.

5. The measures taken to protect the subject's confidentiality are described.

6. If research poses more than minimal risk, any compensation and/or treatment to be given if injury should occur are explained.

7. Contact numbers for the principal investigator and the local IRB are given to the subject.

8. The consent form states that participation is VOLUNTARY; the subject may withdraw at any time, and the consequences of withdrawal, if any, are described.

Source: U.S. Department of Health and Human Services. (1998). Informed Consent Checklist—Basic and Additional Elements. Retrieved on November 16, 2005, from http://www.hhs.gov/ohrp/humansubjects/assurance/consentckls.htm

having sutures instead is described, and she is advised that if she participates, she will need to come back to her doctor's office 3 days after surgery instead of 1 week after surgery. She agrees to participate and signs the form. The resident made sure Mrs. Vaughn understood that she did not have to participate, that she would need to come back earlier than if she did not participate, and that the adhesive may or may not be better than traditional sutures. If she had not understood these differences, then she should not have been enrolled in the study. Therefore, assessing her understanding of the study is very important, and the resident should have asked, "Mrs. Vaughn, would you explain to me, in your own words, what you understand the purpose of the study to be? Would you tell me what the risks are? Would you tell me when you will be expected to come back after the surgery? What questions can I answer for you now?" The resident can then clarify any misunderstandings, and if Mrs. Vaughn is still willing, then she can be enrolled in the study.

Suppose Mrs. Vaughn cannot read, and the resident tells her a little bit about the study but leaves her with written information about the rest of the study's details. When he returns, he asks her if she has any questions, and she shakes her head "no." He presents the form, hands her a pen, and she signs at the "X." Did informed consent occur? Although the resident may not be aware that Mrs. Vaughn cannot read, he did not ask her questions to assess her understanding. If he had, he would have discovered that she had been unable to read the information he had left for her. As a result of the resident's poor assessment, because Mrs. Vaughn is a compliant patient, she signs the form that is thrust in front of her without really understanding what she is signing. The danger in her compliance is that she appears to have consented, but, in fact, she does not know what she signed or what she has agreed to do. Nurses advocate for people involved in research by ensuring their consent is truly "informed."

Informed consent is based on the premise that the people giving consent have the capacity to weigh the risks and benefits of what they are consenting to. The federal government recognizes several classes of subjects who may be vulnerable, for various reasons, and may not be able to give informed consent: women of childbearing age; fetuses and children; elderly people; people who are cognitively impaired; prisoners; hospitalized patients who are in comas or who are terminally ill; minorities; students; employees and healthy volunteers; and people in international settings. A few of these groups will be discussed briefly.

Women of Childbearing Age

Women of childbearing age are considered a special class because of their ability to become pregnant. Especially in cases where research involved drugs or devices that could possibly cause harm to developing fetuses, women traditionally were excluded from research unless they were sterile. The federal government realized that not all findings from research done on men could be extrapolated to women, so they mandated that women be included in clinical research or that justification be given as to why women should be excluded (National Institutes of Health, Office of Human Subjects Research, 1994). Evelyn et al. (2001) showed that, from 1995 to 1999, women were included in drug studies in numbers proportionate to their percentage in the population. It is common, however, for pharmaceutical companies to require women to undergo pregnancy testing prior to enrolling in a study, to use an effective method of contraception during the study, and to notify the sponsor immediately if pregnancy is suspected.

Pregnant Women

Special regulations for pregnant women were added to The Common Rule. These regulations provide guidelines for how IRBs should make decisions about research on pregnant women and for what consents are needed. If research is not aimed at pregnant women but pregnant women may be inadvertently included, IRBs should require investigators to provide statements in the consent forms regarding any possible risks currently unforeseeable to the fetuses. If there are foreseeable risks to the fetuses, the IRB may decide that pregnant women should be excluded from the study.

For research that focuses on the health of pregnant women, such as a study measuring a factor in women's urine that might indicate early signs of pregnancy-induced hypertension, the IRB would determine whether there are any risks to the fetuses. The study only involves collecting urine, so there is no more risk to the fetuses than the risks that the women already encounter in everyday life. The pregnant women can give consent to participate, if they wish, after being fully informed. However, if the study involved first taking a medication and then collecting urine, the risk to the fetuses could be greater than minimal risk, and then the IRBs would evaluate whether the study should be approved. If the study may benefit the woman's health, such as preventing pregnancy-induced hypertension, then the woman's consent is adequate, even though the fetus may be at risk. On balance, though, the fetus is at risk if pregnancy-induced hypertension occurs, so the IRBs would attempt to weigh the risks of exposure to hypertension versus the risks of exposure to the experimental drug.

If a study is focusing on some aspect of pregnancy but is not intended to benefit the health of the mothers, and if there is greater-than-minimal risk to the fetuses, then the IRBs must decide whether they will approve the study, and the study may need to be reviewed at the Department of Health and Human Services level. If approved, both the pregnant women's consent and the fathers' consent may be required. If the father is unknown or is not reasonably available, if the pregnancy resulted from rape, or if the purpose of the research is to protect or improve the health of the women, then the fathers' consents are not required. If the father is known but assumes no responsibility for the fetus, then his consent is not required, but the IRB may require documentation from the pregnant woman to that effect.

Fetuses

A fetus is "An unborn or unhatched vertebrate especially after attaining the basic structural plan of its kind, specifically, a developing human from usually three months after conception to birth" (U.S. National Library of Medicine, 2005). Regulations in this area apply up to birth, the time the fetus becomes an infant (at which point regulations regarding research with children apply). Any risks to the fetus must only be minimal or, if greater than minimal, must be justified in terms of potential benefit to the pregnant woman or fetus. There should be no other means by which the information could be obtained. Chapter 13 discusses fetal surgery-as-research. Closing a neural tube defect in the second trimester of pregnancy is an example of experimental fetal surgery. Chervenak and McCullough (2002) considered any surgery on a fetus as experimental. They maintained that even if a woman has decided to terminate her pregnancy, the risks for the fetus to be in a study must be weighed independent of the decision to terminate the pregnancy.

Fetal tissue transplantation, primarily used in studies evaluating its efficacy in treating Parkinson disease or juvenile diabetes, is the subject of an intense ethical debate. A moratorium on the use of fetal tissue for transplantation was imposed by the assistant secretary of health in 1988, but it was lifted by President Bill Clinton in 1993 on the anniversary of *Roe v. Wade*. There was concern that women might become pregnant for the purpose of aborting the fetus to have the fetal tissue available for transplantation. To eliminate that concern, the federal government prohibits directed donation of fetal tissue.

State statutes regarding the use of fetal tissue must be followed, and a number of states have bans on fetal tissue research. See the website of the National Conference of State Legislatures (2005) for current state law information. The use of fetal tissue is a hot political issue because it is entwined with the abortion debate. Discussions in the President's (George W. Bush) Council on Bioethics about the use of fetal tissue invoked earlier state supreme court decisions that categorized the fetus as a "special entity" or an "interim category" that is neither property nor a person (President's Council on Bioethics, 2004). Although federal regulations may permit fetal tissue research, states may have certain requirements that must be met.

The results of transplanting fetal tissue for the treatment of Parkinson disease have not been encouraging, and one study raised another ethical issue—sham surgery. Based on the argument that placebo-control trials are the gold standard for research, sham surgery was conducted in patients with Parkinson disease. A placebo is an inert or inactive substance; subjects who consent to be in placebo-control trials agree be randomly assigned so they are unaware of whether they are receiving an active or an inactive substance. In the sham surgery study, subjects agreed to be randomized into either an experimental group that would have fetal tissue transplanted into their brains or a control group that would have a hole burred into their skull to mimic the appearance of the same surgery undergone by the experimental group.

Initial findings of this study showed some improvement in subjects younger than 60 years of age (Freed et al., 2001), but a later study showed no difference in the responses between the two groups (Trott et al., 2003). Macklin (1999, p. 5) concluded that sham surgery was unethical "unless the surgery would be recommended solely for therapeutic purposes outside the research context." Although the sham surgery studies were approved by the investigators' IRBs, other IRBs may not approve such studies. According to federal regulations, each IRB has the prerogative to approve or deny studies, and each is guided by the values of the community that they represent.

In Vitro Fertilization/Embryos

All research involving in vitro fertilization (IVF) or embryo transfer must be approved by a national Ethics Advisory Board, but the Board has not been in existence since 1980, resulting in a "de facto moratorium on federal funding for embryo research until 1993" (President's Council on Bioethics, 2004, p. 128). In August 2002, President George W. Bush, in a televised address to the nation, said that federal funding would be permitted for embryo research (specifically stem cell research) that used cell lines that were derived from unused embryos that had been donated for research (National Human Genome Research Institute, 2004). Researchers responded by saying that there were far fewer usable cell lines than originally believed, which would severely limit stem cell research. The President's Council on Bioethics is expected to make further recommendations about the ethics of stem cell and embryo research. However, cloning of humans for the purposes of research has already been prohibited.

Children

The lessons from the Willowbrook hepatitis study and other unethical studies done with children point to the need to protect children even if their parents are willing to enroll them in research. The Common Rule notes several conditions that must be satisfied in order for research involving children to be approved. According to 45 CFR 46 Subpart D, IRBs must consider whether the research poses no greater than "minimal risk" to the child. If it does, then it must also hold the promise of a direct benefit to the child that outweighs the risk.

If there is no promise of a direct benefit and if the risk is greater than minimal, then the IRB can only approve the research study if the risk it poses is no more than a minor increase above minimal, if the research intervention is something the child may encounter in the course of his or her treatment, and if the intervention is likely to yield generalizable information that is vital to the treatment of the child's condition.

The last category under which research with children can be approved covers studies that would otherwise not be approvable but that "present an opportunity to understand, prevent, or alleviate a serious problem affecting the health or welfare of children" (U.S. Department of Health and Human Services, Office for Human Research Protections, 2004b, p. 11). The secretary of the Department of Health and Human Services, in consultation with a panel of experts, must approve any study in this category.

Consent and Assent

Parental permission must be obtained. If the research holds the promise of providing a direct benefit to the child, then only one parent needs to sign the permission form. If there is no direct benefit but the research has been approved, then permission must be obtained from both parents (unless one parent is unavailable, has sole custody, is incompetent, or is unknown). Assent, the affirmative agreement to participate, must be obtained from the child, and the IRB usually requires that the investigator provide a detailed description of how assent will be obtained. Often, investigators provide the children with oral and written information for their appropriate age levels. In a study where children of ages 3 to 13 years can be enrolled, the investigators might prepare oral information for 3 to 5 year olds, one form of written information for the children who are 6 to 12 years old and another form for the children who are older than 12 years of age. Often, the child is asked to sign the information form, indicating assent to participate.

The child's signature, however, should not close the assent process; children should be given explanations of all the procedures they are undergoing, as developmentally appropriate, and their ongoing assent should always be obtained, with the following caveat. If a child refuses to assent to participate in research and if the research is likely to provide direct benefit, then the child's refusal can be overruled by the child's parents. It might be argued that if the child's refusal will not be honored, then it is inappropriate to *ask* the child to participate.

Some states permit adolescents to consent to medical treatment without parental permission. These states may also allow adolescents to consent to participate in research that falls into the same realm as treatment. There may also be certain studies that feasibly could not be done if parental consent was required. Studies examining the lives of adolescent runaways could not be done if parental consent was required; similarly, studies exploring the lives of adolescents who are gay but who have not disclosed this to their parents could not be done if parental consent was required. IRBs must determine whether studies can be conducted without parental knowledge or consent, and, if so, how the adolescents' rights and welfare will be protected.

There may also be situations in which the parents insist the child be enrolled in the study, the child refuses, and there is concern that the parents are not acting in the child's best interests. Much, if not all, of the oncology treatment for children is provided through research protocols. The parents may believe that their child's only hope of cure (or extended life) is through enrollment in a cancer study. The physician/investigator explains to the parents that there is a standard treatment and there is an experimental treatment. The risks and probabilities for a positive response from the experimental treatment are explained to the parents in detail and over several sessions. The physician/investigator tells the parents that their child will be randomized into the standard or the experimental group and that there is a possibility that the child may not improve, no matter which group the child is in. If the child has failed previous treatments and the parents are looking for a cure, it can be very difficult for them to understand the difference between research-intervention and treatment. It can also be very difficult for parents to believe that their child's doctor would suggest that they enroll their child in a study were it not in the child's best interests.

Research and treatment may appear the same to parents, yet research is intended to yield information that, in the aggregate, will help guide treatment for *other children* in the future. So, in cases where the parents want the child enrolled in a study and the child is unwilling to continue cancer treatment, it may be appropriate to have an advocate (or a court-appointed guardian) to represent the child's interests. No parent wants to lose a child, but there may be a point where a palliative approach is more appropriate than a curative approach, and the oncology staff can advocate for the peaceful dying of the child.

Inducements

Another ethical issue associated with research on children is the concern for inducement (or undue influence). For example, a study investigating a vaccine recruits parents in a low-income area and provides them with $25 if they enroll their child in the study. To determine whether this payment will unduly influence parents, the IRB members need to discuss whether they think the parents would enroll their children in the study on the study's merits alone. If they believe the parents will enroll their children only because they will get $25, then the payment is coercive. Likewise, if a study offers CDs, gift certificates, or other desirable items to entice children to enroll in a study in which they otherwise would not participate, then the gifts are coercive.

Paying research subjects is often a means of acknowledging the time and energy they put into participating in the study, and the amount or the type of payment depends on the population. Offering physicians $30 for an hour of time in which samples of their breath are taken is unlikely to be an enticement, but offering a new mother $500 to have her blood drawn every 15 minutes while she nurses her infant over a 6-hour period could be viewed as an enticement. These decisions are relative to the community, and federal regulations empower IRBs to make these decisions. Often, investigators will provide rationales for the payment amounts (or lack of payments) they give to their research subjects.

In the last decade, the Kennedy Krieger Institute of Johns Hopkins University conducted a study on lead abatement in low-income housing in Baltimore. Landlords were given incentives to rent to families with young children, and then the children were recruited into the study. The study required that the children live in the apartment for its duration and that they have their blood drawn periodically. Despite the fact that researchers knew that lead dust was prevalent in low-income housing, even in houses that had lead abatement, and that young children were particularly at risk for lead exposure, they recruited families with young children.

Two parents of children in this study sued the Kennedy Krieger Institute (and the researchers) for negligence in failing to warn them of its dangers. The consent forms, according to the Maryland Court of Appeals, did not clearly indicate that the purpose of the study was to measure the level of lead contamination in their children's blood. The court characterized the experiment as treating the children like "canaries in the mine," comparing the children to the canaries that miners would bring with them into the mines because of the birds' sensitivity to lethal gases that the miners could not otherwise detect. If the canaries died, the miners would be alerted that the lethal gases were present and that they should seek fresh air. The court concluded:

Otherwise healthy children, in our view, should not be enticed into living in, or remaining in, potentially lead-tainted housing, and intentionally subjected to a research program, which contemplates the probability, or at least the possibility, of lead poisoning or even the accumulation of lower levels of lead in the blood, in order for the extent of the contamination of the children's blood to be used by the scientific researchers to assess the success of lead paint, or lead dust abatement measures. Moreover, in our view, parents, whether improperly enticed by trinkets, food stamps, money or other items, have no more right to intentionally or unnecessarily place children in potentially hazardous nontherapeutic research surroundings, than do researchers. In such cases, parental consent, no matter how informed, is insufficient. (Maryland Court of Appeals, 2001, p. 8)

The Court of Appeals overturned an earlier decision that ruled in favor of the Kennedy Krieger researchers, which found that the researchers did not have a special relationship that created a duty to warn the research participants and their parents of the dangers of participation in the study. The Court of Appeals was especially scathing in its criticism of the IRB and its failure to protect the child subjects and instead collude with researchers to circumvent the federal regulations for research with children. It behooves IRBs carefully to assess the risks to the health and welfare of children in comparison to the potential benefits of the research. They should also assess the effect of inducement for participation on conducting research with children. This case also illustrates how IRBs can experience conflicts of interest when their desire to promote research outweighs their primary responsibility to protect the subjects from harm.

Prisoners

As described earlier, prisoners are a convenient population for researchers to target. Federal regulations for research on prisoners, codified in The Common Rule, mandate that any research done with prisoners should pertain to criminal behavior, incarceration, prison life, or other conditions affecting prisoners. There should be no more than minimal risk involved, and if there is greater risk than minimal risk or if the research is nontherapeutic (offering no direct benefit to the subjects), then the secretary of the Department of Health and Human Services must approve the research. In assessing risk, the typical practice of using one's "everyday life" risks to assess minimal risk is not appropriate for prisoners. Their everyday life carries a high risk of harm from fellow inmates; therefore, their "everyday life" risk should not be the standard for their minimal risk. Their allowable risks should be the same as the risks accepted by nonprisoners.

Research with prisoners as subjects can invoke concerns about inducements. Researchers cannot offer potential prisoner-subjects special privileges for participating in research, such as extra outside recreational time. Because the potential subject's decision is based on the desire to obtain the incentive and is not based on a rational decision about the risk involved in participating in the study, it is unethical to offer incentives that are too enticing.

The IRB reviewing any protocols for research with prisoners must have, as a regular member, a prisoner, a prisoner representative, or someone with expertise in criminal justice or in the penal system. Researchers should be aware of the state laws and the Federal Bureau of Prisons' rules and restrictions on research.

People Who Are Cognitively Impaired

Although the authors of The Common Rule recognized the vulnerability of people with cognitive impairments, they could not reach a consensus on regulations to protect them from research harm. This category lumped together groups of people with the common condition of "cognitive impairment," but these impairments had widely varying causes such as mental retardation, mental illness, dementia, traumatic brain injury, drug dependence, and other conditions affecting capacity to consent. Recommendations were offered, but not codified, into The Common Rule. Similar to what was recommended for other vulnerable groups, the recommendations were that a regular IRB member be a person with experience or expertise relative to the diagnostic category of the subjects. If the IRB is reviewing research protocols on schizophrenia, and if the study plans to recruit people with schizophrenia, then the IRB should have a regular member who represents that population, such as a family member who belongs to National Association for the Mentally Ill. If the IRB is reviewing research protocols on exercise physiology in people with Down syndrome (or other persons with intellectual disability), then a regular member should be someone familiar with intellectual disabilities and people who have them. It is necessary to involve people with cognitive impairments in the conducting of research on such people. For example, to learn the therapeutic dosing for people with fragile X syndrome who have extreme anxiety, it is necessary to recruit subjects who have this syndrome, a genetic condition associated with intellectual disability. The critical ethical issue is how to obtain consent.

When a person has a "cognitive impairment" diagnosis such as Alzheimer disease or mental retardation, should capacity to consent be questioned? When someone has been declared legally "incompetent," indicating that the person cannot make decisions, the court appoints a guardian, who gives consent, and the incompetent person gives assent, depending upon their level of understanding and the IRB's requirement.

Short of being declared incompetent, the person's capacity to consent must be assessed, and that assessment process may differ from one group to the next. For example, some people with intellectual disabilities can make choices about living arrangements, purchases, and selection of friends, but they cannot make higher-level or more complex decisions related to health care. They rely on their next of kin to make those decisions. Because they have not been legally declared incompetent, they have the legal authority to consent, but in conversation, they may not be able to explain their understanding of the research process, purpose, risks, benefits, and ability to withdraw from the study, although they may express interest in participating in it. In another example, some people with schizophrenia may anticipate that there may be periods, especially if they are not taking medication, where their decision-making abilities are compromised. A third example would be people who have Alzheimer disease who are interested in participating in a longitudinal study but realize that they may lose their decisional capacity over time, before the study concludes.

Various mechanisms for assessing a person's capacity to consent can be implemented. The National Bioethics Advisory Commission (1998) made a number of recommendations, and the National Institutes of Health, Office of Human Subjects Research (n.d.) provided eight case types and suggestions for protections. The IRB must decide which protections are necessary with each research protocol. The investigator must provide detailed descriptions and rationales for the recruitment method, the target population, the procedures or interventions, their risks and potential benefits (if any), how capacity to consent will be assessed, and, if capacity is lacking, who will give consent and how assent will be obtained.

Depending on the cause of the cognitive impairment, assessment of capacity will vary. In people with psychiatric disorders, a professional (psychiatrist or psychologist) other than the treating professional or researcher will assess capacity. Appelbaum and Grisso (2001) developed an instrument for assessing a person's capacity to consent for research participation, the MCAT-CR, which is useful with the psychiatric population. Another instrument that may be useful for any population is the ACE (Aid to Capacity Evaluation) (Etchells, 1996). With each instrument, the evaluator's clinical judgment is relied on to interpret the responses and decide whether the person has the capacity to make the decision at hand. There is no threshold or cut-off score that indicates capacity.

People with intellectual disabilities (ID) may have the capacity to make a decision about participation in research, but may lack the communication skills to convey their understanding, or they may lack experience in expressing their choice. Organizations like the Roeher Institute in Canada developed a supported-decision model in which people with ID can designate a person to assist them with making decisions (Bach & Rock, 1996). In this respect, they are not designating someone to make the decision for them; rather, they are getting support from a trusted person to assist them in understanding, manipulating, and appreciating information and in expressing a choice. People with intellectual disabilities have a tendency to acquiesce to authority figures or to others who they do not want to disappoint. Researchers need to describe how they will determine whether the consent is genuine or is by acquiescence.

When someone with dementia, such as with Alzheimer disease, is interested in participating in longitudinal research and has decisional capacity, that person may designate a surrogate to give consent for future research when the person loses this capacity, which is the anticipated course of the disease or disorder. This surrogate may also be designated to make treatment decisions, as in the Durable Power of Attorney (DPA) for Health Care. Depending on state statutes for the DPA for Health Care, it may be necessary to specifically include in the agreement that the surrogate may make decisions regarding participation in research.

Other Vulnerable Groups

The federal government recognizes six other groups that may be vulnerable in research: traumatized and comatose patients, the elderly, minorities, students and employees, patients who are terminally ill, and people who participate in international research. There are common points for each group. Inclusion in research of people from these groups should be based solely on the inability to get the information in any other manner. The opportunity for inclusion should be equitable so that minorities in a given community are proportionately represented in the recruitment plan and in the total number of subjects. Justification should be given if the opportunity for inclusion it is not equitable. Coercion should be avoided in specific situations, such as with terminally ill patients and with students and employees of the research institution, yet these groups of potential subjects should be given an opportunity to freely consent if they wish to participate. The researcher should not assume that the elderly lack capacity, but elderly people who are institutionalized or who do lack capacity to consent should have the same protections as the other groups in these categories.

When people come into the emergency department after a trauma and are unconscious, they may be medically treated without their consent, but special criteria must be met before they can be enrolled in research. There is a mechanism by which the IRB can approve the enrollment of these patients in research through a waiving of informed consent. There is a mechanism by which the IRB can approve the enrollment of these patients in research through a waiving of informed consent. For example, the IRB may approve the research if all of the following conditions are present:

- The condition is life-threatening.
- Current treatment is unsatisfactory.
- There is a need to collect evidence to determine the safety and effectiveness of a proposed treatment.
- Consent is not feasible.
- The research holds promise of direct benefit to the subject.
- There is a therapeutic window in which the experimental treatment must be given but a family member cannot be located within that time, so the researchers will have to obtain consent at a later date as soon as possible.
- If other protections of the rights of subjects will be observed (U.S. Food and Drug Administration, 2000).

It is also necessary for a licensed physician to concur that the federal regulations are being met and that, prior to the beginning of the study, there is community consultation and public disclosure. A data monitoring committee may also be required to oversee the study. An example of such a study is the use of a blood substitute in people who need blood but who have a rare blood type for which an adequate supply of blood is not available. Although the IRB can approve the research under specific conditions, an ethical controversy over emergency research exists.

Many U.S. researchers conduct their studies abroad. They must comply with all U.S. regulations and with any regulations that are required by the country in which they are doing their research. Informed consent is a Western practice that may not be common in many other countries. A village elder may be the person who gives consent for someone to participate in a study, or a husband or father may be the person who consents for his wife or daughter to be in a study. These notions are very different from the Western notion of autonomy, yet they are customary practices. An American investigator who is conducting research in another country still must follow U.S. regulations that require informed consent from the subject who is going to participate in the research.

There is also great concern that people in developing countries are considered a more desirable group for research because their standard treatment for some conditions is no treatment at all. For example, consider a South American country in which preterm infants are not given "Surfactant," an artificial lubricant that makes stiff lungs compliant, because it is not available. For a decade or more, it has been the standard treatment in developed countries to give Surfactant to preterm infants shortly after birth. A U.S. manufacturer that would like to market a comparable product selects a neonatal intensive care unit in this South American country in which to test it because the experimental drug will be compared to no drug at all. In the United States, it would be considered unethical to randomize infants into a placebo group and an experimental group and then give the infants in the placebo group an inert substance when Surfactant, which is known to be effective, is available. The ethical question is, is it ethical to test this product in the South American country? This question becomes even more complex if the country where the research is conducted will not benefit from the results (often because of financial constraints), but the country is assuming all the risks. Is it ethical for people in developed countries like the United States to benefit from this research without assuming any of its risks? Does the U.S. manufacturer of the experimental product have any obligation to provide the treatment that is considered standard in the United States to infants in this South American country?

In addition to the Nuremberg Code, researchers conducting international research also need to comply with the Ethical Principles for Medical Research Involving Human Subjects according to the World Medical Association Declaration of Helsinki (2002). Another resource is the Council for International Organizations of Medical Sciences (CIOMS) International Ethical Guidelines for Biomedical Research Involving Human Subjects (2002).

SUMMARY

Whether a nurse is involved in human subject research as a recruiter, a data collector, a subject, or a researcher, he or she needs to be aware of and understand the scope of research ethics in this area. Studies should follow the tenets of the Nuremberg Code, should be approved by the appropriate oversight bodies (usually IRBs), and should provide protections for vulnerable groups as described in the resources in this chapter. However, the protections are only as effective as the integrity of the research team. Each member of the team has an obligation to the research subjects to protect them, and the nurse should keep that obligation uppermost in his or her mind.

CLINICAL EXERCISES

1. Find the Research Office in your academic and/or health care institution, obtain copies of an application for submitting a research proposal, and review it for all the elements of the Nuremberg Code. (*Hint*: Many of these applications are available on the institution's website. If your institution does not have a website, use the website of another institution close to your community.)
2. Obtain a copy of a consent form for a study being conducted in your institution. Examine it for the elements of informed consent and for readability in light of the proposed subject population. (*Hint*: Your word processing program may have a reading-level feature.)

Discussion Questions

1. Suppose that Mrs. Vaughn in the example in this chapter signed the consent form for the research project to test the surgical adhesive, but later, when asked about the research project by the nurse, she could not recall the conversation or that she signed a consent form. When the nurse reviews the specifics of the study with her, Mrs. Vaughn responds that she does not want to be a "guinea pig." What is the nurse's responsibility under these circumstances? What ethical principles are at risk?
2. Randy, a 10-year-old, is a patient on the pediatric unit. He is scheduled to receive chemotherapy consistent with a research protocol. He is refusing his medication. Can you accept his refusal as valid? Suppose Randy is 17 years old and has end-stage osteogenic sarcoma (bone cancer) with metastatic disease to his lungs, brain, and spinal cord. He is refusing further chemotherapy, but his parents want him to receive it because they are hoping to delay his death for as long as possible. Can you accept his refusal as valid and withhold the chemotherapy? Explain your answers.
3. You are asked to collect data about fetal well-being through blood and urine samples from pregnant woman and from measurements of fetal heart rates. If a woman has given her informed consent to participate, do you need the father's consent too? Give the rationale supporting your answer.
4. On a psychiatric unit, a patient is showing signs consistent with an adverse reaction to medication. You report this to his physician, who tells you that the patient is in a study and that you should continue giving the patient the medication as ordered. The patient refuses to take the medication. Can this patient refuse medication? Give your rationale. Can you refuse to give the medication to the patient? What would be your rationale?
5. You have been asked to join your hospital's IRB, and you attend your first meeting. A study to investigate a treatment for endometriosis is proposed. Subjects must undergo a laparoscopy prior to beginning medication and then they must have a second laparoscopy 1 year later. The first laparoscopy is consistent with a routine diagnostic work-up, but the second laparoscopy is strictly for research purposes. It is clearly stated in the consent form that the second laparoscopy is for research purposes only. Would you approve this study? What else do you need to know?

Resources

National Institutes of Health, Office of Human Subjects Research. (1979). The Belmont report: Ethical principles and guidelines for the protection of human subjects of research. Retrieved January 22, 2005, from http://ohsr.od.nih.gov/guidelines/belmont.html

National Institutes of Health, Office of Human Subjects Research. (2001). Regulations and ethical guidelines. Code of Federal Regulations. Title 45. Public welfare. Department of Health and Human Services. Part 46. Protection of human subjects. Subpart C. Additional DHHS protections pertaining for biomedical and behavioral research involving prisoners as subjects. Retrieved January 22, 2005, from www.nihtraining.com/ohsrsite/guidelines/45cfr46.html

National Institutes of Health, Office of Human Subjects Research. (1993). OHSR Information Sheets/Forms. Sheet 10. Research involving children. Retrieved January 22, 2005, from www.nihtraining.com/ohsrsite/info/sheet10.html#kid

References

Annas, G. J., & Grodin, M. A. (1992). *The Nazi doctors and the Nuremberg code: Human rights in human experimentation*. New York: Oxford University Press.

Appelbaum, P. S., & Grisso, T. (2001). *MacArthur Competence Assessment Tool for Clinical Research (MacCAT-CR)*. Sarasota, FL: Professional Resources Press.

Bach, M., & Rock, M. (1996). *Seeking consent to participate in research from people whose ability to make an informed decision could be questioned: The Supported Decision Making Model*. Toronto: Roeher Institute.

Beecher, H. K. (1966). Ethics and clinical research. *New England Journal of Medicine, 274*(24), 1354–1360.

Brody, B. A. (1998). *The ethics of biomedical research: An international perspective*. New York: Oxford University Press.

Burleigh, M. (1994). *Death and deliverance: "Euthanasia" in Germany 1900–1945*. New York: Cambridge University Press.

Chervenak, F. A., & McCullough, L. B. (2002). A comprehensive ethical framework for fetal research and its application to fetal surgery for spina bifida. *American Journal of Obstetrics and Gynecology, 187*(1), 10–14.

Council for International Organizations of Medical Sciences. (2002). *International Ethical Guidelines for Biomedical Research involving Human Subjects*. Geneva: Author.

Etchells, E. (1996). *Aid to capacity evaluation*. Retrieved April 30, 2004, from http://www.utoronto.ca/jcb/

Evelyn, B., Toigo, T., Bank, D., Pohl, D., Gray, K., Robins, B., et al. (2001). Women's participation in clinical trials and gender-related labeling: A review of new molecular entities approved 1995–1999. Retrieved April 30, 2004, from http://www.fda.gov/cder/reports/womens_health/women_clin_trials.htm

Freed, C. R., Greene, P. E., Breeze, R. E., Tsai, W. Y., DuMouchel, W., Kao, R., et al. (2001). Transplantation of embryonic dopamine neurons for severe Parkinson disease. *New England Journal of Medicine, 344*(10), 710–719.

Gaylin, W. (1989). Nazi data: Dissociation from evil: Commentary. *Hastings Center Report, 19*(4), 18.

Hornblum, A. M. (1998). *Acres of skin: Human experiments at Holmesburg Prison*. New York: Routledge.

Jones, J. H. (1993). *Bad blood: The Tuskegee syphilis experiment*. New York: Free Press.

Lederer, S. E. (1995). *Subjected to science: Human experimentation in America before the second world war*. Baltimore: Johns Hopkins University Press.

Levine, R. J. (1986). *Ethics and regulation of clinical research* (2nd ed.). New Haven, CT: Yale University Press.

Lifton, R. J. (1986). *The Nazi doctors: Medical killing. The psychology of genocide.* New York: Basic Books.

Macklin, R. (1999). The ethical problems with sham surgery in clinical research [Electronic version]. *New England Journal of Medicine, 341*(13), 992–996.

Maryland Court of Appeals. (2001). Case numbers 24-C-99-000925 and 24-C-95066067/CL193461. Retrieved April 30, 2004, from http://www.courts.state.md.us/opinions/coa/2001/128a00.pdf

Moe, K. (1984). Should the Nazi research data be cited? *Hasting Center Report, 14*(6), 5–7.

National Bioethics Advisory Commission. (1998). *Research involving persons with mental disorders that may affect decisionmaking capacity.* Rockville, MD: U.S. Government Printing Office.

National Commission for the Protection of Human Subjects of Biomedical and Behavioral Research. (1979). *The Belmont Report.* Bethesda, MD: U.S. Government Printing Office.

National Conference of State Legislatures. (2005). State embryonic and fetal research laws. Retrieved November 14, 2005, from http://www.ncls.org/programs/health/genetics/embfet.htm

National Human Genome Research Institute. (2004). Cloning/embryonic stem cells. Cloning for the isolation of human ES cells: Policy and regulation. Retrieved April 30, 2004, from http://www.genome.gov/10004765

National Institutes of Health, Office of Human Subjects Research. (n.d.). OHSR Information Sheets/Forms. Sheet 11. Inclusion of women and minorities in study populations. Guidance for IRBs and principal investigators. Retrieved January 22, 2005, from http://www.nihtraining.com/ohsrsite/info/sheet11.html

National Institutes of Health, Office of Human Subjects Research. (n.d.). OHSR Information Sheets/Forms. Sheet 7. Research involving cognitively impaired subjects: A review of some ethical considerations. Retrieved April 30, 2004, from www.nihtraining.com/ohsrsite/info/sheet7.html

President's Council on Bioethics. (2004). *Reproduction & responsibility: The regulation of new biotechnologies.* Washington, DC: Author.

Proctor, R. N. (1988). *Racial hygiene: Medicine under the Nazis.* Cambridge, MA: Harvard University Press.

Spiro, H. M. (1985). Nazi research: Too evil to cite. *Hastings Center Report, 15*(4), 31–32.

Trott, C. T., Fahn, S., Green, P., Dillon, S., Winfield, H., Winfield, L., et al., Breeze (2003). Cognition following bilateral implants of embryonic dopamine neurons in PD: A double blind study. *Neurology, 60*(12), 1938–1943.

U.S. Department of Health and Human Services. (1998). Informed Consent Checklist—Basic and Additional Elements. Retrieved on November 16, 2005, from http://www.hhs.gov/ohrp/humansubjects/assurance/consentckls.htm

U.S. Department of Health and Human Services, Office for Human Research Protections. (2004a). IRB Guidebook: Introduction. Retrieved September 29, 2005, from http://www.hhs.gov/ohrp/irb/irb_introduction.htm

U.S. Department of Health and Human Services, Office for Human Research Protections. (2004b). IRB Guidebook: Chapter VI. Special classes of subjects. Retrieved September 29, 2005, from http://www.hhs.gov/ohrp/irb/irb_chapter6.htm

U.S. Food and Drug Administration. (2000). Draft guidance: Exception from informed consent requirements for emergency research. Retrieved January 22, 2005, from http://www.fda.gov/ora/compliance_ref/bimo/err_guide.htm

U. S. National Library of Medicine. (2005). Genetics Home Reference. Glossary. Fetus. Retrieved January 9, 2005, from http://ghr.nlm.nih.gov/ghr/glossary/fetus

World Medical Association Declaration of Helsinki. (2002). Ethical principles for medical research involving humans subjects. Retrieved April 29, 2004, from http://www.wma.net/e/policy/b3.htm

Clinical Ethics
Issues

CHAPTER 11

Nursing of Children and Adolescents

Objectives

At the end of this chapter, the student should be able to:

1. Identify the ethical issues in pediatric clinical cases.
2. Identify the most appropriate decision-maker in each specific situation.
3. Advocate for a child's best interests.
4. Describe the conflicts in determining who speaks for a child.
5. Facilitate adolescent decision-making, when appropriate.
6. Analyze institutional and public policy issues related to children's health care.

KEY WORDS

- Assent
- Baby Doe regulations
- Best interest standard
- Brain death
- Emancipated
- Health Insurance Portability and Accountability Act of 1996
- Intersex
- Mature minor
- Substituted judgment standard

All of the specialties in nursing—medical, surgical, orthopedic, neurological, gastroenterological, and so on—are present in the nursing care of children and adolescents. In the past, the medical approach treated children as though they were just miniature adults. Physically, physiologically, psychologically, emotionally, and socially, however, children are very different from adults. This chapter addresses the ethical issues the nurse might face in caring for children and adolescents in various health care settings, school, and the home.

SECTION 1: *Ethical Themes: Building From the Basic to the Complex*

This section addresses the ethical building blocks described in previous chapters and offers examples of situations that may arise in the nursing care of children.

TRUTH-TELLING

One of the most difficult situations for nurses arises when parents request that their child not be told that he or she is dying. Parents defend their request by saying that they believe it would be too upsetting for the child to know or they fear the child will lose hope. Experienced nurses have found that children often know when their parents are keeping something from them and realize that their parents are trying to protect them. For example, Lisa is a 10-year-old with a brainstem glioma. According to the National Cancer Institute (2005), there is 90% mortality within 18 months of diagnosis of brainstem glioma. She has undergone 18 months of radiation, chemotherapy, and surgery, but the tumor continues to grow. Whether to tell Lisa about her diagnosis and prognosis is an issue of truth-telling. The nurses will rely on the parents' judgment about whether the child should be told, but also may advise the parents, based on the nurses' experiences and their assessment of Lisa's developmental level, maturity, and readiness to hear. Although Lisa's *assent* is required before she can be enrolled in a research project, some nurses may confuse such assent with permission to share the diagnosis and prognosis (see Chapter 10). Assent is the affirmative agreement to participate in clinical research; it is a regulatory requirement for children of certain ages and adults who are incapable of giving informed consent. Nurses may believe that it would be in Lisa's best interests to know her diagnosis and prognosis and be able to talk about her impending death. They can give parents their rationale for wanting to disclose the information to Lisa, but in the end, the parents' wishes are usually respected.

Another issue of truth-telling arises when an adolescent receives treatment without parental consent where this is legal, and the parent seeks information from the health care providers regarding the condition and treatment the child received. Annette, 16, went to a family planning clinic to obtain birth control. She was examined by a nurse practitioner and counseled regarding various methods of contraception as well as education on sexually transmitted infections and psychological aspects of sexual activity. Annette's mother discovers the prescription for oral contraceptives and calls the clinic. She demands to know how her daughter can obtain the "Pill" without her consent. She is invited to attend a parent information session but is told that she cannot receive any specific information about her daughter's visit. Because of patient confidentiality, reinforced by the Health Insurance Portability and Accountability Act of 1996 (HIPAA), Annette's information cannot be released without her written informed consent, not even to her parents. What may seem inconsistent is that if, on examination, it was discovered that Annette had a urinary tract infection, the infection could not be treated without parental consent. Only certain conditions can be treated without parental consent, and each state differs on the permissible conditions to treat. So truth-telling, or, rather, disclosure of the truth, in this instance is not ethically or legally permitted. Even if Annette were pregnant and seeking prenatal care or termination of the pregnancy, in many states her parents could not be notified without her consent.

Nurses realize that situations of withholding or disclosing information can cause a great deal of tension in families. Often the nurse can facilitate communication between parents and children, helping them to decide what to withhold or disclose. Identifying mutual goals of the parents and the children is a beginning. State laws vary regarding a minor's access to services for sexually transmitted diseases (STDs), but all states and the District of Columbia allow minors to consent to STD services, although 11 states have a minimum age requirement (12 or 14 years) (Alan Guttmacher Institute, 2005). It is imperative that nurses be familiar with their state's statutes pertaining to minors' rights.

CONFIDENTIALITY

Children's medical information is kept confidential between the health care providers and the parents. According to some state statutes, children 13 years of age and older must give consent for medical records to be released. Parents must also give consent. Apart from records, other information may need to be kept confidential. Children may tell health care providers information that they do not want shared with their parents. A common example occurs when the child is dying and parents are unable to discuss this with the child. As in the previous example of truth-telling, Lisa, a 10-year-old, has a brain tumor that is not responding to treatment. She tells the nurse working with her that she knows she is going to die but she cannot discuss it with her parents because they are trying to protect her. The nurse can work with Lisa to see whether there is a way to bridge the communication between her and her parents. If Lisa does not want this information shared, the nurse must weigh the obligation to respect the communication with Lisa against the parents' right to know.

Another common example occurs when adolescents seek treatment for specific conditions, such as mental health or substance abuse treatment, contraception, pregnancy or abortion services, or treatment for a sexually transmitted infection. Both ethically and legally, the health care provider must keep the information confidential and not disclose it to the adolescent's parents. The motivation for some states to grant this privacy to adolescents stems from the desire to have these services accessible to them. There is concern that adolescents would refrain from seeking treatment if their parents were informed. What seems incongruent is that a child could not be treated for a relatively minor problem such as acne, but could be treated for a very serious and life-altering condition such as pregnancy. Ross (1998) argued that parents should make decisions for their children until the age of majority and supported the repeal of state laws that permit treatment of adolescents without parental consent.

Bartholome (1995) supported getting the child's assent along with the parents' consent. *Assent* is affirmative agreement; *consent* is the legal concept of agreeing that can only be given by adults or emancipated or mature minors. His treatise on informed consent was adopted by the American Academy of Pediatrics Committee on Bioethics (1995), and stressed the concepts of parental permission as well as child assent. As the child matures, there is the expectation that he or she is developmentally capable of making health care decisions, although Weithorn and Campbell (1982) found children as young as 14 could make decisions for themselves as well as adults could. Just as an adult's capacity to consent should be assessed, so should a child's. Assent should be sought and refusal honored. The age of assent varies, however, and is based on the developmental assessment of the child's capacity to make the decision at hand. Some children at age 6 may be able to give assent, whereas another child at age 13 may not. All children, not just children with developmental disabilities or other known cognitive impairments, should have their capacity assessed. When a child will be treated whether or not he or she agrees, then assent should not be sought, and the child should be given developmentally appropriate information about what is to happen.

There are conditions in which an adolescent who has not yet reached age 18 can give consent, other than in the situations listed previously. If a child meets certain conditions listed in the state statute, a child is considered *emancipated*. For example, a child who marries at age 16 could be considered emancipated in some states, but in other states would only be emancipated if she and her husband did not live with either set of parents and did not depend on them for financial assistance. If an adolescent enters military service, he or she is considered emancipated. An emancipated minor has the same rights as adults in society, but because state statutes vary, the nurse is encouraged to investigate the relevant state statutes for the practice setting. In some states, pregnant adolescents are considered emancipated for the purposes of giving or refusing consent for medical treatment for themselves and the fetuses; however, after the infant is born, the adolescent mother may only make decisions for the infant, not for herself unless she is married (but the nurse should always check the relevant state's statute; some states allow adolescents who are parents to consent for health care for themselves).

A *mature minor* is a child who has been declared mature by a court proceeding for the purposes of giving or refusing consent for medical treatment. Children with chronic conditions or disabilities have interacted with the health care system regularly. This frequent contact gives them experience on which to make decisions, and most pediatric nurses respect a child's right to have information about his or her health care. Unless the child has been declared a mature minor through a court proceeding, the child cannot give or refuse consent for medical treatment unless, through state statute, the child can be treated without parental consent for specific conditions, such as sexually transmitted infections, substance abuse, birth control and pregnancy treatment, and mental health treatment. A child may seek treatment through school-based clinics, and the clinics should have clear policies on what conditions can be treated without parental consent or notification and what conditions cannot. In addition, the child seeking treatment should be made aware of the mandatory reporting statutes. Certain professionals, such as health care providers, teachers, social workers, and police officers, are mandated by state law to report suspected or actual abuse and/or neglect of a child. If a child with immersion burns on his or her hands or with apparent bruises and welts seeks treatment at a clinic, the health care providers should seek information to clarify the source of the injuries, and if the information makes the provider suspicious of abuse, he or she is mandated to report the occurrence to the appropriate state agency. However, until the agency makes a determination, the parent(s) retain custody and must give consent for treatment for the injuries. If the agency determines that the child is in an unsafe situation in the home, it will seek temporary custody and remove the child from the home. According to the state agency's protocol, a legal guardian will be appointed to give consent for any medical treatment.

Often, children are brought to outpatient centers by relatives other than their parents for routine examinations. Occasionally the relative will bring a form that authorizes him or her to give consent for routine procedures, such as laboratory tests or immunizations, but more often, he or she does not have such a form. It is common for children to be raised primarily by their grandparents although the parent retains legal custody. A divorced parent may not be the custodial parent and cannot legally give consent for the child. Nurses in outpatient settings should be aware of the relationship to the child of the adult who brings the child into the office and should clarify authority to consent if there is any question about legal custody. The nurse should consult institutional HIPAA policies about release of information to any adult other than the custodial parent who brings the child for health care.

Confidentiality and HIV Testing in Adolescents

Although the percentage of new HIV infections has decreased in the overall population, the percentage of youth, defined by the Centers for Disease Control and Prevention as ages 13 to 24 years, has increased (Centers for Disease Control and Prevention [CDC], 2005). The American Academy of Pediatrics asserted that half of the newly diagnosed HIV infections in the United States occur in this population (Committee on Pediatric AIDS and Committee on Adolescence, 2001). To combat the epidemic of HIV/AIDS among this population, education on prevention and transmission is needed. Additionally, adolescents who are at risk (have engaged in unprotected sex or shared needles) should have testing.

Although all states and the District of Columbia permit minors to consent to services related to STDs, only 30 states include HIV testing in these services (Alan Guttmacher Institute, 2005). Only one state, Vermont, requires that the health care provider inform the parents if the adolescent tests positive for HIV. Eighteen states allow, but do not require, the physician to inform parents that the adolescent is seeking testing or treatment for STD. Jackson and Hafemeister (2001) acknowledged that there is a dearth of research on the impact of parental consent requirements and HIV testing, but they hypothesized that the effects would be as detrimental as notification requirements on abortion, contraception, and disclosure of homosexuality. It is likely, therefore, that the adolescent would not submit to HIV testing if parental consent or notification was required.

Nurses working in settings where adolescents are seen for STD services should be aware of relevant laws. Nurses can explore with the adolescent whether to inform parents of test results and whether to include parents in future health care decisions the adolescent may face. The lack of parental involvement may feel problematic for nurses who prefer a family-centered approach. In the area of sex education and sexuality of adolescents, many parents have opinions based on their family's values, religious preferences, culture, and personal experiences. Believing that parents should provide guidance in these areas, nurses may feel constrained when they cannot share specific medical information with them. Health care facilities should advise parents that children of a certain age may receive health care services for specific conditions without parental consent, according to state law. There may be a few situations in which the health care provider would breach confidentiality and share privileged information with an adolescent's parents.

Confidentiality and Risk of Harm

If the adolescent poses a threat to himself or herself or to a third party, the health care provider has an ethical and legal obligation to share the privileged information. Because adolescents may receive mental health treatment or treatment for substance abuse, they may, in the course of their treatment, confide that they plan to harm themselves or harm another person. Again, the health care provider should be aware of relevant state law pertaining to disclosure of confidential information. In both inpatient and outpatient settings, adolescents may be treated for mental health conditions or substance abuse. Therefore nurses in all settings should be aware of the limits of confidentiality in special situations.

ADVOCACY

Neonatal Decision-Making

In children's nursing, advocacy involves speaking for the child. From a family-centered care perspective, what is good for the child must be seen in the context of the family. However, there may be times when the child's interests may appear to conflict with the family's interests. In situations like this, the nurse may advocate for the child's interests apart from the family's. Advocacy can be complicated in neonatal intensive care. With the gestational-age margins of viability overlapping with legally permissible pregnancy termination, conflicts of interests between the woman and the fetus emerge. The law helps to define boundaries for when a fetus has legal protections, but nurses may view the fetus as a person worthy of ethical consideration. Consider the woman who is primiparous, 22 weeks pregnant, in preterm labor, and with breech presentation. Despite aggressive treatment to halt labor, the child may be born. Typically for a primiparous woman delivering a preterm infant who is breech, a Caesarean section (C-section) would be recommended. However, for the gestational age of 22 weeks, C-section is not recommended (American Academy of Pediatrics, 2002). After 23 weeks, however, the perinatologist may be more inclined to perform a C-section for fetal indications. If the woman refuses the C-section, should someone advocate for the fetus and force the woman to submit to surgery? Under what conditions, if any, should a woman be forced by court order to have a C-section? (This issue is discussed in more detail in Chapter 13.) The question of whether the fetus needs an advocate other than its mother is an ethical question.

Infants born prematurely and those born with genetic conditions or perinatal complications can pose ethical problems. How aggressively should they be treated? For extremely preterm infants, even with aggressive treatment, data show a range of outcomes (Wood, Marlow, Costeloe, Gibson, & Wilkinson, 2000). Catlin (1998) found that physicians in her study would most likely resuscitate an extremely preterm infant, one weighing less than 500 grams, yet would not want their own preterm infant of the same gestational age resuscitated. The physicians carried a great deal of worry about the responsibility of saving tiny infants who subsequently have significant disabilities, yet they felt compelled to treat them.

Pinch (2002) documented the history of decision-making in the neonatal intensive care unit (NICU) and parental perceptions of decision-making. Prior to the 1980s, decisions to discontinue life support were made between parents and physicians (Duff & Campbell, 1973). In the 1980s, decision-making came under public scrutiny when an infant with Down syndrome and esophageal atresia died of dehydration from nontreatment (Lyon, 1985). The parents of Baby Doe, as he became known, opted to forgo surgical intervention, the case came to the attention of the Secretary for Health and Human Services, and eventually regulations, called the *Baby Doe regulations*, were amended to existing child abuse and neglect laws in every state to prevent discrimination based on a handicapping condition. Practice changed, and there seemed to be an era of "overtreatment" to avoid any perception of discrimination. The propensity to treat first, then evaluate, has become the common approach in neonatal care. There is also the technological imperative, by which one feels morally compelled to provide an intervention if it is technically possible to do so. Parents are often given information about their infant's condition, treatment, and expected course, but not asked to consent to treatment unless a procedure requires written informed consent, such as a blood transfusion, lumbar puncture, or surgery. Harrison (1993), one of the first parents to write of her experience with her prematurely born son, called for increased parental involvement in decisions. Representing the views of many other parents whose children are now significantly disabled, Harrison (2001) believed that parents should "be apprised of all the facts" (2001, p. 247) and should know the "financial and professional incentives for neonatologists to provide intensive care for *other people's* [her emphasis] preterm infants, along with the pain, suffering and undeclared experimentation that constitutes much of this care" (p. 247). An issue not adequately addressed is prognostic uncertainty.

Parents may be given statistics such as "Infants born at this gestational age at this hospital have an 85% mortality rate." National data may be very similar, and parents are told this as well. Are they told which infants died because therapy was not effective or because life support was withdrawn? How is the information presented to them? If parents are told there is a 15% chance of survival with intensive care and a 40% chance the child will be without major disability, are they more inclined to favor treatment? Does the framing of the outcome as the likelihood of survival versus the likelihood of death influence parents toward favoring treatment? Pinch (2002) found that parents often felt they were informed but did not make decisions about their infant's neonatal treatment.

Although family-centered care is the ideal, nurses may sometimes feel torn between advocating for the infant and advocating for the parents. Until 1982, in some areas of the country, infants with Down syndrome (trisomy 21) or myelomeningocele (spina bifida) would be deprived of food and water at their parents' request. The "Baby Doe regulations" resulted from a case in Bloomington, Indiana, in which parents refused surgery for their infant with Down syndrome. The infant had esophageal atresia, a condition in which food and fluid cannot pass into the stomach. He also had a tracheo-esophageal fistula, an opening between the trachea and esophagus, which made oral feedings dangerous. Because of the likelihood of intellectual disability (primarily mental retardation) associated with Down syndrome, the parents decided to forgo lifesaving surgery despite a pediatrician's urging. The Indiana Supreme Court upheld their right to refuse medical treatment for their child, and the infant died before the U.S. Supreme Court could hear the case. The case came to the attention of the director of health and human services and others in the Reagan administration, and the Office of Civil Rights sent hospitals a warning that they could lose federal funding if they withheld food and fluid from "handicapped newborns." Eventually this warning and the subsequent regulations and court ruling became known as the Baby Doe regulations. State child abuse and neglect laws were amended to include forbidding the withholding of food and fluid from newborns unless they met one of three conditions: they were in an irreversible coma, treatment would prolong dying and be futile in terms of survival, or the treatment would be considered inhumane. Because these regulations are vague, health care providers can consider the particulars of each case and decide whether forgoing treatment is consistent with the usual and customary practices in neonatal care (Lyon, 1985).

The nurse advocates for parents by ensuring that they get and understand information for decision-making. It is usually helpful for a nurse to be present when a physician or nurse practitioner gives information to parents. Often parents need time to process the information, and so they may not ask questions at this time, but will have questions later. The nurse who was present can clarify and reinforce information, and may be able to answer questions. For questions the nurse cannot answer, the physician or nurse practitioner can be contacted. The nurse shows respect for the parents' autonomy by facilitating informed decision-making.

Circumcision

Circumcision of the male infant is a common medical procedure, although not without controversy. Opponents of circumcision argue that it is medically unnecessary. Even those who believe it is a matter of parental choice advocate for anesthesia or analgesia for the infant. Both the American Academy of Pediatrics Task Force on Circumcision (1999) and the Canadian Paediatric Society Fetus and Newborn Committee (1996) oppose circumcision as a routine procedure. Some insurance companies will only pay for circumcision if it is performed soon after birth, prior to discharge, as part of the obstetrical delivery services. Infants discharged before circumcision may only have the procedure covered only if there is a medical indication, such as phimosis. The Canadian national health program does not pay for routine neonatal circumcision; less than half the male infants in Canada are circumcised (Canadian Paediatric Society, 1996). As with other health care choices, parents are permitted to have their male infants circumcised.

Female circumcision is quite different, though. Many African, Middle Eastern, and Asian cultures perform various types of circumcision on females between the ages of 6 and the teens. The surgeries may range from removal of the clitoral hood to removal of the clitoris and labia majora and the sewing together of the remaining tissue so only a very small opening is left for urination and menstrual flow (infundibulation). Immigrants to the United States may still wish to continue this custom, but in some states, such as Illinois, it is illegal to perform female circumcision, also referred to as female genital mutilation, on a child (Abused and Neglected Child Reporting Act 325 ILCS 5/3, effective August 16, 2002).

Although parents are given the option of circumcision for their male infants, they are not given the option for female infants. The primary ethical issue in circumcision is informed decision-making and the prevention of harm, based on the parental assessment of what constitutes a harm. Nurses need to ensure that parents have information with which to make an informed decision about male circumcision.

Intersexuality

Infants born with genitalia that do not indicate the infant's gender (ambiguous genitalia) pose clinical and ethical challenges. In the decades prior to 1990, when infants were born with ambiguous or atypical genitalia, physicians decided which gender the child should be assigned. Based on the John/Joan case in the 1970s, John Money maintained that children were born with a neutral sexual identity and could be raised as either a boy or a girl (Colapinto, 2000). It was later learned that this child, who lost his penis through a cautery accident during his circumcision at 7 months of age and was raised as Joan, did not adjust to being a girl. In his adolescence, he assumed a male identity, later had a mastectomy and phalloplasty, married a woman, and adopted children (Colapinto, 2000; Diamond, 1999). Because the failure of his gender reassignment was concealed, then denied by Money, the standard practice was unchanged. Surgery to "normalize" the appearance of the external genitalia was recommended, gender was assigned consistent with the genitalia, and appropriate hormonal therapy at puberty was the standard treatment. Children were not told about their condition or medical history for fear that it would be confusing and emotionally devastating. Treatment decisions were usually based upon the technical abilities of the surgeon to construct as normal-appearing and functional genitalia as possible. Often it was technically easier to convert male genitalia to female genitalia. The ethical underpinning of the decisions was that professionals knew best—a paternalistic approach. Health care professionals, however well intentioned, proceeded with little evidence, so they could not fully inform parents of the enormity of the treatment decisions.

On reaching adulthood, individuals who were born with these conditions describe shame, stigma, and rage over their treatment. Forming a network for support, education, and social change, they began the Intersex Society of North America. They prefer to be referred to as *intersex* individuals rather than by such terms as hermaphrodite, pseudo-hermaphrodite, malformed, defective, or mistake of nature (Diamond & Sigmundson, 1997). Occurrence of the intersex condition is considered rare, but Dreger (1998) maintained that although the incidence is unknown, the condition likely is common. There are numerous conditions in which the genitalia do not appear to be typical, and these can represent a wide variation in anatomical appearance. Designations such as micropenis or clitoromegaly are used when the appearance of the external genitalia do not conform to someone's idea of "typical" or "standard." Conditions such as hypospadias, vaginal agenesis, or ovotestes, usually recognized at birth, fall into the "intersex" category, as do hormonally influenced conditions, such as congenital adrenal hypoplasia, 5-alpha reductase deficiency, and androgen insensitivity syndrome. Klinefelter syndrome (XXY) and other chromosomal variants (not XX and not XY) are also conditions falling within the "intersex" category (Dreger, 1998; Intersex Society of North America, 2005). In a review of the medical literature from 1955 to 2000, Blackless, Charuvastra, Derryck, Fausto-Sterling, Lauzanne, and Lee (2000) found a minimal estimate of 1.728% per live births. They held that "a belief in absolute sexual dimorphism is wrong" (p. 163).

Advocacy is key in the case of an intersex child. Although parents will be acutely distressed that the gender of their infant is difficult to determine, intersex adults and many health care professionals working in the intersex field believe that children should not have surgery to relieve their parents' distress. An evaluation should occur, and parents and professionals should make a provisional assignment of gender without surgically altering the child's genitalia. Peer counseling and psychological counseling by qualified individuals should begin immediately. Because surgical intervention is almost always irreversible, surgery should be postponed until the child (usually after puberty) can decide whether it is desirable.

The issue of informed consent is crucial because the benefits and risks of early surgical treatment have not been well documented, and so are unknown. Diamond and Sigmundson (1997) recommended that surgery should be withheld unless the life of the child is threatened, as in extrophy of the bladder. They also recommended that information be shared with the parents and the child, when cognitively able to understand, and that the child should decide what surgery, if any, should be done. Nurses should facilitate referrals to sources such as the Intersex Society of North America. The American Academy of Pediatrics, in a recent policy statement by the Committee on Genetics, Section on Endocrinology, and Section of Urology, endorses surgery on infants under certain conditions, this policy statement is in conflict with the recommendations of Diamond and Sigmundson (1997), Dreger (1998), the Intersex Society of North America (2005), and a task force convened by the Hastings Center (Frader et al., 2004).

The nurse's role in enabling parents to get information is very important. Not all cases of intersex require surgery, but parents need information to plan for their child's future needs and to understand the challenges the intersex condition may pose; nurses can assist parents to find helpful resources.

Conjoined Twins

There have been widely publicized cases in the popular media of conjoined twins. The most famous are Eng and Chang Bunker (1811–1874), who are considered the original "Siamese" twins. Approximately 1 in 75,000 to 100,000 births results in conjoined twins. Between 40% and 60% are stillborn and 35% survive for 1 day, which means that 5% to 25% live beyond 1 day (Conjoined Twins, 2005). The majority of conjoined twins are joined at the chest and always share the heart (thoracopagus) (35%); the next highest percentage are joined at the lower back (pygopagus) (19%). As many as 68% of pygopagus twins survive separation, but none of the thoracopagus twins survive. Two recent cases, one pediatric and one adult, highlight the ethical issues in separating conjoined twins.

Mary and Jodie Attard were born in August 2000. Their parents traveled to England from Malta during the pregnancy to seek medical care. The girls were fused at the pelvis and shared internal organs. Separation could only be accomplished if one twin was sacrificed. The parents did not want to sacrifice the weaker twin, Mary, for the stronger twin, Jodie, so they refused consent for surgery even if it meant that both twins would not survive. They believed their decision was consistent with the teachings of their faith, Roman Catholicism. The physicians, perhaps motivated by their belief that they could save Jodie, petitioned the court for permission to override the parents' refusal and separate the twins. Two courts in England reviewed the case and supported the physicians' request for surgery. Mary, as expected, died in the operating room. Annas (2001), in his review of the court decision, believed that the physicians should not have separated the twins without parental consent. He did not agree that there was ethical or legal justification for sacrificing Mary for Jodie. He argued that there must be compelling evidence in favor of separation before custody and decision-making can be removed from parents.

The infants Mary and Jodie could not make the decision, but the adult twins Laleh and Ladan Bijani, who were joined at the head, requested separation surgery. In 2003, the 29-year-old Iranian twins traveled to Singapore to be separated. Born attached at the head, the two women wished to pursue separate careers. One wished to go to law school; the other wanted to be a journalist. Despite the 50:50 chance of survival, the twins were reported to be "adamant" about having separation surgery (CNN, 2003). In a 53-hour operation, it was not possible to separate them, and both bled to death during the surgery.

There are two primary ethical issues in this case. The first is the question of informed consent. Can it ever be known whether both twins desired separation or one was influenced (or possibly coerced) by the other? Ordinarily, the health care provider and patient can discuss medical treatment in private and the discussion remains confidential, but in the case of conjoined twins, one can never have privacy. How far should the health care providers go to ensure the individual wishes of each twin? The second ethical issue relates to the first one, that of informed consent. Because this type of surgery is rarely done, should it be considered experimental? One of the surgeons was quoted as saying he learned from this experience what to do differently the next time he attempts this procedure. He was also quoted as saying, "It's a failure only if you do not get anything out of it. . . . Thomas Edison said he knew 999 ways that a light bulb did not work, and yet we have lights today. There's a cleaning formula called 409. The first 408 did not work." (CNN, 2003)

Medical advances depend on learning from failures, but was so little known about the procedure that it should not have been attempted? If there is concern about the adequacy of the Bijani twins' informed consent, that concern is increased when parents, as surrogates, make decisions for their conjoined twins.

When should nurses and other health care providers intervene in their quest to advocate for infants? Parents lose their right to make health care decisions for their infants when abuse and/or neglect is suspected or known and a state agency has assumed medical custody (and sometimes physical custody). Short of abuse and neglect, parents are permitted to give or refuse consent for medical treatment. In the intimate and therapeutic relationships between parents and health care providers, the values of each can become known, and there may be a clash between them. Parental autonomy ordinarily trumps the views and wishes of the health care providers. If the health care provider has a moral objection to the decision of the parents, that provider may seek to transfer the care of the child to another provider who does not have the moral objection. There is a tension for pediatric nurses between their desire to advocate for the child and their desire to advocate for the family. When these desires are incompatible and irreconcilable, the nurse should decide for whom to advocate.

Adolescent Decision-Making

Adolescents may be capable of making informed health decisions (Weithorn & Campbell, 1982), but should make them in consultation with their parents (or legal guardians) (Ross, 1997). Especially for adolescents with chronic conditions, it is important to engage them in the management decisions (Hyun, 2000). As previously discussed, decision-making should consider the benefits of the proposed treatment in relation to the risks and burdens of treatment, and the adolescent should be involved in the decision-making process. For example, a 17-year-old boy is diagnosed with aplastic anemia. Transplantation technology has improved and is a curative treatment option in this case, but it is critical that the boy be willing to meticulously adhere to the medical regimen necessary to prevent rejection. Although a bone marrow transplant could be performed on a 17-year-old without his consent, the likelihood of success of the transplant depends on his cooperation. Suppose that this 17-year-old has an identical twin. Should the twin be compelled to be a bone marrow donor? What if he has a younger sibling who could provide a close but not identical match; should the sibling be compelled to be a donor? Because the donor procedure involves some risk and discomforts but no therapeutic benefit to the donor, can the parent force the sibling or twin to donate bone marrow? The sibling may desire to help the critically ill adolescent, and may donate for altruistic reasons. The pressure to donate, however, cannot be minimized, so the sibling should be able to speak privately and confidentially with health care providers without other family members present. If the sibling does not want to donate but the parents insist, the health care providers should honor the sibling's refusal.

Another consideration for the adolescent who will have a bone marrow transplant is fertility. Preparation for bone marrow transplantation involves chemotherapy, whole-body irradiation, or both, which can temporarily or permanently alter fertility. Adolescents should be counseled about options, such as cryopreservation of gametes, the pursuant risks, benefits, and costs of the harvesting the gametes, and likelihood of successful pregnancy in the future (Dunstan, 1997).

Nurses can advocate for the adolescent by encouraging his or her inclusion in decisions, using understandable language and inquiring to ensure comprehension, allowing the adolescent to have time to contemplate the information and options, and eliciting his or her perception and wishes. The nurse should also be aware of legal avenues available to the adolescent, in terms of *guardian ad litem* or court proceedings for emancipation of a minor.

ALLOCATION OF RESOURCES

Chapter 9 discussed some of the allocation issues pertaining to children. The lack of affordable, accessible, comprehensive health care for children is a serious problem in the United States, with some areas or groups having health indicators like those of Third World countries (Broffman, 1995). Two additional aspects of resource allocation in children's health care will be discussed here: primary and "sick" care, and the concept of *futility*.

Primary care for children consists of well-child examinations, immunizations, vision and hearing testing, dental examination, anticipatory guidance for caregivers, and other specific evaluations at different developmental periods. Immunizations, critical for the health of the entire population, are available through private physicians, clinics, and public health programs, yet in 2001 only 77.2% of toddlers 19 to 35 months of age received the basic series of vaccines (Wood, 2003). Children of minority or ethnic groups living in poverty in an inner-city or rural area were less likely to get their immunizations. There are fewer pediatricians serving these populations, and these groups have no regular source of primary care (Broffman, 1995). Many of these children receive their "sick" care versus their "well" care through their local emergency department (ED), which is an expensive and inappropriate site for pediatric care. Halfon, Newacheck, Wood, and St. Peter (1996) were surprised that the regular use of the ED was not associated with certain specific recurrent health problems, like tonsillitis, asthma, or febrile seizures, or the parents' health insurance status, such as Medicaid. Children who received their well-child care in neighborhood clinics were more likely to get sick care in the ED. Halfon et al. speculated that there were fewer resources in the neighborhood clinics to operate after hours, on weekends, and at other times when the ED is the only available resource. Controlling for income and insurance status, they found that racial disparities in medical care persisted, with blacks more likely to use the ED than whites.

Friedman (1994) also found that income and insurance were not the only barriers to access to care. She found that nonwhite children and adolescents, regardless of their insurance, had less access to care. This may be related to their geographic location (rural or inner city) and poor transportation options, their family situation (lack of child care for other children, inability of a parent to take time off from work, poor parental health, other family crises taking priority over child health care needs), or an "informal, unconscious barrier" to equality (Friedman, 1994, p. 6). She called for statutes such as civil rights acts and the American with Disabilities Act to be enforced in cases of discrimination.

Allocation of resources is a matter of justice. The inappropriate use of resources such as the ED may represent barriers in access, such as discrimination, lack of pediatric health care providers, and the lack of respect for the competing priorities in families. To improve access for children, there needs to be an ethical analysis of the current structure of health care services.

Another source of ethical tension in pediatric health care is the notion of *futility*. As discussed previously, predicting outcomes for children who are born prematurely or at term but very sick is extremely difficult. Even for children with devastating injuries such as near-drowning or traumatic brain injury, it is impossible to know how the family will respond to the child's condition and prognosis. Nurses have expressed discomfort in repeatedly resuscitating a very sick newborn or continuing intensive care for a child who is not expected to ever regain consciousness. In cases like these, the treatment might be considered futile and the resources invested in futile care might be considered wasted. Futility, however, is a negotiated reality (Rubin, 1998). The goals of treatment should be articulated and discussed with the family. The health care providers may have cure or recovery as the goal of treatment, where the family may want survival as the goal. If the child survives but is significantly disabled, then he or she will need extensive support. Most families do not have resources that would totally cover the costs for 24-hour care nursing, therapies, equipment and supplies, surgeries, hospitalizations, and remodeling of the home to accommodate everything the child needs. In cases where the parents win a lawsuit, there is substantial money available for the child's care. Short of that, most parents who face this situation struggle to piece together insurance, other support from federal, state, or local programs, and personal financial resources. Given that the child's functional level may never improve, society might question the value of investing extensive resources in his or her care. The return on the investment will probably not be measurable in terms of future productivity of the child.

In other cultures or civilizations, children who were unlikely to contribute to the family's resources were killed at birth or abandoned. In the United States, that perspective is unacceptable, yet there is still a tension between keeping a child alive in an unresponsive state and withdrawing life-sustaining treatment. Parents are counseled as to the prognosis and are advised about the projected needs of the child. The options available to the parents may influence their decision about continued treatment. When there is disagreement between parents and health care providers, the case is often referred to the hospital ethics committee. Frader and Watchko (1997) recognized the potential conflict of interest in having the hospital ethics committee, usually composed of hospital employees, advise on a case that could have major financial impact on their institution. Savage and Michalak (2002) found that at one point in time, children who were wards of the state could not have a Do Not Resuscitate (DNR) order because the agency authorizing the order was also paying for the child's care, so the state wished to avoid the conflict of interest and the appearance that treatment was discontinued because of the expense to the state. (It is now possible for children who are wards of the state to have a DNR order, but an ethics consultation is required.) The needs of the child cannot be considered in isolation from the available resources, but at least the criteria of social worth and productivity should be excluded from the decision-making process.

Nurses can assist families to make their decisions by carefully listening to their perspective and goals. Directing them to resources so they can make informed decisions is helpful. Learning of community services, state programs, support groups, and advocacy groups or agencies can help parents in their decision-making, as can knowing of palliative care and hospice programs if they are considering withdrawal of treatment. The nurse can also advocate for the family by informing them how to access and prepare for an ethics consultation.

End-of-Life Care

Although there have been improvements in survival from many conditions that were previously fatal, some conditions remain terminal. The Centers for Disease Control and Prevention lists unintentional injury as the leading cause of death in children of ages 1 to 21 years (Table 11-1) (CDC, 2002). The next-leading causes are congenital anomalies (ages 1 to 4 years), malignant neoplasms (5 to 14 years), and homicides (15 to 21 years). The death of a child seems especially difficult, whether it is from an accident or an acute or chronic illness. In the health care system, death is often orchestrated, which means that death occurs because of deliberate decisions to withhold or withdraw life-sustaining treatment. Decisions to withhold or withdraw treatment occur at every age level and in every health care setting.

Different ethical issues in end-of-life situations will be portrayed in the discussion of the following cases. In the pediatric intensive care unit (PICU), for example, there are three patients: a 13-month-old girl with *Haemophilus influenzae* meningitis who is being evaluated for brain death, a 10-year-old girl with a brainstem glioma, and a 17-year-old boy with a severed spinal cord at C-4, which renders him tetraplegic. In each of these cases, technology affords some hope, but death may occur despite treatment. Each of these cases will be discussed in more detail to illustrate the ethical issues the nurse is likely to encounter.

Illustrative Case 11-1

Shaquita, a 13-month-old, has been diagnosed with *H. influenzae* meningitis; her parents have been informed that she has sustained extensive injury to her brain

Table 11-1	Ten Leading Causes of Death, From Birth to 21 Years of Age				
Rank	<1 Year	1–4 Years	5–9 Years	10–14 Years	15–21 Years
1	Congenital anomalies	Unintentional injury	Unintentional injury	Unintentional injury	Unintentional injury
2	Short gestation	Congenital anomalies	Malignant neoplasms	Malignant neoplasms	Homicide
3	Sudden infant death syndrome	Malignant neoplasms	Congenital anomalies	Suicide	Suicide
4	Maternal pregnancy complications	Homicide	Homicide	Congenital anomalies	Malignant neoplasms
5	Placenta cord membranes	Heart disease	Heart disease	Homicide	Heart disease
6	Respiratory distress	Influenza and pneumonia	Benign neoplasms	Heart disease	Congenital anomalies
7	Unintentional injury	Septicemia	Influenza and pneumonia	Chronic low respiratory disease	Cerebrovascular
8	Bacterial sepsis	Perinatal period	Chronic low respiratory disease	Benign neoplasms	Chronic low respiratory disease
9	Circulatory system disease	Benign neoplasms	Cerebrovascular	Influenza and pneumonia	Influenza and pneumonia
10	Intrauterine hypoxia	Cerebrovascular	Septicemia	Cerebrovascular	AIDS

Adapted from Centers for Disease Control and Prevention. (2002). Web-based Injury Statistics Query and Reporting System (WISQARS). Retrieved December 17, 2003, from www.cdc.gov/ncipc/wisqars.

because of the swelling caused by the infection. She has been aggressively treated to preserve brain function, but tests indicate that she has irreversible cessation of function of the entire brain. The tests have been performed in accordance with the standard of care. The diagnosis is brain death (Table 11-2). The parents are counseled that there is no treatment available, that the ventilator and medications are keeping her heart beating, and that if they are discontinued, she will not survive. In as gentle and compassionate way as possible, the parents are told that in situations like this, the child is considered legally dead and all interventions are stopped. A counselor from the local organ and tissue recovery program discusses options with the parents for organ donation, explaining that life support continues until the organs are retrieved. Parents are given time to be with their child. There may be extended family who are out of town and are on their way to the hospital. Parents may want to consult with their family, close friends, minister, or spiritual adviser about the discontinuation of life support.

Practices vary in involving parents in the decision to withdraw life support in cases of brain death. The determination of *brain death* is based on repeated clinical assessments and tests such as an electroencephalogram (EEG) to yield a clinical diagnosis of whole-brain death (Task Force, 1987). However, state statutes vary in their criteria for declaration of death. Some states, using the Uniform Anatomical Gift Act of 1968 or the Uniform Declaration of Death Act of 1980, adopted statutes on how and when death can be declared by neurological criteria. If the child is in a jurisdiction that recognizes brain death, the health care providers inform the parents of the diagnosis and usually allow them time to deal with the

Table 11-2 Differentiation Between Brain Death and Other Neurologic States

Neurologic State	Breathing	Ability to interact	Cranial nerves	Sleep/wake cycles	Purposeful movements	Confirmatory tests
UNCONSCIOUS	Spontaneous	On awakening	Intact	Sleep only	Absent	Examination
COMA						
Reversible	Spontaneous	Depends on cause of coma	Depends on cause of coma	Sleep only	Absent	Examination; BEP; brain imaging; brain function tests
Irreversible	Spontaneous	Unable to interact	May be present	Sleep/wake cycles	Absent	Exam and above tests; repeated over time
MINIMALLY CONSCIOUS STATE	Spontaneous	Intermittent	Present, but may be impaired	Sleep/wake cycles	Intermittent	Exam and above tests; repeated over time
VEGETATIVE STATE (VS)	Spontaneous	Unable to interact	Present, but may be impaired	Sleep/wake cycles	Absent	Exam and above tests; can be diagnosed 1 month after injury
Persistent VS	Spontaneous	Unable to interact	Present, but may be impaired	Sleep/wake cycles	Absent	Exam and above tests; can be diagnosed 3–6 months after injury
Permanent VS	Spontaneous	Unable to interact	Present, but may be impaired	Sleep/wake cycles	Absent	Exam and above tests; can be diagnosed >6 months after injury
BRAIN DEAD	Absent	Unable to interact	Absent	Absent	Absent	Isoelectric EEG; no CBF

BEP, brainstem-evoked potential; CBF, cerebral blood flow; EEG, electroencephalogram; VS, vegetative state.

information before withdrawing life support. If, however, the jurisdiction permits a religious exemption, so that if the concept of brain death is not recognized by the family's religion, the child with brain death cannot be pronounced dead until criteria for cardiorespiratory death are met. Some of the child's organs may not be suitable for transplant if death occurs through cardiorespiratory cessation, but nurses caring for Shaquita should be advocating for her and her family's best interests and not considering salvaging organs if the parents reject the diagnosis of brain death. If the parents have not expressed a religious objection to the diagnosis of brain death, it is important for Shaquita's nurses to refrain from any discussion about organ donation until the parents have met with a representative from the Organ Procurement Organization (OPO). This is to avoid any suggestion of conflict of interest between Shaquita's interests and the interests of the child awaiting an organ.

Ethical Issues With the Diagnosis of Brain Death

Ethical problems that might occur with the diagnosis of brain death are the refusal of parents to accept brain death as the criterion for determining the death of their child, the appearance of conflict of interest when parents are approached about organ donation, and the general confusion about brain death, permanent coma, and other severe brain injuries.

Refusal to Accept the Diagnosis

The diagnosis of brain death is controversial. For centuries, death was accepted when the heart stopped beating and breathing stopped. With resuscitation and mechanical ventilation, breathing continues and the heart continues to beat. A child on a ventilator appears to be sleeping, especially if the brain injury is atraumatic and there are no obvious wounds, as with an accidental asphyxia or drowning. The body is warm because blood circulates, the chest rises and falls with each breath, and urine is created. Parents may have difficulty understanding how the body can appear normal and be considered "dead," and so they may reject the concept of brain death and not agree to the discontinuation of life-supporting technology. Although there are standards for diagnosing brain death in children and neonates, not all physicians may be skilled in performing the clinical evaluation. Some conditions, such as hypothermia or drug intoxication, can mimic brain death, so the child's body temperature should be within a normal range and a toxicology screen should be negative, although not all drugs can be detected. Confirmatory tests to assess electrical activity and blood flow in the brain are sometimes performed. Even with accurate and repetitive data documenting brain death, parents may not accept the diagnosis.

As mentioned previously, parents may be members of a faith that does not recognize brain death as death. Bernat (2002) claimed that all Christian, Jewish, and Islamic religious groups accept brain death except for a small group of Orthodox Jews. He was unaware of positions held by Eastern religions. In states such as New Jersey that allow a religious exemption to the declaration of death by brain death criteria, the family must provide evidence that brain death declaration would violate the patient's beliefs (New Jersey Advance Directive for Health Care Act). In New Jersey it is possible that a child whose parents reject brain death will not be declared dead until cardiorespiratory death occurs.

Parents' objection to brain death criteria is often attributed to their shock, grief, and unwillingness to accept the loss of their child. Because these are appropriate feelings, parents may not accept death until the heart stops and the body cools. Bernat (2002) advised clear, compassionate communication with the family. He added that physicians are not obligated to continue aggressive treatment in children with brain death, and the discontinuation of hemodynamic support may precipitate a cardiovascular death. However, parents may see withdrawal of medication as no different than other life-sustaining treatment and oppose any change that could result in the child's death. Bernat encouraged physicians to inform parents, if relevant, that an insurance company may not cover any costs after brain death has been declared.

Appearance of Conflict of Interest

Many states and/or institutions have specific policies regarding who may approach a family to discuss organ donation. The institution may have a counselor from their organ transplant program or someone from the OPO meet with the family after a diagnosis of brain death has been made. Parents must be assured that their child's health care providers are acting in their child's best interests and not in the interests of another child in need of an organ, so the request for donation should come from someone not directly involved in the child's care. Therefore, nurses should not discuss organ donation with the parents before the OPO representative's discussion with the parents. After that, however, nurses can share and clarify information about organ donation.

General Confusion Regarding Brain Death/Injuries

The public may not understand the differences among unconsciousness, coma, irreversible coma, vegetative state, minimally conscious state, and brain death. The distinctions are crucial for ethical decision-making. When the child is not brain dead, treatment options are based on accurate diagnosis and prognosis (Table 11-2). Decisions also may depend on the resources available to the family. The nurse and other members of the health care team can assist families to identify resources, such as home health programs, rehabilitation centers, and government agencies providing financial and other assistance. Accessibility to necessary resources will influence treatment decisions, which, in turn, will influence ethical decision-making by the parents.

Illustrative Case 11-2

Lisa is a 10-year-old girl with a brainstem glioma. Her parents desire every possible treatment to combat the cancer and extend her life. She has undergone several chemotherapy regimens, radiation, and high-dose steroids. A ventriculo-peritoneal shunt was placed to treat obstructive hydrocephalus. She required a tracheostomy and gastrostomy because the tumor affected her ability to swallow and protect her airway. Her parents realize she is dying, but want all life-sustaining treatment to be given. They also do not want anyone to tell her she is dying. This poses a problem for the health care providers who believe she should be told if she asks. Some of the staff believe that she would be more comfortable if a palliative approach versus a curative approach were to be taken. In conversations with the parents, the staff suggested a palliative approach, including a DNR order, but the parents stated that to abandon the attempt to cure would feel like they were giving up hope. Some institutions require the parents to sign a document indicating their consent for withdrawal of life support and to consent to a DNR order. Parents have remarked about the great difficulty in signing a "death warrant" for their child, so institutions should re-evaluate their policies in forcing parents to sign such a document. The staff also argued among themselves about whether she should be in the PICU because she is not going to survive. To address the ethical concerns of the staff (truth-telling, advocacy, allocation of resources) an ethics consultation was requested.

The ethics consultant met with the family, then met with the staff, and suggested a joint meeting. At the meeting, the goals of Lisa's care were discussed. All parties believed they were advocating for Lisa's best interests. Her parents believed they must fight for her to be kept alive; the staff believed Lisa's treatment was painful to her and futile in terms of survival to discharge. They believed that no further life-sustaining treatment should be provided and she should receive maximal comfort care. The parents believed that if Lisa was told that she is dying, she would give up hope and die sooner than if she was not told. The staff believed Lisa was aware she was dying and should have an opportunity to ask questions and prepare for death. The parents expressed a concern that Lisa would be "abandoned" by the staff if she had a DNR order; they also viewed any transfer out of the PICU as abandonment. The ethics consultant facilitated communication between the parents and the PICU staff, and goals for Lisa's care were negotiated. After exploring other options including hospice and home hospice, it was decided that Lisa would remain in the PICU with all her treatments continued, but would not be resuscitated. The family's minister and pediatric oncology clinical nurse specialist would help the parents talk to Lisa about dying when she showed a readiness to discuss it. This plan respects parental autonomy in decision-making for Lisa, but also addresses the moral distress of the staff.

Illustrative Case 11-3

Bobby is a 17-year-old whose spinal cord was incompletely severed during a collision with another player on the ice at a hockey game. His cord was damaged at the C-4 level, and so he has a loss of movement and intermittent sensation below his shoulders. He requires a ventilator at this time, but may be successfully weaned in the future. He has repeatedly asked his parents to stop his ventilator so that he may die; he says he does not want to live if he cannot play hockey. His father has asked the health care team to acquiesce to his son's wishes. His mother does not want the ventilator discontinued, and says she will go to court to prevent it, if necessary. The pediatric subspecialists who are involved in Bobby's care indicate that it is possible that Bobby will live another 25 years, and he could be somewhat independent with assistive devices. They also suggest that research may afford some improvement in function over the next 25 years. The pediatric intensivists believe Bobby's reaction is not unusual, and that his request for withdrawing the ventilator should be denied at this time. Paternalism in pediatrics is common; authority figures, such as parents and health care professionals, often act against the wishes of the child, who they believe is not capable of making health care decisions. In Bobby's situation, however, his father supports Bobby's decision to withdraw the ventilator. If parents are the surrogates with regard to their child's autonomy, how is the decision to be made when the parents are in conflict?

The health care team opposes withdrawal of the ventilator. They believe that Bobby's reaction is transient and he will eventually adapt and be thankful that he did not die. Because they believe he will likely recover the ability to breathe without the ventilator, they feel withdrawal is tantamount to assisting his suicide. Bobby and his father believe his quality of life, if he cannot play hockey, will be intolerable. He cannot imagine someone tending to his bodily functions, he cannot envision ever having a sexual relationship, he does not see how he could attend college (he was planning to earn an athletic scholarship), or how he could work in marketing. Despite the efforts of the health care team to dispel Bobby's fears and present him with factual information, Bobby and his father ask that the ventilator be withdrawn. Can and should the health care team advocate for keeping Bobby on the ventilator, against his and his father's wishes?

Rehabilitation specialists often see patients who initially react to their situation with shock and horror. With adults, they would carefully assess decision-making capacity and negotiate with the adult who is refusing treatment for a trial of therapy. This apparent challenge to the patient's autonomy is warranted because the decision to forgo treatment does not allow room for error. With children such as Bobby, it is even more complex to ascertain his wishes and his parents' wishes and determine the right course of action. It would be precipitous to discontinue Bobby's treatment at this point, but he and his father are requesting this. His mother, however, objects, so the physicians may insist on consensus in the family. Even then, however, the physicians might resist discontinuing life-sustaining treatment until they allow Bobby and his parents some time to adjust and deliberate on the request to withdraw treatment. *Rescuing Jeffrey* is a short book describing the diving accident of a 17-year-old boy and his father's quest to have his son's life support discontinued (Galli, 2000). The book is an account of the 10 days following the accident from the father's perspective. The difference between the previous scenario and Jeffrey's situation lies in the extent of the injuries (Jeffrey's injury was more extensive and his paralysis greater) and the fact that Jeffrey's father did not consult with his son about discontinuing life support. The book is highly recommended for nurses to give them the view of a parent facing a decision about life-sustaining treatment.

SUMMARY

Nurses should continue to work with parents who are in conflict over their child's treatment decision, and often can facilitate communication through patient-care conferences. Clarification of goals and the child's interests seem obvious, but often are not explicitly stated and discussed. If parents remain in conflict and it becomes necessary to have a decision made (such as when surgical consent is needed), one of the parents may have to go to court to seek custody for purposes of health care decision-making.

CLINICAL EXERCISES

1. Investigate your state's law on adolescent consent for medical treatment. Compare with your institution's policies on treating adolescents without parental consent.
2. Investigate your clinical agency's policy on disclosing information related to children to adults other than the parents. Does this policy address non-custodial parents and other family members, such as grandparents or adult siblings who accompany the child to see the health care provider?
3. Investigate whether your clinical agency has a policy on HIV testing in children and adolescents. How are the results of testing communicated to the child?
4. Investigate your clinical agency's circumcision consent practices. When assigned to a mother/baby boy/father, observe how circumcision is discussed. Were the elements of informed consent present?

Discussion Questions

1. Mutan, a 13-year-old girl, is in the clinic today for a school physical. A male nurse practitioner introduces himself and explains he will be performing her school physical. She refuses to undress. Her father insists on a female nurse practitioner or a female physician. How should this situation be handled? What are the ethical issues involved?

2. Daphne, 17, is hospitalized for probable pyelonephritis. She denies being sexually active, but her tests reveal she has pelvic inflammatory disease and chlamydia and not pyelonephritis. Her mother asks you, the nurse caring for Daphne, whether the tests are back yet and, if so, what they showed. You have seen the test results. What do you tell Daphne's mother?

3. How would you respond if the father of a 3-day-old preterm baby with respiratory distress syndrome and intraventricular hemorrhage asks you, "How aggressive do we have to be? Do we have to agree to every treatment, just because this hospital has the technology?"

4. For part of your pediatric rotation, you are spending the day in a school-based clinic at a local grade school. You are doing the initial assessment for an 8-year-old girl who presents with a stomachache. The girl asks you, "Will you promise not to tell my mom if I tell you something?" How would you respond?

SECTION 2: *Decision-Making*

One primary difference between ethical issues in adult care and in the care of children is how autonomy is exercised. Children are not considered autonomous, although they may have the requisite abilities for making health care decisions by adolescence. Central to most of the ethical issues involving children is the determination of who speaks for the child. The law endorses the parents as the party responsible for the child's welfare, and gives them the authority to make decisions for the child. Parents get wide latitude for making decisions related to health, education, and childrearing. Parents can reject mandatory programs, such as newborn screening, immunizations, and public education, if they do not fit with their childrearing practices. Even decisions to forgo life-sustaining medical treatment can be made by parents. Only in the case of suspected or proven child abuse and/or neglect is parental authority abrogated to another surrogate.

SURROGATE DECISION-MAKING

There are two standards employed in surrogate decision-making: the substituted judgment and the best interests standard.

Decision-Making Using Substituted Judgment Standard

The surrogate for an adult is expected to use a *substituted judgment* standard (President's Commission for the Study of Ethical Problems in Medicine and Biomedical and

Behavioral Research, 1983), in which the surrogate makes the decision that the incapacitated adult would make. If Mr. Akbar, an adult who has had a stroke and is in a coma, needs surgery, the surrogate would be the person Mr. Akbar designated in his durable power of attorney for health care (DPAHC). If he does not have a DPAHC, the state may have an applicable statute that identifies a surrogate for the purposes of consenting or refusing medical treatment. For example, in the state of Illinois, the Health Care Surrogate Act permits a surrogate to be selected from a prioritized list (see Chapter 12, Box 12-5, for this act), which includes, in hierarchical order, legal guardian, spouse, adult son or daughter, parent, adult sibling, adult grandchild, close friend, and guardian of the person's estate (755 ILCS 40/25, Section 25, Paragraph 1, 2003). The surrogate must make the decisions he or she believes the incapacitated patient would make. In Mr. Akbar's case, his wife is identified as his surrogate. The surrogate exercises autonomy on behalf of the patient because he is incapacitated. The health care team gives her the information regarding Mr. Akbar's condition and why surgery is being recommended. Based on how she believes her husband would make the decision, Mrs. Akbar will either consent to or refuse treatment. She may want the surgery to be done, but the decision is based on whether she thinks Mr. Akbar would want it done.

Decision-Making Using Best Interests Standard

There is an assumption that children have not reached a maturational level required to make many of their own decisions. Children have an emerging autonomy as they develop and mature. Parents are appropriately paternalistic; they make decisions by deciding what they believe is best. They may allow their children to make some decisions, such as which musical instrument they want to learn, what sport or hobby they would like to pursue, or how they want their room decorated, but they usually do not allow a child to decide whether to have surgery, take medicine, or forgo other recommended medical treatment. There are exceptions, which will be discussed later in this chapter. Substituted judgment is inappropriate or impossible to carry out in most cases in pediatrics because the child does not have a clear or well-defined values system. Exceptions may be older adolescents (e.g., 17-year-olds) and children who are more mature than typical for their age due to life experiences, such as a severe illness or trauma, or who have been exposed to the death of loved ones. Therefore, parents (or legal guardians) are expected to use the *best interests* standard (President's Commission for the Study of Ethical Problems in Medicine and Biomedical and Behavioral Research, 1983). According to this standard, the surrogate makes a decision that will "promote the patient's good" (p. 179). Parents consider what is in their child's best interests. What are the goals of the proposed treatment? What are the likely benefits and burdens associated with the treatment and the sequelae? What will the child's life be like if the treatment is given, or not given? What is the likelihood of success of the treatment? What other treatment decisions will need to be made after this one; in other words, will the treatment decision be the first on a trajectory of decisions? Depending on the child's ability to express an opinion, should the child's preferences be elicited? How much weight should those preferences have? As discussed previously, the child's developmental level, as assessed in relation to a specific decision to be made, determines whether he or she is included in the decision-making process.

Parents are given information, usually on more than one occasion, have their questions answered, and can consult with those people whose opinions they value, such as relatives, friends, or spiritual advisors. How the information is shared with parents can influence their decision. Health care professionals who believe a treatment should be given usually use language that reveals the decision they favor. Parents seek the advice of professionals, who are expected to give their best judgment, but parents then must decide whether the treatment will be in their child's best interests.

For example, Barbara is a 20-month-old with a history of frequent ear infections. Her parents have had her seen by the pediatrician numerous times. Because her language is developing very slowly, her pediatrician recommended that she see a pediatric otolaryngologist, or ear-nose-and-throat (ENT) physician. The ENT physician recommends insertion of pressure-equalizing (PE) tubes, or middle-ear ventilating tubes, to reduce the fluid in the middle ear. The fluid interferes with hearing, thereby interfering with Barbara's language development. The risks and potential benefits of the procedure are explained to Barbara's parents. They are advised that this is a critical learning period for Barbara, so improving her hearing at this time is very important. They consult with their pediatrician and talk to other parents who faced the same decision. Deciding that the potential benefits outweigh the risks, they agree to the procedure. They did not ask Barbara, who is too young to understand. They believe that having PE tubes inserted in Barbara's tympanic membranes is in her best interests.

Suppose that, instead of ear infections, Barbara has a hearing loss that may be treated with a cochlear implant. The efficacy of the implant is debatable, and there is more risk with this surgery than with PE tubes. Parents consider the goals of surgery: Barbara will be able to hear better than she does now. The risks are those associated with neurosurgery and anesthesia. There is also the risk that the implant will not work or will have side effects that outweigh the benefits. Parents are given the latitude to decide whether the potential benefits outweigh the risks. They may talk to people who had the surgery and to parents of children who either decided to have the surgery or opted not to. Barbara's parents also may want to consult with the communication specialists who work with Barbara and get their opinion of the cochlear implants. If the parents peruse the Internet, they may find a myriad of opinions on cochlear implants. Again, the decision is solely the parents.

Now suppose that Barbara's parents are deaf. They are part of a deaf culture in which the ability to hear is unimportant. They do not accept a cochlear implant for their child. Barbara's speech therapist, who has been teaching her sign language, believes that Barbara would be able to hear if she had the cochlear implant. Parents still have the right to decide what is in their child's best interests. To change this scenario slightly, imagine that Barbara had a hearing loss amenable to external hearing aids. Should her parents be able to prohibit Barbara from using hearing aids because they want her to remain deaf? There may be compelling reasons why the speech therapist believes Barbara should use a hearing aid, but the parents have the right to prohibit the use of the hearing aid on Barbara. The speech therapist believes it is in Barbara's best interests to use hearing aids to improve her hearing; her parents believe it is in Barbara's best interests for them to reject hearing aids because being deaf is more desirable in their culture. There is a clash of values between the speech therapist, who values hearing, and the parents, who do not.

Child's Best Interest Versus the Family's Best Interest

The speech therapist may believe that the parents are making the decision in their interests, not in Barbara's best interests. However, the parents believe they are making the decision in the best interests of their family, which includes Barbara. Should the child's interests be made in isolation from the family's interests? Let's say that Barbara's family supports the surgery for the implant, but cannot afford it. Should the parents be able to decide based on the allocation of their resources? Should Barbara be removed from the family so she can get an implant? It seems drastic to separate a child from her parents for a non–life-threatening condition. In rare cases, children are removed from their parents' custody for medical treatment. When treatment is life-saving and clearly efficacious, the courts have awarded temporary custody to the physician (or hospital administrator) for the purposes of consenting to medical treatment. Refusal of treatment based on religious reasons, such as refusal of blood by Jehovah's Witnesses, is an example.

Assent

If Barbara were an adolescent, her preferences might be solicited. If she wanted the implant but her parents refused, she might want to petition the court to become a mature minor so that she could give consent for herself. Assent is a very important concept in the care of children. Historically, children were considered chattel of their parents. Although infanticide was illegal, it was not vigorously prosecuted. Children were used in the labor force until child labor laws were passed. The old adage, "Children should be seen and not heard," represents the paternalism that was pervasive in U.S. culture up until the 1960s. As the consumer movement, the women's movement, and the patients' rights movement progressed, attention was focused on children's rights. W. G. Bartholome was among the first pediatricians and ethicists to call for inclusion of children in decision-making. He was instrumental in drafting the American Academy of Pediatrics (AAP) Position Statement on Informed Consent, Parental Permission, and Assent in Pediatric Practice (American Academy of Pediatrics Committee on Bioethics, 1995). *Assent* is affirmative agreement; *consent* is the legal concept of agreeing, and can only be given by adults or emancipated or mature minors. Parents give or refuse their permission (proxy consent) for their children to accept treatment. Children are asked to give their assent for interventions; parents are asked to give *informed permission*.

After the position statement was published, though, Bartholome (1995) sent a letter to the editor of *Pediatrics* detailing some concerns. He found some of the additions to the statement worrisome, such as the statement that physicians and parents could exclude children from the decision-making process for "persuasive reasons." His worry was that this excuse would be used routinely to exclude children. It might reflect parents' discomfort or inexperience in discussing life-and-death issues with their children or a lack of respect for the child's right to participate in health care decision-making. Bartholome advocated always including children in the decision-making process according to their capacity and willingness to participate.

His second concern was a statement declaring that an impasse between parents and children is rare, whereas he thought that impasses are common and harmony was rare. The view that parents and children often agree is "hopelessly romantic" (Bartholome, 1995, p. 981). The health care provider, then, has a role in facilitating discussion between the parents and children. In those instances where the child's refusal would not be honored, Bartholome disagreed with the policy statement that recommended not seeking assent if this were the case. Assent should be sought and the dialogue should continue. A compromise may be possible, or if the intervention must be performed, Bartholome argued that the pediatrician should inform the child and apologize for having to "force" the intervention on him or her. He acknowledged that this level of respect toward children is unusual, but believed society should move in that direction.

Zawistowski and Frader (2003) (the latter author contributed to the 1995 AAP Position Statement on Informed Consent, Parental Permission, and Assent in Pediatric Practice) endorsed Bartholome's views of assent and cited evidence that older children and adolescents, especially those with chronic illnesses, may be capable of participating in their health care decisions. They urged pediatric intensivists to assess a child's ability to participate and to obtain assent, even with younger children, if they are capable and willing to participate.

The movement to recognize the rights of children to participate in decision-making is not uniquely American. In 1999, a 15-year-old girl refused a heart transplant, but her decision was overruled by the United Kingdom's High Court, and she underwent the transplant against her will. Dixon-Woods, Young, and Heney (1999) observed that the courts are not in sync with the growing movement for children's rights. They called for research to investigate:

1. The outcomes of joint decision-making with children.
2. Vehicles for assessing decision-making capacity.
3. The creation of developmentally appropriate informational materials.
4. Models of decision-making involving a family perspective.

The reader can see how the ethics of the situation changes as the details change. Terms like "best interests" are subject to interpretation. Furthermore, children can be included in the decision-making process depending on their maturational level and experience with decision-making and their parents' preferences for including them.

SUMMARY

Children's autonomy is exercised by their parents, or, in some cases, a legal guardian because children are assumed to lack the abilities to make health care decisions. As children grow and mature, they acquire language and reasoning skills, but still may lack the judgment and wisdom to make decisions. As part of the maturational process, over time parents give children choices of increasing importance. Penticuff (1990) referred to the nurse's role in protecting a child's "determining self," which she described as the potential for the child to understand his or her circumstances and formulate goals within the family context. Experiences within the health care system that a child with a chronic illness or disability often has may accelerate the acquisition of decision-making abilities. However, both a child's ability to participate in decision-making and the parents' willingness to include the child should be assessed. Paternalism continues to be arguably appropriate in pediatrics. Nurses have a role in facilitating informed decision-making in families, thereby honoring the child's autonomy as exercised by the parents.

CLINICAL EXERCISES

1. What is your institution's policy on Do Not Resuscitate orders? Is there a policy permitting family members to be present during resuscitation? How

do the nurses on your unit feel about family presence during resuscitation?
2. When rotating through a pediatric clinical setting, observe how the staff nurses and/or physicians assess assent from children.
3. Contact your clinical agency or university/college Institutional Review Board to see a copy of the standardized language they require for obtaining a child's assent to participate in research.

Discussion Questions

1. Javon, a 15-year-old who has end-stage renal disease, has been on dialysis and is now requesting that his dialysis be stopped. Discuss the process for determining whether his request should be honored.
2. As a nurse on the pediatric unit, you are assigned to a 6-year-old male child from a Latin American country, who is diagnosed with a terminal illness. He and his parents immigrated two years ago and speak some English. Once it is predicted by his health care team that he has only a couple of days to live, what factors need to be considered and how would you approach the parents regarding organ donation?

SECTION 3: *The Moral Status of Children*

From the moment the umbilical cord is cut, the child is an independent person with a moral and legal standing in society. Parents and society have a duty to provide for children so they may grow and develop. Unlike in past centuries, children are not considered the property of their parents. Although parents have the liberty of making decisions for their children, there is a threshold that parents must meet in taking care of them (food, clothing, shelter). Community standards may vary, but reasonable people should agree on what constitutes neglect and abuse. Many of the rights that children have are negative rights—the rights not to be abused or neglected. Nurses are mandatory reporters, that is, if a nurse suspects abuse or neglect, he or she is mandated to report it to the appropriate authorities. Parents have wide latitude in raising children. They may choose whether or not to have their children immunized, send them to public school, or use corporal punishment as discipline. Parents may also decide whether to accept or refuse life-sustaining treatment for their sick or injured child.

The moral status of the child evolves with the child's development. As a fetus the child has no legal standing, and has legal protections only once viability is reached. There have been cases where a fetus has been harmed by the mother's actions, such as ingestion of illicit substances. Women have been prosecuted for the deaths of their full-term fetuses. Drastic measures have been taken such as imprisoning pregnant women to protect their fetuses from the mother's drug use, but these measures have been unsuccessful and declared unconstitutional (*Ferguson et al. v. City of Charleston et al.*, 2001). Children have been afforded more legal protections, which reveal society's view of their moral status. Child labor laws and laws requiring that children give consent regarding access to their medical records and assent in clinical research represent progress in recognizing the moral status of children. A pluralistic society that embraces and tolerates all kinds of child-rearing practices needs to be vigilant to protect vulnerable children. Under certain conditions, children may have their moral status as persons questioned, as when disabilities are present or likely to evolve after illness or injury. We will discuss a number of these conditions.

PERSONHOOD

One is likely to get a variety of responses to the questions of what constitutes a person and what characterizes personhood. Is being a human being the same as being a person? The animals classified as primates include humans, apes, and other nonhuman species. Without delving into issues relating to the moral status of nonhumans, we can state that they do not have the same moral status as humans. Although in many Western cultures nonhuman primates are not consumed as food, they are used in medical research and when no longer needed destroyed like property. Despite the efforts of groups supporting the moral equivalence of nonhuman animals to humans, in most cultures even highly intelligent animals do not have the moral status of personhood.

Thus, one criterion of personhood is membership in the species *Homo sapiens*. With the ability to identify DNA, one can identify an embryo as being of the human species versus another species. Do the ovum and the sperm constitute a person at the moment they unite? Or is the entity a person at the embryo, fetus, or newborn stage? The assignment of personhood rests with the beholder. Certain religious faiths view the conceptus, even prior to implantation, as a person, whereas others do not accept the personhood of an infant until day 28 of life. Is the concept of personhood relative? Fletcher (1972), a philosopher and ethicist, proposed criteria for humanhood for the purposes of stimulating debate. He used the terms "humanhood" and "personhood" interchangeably. Box 11-1 summarize his positive and negative criteria for humanhood.

Fletcher did not suggest that to be a person, one must fulfill all the positive and negative criteria he mentioned, but merely offered them for debate. From a practical point of view, some authors have argued that if a human lacks personhood, it is acceptable to withhold resources, such as life-sustaining treatment, and their reasoning is reflected in clinical decisions.

Three philosophers have supported withholding life-sustaining treatment from certain infants. Singer (1979), whose appointment as a professor in philosophy at Princeton was vigorously protested by disability activists, has long maintained that it should be morally permissible to kill a newborn who has disabilities. Because certain disabled newborns lack the capability of becoming sentient, Singer believed that their parents should have the option of killing them. Furthermore, as an animal liberation activist, Singer argued that it is "speciesism" to discriminate against animals because they are not members of the human species. Human newborns do not have the ability to communicate, as do some adult apes, so if personhood relies on the ability to communicate, then, Singer argued, apes should have the moral status of persons whereas newborns should not. Tooley (1983) sought consistency between the ethical justification for aborting an infant who has or is at risk for a disability and killing a newborn who has or is at risk for a disability. He also attempted to describe criteria for personhood and believed that the use of language is critical to personhood, which would leave many infants and young children in limbo until their

BOX 11-1

Positive and Negative Criteria for Personhood

Positive:

Minimal intelligence

Self-awareness

Self-control

A sense of time

A sense of futurity

A sense of the past—memory

Capability to relate to others

Concern for others

Communication

Curiosity

Change and changeability

Idiosyncrasy

Neocortical function

Negative (i.e., humans are not):

Antitechnology (e.g., in vitro fertilization is OK)

Essentially sexual (e.g., cloning)

A bundle of rights (e.g., rights are relative)

Compelled to worship (e.g., it's a choice)

Source: Fletcher, J. (1972). Indicator of humanhood: A tentative profile of man. *Hastings Center Report*, 2, 1–4.

language skills developed. Another philosopher to exclude newborns as persons is Englehardt (1975), who argued that having a self-concept is critical to personhood, and newborns lack a self-concept.

Secular philosophers as well as sectarian philosophers separate the infant and young child from the older child in determining personhood. Richard McCormick (1974), a priest and Catholic theologian, also supported the position that it was permissible to withhold life-sustaining treatment from infants who are "abnormal" and unlikely to develop human relationships. The philosophers who believe that treatment can be withheld from certain newborns base their positions on the limited cognitive abilities of these newborns. If the newborn lacks the cognitive abilities to think, reason, and plan and will likely never develop them, then these philosophers would find it permissible to withhold or withdraw treatment. Some, such as Singer and Tooley, might go one step further and permit actively taking the life of the newborn who is cognitively impaired or at risk of impairment. Their arguments are primarily utilitarian, based on the view that resources should be invested to maximize utility. If the cognitive impairments cannot be corrected or sufficiently ameliorated, then the investment of resources for these newborns would be unwise because it does not maximize utility. Categorizing these newborns as "nonpersons" justifies, to those who subscribe to this reasoning, the utilitarian allocation of resources. From a deontological perspective, human worth cannot be measured. A utilitarian might argue that society does not have the same obligations to nonpersons and that there may be value in using the organs of a nonperson to transplant into a person. A deontologist such as Kant would argue that a person should never be a means to someone else's end. Would Kant have accepted that newborns are not persons? Newborns with anencephaly may be the type of case that raises the question of personhood.

Newborns with Anencephaly

Early in gestation, if the neural tube fails to close, a defect occurs in which the brain matter is exposed and the cerebral cortex is absent. This defect is called *anencephaly*. It can be diagnosed with prenatal screening through the use of maternal serum or amniotic alpha-fetoprotein and with ultrasound confirmation. When the condition is discovered prenatally, most such pregnancies are aborted; half of the pregnancies that go to term result in stillborns (Bernat, 2002). Although infants with anencephaly behave similarly to other newborns (e.g., they can suck, swallow, cry, and have intact spinal reflexes), the condition is considered terminal. Death usually results from non-treatment of apnea or infection. With the failure of xenotransplantation for newborns and the early disappointing results in treating hypoplastic left heart syndrome, interest grew in using infants with anencephaly as organ donors. The problem is that if one waits until the infant meets brain death criteria, the organs will likely suffer hypoxia and be unusable. Efforts to have infants with anencephaly declared brain dead at birth or to declare that they are not persons and could be sacrificed have met with opposition. The American Medical Association Council on Ethical and Judicial Affairs (1995) issued a policy statement in support of using infants with anencephaly as multiple-organ donors, but because of intense criticism and opposition, it reverted to its previous position opposing their use. Because infants with anencephaly lack the physiological substrate—the brain tissue—to ever satisfy Fletcher's criteria, is it permissible to withhold or withdraw life-sustaining treatment? There are two cases in the ethics literature regarding infants with anencephaly, in which the cranium and cortex were missing although the brainstem and spinal cord were present.

Baby K. was born in October 1992 in Virginia. Her case was thrust into the media spotlight because of a dispute between her mother and the health care providers at a local hospital (*In the Matter of Baby "K,"* 1994). When her respiratory effort began to fail, which was expected with anencephaly, Baby K was placed on a ventilator. Her physicians counseled her mother that Baby K would die in a few days from this brain defect, so "aggressive treatment would serve no therapeutic or palliative purpose" (p. e3). However, the mother did not agree, and aggressive treatment was continued. Baby K was weaned from the ventilator and transferred to a nursing home, but was brought back to the hospital three times because of respiratory distress. The hospital sought a court order to refuse treatment for Baby K, and, on not receiving it, appealed. The court of appeals affirmed the lower court ruling that the hospital was legally bound to stabilize the infant, based on the Emergency Medical Treatment and Active Labor Act (EMTALA). The courts were not willing to comment on the appropriateness or inappropriateness of aggressive treatment for infants with anencephaly, but an affirmation of such an infant's right to treatment under EMTALA signifies the legal personhood of the infant.

The second case is that of Baby Theresa Campo, born in Florida in the same year as Baby K. Baby Theresa's parents were aware since the eighth month of gestation that she had anencephaly. On the advice of their physicians, they planned for delivery via Caesarean section at term so that the baby's organs could be harvested for donation to other infants. Because anencephaly does not mean brain death, the health care providers feared prosecution if they retrieved Baby Theresa's organs before she was declared dead. The parents sought judicial determination that anencephaly qualified as legal death. Three courts, including the Supreme Court of Florida, refused to equate anencephaly with death and stated that it would have been illegal to take Baby's Theresa's organs prior to her whole-brain death (*In RE T.A.C.P.*, 1992). She died at 9 days of age, and her organs were not harvested for donation. Again the court upheld the legal personhood of the infant with anencephaly. The court also acknowledged in its deliberations that there is concern for the "slippery slope," that is, the use of infants with anencephaly as organ donors could lead to the use of other infants with less severe brain disorders.

Although anencephaly is the most severe brain malformation, there are other neurological conditions in which the cortex is absent or malformed. These infants can often survive with careful medical and nursing care, but do not develop and mature. Current methods of measuring cognitive function indicate that these infants remain at the developmental level of a newborn. They gain weight and grow in length, but do not acquire the developmental skills required to roll over, sit unsupported, stand, or communicate. Are they persons in the moral sense? Although some philosophers would argue against the view that they are not persons, Veatch (1975) proposed that neocortical death should be considered a form of legal death. He argued that the cortex holds the essential nature of a person and its irrevocable loss is equivalent to death. Infants with anencephaly and children with irreversible loss of cortical functioning would fall into this category. Infants with hydranencephaly or holoprosencephaly, where the cortex is missing and replaced with cerebrospinal fluid, might also fall into Veatch's category. His proposal, however, has not received much support. Questions abound, such as how could death occur so that organs could be usable because there is no life support to withdraw other than nutrition and hydration, and how much time should elapse before there is certainty about the irreversibility of the loss of cortical functioning? If neocortical death was adopted as another definition of legal death, does that mean that the thousands of people now living in a vegetative state would be considered dead? Should people with dementia or a brain disorder of the cortex that drastically and irreversibly alters their cognitive functioning fall into this category of neocortical death? Although these might seem like questions out of a science fiction story, the use of neocortical death as a criterion for organ donation recently has been proposed.

Accepting that the "continuum from near brain death to brain death is murky," Ferguson and Zuk (2003, p. 219) advocated obtaining organs from children in their PICU for whom withdrawal of treatment is planned (with parental consent). Given that the incidence of brain death in children is on the decline, they believe the donor pool could be markedly increased (they estimated a 72% increase in their unit) by the inclusion of children with "isolated head injury." The decision to withdraw life-sustaining treatment is made independent of the discussion of organ donation. They recognize that the existence of a policy like this could affect decision-making regarding futility of life-sustaining treatment. Initial reaction to this so-called Pittsburgh Protocol when it was aired on a segment of CBS's *60 Minutes* newsmagazine revealed that the public might not be ready for non-heart-beating donation (now referred to as donation after cardiac death), and such a proposal furthers the perception that critically ill people may not be effectively treated if the institution desires to increase its donor pool.

There have been descriptions of categories of personhood: potential persons, former persons, and nonpersons. A *potential person* is a fetus, embryo, or fertilized ovum that has the potential to develop into a human person. A *former person* is someone who was once a person but lost the cognitive capacity required to be a person. Permanent loss of the cortical functions of the brain might render a person a former person. People in irreversible coma or in a persistent vegetative state are former persons. *Nonpersons* are those humans who never acquired the capacity to be a person. Children with anencephaly, hydranencephaly, or other neurological conditions fall into the nonperson category. The obligations to a potential person are different than those to a person; the same goes for the former person and the nonperson. The language may offend some, but it reflects the harsh reality of allocation decisions.

Infanticide

Some people bristle at the characterization of withholding or withdrawing treatment of newborns as infanticide. Some consider withholding life-sustaining medical treatment for an infant with or at risk of a disabling condition as infanticide (Gross, 2002). Gross (2002) believed that the practice is not uncommon in U.S. neonatal intensive care units. Others view the practice of withholding or withdrawing as removing unwanted medical treatment, and therefore allowing the dying process to proceed. Infanticide, however, does occur outside of hospitals.

During 1989 to 1998, the infant murder rate in the United States was 8.3 per 100,000 person-years. The majority (95%) of infants who are murdered on the day of birth or within the first few days of life are born outside hospitals. The perpetrators are usually adolescent mothers with a history of mental illness. The CDC speculated that there might be more murders that go unreported because the deaths are attributed to unintentional injuries or sudden infant death syndrome (CDC, 2002). Whereas female infanticide is more prevalent in countries, such as India and China, infanticide in industrialized countries does not seem to be gender-specific. Some states have instituted infant abandonment laws that encourage a safe, confidential procedure for mothers to anonymously relinquish their infants to state custody rather than abandon them (Dailard, 2000). Critics of these laws call them overly simplistic and suggest that prevention of unwanted pregnancies and improved social support for mothers would be a better solution.

In developing countries, female infanticide occurs more often than male infanticide. In China, for example, the female infanticide rate is 15.5 per 100,000 person-years compared with 8.3 per 100,000 person-years for male infants. Sons are preferred, and with the one-child policy, female infants are murdered so that the couple can try again to bear a son. When a woman marries, she leaves her family and joins her husband's family and cares for her in-laws through their elder years. Having a son is insurance for care through one's own old age. In India, ultrasound and subsequent abortion of females may replace infanticide. It is very difficult for a bride's family to afford her wedding expenses and dowry, which can cost as much as ten times a father's annual income. Both China and India now are seeing a disproportionate number of males to females in the population, which will pose problems when the men search for women to marry. Discounting the value of females in infancy will have a far-reaching effect on these societies (Gendercide Watch, 2005).

SUMMARY

Children do not have the same moral status as adults, as evidenced by their treatment in infancy or when they lack certain attributes. Assigning personhood is one way of determining what obligations are owed and what resources should be allocated. If there were no scarcity of resources, would society bother with the categorization of some humans as nonpersons or former persons?

Moral status is not an "all or none" phenomenon. Moral status, signified by the exercise of autonomy, is an evolving process. As discussed in this section, children acquire the capacities for decision-making as they grow and mature. Their parents still maintain decision-making authority, but may inform their children and attempt to elicit their assent for participation in health care activities. This respect for their preferences confers a moral status on children as persons.

There may also be a conflation between the moral status of the fetus and the moral status of the child once born. Arguably the fetus has some rights (discussed in Chapter 13), and when maternal rights are in conflict with fetal rights, maternal rights usually supersede those of the fetus. Because abortion on demand in the first trimester (1 to 12 weeks postconception) is legal in the United States, the fetus is treated like the property of the pregnant woman. In the second trimester (12 to 24 weeks postconception), abortion can also be performed for genetic reasons or if the mother's life is in danger. If an infant is born prematurely at 22 weeks of gestation, there is a risk that the infant will eventually display impairments because of complications of prematurity. Yet there is no consensus on whether the mother (or both parents) could request that the infant not be resuscitated. A woman can terminate a 22-week pregnancy if the fetus has a genetic condition such as Down syndrome (trisomy 21), but if she asks that a 22-week-gestation infant not be resuscitated, her request might not be honored. Some health care providers might view the infant as having rights, and unless there are clinically compelling reasons not to resuscitate, they believe they are morally (and perhaps legally) obligated to resuscitate a 22-week gestation infant. Recently the Supreme Court of Texas ruled that the decision to resuscitate an extremely preterm infant in the delivery room should be made by the physician at the moment of birth, and that there is not enough time in the moments following birth to seek informed consent from the parents or obtain a court order should the parents disagree with the physician that the infant should be resuscitated (*Miller, Sidney Ainsley v. HCA, Inc.*, 2003). Is there a substantive moral difference between a 22-week-gestation fetus and a 22-week-gestation infant? If the mother can terminate a 22-week-gestation pregnancy, why can not she request life-sustaining treatment (resuscitation) be withheld from her 22-week-gestation infant?

CLINICAL EXERCISES

1. Investigate whether your clinical agency has a policy regarding newborns with anencephaly being organ donors.
2. When assigned to labor and delivery and/or the newborn or special care nursery, talk to the staff nurse about his/her experiences with newborns with anencephaly, especially related to treatment decision-making and end-of-life care.

Discussion Questions:

1. Just as an exercise, apply Fletcher's (1972) Indicators of Humanhood criteria to the infant/child you provided care for most recently. According to the criteria, would you consider the infant/child a "person"? Explain why or why not.
2. Divide the clinical practicum group into two groups to debate the ethical justifications for and against harvesting Baby Theresa's organs for donation.

SECTION 4: *Genetics*

EUGENICS

With the understanding of the genetic basis of many human conditions, there has been the hope that genetic testing, gene manipulation, and gene therapy will someday cure and/or prevent many unwanted conditions. The use of genetic testing is not without controversy, and the history of the eugenics movement compels us to carefully consider the implications of advancing genetic technology. Even before molecular genetics, patterns of inheritance were recognized. Some characteristics appeared to be dominant, such as brown eyes over blue eyes, although if two brown-eyed parents each had the recessive gene for blue eyes, then they could have a child with blue eyes. There were also misconceptions about what was genetically determined. Along with immigration laws to keep people considered "undesirable" from entering the country, eugenicists in the late 1800s and early 1900s promoted sterilization laws. They focused on people in lower socioeconomic classes and people they considered to have lower moral character, for example, those who smoked, drank alcohol, and had illicit sexual relations. Eventually the sterilization laws included people who were "feebleminded," one of the labels for people with intellectual disabilities.

In late 1920s sterilization laws were being constitutionally challenged, so eugenicists from Virginia decided to press a case, *Buck v. Bell*, to clarify the issue. Carrie Buck was a 17-year-old whose mother had lived in the Virginia Colony for Epileptics and Feebleminded since 1920; Carrie was now being committed to the same institution. She had a baby out of wedlock shortly before she was committed, and the child was placed in a foster home. The board of directors of the institution ordered her to be sterilized, and her court-appointed guardian appealed, thus paving the way for Supreme Court review. An official of the Eugenics Record Office who never examined Carrie or her mother reviewed the records and attested that Carrie and her family "belong to the shiftless, ignorant, and worthless class of anti-social whites of the South" (Kevles, 1995, p. 110). A Red Cross worker testified that she had seen Carrie's baby when the baby was 7 months old and thought that she did not look "quite normal" (Kevles, 1995, p. 110). The Court ruled that sterilization was constitutional, with Justice Holmes stating, "Three generations of imbeciles are enough." Carrie was sterilized; her daughter, who died at the age of 8, finished the second grade and was reported to be very bright (Kevels, 1995, p. 112). It was not until the 1960s that states began to repeal compulsory sterilization laws, but even then, coerced "voluntary" sterilization was done (Kevels, 1995, p. 275).

Forced sterilization occurred in concentration camps in Europe during World War II, and eugenics took on an even more sinister meaning. [For a history of the eugenics movement in the United States, see the Image Archives on the American Eugenics Movement (2005).] Although the term "eugenics" fell into disrepute, efforts to understand inheritance and to attempt to reduce genetic defects persist. There is more discussion on prenatal genetic counseling in Chapter 13.

In 1990, the U.S. National Institutes of Health and the Department of Energy combined to embark on a 15-year international project to map the entire human genome. Rapid progress was made, and the genome was completely mapped by April 2003. The clinical purpose of mapping the human genome was to diagnose, treat, and prevent genetic diseases. Now genomic research focuses on the expressivity of genes, variations in gene sequencing and phenotypes, and clinical applications of genetic knowledge.

Since the successful mapping of the human genome, efforts have been devoted to identifying markers of genetic conditions or markers indicating risks of developing particular conditions. Since the development of the Guthrie test for diagnosing and treating phenylketonuria (PKU), genetic testing has been applied in pediatrics. Because it has been in existence for many years, most pediatric nurses may be very comfortable with genetic testing. Chromosomal analysis to diagnose Down syndrome has been available for nearly three decades, and techniques have improved considerably. There are numerous ethical issues regarding genetics and children. When should a child have genetic testing? Should children be tested for genetic conditions for which there is no treatment? Should a child be tested for a condition that will not manifest until adulthood? If a blood relative's genetic condition may be revealed by testing a child, should consent be obtained from that blood relative, or if the test is done without the blood relative's knowledge, is there a duty to inform the relative of the test results? Should consent be obtained from parents before a newborn screening test is done?

GENETIC TESTING

Genetic testing has become much less invasive; a gentle swab inside the cheek can obtain all the necessary cells for analysis and replace the need for a venipuncture for a tube of blood. Often in pediatrics a broad, screening approach is taken when a child presents with delayed development. Depending on the presenting signs, the work-up might include history and physical exam and routine laboratory tests such as complete blood count and blood chemistries. In addition, screening for metabolic diseases can be done using urine or blood. Imaging can be done if there is a concern about structural anomalies in the brain. A number of conditions can be diagnosed through DNA analysis, and that number is increasing (Human Genome Project Information, 2004). Boys with delayed development, an elongated facies, and prominent ears may have Fragile X syndrome, and a chromosome analysis for this syndrome can be done. Even though a genetic condition cannot be "cured," from a clinical perspective, it is useful to identify the condition so that parents and children can know what to expect based on what is known about others with the condition. Clinicians can evaluate for other clinical features associated with a given syndrome, such as congenital heart problems or orthopedic problems, and monitor for leukemia, for example, in people with Down syndrome. Testing is warranted when there is a medical benefit to the child, such as identifying the condition, limiting its severity, or avoiding secondary disabilities or complications. The value in identifying genetic conditions early in life is to begin treatment if possible, such as in the case of PKU, which is treated with a special diet without phenylalanine. Another value is in suggesting supportive care and early intervention to promote development and adaptation when the condition cannot be physiologically altered. Children with cystic fibrosis can begin a regimen of aggressive health maintenance to stay as healthy as possible. Parents can anticipate the needs of a child with spinal muscular atrophy and plan for future needs. The use of genetic testing for this purpose is not controversial. Testing for carrier status or for late-onset conditions, however, is controversial.

Consider the case of Mrs. Pfister, a 32-year-old recently diagnosed with breast cancer, whose mother and maternal aunts also had breast cancer; she wants to have her 10-year-old daughter tested for the BRCA1/BRCA2 breast cancer genes. The American Academy of Pediatrics (2001) and the American Society of Human Genetics and the American College of Medical Genetics (1995) discourage testing children for adult-onset conditions. There has been no reduction in morbidity and mortality based on identifying children at risk for adult-onset conditions. Having parents consent to the testing negates the child's opportunity to make an informed decision about genetic testing on reaching adulthood. Because Mrs. Pfister has a strong family history of breast cancer, she can discuss with her daughter's pediatrician whether there are any measures her daughter can follow to reduce her risk of developing breast cancer. The usual surveillance for high-risk individuals should be instituted, but genetic testing is not advised because of the risk of psychological harms of anxiety, negative effect on the child's self-esteem, stigma, and discrimination in insurability and employment. There are exceptions, however.

Kodish (1999) suggested that the rule of earliest onset be followed, so that genetic testing for cancer risk should not be done at an age earlier than the first possible onset of disease. He gave colon cancer as an example; cases of familial adenomatous polyposis (FAP) have been seen in children as young as 10. Thus, children with the genetic mutation for FAP should have annual colonoscopies after age 10. Another form of colon cancer, hereditary nonpolyposis colon cancer (HNPCC), presents after age 20, and usually in the mid-40s. Different surveillance recommendations are made for this type of colon cancer. Children with family histories of colon cancer may benefit from genetic counseling to determine whether genetic testing should be done. Testing for FAP may provide a medical benefit to the child; testing for HNPCC may not confer a benefit.

Adolescents may seek genetic testing for adult-onset conditions; with parental permission and genetic counseling, it may be appropriate to honor the request if the adolescent is making an informed decision. A 17-year-old may want to know if he is carrying the gene for Huntington disease (HD) because he is aware that one parent has the gene. Numerous groups have issues guidelines for pretest counseling and evaluation because of the psychological impact of testing (Anonymous, 1994a, 1994b). The minimum age recommended for testing is 18, but neurological and psychiatric evaluation, and genetic counseling prior to testing will determine whether testing should proceed on an adolescent who is requesting it.

Davis (2001) argued that a child has a right to an open future, meaning that making certain decisions for a child precludes him or her making later decisions. A dramatic illustration would be a decision to sterilize a child, which would preclude the child, at a later age, deciding whether to have children. A more common example in pediatrics involves blood transfusions and children of Jehovah's Witnesses. In most hospitals across the country, if a child has a life-threatening condition for which the standard of care is a blood transfusion, the treating physician or hospital administrator will seek a court order to administer a lifesaving blood transfusion if the parents refuse based on religious objection. The decision to override the parental objection leaves the child's future "open" to make his or her decision on reaching adulthood. To honor the parents' objection and risk the death of the child renders the child's future "closed."

LINKAGE ANALYSIS

Sometimes a linkage analysis can be done for diseases for which there is no direct test for a specific gene. Several members in different generations of the same family are tested for a specific DNA marker that is associated with a specific disease. Identifying the genetic sequence of the affected person and comparing that sequence to others in the same family assists in locating the area of the responsible gene. For example, researchers used linkage analysis in searching for the gene responsible for celiac disease, a familial autoimmune condition in which specific types of foods cannot be digested, but were unable to identify the likely candidate gene (Neuhausen, Feolo, Farnham, Book, & Zone, 2001). However, genetic testing of children occurred in this study. The testing might not have conferred a direct benefit to the children, but there may have been a benefit to another family member, and the testing posed no more than minimal risk to the children. (For a more detailed discussion of research ethics, see Chapter 10.)

One risk with linkage analysis testing is that paternity is determined; if the legal father is not the biological father, who should get that information? In clinical practice, when human leukocyte antigen (HLA) testing is used to identify matches for bone marrow transplantation, the risk of paternity identification should be discussed with the mother privately and any findings shared with her privately. Whether to share the findings with other parties, such as the legal father and the biological father, is more complex and beyond the scope of this chapter. It is apparent that genetic testing of one individual can affect that person's family.

IMPLICATIONS FOR THE FAMILY

Genetic testing sometimes reveals information about a relative of the person being tested. For example, Huntington disease is an autosomal dominant disease, meaning there is a 50:50 chance that each offspring will inherit the HD gene, and if the gene is inherited, the disease will eventually manifest itself. If a mother with a family history of Huntington disease (a paternal uncle has the disease) wants to know whether her child has the Huntington gene, but does not want to know her own status, a positive finding will show that the mother has passed the gene onto her child. A negative finding does not assure the mother that she does not have the HD gene. She would need to have the testing herself to determine whether she has the gene if her child does not. In addition, if prenatal genetic testing is done to identify a particular gene (or absence of a gene), the mother's genetic risk may also be identified. In the example, the woman may want to know whether she is carrying a child with the HD gene, but will risk learning whether she has inherited the HD gene. She should be fully informed of this risk prior to submitting to prenatal testing.

In this situation, if the fetus has the HD gene, then the woman likely has the gene and her father does as well. Suppose, however, her father has never been tested and does not want to be tested. The result of testing the fetus can imply the grandfather's genetic status, unless the fetus' biological father has the HD gene. Does the mother or the genetics counselor have a duty to inform the woman's father that he has the HD gene? Because he is not seeking testing and has indicated he does not want to know, he should not be informed of the test results. If, however, he is employed in an occupation where manifestations of HD could compromise the safety of others, say as a bus driver, does that require a duty to inform him, or others, such as his employer? Again, genetics associations have wrestled with this issue, and the reader is referred to the position statement on familial disclosure of the American Society of Human Genetics (ASHG) Social Issues Subcommittee on Familial Disclosure (1998).

NEWBORN SCREENING

Another area of genetic testing involves the newborn screening programs conducted in every state. Most states screen for phenylketonuria, congenital hypothyroidism, galactosemia, sickle cell disease, congenital adrenal, hyperplasia, biotinidase deficiency, maple syrup urine disease, and homocystinuria (U.S. Government Accounting Office, 2003). Early identification and treatment of these disorders may prevent disability or death of a child with one of these conditions. In most states, testing is mandatory and parental consent is not required. Thirty-three states permit parents to forgo screening based on religious reasons, 13 states permit parents to forgo screening for any reason, and 5 states do not allow any exemption to the screening for any reason. The Health Insurance Portability and Accountability Act of 1996 (HIPAA) and state genetic privacy laws determine what information can be shared from newborn screening tests, but primarily, positive test results are reported to the physician of record, either from the hospital where the screening was done or the hospital where the child was born (or where testing was done, if the hospital is different than the birth hospital). The responsibility of notifying parents is the physician's or hospital's, although some states notify parents of abnormal results through a letter. From the public health standpoint of preventing secondary disorders and complications, newborn screening is a social good. The potential harm is in the abrogation of parental authority by having mandatory testing for which a parent must request exemption. The American Academy of Pediatrics supports the mandatory offering of the newborn screening to parents and the establishment of an informed consent process that will educate parents as to the purpose of screening and follow-up if results are positive (American Academy of Pediatrics, Committee on Bioethics, 2001). As genetic testing becomes more widespread and testing for more disorders becomes available, states will need to evaluate the benefits and costs of expanding or otherwise modifying newborn screening programs.

There are other issues in genetics that pose ethical questions, such as gene therapy, genetic enhancement, banking of cord blood, and genetics research. These will be addressed in later chapters.

SUMMARY

Nursing for children and adolescents poses unique ethical challenges. To face them, it is helpful for nurses to know their institution or agency mechanism for assisting patients and families in resolving ethical issues. Knowing what resources are available to nurses, such as ethics committees or ethics consultants, is also very important. Ethical decision-making, like the nursing process, begins with gathering data, identifying the clinical problems and ethical issues, identifying the key players and their positions, and clarifying information and facilitating communication. A nurse may help a family to explore its options and their ethical ramifications and then make a decision. The nurse can then reflect on the ethical decision-making process, both the role that he or she played and the role of others, and decide what he or she might do differently the next time. Whether the situation involves a dying child, a 500-gram preterm infant, a child with developmental disabilities, a sexually active adolescent, or a family with values in conflict with those of the health care providers, the nurse can employ an ethical decision-making process to advocate for the child in a family-centered way.

CLINICAL EXERCISES

1. Investigate your state's law on sterilization of minors. Compare the state law with your institution's policies on treating adolescents without their assent.
2. Investigate your institution's policy on genetic testing of children. Does it address testing for adult onset disease or disclosure of paternity?

Discussion Questions

1. Daniel, 3, has leukemia and is a candidate for a bone marrow transplant. He has an 8-year old brother, Phillip, who is a close match. Phillip is extremely frightened of needles and does not want to be a donor. What are the ethical issues in having Phillip as a bone marrow donor for his brother?
2. Divide your clinical group into two groups to debate the ethical issues/justifications for and against a DNR order for the following patient who is currently hospitalized but normally resides in a long-term care facility.

   Jim is currently receiving aggressive treatment in the pediatric intensive care unit and has a full-code status. The health care team and his parents are faced with decisions about how aggressively to treat Jim now since he experienced a 20-minute arrest requiring CPR prior to this hospital admission. Jim has Canavan's disease, a degenerative leukodystrophy, complicated by a perforated ulcer, bleeding, shock, and cardiac arrest. Jim is 10 years of age. The health care team and Jim's parents must determine what level of treatment is appropriate for Jim in light of his response to resuscitation (he does not respond to any stimuli and his pupils are fixed) and his degenerative neurological condition. It is predicted that Jim will not regain his previous level of functioning.

   What additional information do you need to know about Canavan's disease? See www.canavan.org.
   What else do you need to know about Jim's functional level prior to the arrest? Does it matter if he functioned as a "normal" 10-year-old or at the level of a 1-year-old? Why or why not?

Resources

Guidelines for Predictive Testing for HD (Huntington's Disease). Retrieved April 4, 2004, from www.circ.uab.edu/sergg/s95/guid.htm

Image Archives on the American Eugenics Movement. Retrieved April 1, 2004, from www.eugenicsarchive.org/eugenics

Infanticide. Retrieved February, 13, 2004, from www.gendercide.org/case_infanticide.html

Intersex Society of North America. (2005). How common is intersex? Retrieved October 6, 2005, from www.isna.org/faq/frequency.html

The Sperm Bank of California. (2004). The Identity-Release[SM] Program. Retrieved October 6, 2005, from www.thespermbankofca.org/idrelease.html

References

Alan Guttmacher Institute. (2005). State policies in brief: Minors' access to STD services. Retrieved June 4, 2005, from www.guttmacher.org/statecenter/spibs/spib_MASS.pdf

American Academy of Pediatrics. (2002). *Perinatal care at the threshold of viability*. Retrieved November 11, 2002, from www.aap.org/policy/010107.html

American Academy of Pediatrics Committee on Bioethics. (1995). Informed consent, parental permission, and assent in pediatric practice. *Pediatrics, 95*(2), 314–317.

American Academy of Pediatrics Committee on Bioethics. (2001). Ethical issues with genetic testing in pediatrics. *Pediatrics, 107*(6), 1451–1455.

American Academy of Pediatrics Task Force on Brain Death in Children. (1987). Report of special task force: Guidelines for determination of brain death in children. *Pediatrics, 80*(2), 278.

American Academy of Pediatrics Task Force on Circumcision. (1999). Circumcision policy statement. *Pediatrics, 103*(3), 686–693.

American Medical Association Council on Ethical and Judicial Affairs. (1995). The use of anencephalic neonates as organ donors. *Journal of the American Medical Association, 273*, 1614–1618.

American Society of Human Genetics and American College of Medical Genetics. (1995). Points to consider: Ethical, legal, and psychosocial implications of genetic testing in children and adolescents. *American Journal of Human Genetics, 57*, 1233–1241.

Annas, G. (2001). Conjoined twins—the limits of law at the limits of life. *New England Journal of Medicine, 344*(14), 1104–1108.

Anonymous. (1994a). International Huntington Association and the World Federation of Neurology Research Group on Huntington's Chorea. Guidelines for the molecular genetics predictive test in Huntington's disease. *Journal of Medical Genetics, 31*(7):555–559.

Anonymous. (1994b). Guidelines for the molecular genetics predictive test in Huntington's disease. International Huntington Association (IHA) and the World Federation of Neurology (WFN) Research Group on Huntington's Chorea. *Neurology, 44*, 1533–1539.

ASHG Social Issues Subcommittee on Familial Disclosure. (1998). Professional disclosure of familial genetic information. *American Journal on Human Genetics, 62*, 474–483.

Bartholome, W. G. (1995). Informed consent, parental permission, and assent in pediatric practice. *Pediatrics, 96*(5), 981–982.

Bernat, J. L. (2002). *Ethical issues in neurology* (2nd ed.). Boston: Butterworth-Heinemann.

Blackless, M., Charuvastra, A., Derryck, A., Fausto-Sterling, A., Lauzanne, K., & Lee, E. (2000). How sexually dimorphic are we? Review and synthesis. *American Journal of Human Biology, 12*, 151–166.

Broffman, G. (1995). How can pediatric care be provided in underserved areas? A view of rural pediatric care. *Pediatrics, 96*(4), 816–821.

Canadian Paediatric Society Fetus and Newborn Committee. (1996). Neonatal circumcision revisited. *Canadian Medical Association Journal, 154*(6), 769–780.

Case study: Female infanticide. Retrieved February 13, 2004, at www.gendercide.org/case_infanticide.html

Catlin, A. J. (1998). *Physicians' perceptions of the dilemma of neonatal resuscitation for extremely low birth weight preterm infants.* Doctoral dissertation, Rush University College of Nursing.

Centers for Disease Control and Prevention. (2002). Web-based Injury Statistics Query and Reporting System (WISQARS). Retrieved December 16, 2003, from www.cdc.gov/ncipc/wisqars

Centers for Disease Control and Prevention. (2005). HIV/AIDS in youth. Retrieved June 5, 2005, from www.cdc.gov/hiv/pubs/facts/youth.htm

CNN. (2003). Complication almost stopped separation surgery. Retrieved October 6, 2005, from www.cnn.com/2003/HEALTH/07/11/conjoined.twins/

Colapinto, J. (2000). *As nature made him: The boy who was raised as a girl.* New York: Harper-Collins.

Committee on Pediatric AIDS and Committee on Adolescence. (2001). Adolescents and human immunodeficiency virus infection: The role of the pediatrician in prevention and intervention. *Pediatrics, 107*(1), 188–190.

Conjoined Twins. (2005). Retrieved October 6, 2005, from www.conjoined-twins.i-p.com

Dailard, C. (2000). The drive to enact "Infant Abandonment" laws—A rush to judgment? *The Guttmacher Report on Public Policy, 3*(4). Retrieved March 22, 2004, from www.agi-usa.org/pubs/journals/gr030401.html

Davis, D. S. (2001). *Genetic dilemmas: Reproductive technology, parental choices and children's futures.* New York: Routledge

Diamond, M. (1999). Pediatric management of ambiguous and traumatized genitalia. *Journal of Urology, 162*(3-II), 1021–1028.

Diamond, M., & Sigmundson, H. K. (1997). Management of intersexuality: Guidelines for dealing with individuals with ambiguous genitalia. *Archives of Pediatrics and Adolescent Medicine, 151*, 1046–1050.

Dixon-Woods, M., Young, B., & Heney, D. (1999). Partnerships with children. *BMJ, 319*(7212), 778–780.

Dreger, A. D. (1998). Ambiguous sex—or ambivalent medicine? Ethical issues in the treatment of intersexuality. *Hastings Center Report, 28*(3), 24–35.

Duff, R. S, & Campbell A. G. M. (1973). Moral and ethical dilemmas in the special-care nursery. *New England Journal of Medicine, 289*, 885–890.

Dunstan, G. R. (1997). The ethics of organ donation. *British Medical Bulletin, 53*(4), 921–939.

Engelhardt, H. T. (1975). Ethical issues in aiding the death of young children. In M. Kohl (Ed.). *Beneficent euthanasia.* Buffalo, NY: Prometheus.

Ferguson, M., & Zuk, J. (2003). Organ donation after cardiac death: A new trend in pediatrics. *Journal of Pediatric Gastroenterology and Nutrition, 37*(3), 219–220.

Ferguson et al. v. City of Charleston et al. No. 99-936. (U. S. Supreme Court, December 21, 2001). Retrieved December 3, 2005, from http://laws.findlaw.com/us/000/99-936.html

Fletcher, J. (1972). Indicators of humanhood: A tentative profile of man. *Hastings Center Report, 2*, 1–4.

Frader, J., Alderson, P., Asch, A., Aspinall, C., Davis, D., Dreger, A., et al. (2004). Health Care Professionals and Intersex Conditions. [Editorial] *Archives of Pediatrics & Adolescent Medicine. 158*(5), 426–428.

Frader, J., & Watchko, J. (1997). Physicians and medical futility: Experience in pediatrics. In M. B. Zucker, H. D. Zucker, A. Capron (Eds.). *Medical futility and the evaluation of life-sustaining interventions.* New York: Cambridge University Press.

Friedman, E. (1994). Money isn't everything: Nonfinancial barriers to access. *JAMA, 271*(1), 1535–1538.

Galli, R. (2000). *Rescuing Jeffrey.* Chapel Hill, N.C.: Algonquin Books of Chapel Hill.

Gendercide Watch. Retrieved December 3, 2005, from http://www.gendercide.org/case_infanticide.html

Gross, M. L. (2002). Abortion and neonaticide: Ethics, practice, and policy in four nations. *Bioethics, 16*, 202–230.

Halfon, N., Newacheck, P. W., Wood, D. L., & St. Peter, R. F. (1996). Routine emergency department use for sick care by children in the United States. *Pediatrics, 98*(1), 28–34.

Harrison, H. (1993). Special article: The principles for family-centered neonatal care. *Pediatrics, 92*(5), 643–650.

Harrison, H. (2001). Making lemonade: A parent's view of "quality of life" studies. *Journal of Clinical Ethics, 12*(3), 239–250.

Human Genome Project Information, (2004). Retrieved December 3, 2005, from http://www.ornl.gov/sci/techresources/Human_Genome/home.shtml

Hyun, I. (2000). When adolescents "mismanage" their chronic medical conditions: An ethical exploration. *Kennedy Institute of Ethics Journal, 10*(2), 147–163.

Image Archives on the American Eugenics Movement. (2005). Available at www.eugenicsarchive.org/eugenics

In Re T.A.C.P. Supreme Court of Florida: In the matter of Theresa Ann Campo Pearson. 609 So. 2d. 588 17 Fla. L. Weekly S 691 November 12, 1992 Decided.

In the matter of Baby "K." U.S. Court of Appeals for the Fourth Circuit, 16 F. 3d. 590; 1994 U.S. App. LEXIS 2215; 3 Am. Disabilities Cas. (BNA) 128.

Intersex Society of North America. (2005). How common is intersex? Retrieved October 6, 2005, from www.isna.org/faq/frequency.html

Jackson, S., & Hafemeister, T. L. (2001). Impact of parental consent and notification policies on the decisions of adolescents to be tested for HIV. *Journal of Adolescent Health, 29*, 81–93.

Kevles, D. J. (1995). *In the name of eugenics: Genetics and the uses of human heredity.* Cambridge, MA: Harvard University Press.

Kodish, E. D. (1999). Testing children for cancer genes: The rule of earliest onset. *Journal of Pediatrics, 135*(3), 390–395.

Lyon, J. (1985). *Playing God in the nursery.* New York: Norton.

McCormick. R. (1974). To save or let die: The dilemma of modern medicine. *Journal of the American Medical Association, 229*(8), 172–176.

Miller, Sidney Ainsley v. HCA, Inc. (Hospital Corporation of America and Columbia/HCA Healthcare Corporation). Texas Supreme Court, Case no. 01-0079, opinion rendered September 30, 2003. Retrieved December 1, 2003, from http://caselaw.lp.findlaw.com/data2/texasstatecases/sc/010079p.pdf

National Cancer Institute. (2005). Childhood brain stem glioma (PDQ®): Treatment. Retrieved June 5, 2005, from www.nci.nih.gov/cancertopics/pdq/treatment/child-brain-stem-glioma/HealthProfessional/page5

Neuhausen, S.L., Feolo, M., Farnham, J., Book, L., & Zone, J. J. (2001). Linkage analysis of HLA and candidate genes for celiac disease in a North American family-based study. *BMC Medical Genetics, 2*(12). Retrieved April 4, 2004, from www.biomedcentral.com/1471-2350/2/12

Penticuff, J. H. (1990). Ethics in pediatric nursing: Advocacy and the child's "determining self." *Issues in Comprehensive Pediatric Nursing, 13*(3), 221–229.

Pinch, W. J. E. (2002). *When the bough breaks: Parental perceptions of ethical decision-making in NICU.* New York: University Press of America.

President's Commission for the Study of Ethical Problems in Medicine and Biomedical and Behavioral Research. (1983). *Deciding to forego life-sustaining treatment.* Washington, DC: U. S. Government Printing Office.

Ross, L. F. (1997). Health care decision making by children: Is it in their best interest? *Hasting Center Report, 27*(6), 41–45.

Ross, L. F. (1998). *Children, families and health care decision making.* New York: Oxford University Press.

Rubin, S. B. (1998). *When doctors say no: The battleground of medical futility.* Bloomington, IN: Indiana University Press.

Savage, T. A., & Michalak, D. R. (2002). Finding agreement to limit life-sustaining treatment for children who are in state custody. *Pediatric Nursing, 27*(6), 594–597.

Singer, P. (1979). *Practical ethics*. New York: Cambridge University Press.

Tooley, M. (1983). *Abortion and infanticide*. New York: Oxford University Press.

U.S. Government Accounting Office. (2003). Newborn screening. Retrieved April 4, 2004, from www.gao.gov/new.items/403449.pdf

Veatch, R. M. (1975). The whole-brain oriented concept of death: An outmoded philosophical formulation. *Journal of Thanatology, 3*, 13–30.

Weithorn, L. A., & Campbell, S. B. (1982). The competency of children and adolescents to make informed treatment decisions. *Child Development, 53*, 1589–1598.

Wood, D. L. (2003). Increasing immunization coverage. *Pediatrics, 112*(4), 993–996.

Wood, N. S., Marlow, N., Costeloe, K., Gibson, A. T., & Wilkinson, A. K. (2000). Neurologic and developmental disability after extremely preterm birth. EPICure Study Group. *New England Journal of Medicine, 343*, 378–384.

Zawistowski, C. A., & Frader, J. E. (2003). Ethical problems in pediatric critical care: Consent. *Critical Care Medicine, 31*(5, Supplement), S407–S410.

CHAPTER 12

Nursing of the Adult

Objectives

At the end of this chapter, the student should be able to:

1. Analyze special threats to the adult patient's confidentiality.
2. Explain mechanisms for promoting truthfulness when providing care for adult patients.
3. Describe actions a nurse can take in advocating for vulnerable adult patients.
4. Articulate the ethical justifications for allocation decisions related to organ transplantation.
5. Analyze ethical cases pertaining to the care of the adult patient.
6. Discriminate between a legal advance directive and The Medical Directive Form.
7. Discuss end-of-life decision-making preferences with another person.
8. Use the decision analysis model to facilitate ethical decision-making.
9. Identify threats to patient autonomy during end-of-life decision-making.
10. Discuss end-of-life decision-making preferences with a patient.
11. Assist others to complete a written advance directive and The Medical Directive Form.
12. Differentiate between withholding and withdrawing treatment, and between assisted suicide and euthanasia.
13. Recognize and discuss personal values that influence end-of-life choices.
14. Debate the moral rationale supporting and negating end-of-life choices.
15. Identify the nurse's professional responsibility to act as an advocate during end-of-life choices.
16. Identify ethical issues related to presymptomatic genetic diagnosis.
17. Discuss values that influence an individual's decisions concerning presymptomatic genetic diagnosis.
18. Identify communication strategies for remaining nondirective and morally neutral during discussions about presymptomatic genetic diagnosis.
19. Discuss whether the individual or the family owns genetic data.

- *Adult-onset genetic disease*
- *Advance directive*
- *Age of majority*
- *Altruism*
- *Artificial nutrition and hydration*
- *Assisted suicide*
- *Cadaver organ donation*
- *Comfort care*
- *CPR (cardiopulmonary resuscitation)*
- *Decisional capacity*
- *Durable power of attorney for health care*
- *Elder abuse*
- *End-of-life choices*
- *Futile treatment*
- *Genes*
- *Genetic marker*
- *Human Genome Project*
- *Life-sustaining treatment*
- *Linkage analysis*
- *Living organ donation*
- *Living will*
- *Mandatory reporting*
- *Morally neutral*
- *Nondirective*
- *Pedigree*
- *Persistent vegetative state*
- *Placebo*
- *Presymptomatic diagnosis*
- *Suicide*
- *Terminal condition*
- *United Network for Organ Sharing (UNOS)*
- *Withdrawing treatment*
- *Withholding treatment*

SECTION 1: *Ethical Themes: Building From the Basic to the Complex*

The basic ethical themes (confidentiality, truth-telling, advocacy, and allocation of resources) become more complex depending on the adult patient's ability and willingness to engage in ethical decision-making. In addition, adult patients and their nurses may experience ethical situations in which the needs of the adult may conflict with the needs of others or society.

CONFIDENTIALITY

Nurses have an obligation to ensure that patient information remains confidential and is shared with only those individuals who have a demonstrated right to it. This section expands the concept of confidentiality and discusses the nurse's role in minimizing common threats to maintaining the confidentiality of adults.

Changes in the Patient's Legal Status

Sometimes a person's right to access confidential information may change as a result of changes in the patient's life, including reaching the age of majority (i.e., 18 years of age) or marital status. In addition, some states may have special protections or disclosure mechanisms for specific information, such as HIV status or the presence of sexually transmitted infections.

Reaching the Age of Majority

The patient's legal status may influence how or if information may be disclosed. For example, when an adolescent reaches his or her eighteenth birthday, the adolescent legally becomes an adult and can give or refuse consent for any medical procedure. As a result, his or her parents lose their legal right to access their child's information and consent to treatment. For example, two high school students are taken to the emergency department after an automobile accident. Both students have a tibia fracture that requires surgery. Because the first student is 16 years old and not in any imminent danger, his parents are informed of his status and are asked to sign the surgical consent form.

However, the second student is 18 years old. Thus, the health care team members must discuss his condition directly with him, and he, rather than his parent, will be required to sign the surgical consent. When the 18-year-old student's parents arrive, he needs to be asked whether he wants them to be included in the discussions about his health care and treatment. The possibility exists for the parents to assert a right to access their 18-year-old son's health information if he is included in their health insurance plan. However, financial support is not sufficient justification for disclosing confidential information. Thus, the nurse may need to provide emotional support while the parents cope with their son's attempts at independence. If the student and/or parents display anger or fear, a referral to counseling may be beneficial in assisting them through this role transition.

Persons Lacking Decisional Capacity

Most adolescents who reach the age of majority have the mental and emotional skills needed for making autonomous decision-making. However, adolescents with significant developmental and/or maturational problems may not be able to assume control of their health care information and decision-making. When an adolescent is unable to assume responsibilities for decision-making, a guardian needs to be legally appointed by a judge because parents no longer have the legal right to consent when their child reaches 18 years of age. Thus when working with a young adult (18 years or older) with limited decisional capacity, the nurse needs to determine who, if anyone, has a legal right to the patient's information and to consent for treatment. Again, the nurse will need to be sensitive to the parents' emotions in the event that the parents perceive questions about guardianship as a challenge to their motivations and commitments to their child's best interests.

A loss of decisional capacity can also affect the protection of patient confidentiality when an adult suffers from dementia or changes in mental capabilities secondary to a disease process, such as encephalopathy, delirium tremors, or sepsis. In the event that the patient loses the ability to participate in decision-making, the nurse will need to be aware of the state's or province's laws regarding how a surrogate decision-maker is identified. The nurse must be cautious not to disclose confidential patient information to others just because the person is "family" and present at the patient's bedside.

For example, a friend brings an unresponsive 76-year-old man to the hospital. The man is admitted to the critical care unit. The physician repeatedly dials the contact phone number, but eventually concludes that this number is to the patient's home. In the absence of information about this patient, the health care team members must be especially diligent in acting to protect the patient's confidentiality and autonomy when visitors come to see the patient. The temptation is great to assign the surrogate role to the individual who visits most (e.g., the friend visits everyday), but this may not be consistent with state legislation.

Discussion Exercises 12-1

After not being seen by friends for 4 days, Mr. Kwak was found unresponsive in his apartment. His admitting diagnosis was subarachnoid hemorrhage secondary to cocaine use. On his fifth hospital day, Mr. Kwak is alert and follows commands, but rarely speaks due to expressive aphasia. Three men arrive during visiting hours and identify themselves as his brothers; however, Mr. Kwak neither confirms nor denies this relationship. One "brother" states, "We just heard he was in the hospital. How long has he been here? What happened to him? Is he going to be ok?"

1. How would you respond to these questions?
2. After your initial response, one brother states in an aggressive manner, "I need to know what is going on and you do not seem to know anything!" How will you deal with this statement?
3. The next day, a different man visits, stating "I am his brother." How will you respond to his requests for information?

TRUTH-TELLING

Establishing a strong patient–provider relationship requires mutual respect that is built on trust and veracity. However, situations may arise that challenge the nurse's and/or patient's ability to communicate truthfully.

HIV Disclosure

By Seropositive Individuals

Disclosure of one's HIV-positive status is often based on a commitment to prevent transmission of the virus to others. This commitment is illustrated when a patient who is HIV+ reminds a nurse to put on gloves before beginning a procedure where the nurse might come into contact with body fluids, such as drawing blood or changing a dressing. Whereas most persons who are HIV+ are very conscientious about truthfully disclosing their status to protect health care workers from exposure, situations have occurred where persons who are HIV+ have not truthfully disclosed their status. This lapse in veracity may be related to fear.

The fear of loss of confidentiality, stigmatization, or rejection may keep a person living in a community from truthfully disclosing his or her HIV serostatus based on a fear that personal or professional relationships with other residents in their locality would be negatively affected (Vazquez, 2001). For example, an individual may not respond truthfully when asked about his HIV status during an appointment at an orthopedic clinic after he realizes that he attends church with the physician, the billing clerk is his son's best friend's mother, and the office manager is married to a co-worker.

Unfortunately, incidents have occurred where a person who is HIV+ has purposely not disclosed based on a desire for retribution. For example, a man who became infected during a sexual experience with a female sex worker may fail to disclose his HIV status to future sexual partners, especially professional sex workers, based on the belief that "No one cared about me, why should I care about them"? Based on a commitment to prevent harm, many states have enacted legislation requiring individuals to fully disclose their HIV+ status prior to engaging in sexual activities (American Civil Liberties Union, 2000).

Discussion Exercises 12-2

Mr. Dunn, a 35-year-old man, is admitted with *Pneumocystis carinii* pneumonia secondary to advanced AIDS. His mother lives 1500 miles away and has flown into town after being notified of her son's hospitalization. On arriving at the hospital, she approaches Mr. Dunn's nurse and asks, "I just do not understand how he can be so sick. How is he breathing now? What medicines is he taking? Why is he on the infectious disease unit?"

1. If you were Mr. Dunn's nurse, how would you reply to his mother's questions?
2. What rights does Mr. Dunn's mother have?
3. Would your response to questions 1 and 2 change if the person was a former co-worker of Mr. Dunn's who acknowledges a previous sexual relationship with Mr. Dunn? Explain.

By Health Care Providers About a Patient

At times nurses might find themselves in the position of being asked about a patient's HIV status. (The disclosure of a nurse's HIV status is discussed in Chapter 16.) For example, a 35-year-old, seropositive homosexual male is admitted to the hospital. His mother, who lives out of state, visits and says to the nurse, "I do not understand why he is so sick. What are those purple spots on his face?" Although the best response, based on patient autonomy and confidentiality, would be for the nurse to reply, "At this time, I am not able to discuss your son's medical care with you. You will need to ask your son these questions," the nurse should be diligent to avoid making comments that are untruthful or inaccurate, such as, "I do not know what is wrong with your son," because comments like this can diminish the family's trust in the nurse's abilities and ultimately the patient's safety.

In addition, health care professionals should be aware of their state's current legislation concerning when or if a health care professional can or may disclose a patient's HIV status to another person. For example, in Illinois (Illinois Public Health Communicable Diseases AIDS Confidentiality Act, 1997), a physician may, but is not obligated to, disclose a patient's HIV+ status to a spouse, but not other sexual partners, if the patient refuses. Because of this law, Illinois nurses have experienced moral distress when, for example, a patient with a history of intravenous drug use tested positive for the HIV, but refused to disclose this information to his girlfriend with whom he lives. This law illustrates how legislation can lag behind or not clearly reflect current societal morals. The law also does not prevent the commission of a crime, for example, failure of the person with HIV to disclose his or her HIV status to a sexual partner but failure to disclose is illegal and prosecutable.

One way in which nurses have maintained their commitment to truthfulness, confidentiality, and beneficence is through education. In the previous illustration, the patient wanted his girlfriend to be present when discussing drug rehabilitation. During this session, the nurse discussed the fact that anyone engaging in risky behavior, such as intravenous drug use, is risking exposure to HIV or other infectious diseases and thus should be tested. At the end of this session, the girlfriend verbalized her intentions to be tested. In her documentation, the nurse noted that the girlfriend was present per the patient's request and that the patient's HIV status was not discussed, thus, reflecting her commitment to truthfulness and confidentiality as well as beneficence. Nurses must keep current with legislation regarding HIV disclosure in their practice state.

Placebos

A placebo is an inert substance, such as a sugar pill or intravenous saline flush, that is presented as if it were an active medication. The use of placebos is common practice in pharmaceutical research where researchers are attempting to ascertain whether a new drug is more effective and/or has increased side effects than no treatment. In the clinical setting, patients are rarely informed whether their plan of care includes the use of a placebo; thus, when administering a placebo the nurse is not being truthful with the patient about the mode of action of the "drug" being administered.

McAffery and Beebe (1989) defined pain as "whatever the person experiencing it says it is" (p. 7). However, sometimes health care team members may doubt the veracity of a patient's complaints. In these situations, health care team members may debate using a placebo. For example, a 56-year-old man is readmitted to the hospital with a complaint of chest pain 2 days after an extensive cardiac work-up found no cardiac disease. The physician orders include "Administer 1 cc of sterile saline intravenously for complaint of chest pain. If no pain relief within 5 minutes administer 2 mg of morphine sulfate intravenously." In this example, the physician may be attempting to identify whether this patient's chest pain has a psychological component.

When the patient complains of chest pain, the nurse has an ethical obligation to completely assess the patient's condition before deciding to administer a placebo. If the nurse decides to administer the placebo and thus engage in an act of deception, he or she should be as truthful as possible with the patient. For example, the nurse could state, "I have the injection the physician ordered for your chest pain." However, the nurse needs to be prepared for the possibility that the patient will ask to know the specific name of the medication. Although some patients may not realize that saline is salt water, many patients will be knowledgeable and may confront the nurse, thus putting a stop to the deception.

Because the ethical issue with the use of placebos is that of deception, actions could be taken to obtain the patient's consent for incorporating the use of placebos into a treatment plan. In the previous illustration, after the patient is readmitted to the hospital, the physician could say to him, "The cause of your chest pain is not clearly understood. I would like your permission to try a variety of treatments to see which works best. I expect that some drugs and/or dosages will work better than others." Through this honest explanation, the patient is included in the plan of care, deception is minimized because the patient consents to try treatments that may not be effective and the patient–provider relationship is honored.

Each nurse assigned to the patient will need to make an individual decision regarding his or her willingness to participate in the use of placebos. Nurses opposed to the use of placebos would need to express their refusal following the agency's policy. Conscientious objection is discussed in greater detail in Chapter 16. In addition, the use of placebos in research studies is discussed in Chapter 10.

ADVOCACY

Nurses working with adults need to be attentive to situations that are or have the potential of placing their patients in harm's way and/or limit a patient's ability to promote his or her own interests. Section 2 of this chapter discusses in greater detail the nurse's advocacy role in promoting the patient's autonomy through the use of advance directives.

Mandatory Reporting of Elder Abuse

In an ideal world, everyone, especially family members, would always act to promote good and prevent harm toward other family members, but unfortunately not every family or relationship is a loving, positive experience. Whereas anyone can become the recipient of abuse, the elder members of society may be more vulnerable because of social isolation, diminished or compromised senses, cognition, mobility, or financial dependence. Elder abuse is "any knowing, intentional, or negligent act by a caregiver or any other person that causes harm or serious risk of harm to a vulnerable adult" (National Center on Elder Abuse, 2003, p.1) and includes physical, emotional, and sexual abuse as well as exploitation, neglect, and abandonment.

As advocates, nurses have an obligation to identify vulnerable persons and assist them to improve their situation, increase their autonomy, and decrease their vulnerability. For example, nurses, especially parish and home health nurses, can assist individuals to identify safe housing, implement financial and health care durable power of attorneys, lessen social isolation through involvement in religious and community activities, and understand their self-determination rights (National Center on Elder Abuse, 2003).

Because of the profession's commitment to advocacy, nurses may be required to act to protect a vulnerable person when abuse or neglect is suspected. In fact, most states have laws mandating health care professionals to report elder abuse to the police or local adult protective service agency. In addition, nurses should be involved in community educational efforts regarding community resources and ombudsman available to assist individuals who feel their autonomy and safety are being limited because of another person's abusive or negligent actions.

Discussion Exercises 12-3

Ms. Barry is the matriarch of her family. She owns a three-flat apartment building. She lives in the first-floor apartment and her adult children and grandchildren occupy the other two apartments. Her family assumed responsibility for her care after Ms. Barry experienced a massive stroke that left her unable to communicate her wishes or move independently. After being at home for less than 1 month, Ms. Barry is readmitted to the hospital with stage III decubitus ulcers, pneumonia, and dehydration. The family is advised that Ms. Barry will not be able to return home, but rather will need placement in a long-term care facility. Because of Ms. Barry's financial status, she will be required to sell her building. When the utilization management nurse discussed these plans with Ms. Barry's family, the children replied, "If you do that all of us will be homeless! We will just keep caring for her at home."

1. Does Ms. Barry's situation fit the criteria for elder abuse? Explain.
2. What obligations, if any, does Ms. Barry have toward her family?
3. What obligations, if any, does Ms. Barry's family have toward her?
4. What options exist for resolving this difficult situation?

ALLOCATION OF RESOURCES

Nurses who provide care for adult patients may experience situations in which the nurse asks "Why are we doing this to this patient, it is not helping him?" or "This patient is going to die soon. Why are we doing this costly procedure?" These questions illustrate the dissonance a nurse can experience between his or her moral commitment to promote the goals of the community at large as well as those of the individual patient. Renal transplantation will be used as a prototype in this discussion.

Organ Transplantation: End-Stage Renal Disease

Dialysis

In the early 1960s, when renal dialysis technology became available, there were more patients who could benefit from this technology than the number of dialysis machines available. Institutions were faced with deciding who should be provided with this scarce technological resource. In response to this dilemma, hospitals created committees made up of health care professionals and community members. These committees used social criteria, such as occupation, marital status, potential to contribute to society, and/or emotional stability, to determine who would ultimately receive dialysis. Despite their good intentions, these committees were widely criticized for the use of subjective social criteria that appeared to favor married adults younger than 45 years of age with children and of modest income who attended religious activities. Fortunately, there is no longer a shortage of dialysis services; however, questions continue to arise regarding a dialysis clinic's obligation to provide care for persons with histories of noncompliance or combative behavior (Pence, 1995).

Renal Transplantation

Rather than undergo lifelong renal dialysis, many individuals pursue the option of renal transplantation. Kidneys for transplantation can be procured in two ways: from cadavers and living donors. Kidneys from cadaveric donors are coordinated through the United Network for Organ Sharing (UNOS), which coordinates the matching of organs for donation to individuals waiting for transplantation. Organs are matched to waiting recipients via a computer algorithm that considers blood type and body size among other variables as a means for preventing preferential allocation of organs to individuals who are lower on the waiting list. The UNOS system is an example of allocation of a scarce resource based on need rather than social criteria, such as actual or potential contribution to society, as was implemented by the early dialysis committees.

Because the number of individuals listed for kidney and other organ transplants far exceeds the number of available cadaveric organs, many individuals pursue the identification of a living donor.

To qualify as a living organ donor, the person must be in good health (i.e., normal blood pressure, no heart disease, kidney disease, diabetes, or cancer) and have a blood tissue type that is compatible with that of the recipient. Because a living donor does not have to be a genetic or ethnic match with the recipient, the possibility exists for those with lower social or financial standing (the homeless, college students, immigrants) to be exploited.

Although the sale of organs is illegal in the United States, the possibility exists for "under the table" financial or other types of compensation (e.g., employment or housing) to occur as an act of appreciation for donation. For example, an affluent young businessman whose family was originally from a developing country advertised in an U.S. newspaper for a donor. A 19-year-old woman whose family originated from the same geographical region as the businessman volunteered to undergo evaluation as a living donor. Several ethical issues were identified by the transplant team regarding this selection. First, the team questioned why the daughter was selected/volunteered rather than one of her three brothers. Second, questions about potential coercion were raised because the potential donor's family was of a lower social status than the recipient's family. Did the donator's family hope that donating might result in financial reimbursement or elevation in social status through an arranged marriage if a donation occurred? Third, was this young woman making a voluntary, informed altruistic act?

Altruism is an example of a beneficent act and is "defined as an unselfish concern for the welfare of others" (Steinberg, 2003, p. 21). Altruistic acts are sometimes referred to as saintly acts that go above and beyond the expectations society holds for individuals. Examples of altruistic acts include the "women and children first" philosophy when evacuating a sinking ship or a soldier placing himself in the line of fire to protect an injured buddy. When attempting to explain why an altruistic act was implemented, individuals often explain, "I felt called to do this," or, "I could not live with my self if I did not come forward."

Usually altruistic acts occur between individuals with an existing interpersonal relationship, such as donation of a kidney to a sibling or one's best friend. However, examples of donations where the donor is completely unknown to the recipient are becoming more common. Although many of these cases are clearly examples of altruism, the possibility does exist that the individual is volunteering because of either secondary reasons that may not be as readily apparent, such as the resultant attention and praise, or a psychological deficit in the volunteer's personality. Thus, an interdisciplinary team approach is beneficial when evaluating any person's decision to become a living organ donor.

Discussion Exercises 12-4

Mr. Jagmin is admitted to an academic medical center in renal failure secondary to a history of hypertension and a 30-year history of substance abuse. He is 45 years old and unemployed. His outpatient health care has been covered by a state general assistance grant through the state Welfare Office. This grant provides financial reimbursement for outpatient care and prescription medications, but does not cover in-patient hospitalization or outpatient dialysis costs. The hospital social worker has helped Mr. Jagmin complete the paperwork for Medicaid coverage. The social worker does not anticipate any problems with his application, based on the fact that Mr. Jagmin has a general assistance grant; however, it generally takes 2 to 3 months for the state to process applications. The discharge planning nurse is attempting to refer Mr. Jagmin in an outpatient dialysis center. The center affiliated with the medical center has refused to accept him. The admission nurse stated, "The center has gotten burned too many times with these patients who are waiting for Medicaid approval. Something always seems to go wrong with the application and we get left without any reimbursement for services already rendered." The discharge planning nurse tells the social worker, "This is not right. The dialysis center is labeling Mr. Jagmin based on experiences with other people. How can a dialysis center affiliated with the medical center refuse to accept one of our patients? This just does not seem fair!"

1. What ethical issues are involved in this case?
2. Does the dialysis center have an ethical obligation to accept Mr. Jagmin as an outpatient?
3. When reviewing Mr. Jagmin's patient record in more detail, the admission nurse for the dialysis center notices nursing progress notes that state:

   - "Dialysis stopped after 3 hours per patient request."
   - "Refused to go to dialysis, stating 'my brother is coming to visit and I want to be there.'"
   - "Affect flat. Appears depressed. Does not initiate conversation."

The admission nurse recontacts the discharge planning nurse and states, "The center is not obligated to accept a patient that is noncompliant with treatment." What actions or comments should the discharge planner nurse implement as Mr. Jagmin's advocate?

SUMMARY

When providing nursing care for adult patients, situations will arise that challenge the nurse's commitment to maintaining confidentiality and truthfully communicating with the patient. As patient advocates, nurses have a legal as well as moral obligation to protect vulnerable adults from abuse and neglect. Finally, treatment decisions, such as organ transplantation, may force the nurse to examine resource allocation issues and work for social justice through his or her professional organization as well as political avenues.

CLINICAL EXERCISES

1. Talk with a staff nurse about his or her experiences with administering placebos to a patient.
2. Identify your state or province's legal position on disclosure of HIV status to spouses, sexual partners, family members, or persons accidentally exposed to a patient's blood or body fluids.
3. Identify whether your state or province has mandatory reporting of elder abuse. If so, what steps must be followed?

Discussion Questions

1. Current travel policies can restrict the travel of persons with communicable diseases (American Nurses Association [ANA], 1991).

    a. What ethical principles can be used to justify this policy?
    b. What actions or comments should a nurse make when a recent immigrant traveler who was admitted to the hospital with sudden adult respiratory syndrome (SARS) states "I lied when I came through Immigration. I told them that I felt fine and no one around me had been sick before I left home."

2. Consider the following two situations:

    a. Allow college students to be paid for donating a kidney for transplantation.
    b. Allow college students to be paid for donating ova (eggs) for use by clinics providing assisted reproduction.

    For each situation, identify the ethical reasoning that supports or opposes the action. What are the ethical differences between the two situations?

3. The family of a patient with traumatic brain injury has decided to terminate life-supporting treatments and is approached about the possibility of donation after cardiac death (DCD) in which heparin is administered intravenously to increase the likelihood that the liver will be viable for transplantation. However, administering heparin ante mortem has no medical benefit for the patient while posing numerous potential harms, such as bleeding or quickening of the person's dying process.

    a. In your opinion, does the potential for retrieving a viable liver for transplantation outweigh the actual and potential harms to the patient? Support your answer with ethical justification.
    b. Identify whether your clinical agency has a policy on administering heparin to promote the retrieval of organs for transplantation from a brain-dead patient.

SECTION 2: *Nursing of the Adult: Advance Directives*

This section provides an overview of advance directives, discusses the nurse's role during discussions of end-of-life decisions, and identifies ethical issues related to the use of advance directives.

AUTONOMY

Until the 1970s, Western health care was based on a paternalistic model in which the doctor knew best. The idea that a patient had a right to make autonomous health care decisions was not recognized until the American Hospital Association (AHA) drafted the Patient Bill of Rights in 1973. In 2001, the American Hospital Association replaced this document with The Patient Care Partnership: Understanding Expectations, Rights and Responsibilities. With this new document, the AHA acknowledged that the patient and the health care provider share the responsibility for protecting the patient's rights.

Despite more than a 30-year history of publications about patient rights, many older individuals (both lay persons and health care professionals) may not be fully aware of how patient autonomy should guide health care decisions. Informed consent/refusal is a process that is grounded in the principle of autonomy, which requires that decisions be made voluntarily and that information be communicated in a jargon-free manner in the person's preferred language. Informed consent/refusal requires that four steps must be fulfilled:

1. The person must be aware of and understand the problem and the decision to be made.
2. The person must be aware of all possible options or alternatives.
3. The person must be aware of all potential and actual consequences (both positive and negative) of each possible option (positive and negative consequences may be referred to as benefits and risks).
4. The person must be able to explain why a particular option was selected.

This list creates a high level of expectation. Is it realistic to expect that anyone (either the person who needs to make the decision or the health care provider) can ever know every possible option or consequence?

Theoretically, the person who knows the most about the decision needing to be made should assess for the presence of informed consent/refusal. Therefore, the surgeon would seek informed consent before surgery and an endocrinologist would determine the patient's consent/refusal before beginning an insulin pump. Nurses are often the best individual for assessing a patient's informed consent/refusal related to activities of daily living, such as getting out of bed, eating, turning, refusing medication, physical hygiene decisions, and so on. Nurses can also assess the patient's understanding of what the physician told them and notify the physician if the patient does not understand/misunderstands the information or has questions.

Illustrative Case 12-1

After being treated for impaired renal function for several years, Ms. Gann, a 68-year-old woman, is hospitalized with a diagnosis of end-stage renal disease (ERSD). The nephrologist meets with Ms. Gann to discuss beginning hemodialysis. After an extensive patient education session, Ms. Gann states, "I know my kidneys are not doing good, but I do not want dialysis. No one is ever helped by dialysis." The nephrologist assumes that Ms. Gann does not have an adequate understanding of the consequences associated with renal dialysis, and therefore additional patient education is conducted by the renal clinical care nurse specialist. Despite multiple patient education sessions, Ms. Gann claims she cannot identify a single positive benefit from receiving hemodialysis. Based on her repeated statements that no one ever benefits from having renal dialysis, the nephrologist suspects that Ms. Gann is unable to meet the criteria for providing informed consent or refusal for treatment of her renal failure. Because Ms. Gann lacks decisional capacity, the nephrologist initiates actions for identifying a surrogate decision-maker for Ms. Gann.

Illustrative Case 12-2

A 20-year-old fashion model seeks care in the emergency department for acute abdominal pain. Based on the physical examination and laboratory tests, the physician makes a diagnosis of probable appendicitis and contacts the on-call surgeon. The surgeon meets with the patient and explains the need for emergent surgery to remove the appendix before it ruptures. The patient verbalizes an accurate understanding of her medical condition as well as the two available options (surgery or no surgery). She states, "I know that if my appendix bursts I could die; however, I cannot make this decision now. Being a model is my whole life. I need time to think about how this will impact my career." As she is admitted to the general surgical unit for observation, the woman tells the nurse, "I'll give you my final decision in the morning." Based on respect for patient autonomy, the nurse should respect the patient's decision and refrain from asking further questions (unless the patient's condition changes or the patient initiates the discussion), but reinforce the time constraints.

In this example, the woman demonstrates an understanding of the severity of her medical condition and the available options. In addition to the potential and actual consequences identified by the surgeon, the patient has identified another potential consequence from having surgery, that is, "Will having an abdominal scar have a negative impact on my career?" Rather than making a final decision without completely considering this potential long-term consequence, the patient, by delaying, has in fact made a default decision to refuse surgical intervention. Although the surgeon did not agree with her decision and engaged her in repeated educational discussions, her decision was respected because she demonstrated her ability to fulfill all criteria for an informed refusal of treatment. Failure to respect the woman's informed refusal by forcing her to have surgery would be an illustration of battery.

BEFORE THE ADVENT OF ADVANCE DIRECTIVES

Baby Boomers and persons belonging to Generation X and subsequent generational cohorts have lived most of their lives hearing about cardiopulmonary resuscitation, ventilators, and intensive care units; however, this was not always the case. Before this technology and the use of antibiotics and feeding tubes, patients who experienced major physical insults, such as pneumonia, stroke, heart attack, or trauma, often died from infection or dehydration. Often the family would opt to care for their ill family member at home, perhaps with the assistance of a private duty nurse. Thus in the first half of the twentieth century, deaths generally occurred at home in the midst of loved ones and were viewed as an expected natural part, that is, ultimate outcome, of the life process.

Cardiopulmonary Resuscitation

Although various versions of mouth-to-mouth resuscitation have existed since biblical times, it was not until the 1950s that it began to be used by health care professionals and lifeguards. In 1960, Drs. W. B. Kouwenhoven, G. G. Knickerbocker, and J. R. Jude (History of CPR, n.d.) merged chest compressions with mouth-to-mouth ventilation to create cardiopulmonary resuscitation (CPR). Originally, only physicians and military personnel performed CPR. Nurses and even medical students were prohibited from performing CPR until the late 1960s. However in 1973, the American Heart Association began teaching CPR to lay persons (University of Washington School of Medicine, 2003).

The original purpose of CPR was to revive an otherwise healthy person's heart after a witnessed cardiac arrest. However, as the possibilities of CPR became known to health care professionals and lay persons, it began to be implemented when a hospitalized patient or a person not in a hospital was found to be without cardiac and/or respiratory functions. Thus, the original intent for CPR has been expanded, and it is now performed on persons of all ages regardless of their health status or whether cardiac or respiratory arrest was witnessed. One ethical justification for expanding the use of CPR is the principle of justice, according to which equals (all persons without a pulse or breathing) should be treated equally, or, in other words, receive CPR.

Although the expectations for CPR are optimistic, the reality is that fewer than 10% of hospitalized persons who receive CPR eventually leave the hospital alive. Based on this statistic, one could argue that CPR is a futile intervention for the majority of hospitalized patients experiencing a cardiac or pulmonary arrest. However, this argument is generally countered with something like, "Does not even a 1 percent or less chance for maintaining someone's life justify the effort? Do not you think we should at least try?" The majority of U.S. hospitals have a policy stating that CPR (or calling a "code") must be performed on any patient found in cardiac or respiratory arrest unless there is a physician order to withhold specific resuscitative measures. The question therefore must be raised whether CPR has become a basic health care obligation for every hospitalized patient.

OTHER LIFE-SAVING INTERVENTIONS

The 1960s and 1970s saw rapid developments in medical technology and dramatic changes in how health care was provided as well as improvements in patient outcomes. For example, critical care and burn units were created, arterial blood gases (ABGs) and renal dialysis were developed, and marked improvements were made in respiratory technology and enteral and parenteral nutrition. Because of these new technologies, persons who traditionally would have died from their disease or illness (e.g., renal failure or burns) survived. However, this ability to save and/or extend life did not occur without concurrent problems. For example, health care professionals sometimes question whether technology must be used simply because the technology exists. The ability to prolong life and delay death has initiated discussions about whether these life-prolonging interventions are always welcome, leading to debates over the "right to die" and whether "quality of life" should be considered over "quantity of life. Thus, patients and their families often are required to make decisions about whether to initiate specific technology that less than 30 years ago was not an option. The manner in which a person dies in the United States has changed over the last 30 years.

Pivotal Points in History

Karen Ann Quinlan

The ethical discussion surrounding a person's right to die originated after Karen Ann Quinlan's parents sought legal approval to disconnect her ventilator in 1975. Earlier that year, she had been found not breathing after taking diazepam (Valium) together with alcohol. A policeman resuscitated her, and she was left in what is now called a *persistent vegetative state* (PVS). The court permitted disconnecting her ventilator; however, rather than disconnecting immediately, the health care team aggressively weaned her from the ventilator over a 4-month period. She lived for more than 10 years after being weaned off the ventilator (Pence, 1995).

Nancy Cruzan

In 1983, 24-year-old Nancy Cruzan was thrown out of her car after skidding off an icy Missouri county road. The paramedics found her without a pulse and with her face submerged in a ditch full of water. Although she was resuscitated at the site, she was left in a persistent vegetative state. She was discharged from the hospital and moved to a nursing home, where she required a feeding tube to provide nutrition and hydration (Pence, 1995).

After 7 years, Nancy's parents requested legal permission to discontinue her feeding tube (*Cruzan v. Director, Missouri Dep't of Health*, 1990), which raised the question, "legally or morally, is a PVS patient 'owed' food and water?" (Pence, 1995, p. 17). The Missouri Supreme Court reversed the initial probate court's decision granting the parents' 'quality of life' request on the grounds that "the state had an interest in preserving life—regardless of quality of life—and that before medical support could be withdrawn from an incompetent patient, there must be *clear and convincing evidence* of the patient's wishes" (Pence, 1995, p. 18).

Based on the *Cruzan v. Director* decision, a competent person's right to refuse medical treatment even if death would result was recognized by the U.S. Supreme Court, which said that states could decide the threshold for evidence and that Missouri had a clear and convincing standard, although other states may have less rigorous standards. The Supreme Court did not rule on the right to refuse treatment. Linda Greenhouse (1990), a reporter for the *New York Times*, noted the irony of this decision: "the framers of the Constitution, who prohibited the Government from depriving a person of 'life' or 'liberty' without due process of law, had little reason to envision a day when the very act of sustaining a life might itself be a deprivation of liberty" (p. A1). The right to life and the right to die are discussed further in Section 3 of this chapter.

These legal decisions were debated widely in the media, and the fact that Nancy Cruzan was divorced became known. Friends who knew her by her married name before her divorce came forward and provided testimony that provided clear and convincing evidence that Nancy would not want to be kept alive by a feeding tube. Her feeding tube was withdrawn, which allowed her to die. At that point in time, "twenty states had recognized the right of competent patients to refuse medical life support, and all these states (with the exception of New York and Missouri) had recognized the rights of surrogates to make decisions for incompetent patients" (Pence, 1995, p. 17).

Terri Schiavo

Terri Schiavo experienced cerebral hypoxia following a cardiac arrest secondary from unknown causes on February 25, 1990. After this arrest, Ms. Schiavo was left in a presumed persistent vegetative state. She did not have a written advance directive and had never stipulated who she would want to serve as her decision-maker. In 1994, as her guardian, her husband requested that treatments be stopped; however, her parents (the Schindlers) and the extended care facility where she was living objected.

Thus began an 11-year dispute about who should serve as surrogate decision-maker and whether life-prolonging interventions (specifically a feeding tube) should be withdrawn for the express purpose of allowing Terri Schiavo to die.

In October 2003, Schiavo's feeding tube was removed, but was reinserted after Florida passed "Terri's Law" and Governor Jeb Bush issued an executive order requiring that the tube be reinserted. Subsequently, the Florida Supreme Court ruled "Terri's Law" to be unconstitutional. On March 21, 2005, President George W. Bush signed the "Palm Sunday Compromise" into law, which transferred the Schiavo case to federal jurisdiction. However, all federal appeals by the Schindlers were denied, and Terri Schiavo died on March 31, 2005, 13 days after her feeding tube had been removed (Wikepedia, 2005). Besides illustrating the need for a written advance directive, this case also raises many questions about the role special-interest groups, politics, and /or the government should have during individual bedside decision-making. This case is also discussed in Chapter 3.

THE PATIENT SELF-DETERMINATION ACT OF 1990

In 1990, the U.S. Congress passed the Federal Patient Self Determination Act (PSDA). The intent of this law was to promote patient participation and knowledge about health care options available for treatment. However, an unspoken intent may have been to decrease Medicare spending in the hope that a significant number of elderly persons would refuse aggressive treatment at the end of life. Box 12-1 provides further information.

The PSDA does **not**:

1. Provide an advance directive that is accepted universally by every state.
2. Force health care professionals to talk more candidly with patients.
3. Prompt consumers to initiate discussions with their providers.
4. Resolve issues arising from the provision of care for patients without a written advance directive.
5. Deal directly with issues of physician-assisted suicide and euthanasia.

BOX 12-1

The Patient Self-Determination Act

The Patient Self-Determination Act requires every institution that receives Medicare and Medicaid monies to:

1. Provide written information to patients about their right to make decisions, refuse treatment, and complete an advance directive and the institution's written policies concerning the implementation of these rights.

2. Document in the patient's medical record the presence or absence of a written advance directive.

3. Not discriminate based on whether or not an advance directive has been completed.

4. Ensure compliance with state laws concerning advance directives.

5. Provide education to health care professionals and the community on advance directives.

ADVANCE DIRECTIVES

Western society places great importance on a person's right to self-determination even when he or she is unable to participate in decision-making due to dementia or other medical conditions. However, many important, expensive, and complex medical decisions are made during the last month of a patient's life. Often, the person is not able to participate in these decisions because of acute illness or cognitive impairment.

One major decision that is often avoided by patients, family members, and health care professionals is related to end-of-life decision-making. Discussion of this topic is postponed because of fear of death, unwillingness to negate hope, being too busy, and discomfort with discussing values and beliefs. Unfortunately, decisions about end-of-life care are often postponed until the patient is unable to participate in the decision-making, thus negating his or her autonomy.

One proposal for promoting patient autonomy during end-of-life decision-making is to have him or her complete an advance directive to document his or her wishes about the aggressiveness of treatment and values to consider if he or she is unable to participate in the decision-making process. In the United States, there are two commonly recognized legal advance directives: a living will and a durable power of attorney for health care. However, other methods for noting one's health care preferences exist, about which nurses should be aware, such as the *Five Wishes* (n.d.).

Unfortunately, only approximately 15% of all adults have a written advance directive (Tilden, 2000). Many discussions on why Americans are reluctant to complete an advance directive have been held by professional as well as ethics organizations. They usually conclude that the process needs to be overhauled. Suggestions include simplifying the language used on the forms, increasing communication and trust between patients and their primary care providers, and including discussions of advance directives as part of the ongoing health care plan as a means for empowering the patient's decision-making. Because of the 24/7 nature of acute and long-term nursing care, nurses are actively involved in educating patients and their significant others about advance directives and, depending on the individual state law and/or agency policy, may assist the patient to complete a written advance directive.

Verbal Advance Directives

When Nancy Cruzan's friends provided testimony about her wishes, they described her statements on this subject; some may consider these statements verbal advance directives. Verbal advance directives are often related to a specific event that was significant to the individual. Not all institutions recognize verbal advance directives, so patients should be advised to complete written advance directives as well as share their views with significant others. For example:

- After the death of a loved one, a person might state, "I never want to be kept alive by dialysis and a ventilator like Joe was."
- During a significant change in a person's health, say an elderly woman, she might state, "I'd rather die here at home than go back to the hospital."
- A significant current event (like the Terri Schiavo case) might stimulate people to discuss whether they believe tube feedings are part of basic care and thus should never be stopped.

VALUES CLARIFICATION

Values clarification is a process that is frequently conducted to help the patient and subsequently the patient's health care team and significant others to better understand what is important to the patient and what factors he or she considers when making decisions.

Values are learned through socialization. For example, beginning nursing students during their first clinical nursing course are socialized to value professionalism, respect for persons, caring, and veracity. Similarly, children are socialized into the values held by their family, school, and community. An individual's value set will be influenced by the various experiences as well as lack of experiences to which he or she is exposed. Therefore, two individuals may share many similar values as well as have dissimilar values. Examples of personal values are those relating to fidelity, love, family, physical fitness, religious faith, health, and beauty.

Whereas everyone has a set of personal values, some individuals may have difficulty expressing them because of fear, shyness, or limited exposure to the values clarification process. A variety of values clarification exercises can be found in the literature and through the Internet, and are designed to promote self-awareness about what matters most and what priorities are guiding the person's life and decision-making. The decision analysis model presented in Chapter 5 includes values clarification.

Another values clarification exercise (Figure 12-1) uses the metaphor that one's life is like a jigsaw puzzle. When putting a puzzle together, one generally starts with the corners and borders and then fills in the middle section. Following this metaphor as a values

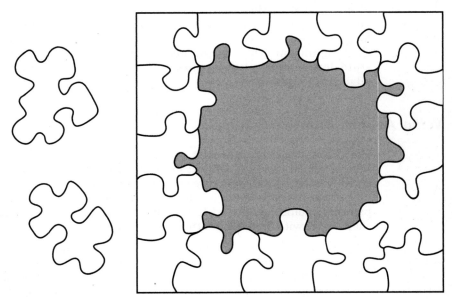

Figure 12-1
Values clarification exercise.

clarification exercise, the person would label the four corners with his or her most fundamental values and the remaining border pieces with other top values that provide meaning to life. The inner pieces would then be labeled with values of lower importance.

Once a person has identified his or her values using the puzzle, the next step is to test the robustness of these values and their ability to withstand life's trials. The reader should complete his or her values puzzle and mark off any identified value that would not withstand the following experience: You are in an automobile accident. Your entire immediate family is killed and you are left tetraplegic. Ideally, your corner or foundational values and the majority of border values should remain intact despite this tragic event. The more values that are threatened by an experience, the more difficulties the person may have coping with the situation. What values would you need to add to cope with this experience?

| Illustrative Case 12-3 |

An 86-year-old woman who has never been married has colon cancer that has metastasized to the liver; she repeatedly states, "I do not want to go to the nursing home. I want to stay in my home." Knowing that her aunt's life expectancy may only be a few weeks, her niece asks the aunt whether she would like to sort through some of her belongings. The aunt immediately replies, "No, I want to keep all of my things with me as long as I live." After this conversation, the niece recognizes that her aunt's experiences growing up during the Depression when the bank foreclosed on the family farm caused her to value the security of home. The niece says to her (the niece's) siblings, "We are going to have to maintain Auntie's home in its current state as long as Auntie lives because having a home is so important to her and makes her feel secure."

Medical Directive Form

To promote better-informed consent regarding end-of-life decision-making, Drs. L. L. and E. J. Emanuel developed an instrument called the Medical Directive Form (MDF). This form is not a legal advance directive, but is proposed as a method for getting patients to think about end-of-life issues and promote dialogue with the health care team. Although it is not a legal document, health care institutions usually honor the values and intentions in a Medical Directive Form in the event that the patient becomes unable to assist in making health care decisions. This form is shown in Box 12-2.

The Medical Directive Form provides a person with a pragmatic opportunity to consider the various steps required for informed consent/refusal regarding treatment options by providing various vignettes or scenarios for consideration. This consideration process should assist the individual to consider the benefits, burdens, and/or futility of aggressive life-sustaining treatment. Many of the technology options included in the MDF are relatively new and have only been available for 30 years or less. Most non-health care personnel have not had any experience with feeding tubes, ventilators, or dialysis beyond what they have seen on television. As a person looks at the various situations posed in the MDF, he or she begins to consider values and beliefs related to life, suffering, and death. The communication of these values and beliefs is important in the event that someone needs to make a surrogate medical decision for that person.

Text continues on p. 250

BOX 12-2

The Sample Medical Directive

Introduction

As part of a person's right to self-determination, every adult may accept or refuse any recommended medical treatment. This is relatively easy when people are well and can speak. Unfortunately, during serious illness they are often unconscious or otherwise unable to communicate their wishes—at the very time when many critical decisions need to be made.

The Medical Directive allows you to record your wishes regarding various types of medical treatments in several representative situations so that your desires can be respected. It also lets you appoint a proxy, someone to make medical decisions in your place if you should become unable to make them on your own.

The Medical Directive comes in effect only if you become incompetent (unable to make decisions and too sick to have wishes). You can change it at any time until then. As long as you are competent, you should discuss your care directly with your physician.

Completing the Form

You should, if possible complete the form in the context of a discussion with your physician. Ideally, this should occur in the presence of your proxy. This lets your physician and your proxy know how you think about these decisions, and it provides you and your physician with the opportunity to give or clarify relevant personal or medical information. You may also wish to discuss the issues with your family, friends, or religious mentor.

The Medical Directive contains six illness situations that include incompetence. For each one, you consider possible interventions and goals of medical care. Situation A is permanent coma; B is near death; C is with weeks to live in and out of consciousness; D is extreme dementia; E is a situation you describe; and F is temporary inability to make decisions.

For each scenario you identify your general goals for care and specific intervention choices. The interventions are divided into six groups: (1) cardiopulmonary resuscitation or major surgery; (2) mechanical breathing or dialysis; (3) blood transfusions or blood products; (4) artificial nutrition and hydration; (5) simple diagnostic tests or antibiotics; and (6) pain medications, even if they dull consciousness and indirectly shorten life. Most of these treatments are descibed briefly. If you have further questions, consult your physician.

Your wishes for treatment options (I want this treatment; I want this treatment tried, but stopped if there is no clear improvement; I am undecided; I do not want this treatment) should be indicated. If you choose a trial of treatment, you should understand that this indicates you want the treatment *withdrawn* if your physician and proxy believe that it has become futile.

The Personal Statement section allows you to explain your choices, and say anything you wish to those who may make decisions for you concerning the limits of your life and

(Continued)

BOX 12-2 (CONTINUED)

the goals of intervention. For example, in situation B, if you wish to define "uncertain chance" with numerical probability, you may do so here. . . .

What to Do With the Form

Once you have completed the form, you and two adult witnesses (other than your proxy) who have no interest in your estate need to sign and date it.

Many states have legislation covering documents of this sort. To determine the laws in your state, you should call the state attorney generals office or consult a lawyer. If your state has a statutory document, you may wish to use the Medical Directive and append it to this form.

You should give a copy of the completed document to your physician. His or her signature is desirable but not mandatory. The Directive should be placed in your medical records and flagged so that anyone who might be involved in your care can be aware of its presence. Your proxy, a family member, and/or a friend should also have a copy. In addition, you may want to carry a wallet card noting that you have such a document and where it can be found.

An earlier version of this form was originally published as part of Emanuel, L.L., and Emanuel, E.J. (1989). The Medical Directive: A new comprehensive advance care document, *Journal of the American Medical Association, 261*, 3288–3293. It does not reflect the official policy of the American Medical Association. Adapted with permission. Complete copies may be ordered at http://www.medicaldirective.org/current/order_options.asp

(Continued)

BOX 12-2 (CONTINUED)

MY MEDICAL DIRECTIVE

This Medical Directive shall stand as a guide to my wishes regarding medical treatment in the event that illness should make me unable to communicate them directly. I make this Directive, being 18 years or more of age, of sound mind, and appreciating the consequences of my decisions.

Situation A

If I am in a coma or a persistent vegetative state and, in the opinion of my physician and two consultants, have no known hope of regaining awareness and higher mental functions no matter what is done, then my goals and specific wishes — if medically reasonable — for this and any additional illness would be:

☐ prolong life; treat everything
☐ attempt to cure, but reevaluate often
☐ limit to less invasive and less burdensome interventions
☐ provide comfort care only
☐ other *(please specify)*: _____
   _____

Please check appropriate boxes:

	I want	I want treatment tried. If no clear improvement, stop	I am undecided	I do not want
1. Cardiopulmonary resuscitation (chest compressions, drugs, electric shocks, and artificial breathing aimed at reviving a person who is on the point of dying).		*Not applicable*		
2. Major surgery (for example, removing the gallbladder or part of the colon).		*Not applicable*		
3. Mechanical breathing (respiration by machine, through a tube in the throat).				
4. Dialysis (cleaning the blood by machine or by fluid passed through the belly).				
5. Blood transfusions or blood products.		*Not applicable*		
6. Artificial nutrition and hydration (given through a tube in a vein or in the stomach).				
7. Simple diagnostic tests (for example, blood tests or x-rays).		*Not applicable*		
8. Antibiotics (drugs used to fight infection).		*Not applicable*		
9. Pain medications, even if they dull consciousness and indirectly shorten my life.		*Not applicable*		

(Continued)

BOX 12-2 (CONTINUED)

Situation B

If I am near death and in a coma and, in the opinion of my physician and two consultants, have a small but uncertain chance of regaining higher mental functions, a somewhat greater chance of surviving with permanent mental and physical disability, and a much greater chance of not recovering at all, then my goals and specific wishes — if medically reasonable — for this and any additional illness would be:

☐ prolong life; treat everything
☐ attempt to cure, but reevaluate often
☐ limit to less invasive and less burdensome interventions
☐ provide comfort care only
☐ other *(please specify):* _____
_____

Situation C*

If I have a terminal illness with weeks to live, and my mind is not working well enough to make decisions for myself, but I am sometimes awake and seem to have feelings, then my goals and specific wishes — if medically reasonable — for this and any additional illness would be:

☐ prolong life; treat everything
☐ attempt to cure, but reevaluate often
☐ limit to less invasive and less burdensome interventions
☐ provide comfort care only
☐ other *(please specify):* _____
_____
_____

*In this state, prior wishes need to be balanced with a best guess about your current feelings. The proxy and physician have to make this judgment for you.

I want	I want treatment tried. If no clear improvement, stop.	I am undecided	I do not want	I want	I want treatment tried. If no clear improvement, stop.	I am undecided	I do not want
	Not applicable				*Not applicable*		
	Not applicable				*Not applicable*		
	Not applicable				*Not applicable*		
	Not applicable				*Not applicable*		
	Not applicable				*Not applicable*		
	Not applicable				*Not applicable*		

(Continued)

BOX 12-2 (CONTINUED)

<table>
<tr><td colspan="5">

Situation D

If I have brain damage or some brain disease that in the opinion of my physician and two consultants cannot be reversed and that makes me unable to think or have feeling, *but I have no terminal illness,* then my goals and specific wishes — if medically reasonable — for this and any additional illness would be:

☐ prolong life; treat everything
☐ attempt to cure, but reevaluate often
☐ limit to less invasive and less burdensome interventions
☐ provide comfort care only
☐ other *(please specify):* _____
_____

</td><td colspan="5">

Situation E

If I . . .
(describe a situation that is important to you and/or your doctor believes you should consider in view of your current medical situation):

☐ prolong life; treat everything
☐ attempt to cure, but reevaluate often
☐ limit to less invasive and less burdensome interventions
☐ provide comfort care only
☐ other *(please specify):* _____
_____

</td></tr>
<tr>
<th>I want</th>
<th>I want treatment tried. If no clear improvement, stop.</th>
<th>I am undecided</th>
<th>I do not want</th>
<th></th>
<th>I want</th>
<th>I want treatment tried. If no clear improvement, stop.</th>
<th>I am undecided</th>
<th>I do not want</th>
</tr>
<tr><td></td><td>*Not applicable*</td><td></td><td></td><td></td><td></td><td>*Not applicable*</td><td></td><td></td></tr>
<tr><td></td><td>*Not applicable*</td><td></td><td></td><td></td><td></td><td>*Not applicable*</td><td></td><td></td></tr>
<tr><td></td><td></td><td></td><td></td><td></td><td></td><td></td><td></td><td></td></tr>
<tr><td></td><td></td><td></td><td></td><td></td><td></td><td></td><td></td><td></td></tr>
<tr><td></td><td>*Not applicable*</td><td></td><td></td><td></td><td></td><td>*Not applicable*</td><td></td><td></td></tr>
<tr><td></td><td></td><td></td><td></td><td></td><td></td><td></td><td></td><td></td></tr>
<tr><td></td><td>*Not applicable*</td><td></td><td></td><td></td><td></td><td>*Not applicable*</td><td></td><td></td></tr>
<tr><td></td><td>*Not applicable*</td><td></td><td></td><td></td><td></td><td>*Not applicable*</td><td></td><td></td></tr>
<tr><td></td><td>*Not applicable*</td><td></td><td></td><td></td><td></td><td>*Not applicable*</td><td></td><td></td></tr>
</table>

(Continued)

BOX 12-2 (CONTINUED)

Situation F

If I am in my current state of health (describe briefly):

_____

_____

and then have an illness that, in the opinion of my physician and two consultants, is life threatening but reversible, and I am temporarily unable to make decisions, then my goals and specific wishes — if medically resonable — would be:

☐ prolong life; treat everything
☐ attempt to cure, but reevaluate often
☐ limit to less invasive and less burdensome interventions
☐ provide comfort care only
☐ other *(please specify):* _____

_____

_____

I want	I want treatment tried. If no clear improvement, stop.	I am undecided	I do not want
	Not applicable		
	Not applicable		
	Not applicable		
	Not applicable		
	Not applicable		
	Not applicable		

Please check appropriate boxes:

1. **Cardiopulmonary resuscitation** (chest compressions, drugs, electric shocks, and artificial breathing aimed at reviving a person who is on the point of dying).

2. **Major surgery** (for example, removing the gallbladder or part of the colon).

3. **Mechanical breathing** (respiration by machine, through a tube in the throat).

4. **Dialysis** (cleaning the blood by machine or by fluid passed through the belly).

5. **Blood transfusions or blood products.**

6. **Artificial nutrition and hydration** (given through a tube in a vein or in the stomach).

7. **Simple diagnostic tests** (for example, blood tests or x-rays).

8. **Antibiotics** (drugs used to fight infection).

9. **Pain medications, even if they dull consciousness and indirectly shorten my life.**

(Continued)

BOX 12-2 (CONTINUED)

MY PERSONAL STATEMENT
(Use back page if necessary)

Please mention anything that would be important for your physician and your proxy to know. In particular, try to answer the following questions: 1) What medical conditions, if any, would make living so unpleasant that you would want life-sustaining treatment *withheld?* (Intractable pain? Irreversible mental damage? Inability to share love? Dependence on others? Another condition you would regard as intolerable?) 2) Under what medical circumstances would you want to stop interventions that might already have been started? 3) Why do you choose what you choose?

If there is any difference between my preferences detailed in the illness situations and those understood from my goals or from my personal statement, I wish my treatment selections/my goals/my personal statement *(please delete as appropriate)* to be given greater weight.

When I am dying, I would like — if my proxy and my health care team think it is reasonable — to be cared for:

☐ at home or in a hospice
☐ in a nursing home
☐ in a hospital
☐ other *(please specify):* _____

Written Advance Directives

The legal recognition of written advance directives varies from state to state. Typically two types of written advance directives exist: the living will and the durable power of attorney for health care.

Living Will

The living will (LW) was the first written advance directive (AD) developed; however, how this document is operationalized varies from state to state. The purpose of the LW is to allow a patient to reject death-delaying procedures in the event that he or she is imminently dying of a terminal illness. Thus, this AD does not apply to patients in a PVS or to conditions that are life-limiting but not terminal. In addition, an agent or surrogate decision-maker is not identified. The usefulness of the living will is compromised by the use of vague language, such as *imminent and terminal illness.* An example of an Illinois living will is given in Box 12-3.

Durable Power of Attorney for Health Care

A durable power of attorney (DPOA) for health care is a more comprehensive document than a living will. A DPOA allows for the same provisions as a living will and also

BOX 12-3

Living Will Declaration

This declaration is made this _____ day of _____, 20 _____ (month, year). I _____, being of sound mind, willfully and voluntarily make known my desires that my moment of death shall not be artificially postponed.

If at any time I should have an incurable and irreversible injury, disease, or illness judged to be terminal condition by my attending physician who has personally examined me, and has determined that my death is imminent except for death delaying procedures, I direct that such procedures which would only prolong the dying process be withheld or withdrawn, and that I be permitted to die naturally with only the administration of medication, sustenance, or the performance of any medical procedure deemed necessary by my attending physician to provide me with comfort care.

In the absence of my ability to give directions regarding the use of such death delaying procedures, it is my intention that this declaration shall be honored by my family and physician as the final expression of my legal right to refuse medical or surgical treatment and accept the consequences from such refusal.

Signed _____

City, County, and State of Residence _____

The declarant is personally known to me and I believe him or her to be of sound mind. I did not sign the declarant's signature above for or at the direction of the declarant. At the date of this instrument I am not entitled to any portion of the estate of the declarant according to the laws of intestate succession or to the best of my knowledge and belief, under any will of declarant or other instrument taking effect at declarant's or directly financially responsible for declarant's medical care.

Witness _____

Witness _____

allows for the identification of a surrogate decision-maker. The purpose of a DPOA is to identify a surrogate to make decisions whenever the patient lacks decisional capacity and is unable to guide his or her own decision-making. This surrogate can direct the initiation and withdrawal of any medical treatment. The one limitation of the DPOA is the difficulty in determining whether the surrogate is making decisions based on the patient's values and prior expressed wishes (substituted judgment) or the surrogate's interests are also being weighed in the decision. The law requires a substituted judgment standard be used. Yet it is unrealistic to expect that the surrogate, usually a spouse or other relative, would not consider the effect a decision would have on his or her own life. An example of the Illinois DPOA for health care is given in Box 12-4.

When discussing a DPOA with patients, a nurse needs to be cognizant of the difference between a power of attorney (POA) for finances and a DPOA for health care. These are two separate and distinct concepts and documents. A POA for finances gives

Text continues on p. 253

BOX 12-4

Durable Power of Attorney for Health Care

POWER OF ATTORNEY made this _____ day of _____ 20 _____.

1. I, the undersigned, hereby appoint (insert name and address of agent) _____

as agent to act for me and in my name to make any and all decisions for me concerning my personal care, medical treatment, hospitalization and health care and to require, withhold or withdraw any type of medical treatment or procedure, even though my death may ensue. My agent shall have the same access to my medical records that I have, including the right to disclose the contents to others. My agent shall also have full power to make a disposition of any part or all of my body for medical purposes, authorize an autopsy and direct the disposition of my remains. (Neither the attending physician nor any other health care provider may act as your agent.)

2. The powers granted above shall be subject to the following rules or limitations (if none, leave blank):

_____

_____

(The subject of life-sustaining treatment is of particular importance. For your convenience in dealing with that subject, some general statements concerning the withholding or removal of life-sustaining treatment are set forth below. If you agree with one of these statements, you may initial that statement; but do not initial more than one.)

_____ I do not want my life to be prolonged nor do I want life-sustaining treatment to be provided or continued if my agent believes the burdens of the treatment outweigh the expected benefits. I want my agent to consider the relief of suffering, the expense involved and the quality as well as the possible extension of my life in making decisions concerning life-sustaining treatment.

_____ I want my life to be prolonged and I want life-sustaining treatment to be provided or continued unless I am in a coma which my attending physician believes to be irreversible, in accordance with reasonable medical standards at the time of reference. If and when I have suffered irreversible coma, I want life-sustaining treatment to be withheld or discontinued.

_____ I want my life to be prolonged to the greatest extent possible without regard to my condition, the chances I have for recovery or the cost of the procedures.

3. This power of attorney shall become effective on _____

4. This power of attorney shall terminate on _____

5. If any agent named by me shall die, become legally disabled, resign, refuse to act or be unavailable, I name the following (each to act alone and successively, in the order named) as successors to such agent:

_____

_____

(Continued)

BOX 12-4 (CONTINUED)

6. If a guardian of my person is to be appointed, I nominate the following to serve as such guardian (if same as agent, leave blank):

_____

7. I am fully informed as to all the contents of this form and understand the full import of this grant of power to my agent.

Signed _____
(Principal)

The principal has had an opportunity to read the above form and has signed the form or acknowledged his or her signature or mark on the form in my presence.

_____   Residing at _____
(Witness)

(You may, but are not required to, request your agent and successor agents to provide specimen signature below. If you include specimen signature in this Power of Attorney, you must complete the certification opposite the signatures of the agents.)

Specimen signature of agent   I certify that the signature of my agent (and
(and successors)   successors) are correct.

_____   _____
(Agent)   (Principal)

_____   _____
(Successor Agent)   (Principal)

_____   _____
(Successor Agent)   (Principal)

---

an agent power to handle the person's finances (e.g., pay bills, invest financial resources), but this legal document does not provide the agent with the power to make health care decisions. The reverse is also true. A person exercising a DPOA for health care can make health care decisions when the patient lacks decisional capacity, but, unless this is stipulated separately on a POA for finance form, cannot handle the patient's finances. The authority of the surrogate/agent can be revoked at any time by the person, upon regaining decisioned capacity, who designated the surrogate/agent by either destroying the original document, creating a new document, or verbally expressing this decision.

The *durable* part of the DPOA means that when a person regains decisional capacity, all authority to make health care decisions reverts back to the person. For example, Mr. Knight is unconscious from a head injury, and according to his DPOA, his wife is his surrogate. As Mr. Knights's surrogate, his wife is able to make all decisions related to his health care. Should Mr. Knight recover and after careful assessment be found to have regained decision-making capacity, he would no longer require a surrogate decision-maker and would resume making his own health care decisions.

BOX 12-5

Illinois Health Care Surrogate Act—Physician Certification

It has been determined that patient _____
has one or more of the following conditions:

☐ terminal condition
☐ permanent unconsciousness
☐ incurable or irreversible condition
☐ lacks decisional capacity only

The cause and nature of the condition(s) is summarized as follows: _____
_____
_____

After personally examining the above-noted patient, it has also been determined to a reasonable degree of medical certainty that the patient lacks decisional capacity to decide whether to forgo life-sustaining treatment or consent to medical treatment. The cause, nature and duration of the lack of decisional capacity is summarized as follows:

_____
_____
_____

In conformance with the Illinois Health Care Surrogate Act, the patient has been informed and has not objected to the above determinations, the identity of the surrogate decision maker and the decision made by the surrogate as to whether to forgo life-sustaining treatment or receive medication treatment. The decision and the substance of discussions before making the decision is summarized as follows (include information as to date, time, location and whether decision by surrogate was received in person, by telephone, or in writing):

_____
_____
_____
_____

Surrogate Decision Maker:

_____   _____
Attending Physician   *Date*

_____
Name   I concur in the determination that the above-noted patient
                                     has a qualifying condition and lacks decisional capacity.

Address:_____
_____   _____   _____
                                     Concurring Physician   *Date*

Telephone No.: ( ) _____   I have witnessed the discussion between the attend-
              ( ) _____   ing physician and surrogate decision maker and the
                                     decision expressed by the surrogate as to forgoing life-
                                     sustaining treatment on behalf of the above-noted
                                     patient.

Relationship to Patient:_____
                                     _____   _____
                                     Witness   *Date*

Surrogate Acts

In the absence of a written advance directive, health care professionals and families are often required to go to court (like the Quinlan and Cruzan families) to obtain permission to withdraw life-sustaining treatment. This process takes time and can be expensive (often the minimum charge for going to court is $500). Thus, some states have created health care surrogate acts. Illinois was the first state in the country to implement such an act. Surrogate acts apply to patients lacking decisional capacity who do not have a written advance directive. Generally, such acts legalize a next-of-kin statute for identifying a surrogate decision-maker following a designated hierarchical order. The creation of this type of act may limit the ability of a health care professional to provide care without surrogate consent to only those rare emergency situations where injury or death would result if immediate intervention were not provided. The Illinois Health Care Surrogate Act is shown in Box 12-5.

DO NOT RESUSCITATE ORDERS

Do not resuscitate (DNR) orders are directives by a physician stating that in the event of cardio and/or pulmonary arrest, specific resuscitative measures, such as cardiac medications, external cardiac compressions, defibrillation, endotracheal intubation, and ventilator assistance, should be withheld. The creation of a DNR order is a separate decision from other advance directive decisions. One should not assume that because a person has an advance directive, he or she should not be resuscitated. There are opposing views on whether DNR orders can be issued without the patient's consent. Some believe that patient awareness of a DNR order is desirable. However, in some institutions, the physician may be able to make a DNR decision without the patient's input. This decision may be made based on the physician's medical judgment of the futility associated with conducting CPR, for example, on a 90-year-old man with an ejection fraction of 20% or a patient with AIDS experiencing severe wasting syndrome and a CD4 count of zero. In those institutions that permit unilateral issuance of a DNR order where these difficult decisions are made without the patient's awareness or input, the physician should document his or her decision-making clearly in the patient's record. At times, nurses may conclude that the physician is acting paternalistically when making a unilateral DNR decision when in fact the physician believes he or she is acting on information gathered over a long relationship with the patient. For example, when asked about why a patient was not involved in a DNR decision, a physician may explain, "Mrs. Smith always told me, 'When you think my time is up, I do not want you to do anything to keep me alive, but I do not think I could handle knowing that I could be imminently dying.'"

In contrast, some states, such as Indiana, have DNR legislation that provides residents of that state the right to initiate and make DNR decisions. Many states have community DNR laws that require documentation of DNR order; otherwise, if called, an emergency responder is required to initiate CPR. Thus, every nurse should be aware of his or her state's current legislation concerning advance directives and DNR orders. See Figure 12-2 for a sample DNR.

According to Rubin (1998), futility is a negotiated reality in which the health care providers, patient, and significant others discuss the goals of treatment and explore each person's definition of the concept.

State of New York
Department of Health
Nonhospital Order Not to Resuscitate (DNR Order)

Person's Name:_____

Date of Birth: _____ / _____ / _____

Do not resuscitate the person named above.

Physician's Signature _____

Print Name _____

License Number _____

Date _____ / _____ / _____

It is the responsibility of the physician to determine, at least every 90 days, whether this order
continues to be appropriate, and to indicate this by a note in the person's medical chart.
The issuance of a new form is **NOT** required, and under the law this order should be
considered valid unless it is known that it has been revoked. This order remains valid and
must be followed, even if it has not been reviewed within the 90 day period.

Figure 12-2
Sample Do Not Resuscitate community order. Retrieved December 6, 2005, from
http://www.health.state.ny.us/nysdoh/ems/pdf/doh3474.pdf

Illustrative Case 12-4

Mr. Ripple is a 60-year-old with post-polio syndrome and requires ventilator support at
night. He has pneumonia, has been admitted to the ICU and sedated, and is receiving
ventilator support. Before this illness, he was a full-time university professor. A medical resident tells Mrs. Ripple that because the underlying problem (post-polio syndrome) cannot be cured, Mr. Ripple may remain ventilator dependent. Because the resident holds the belief that no one would want to be ventilator dependent, the resident

recommends a DNR order be established because being left ventilator dependent would be the best outcome possible from a resuscitation attempt. Mrs. Ripple counters that Mr. Ripple knows many people who use ventilators, that Mr. Ripple used one at night routinely, and that when he awakens from sedation he will decide whether he wants a DNR order written. In this scenario, the resident's definition of futility is not the same as Mrs. Ripple's.

Slow Code

In the past, when nurses did not have moral standing in patient care discussions and physicians were reluctant to write DNR orders, certain misguided, unethical actions on the part of nurses occurred. In describing these, we hope to demonstrate the progress that has been made in having nurses advocate for patients, clarify treatment goals, and provide excellent end-of-life care.

A slow code is performing the acts of resuscitation without intending to revive the patient. By delaying the initiation of CPR, the nurse for all practical purposes is guaranteeing that the CPR will be ineffective and the patient will die. A slow code fails to meet the moral obligations associated with a nurse's commitments to non-maleficence and beneficence. Thus, taking one's time before calling the code (hence the term *slow code*) does not fulfill the ethical obligation to perform one's duties to the best of one's abilities and is arguably malpractice.

> **Illustrative Case 12-5**

During the intershift nursing report, Nurse Amanda Swift explained to Sally Kent, who graduated from nursing school 2 months previously, "Mr. Jobe is a 91-year-old with an extensive cardiac history and he has been experiencing significant bradycardia this evening. However, Dr. Downs refuses to make Mr. Jobe a DNR. If you were to find him without a pulse, I would recommend calling the code from the nurse's station and be sure to get a long drink of water before you make the call. In other words, I'd do a *slow code*."

Similarly, nurses may discuss the implementation of a "show code." For example, during the intershift nursing report, a nurse might suggest, "The family is having a difficult time letting go. If the family is here when the patient arrests, you may want to think about giving a few chest compressions and some IV medications just to make the family feel better." Like a slow code, a *show code* is not initiated with the expectation of reviving the patient. Thus, attempts to justify slow and show codes are generally not associated with the patient, but rather as acts of nonmaleficence to the patient's family. Nevertheless, slow and show codes are unethical behaviors and should never be done.

THE NURSE'S ROLE

Nurses are frequently present when patients and significant others are faced with difficult decisions and thus can have a key role in assisting patients and their significant others to identify values that are important to clarify during future decision-making and to provide patient education about available advance directive options.

Illustrative Case 12-6

A parish nurse was approached by Mr. Lynch, a 50-year-old man with a new diagnosis of pancreatic cancer. He stated, "My doctor told me I need to complete an advance directive but I do not know anything about them. Can you help me?" The parish nurse met with Mr. Lynch and his wife. The nurse educated them about their state's Living Will and Durable Power of Attorney for Health Care (DPOA) forms. Mr. Lynch expressed an interest in completing the DPOA but was unsure as to what directions he wanted to stipulate. The nurse explained, "Sometimes people like to identify values that have been important to them throughout their lives as they made other important decisions, especially decisions regarding their health. For example, some people list that they value being able to interact with others or they are concerned about not exhausting their family's financial resources, while others discuss that they value being comfortable over having their life extended." After further conversation, the man completed his DPOA. Mr. Lynch named his wife as his surrogate decision-maker and stated that he would like his health care decisions to be guided by a commitment to promoting comfort and decreasing pain even if this meant that his life expectancy would be shortened. Finally, he indicated that he did not want his life prolonged by the use of life-sustaining interventions.

When the form was completed, the parish nurse validated that completing the form was something Mr. Lynch was doing voluntarily and that the information accurately reflected his wishes. The nurse then asked Mrs. Lynch if she understood her husband's wishes and verified that Mrs. Lynch believed that she could if necessary make future decisions based on her husband's expressed wishes. The nurse encouraged Mr. Lynch to keep the original form somewhere where Mrs. Lynch could easily access it (i.e., not in a safety deposit box), give a copy to his physician, and take a copy with him if he were to be hospitalized in the future.

Three weeks later, Mr. Lynch died in the hospital. Mrs. Lynch called the parish nurse the next day and said, "I am so glad that you helped my husband fill out the DPOA. The last few days he was so uncomfortable and could not talk. The doctor wanted to do an intervention. I remembered the form and asked him, 'Will this procedure make him more comfortable?' The doctor replied, 'No, but it should help him to live longer.' The decision was easy to make since I knew that my husband wanted to be kept comfortable rather than kept alive. You'll never know how much your help has meant to us."

Advance directives have their limitations. Suppose that early in this course of Mr. Lynch's illness, he contracts the flu and becomes very ill. His primary care physician admits him to the hospital, and when his condition worsens, he is transferred to the ICU. The intensivist believes Mr. Lynch requires ventilator support for 2 to 3 days. Although Mr. Lynch's advance directive states that he wants no life-sustaining treatment, the intensivist believes that Mr. Lynch's request is related to the terminal diagnosis (pancreatic cancer). Because Mr. Lynch's current pulmonary compromise is reversible, should he receive ventilator assistance? If this issue cannot be discussed with Mr. Lynch or his wife, the advance directive provides guidelines, but one should not assume that, given new information, the patient or surrogate would not want to change his or her mind.

Sometimes nurses have significant conversations with a patient when no one else is around, for example, at 2 A.M. on a Saturday morning, regarding the patient's perceptions of his or her illness and view about end-of-life care. When these conversations occur, the nurse should document the conversation in the patient's hospital record, especially if the patient is unable to complete an advance directive at that time (e.g., the state—such as Indiana—requires that a lawyer draft the DPOA, or the patient wants to discuss the DPOA with his children prior to completing the form). The nurse's note should describe the circumstances around the conversation, questions or fears raised by the patient, and any values, beliefs, or desires expressed by the patient. The possibility exists that the nurse's note may provide necessary evidence of the patient's verbal advance directive in the event that the patient experiences an emergent change in condition and is unable to participate in decision-making.

SUMMARY

Advance directives provide a method for promoting the patient's autonomous decisions in the event that he or she loses his or her ability to participate in future decisions. Occasionally, health care institutions or practitioners may attempt to establish a "100% advance directive completion rate"; however, such a goal negates the concept of voluntariness that is a key element of autonomy. A better goal would be "100% documentation of an informed decision to complete or refuse to complete an advance directive."

Nurses are often involved in initiating discussions on advance directives and assisting patients to document their wishes. Every nurse should develop skills in values clarification and be cognizant of current legal as well as institutional, state or province, and national legislation regarding end-of-life care and advance directives. Nurses should also be aware of the limitations of advance directives and their limited use as communication tools expressing a person's past thoughts about an issue. New information may change a person's decisions, and thus advance directives should be revisited routinely and revised to reflect any new decisions.

CLINICAL EXERCISES

1. Identify whether your clinical agency has a policy and procedure for:

   - Advance directives (living will, durable power of attorney for health care, surrogate decision-making).
   - Futile care/futility policy.
   - Do not resuscitate orders (in-hospital and/or community orders).

2. Identify the procedure your clinical agency implements to meet the requirements stipulated by the Patient Self Determination Act.

   - Obtain and read all relevant forms and booklets.
   - Monitor your patient's chart for how information required by the PSDA is documented.
   - With your instructor's guidance, talk with your patient and/or surrogate decision-maker about their perceptions of the agency's process for meeting the PSDA requirements. What are their perceptions of the written materials?

3. Talk with the nurses at your clinical agency about how the agency has fulfilled its responsibility to educate employees and the public about advance directives and the PSDA.

Discussion Questions

1. Describe a situation that you were involved in or witnessed professionally during your clinical experience that illustrates patient autonomy/informed consent regarding end-of-life decision-making.
2. Complete the decision analysis model to reflect the possible options and values expressed by the patient in Illustrative Case 12-2.
3. During the admission process, the patient tells you, "I started to fill out a Durable Power of Attorney for Health Care, but I did not know how to answer the line that read *The powers granted above shall be subject to the following rules or limitations*. What kinds of things do people usually say?" Identify three rules or limitations that could be appropriate to list.
4. Identify a verbal advance directive that one of your significant others has shared with you.

   a. What were the circumstances that led the person to make the statement?
   b. Would you be able to support the implementation of this verbal advance directive? Explain your position.

5. Do you believe that CPR should be automatically administered to every hospitalized patient? Explain your position.
6. A 55-year-old woman is admitted with severe cardiac myopathy. During your initial nursing assessment, the woman tells you, "I have a Living Will. If my heart were to stop I do not want CPR." Despite several attempts, you are unable to contact the attending physician. Your hospital policy states that only the patient's attending physician can write a DNR order. What would you do if the patient began to deteriorate and cardiac arrest was imminent? Provide your rationale.
7. Refer to your state's advance directive form(s).

   a. Is the document easy for a lay person to read?
   b. Are there areas that you believe a lay person might have difficulty understanding or completing?
   c. List three strategies or comments you could use in response to the difficulties you have just identified.

SECTION 3: *Nursing of the Adult: End-of-Life Choices*

The capability exists for persons to live longer, but not necessarily healthier lives due to recent advances in medical technology. In addition, medical technology is able to sustain the lives of individuals who previously would never have survived. Thus, patients, surrogate decision-makers, and health care professionals may be faced with questions about when life should end and when the dying process should not be interrupted. End-of-life choices may be limited by legal prohibitions. Nurses need to be aware of the various end-of-life choices, legal restrictions, and their role and responsibilities during decision-making about end-of-life choices.

AUTONOMY AND END-OF-LIFE CHOICES

Patient autonomy is the foundation of health care in Western society. Over the 30 years since the inception of the American Hospital Association's Patient Bill of Rights (1973, 1992), consumers and health care professionals have debated the scope of patient autonomy and whether the right to make autonomous decisions includes the right to decide when to die.

Right to Life

Traditionally, Western governments have recognized a right to life. In fact, in 1776 the Declaration of Independence proclaimed, "We hold these truths to be self evident, that all men are created equal, that they are endowed by their Creator with certain unalienable Rights, that among these are Life, Liberty and the pursuit of Happiness." The government's position supporting the right to life intuitively makes sense because without citizens a government is unnecessary. Based on the premise that a right to life exists, governments have established a variety of laws related to murder, manslaughter, and justifiable homicide designed to protect the lives of citizens.

Similarly, nurses and other health care professionals have recognized the right to life through a commitment to "promote, preserve and protect human life" (American Nurses Association [ANA], 1994a).

Right to Die

Despite the pervasive acceptance of the right to life, arguments have been put forth proposing a coexisting right to die. Historically, in some cultures, such as those of certain native Alaskan or Native American peoples, there was an expectation that the sick, elderly, and/or widows would separate from their group/community and await death from exposure and/or dehydration. Despite these historical roots, recognition of both a right to life and a concurrent right to die appears to be contradictory. How can a nurse support a person's right to die when simultaneously supporting the person's right to life?

Traditionally, if a person has a right, then he or she has a corresponding duty to act in such a manner as to protect and carry out the acknowledged right. For example, in the United States there is a recognized legal right to vote, and thus citizens are urged to act on this right and participate in elections. Applying this reasoning to the right to life is intuitively easy. Because I have a right to life, I should act in ways to protect my life; therefore, I should obey the speed limits, take medications only as prescribed, and eat nutritious meals. However, this line of reasoning does not hold when applied to a right to die because if this right is recognized, the individual would be required to act to cause his or her death. Thus, there is no pervasive right to die that applies to every individual in every situation. However, one must ask whether there are specific circumstances or situations in which (such as historically in the Native American culture) acts to promote one's death would be appropriate and perhaps expected and welcomed by others. Thus, debates continue about the moral and legal status of various end-of-life choices.

End-of-Life Choices

End-of-life choices involve decisions about preferences for how a person should die. The various options differ as to the circumstances and intent and who is the decision-maker.

Moral Arguments

End-of-life choices are an extremely controversial topic because of the variety of emotional responses they invoke and the moral issues they raise. Depending on what role the individual assumes during end-of-life choices, the type of emotion experienced may differ. For example, the "dying" person may experience despair, abandonment, anger, frustration, envy, hope, and/or love. An observer's emotional experience may be similar, but may be attributed to different reasons. For example, a dying person might feel abandoned if health care providers and loved ones become distant when treatment does not provide adequate pain relief. However, an observing loved one may feel abandoned when the dying person professes a desire to die because life (including personal relationships) is no longer meaningful or worth experiencing. The observing person may experience different emotions when making an end-of-life choice and after the decision has been implemented. Therefore, nurses need to also address the family's feelings of loss when end-of-life choices are being made.

One moral argument that continues to be debated involves the scope of a health care professional's (HCP's) obligation to benefit a patient. If a HCP has an obligation to benefit a patient, does this obligation include relieving suffering by hastening the person's death (Welie, 2002)? If this claim is true, does it not send a mixed signal to patients? If a HCP's obligations include relief of suffering through hastening death, society may lose trust in the fundamental commitments of HCPs. Thus, the possibility exists that persons may avoid contact with HCPs out of fear that they may opt to hasten the person's death rather than act to promote the person's health.

Assisted suicide and euthanasia also invoke debates associated with potential long-term negative consequences. Specifically, does acceptance of various end-of-life options result in what philosophers call the "slippery slope towards murder or genocide" (Castledine, 2001, p. 550)? The *slippery slope* is a metaphor used to illustrate the idea that once a step is taken, then one might not be able to stop the course of movement, and thus a smaller issue could become a giant problem. For example, if one is driving a car down an icy incline, the car will pick up momentum, begin to slide, and become an uncontrollable object that could cause damage to itself and to other objects located in its path. Opponents of assisted suicide and euthanasia fear that acceptance of actions to hasten death may result in an expectation that death should be hastened for specific groups, such as the elderly, those with disabilities, or persons who require a large share of health resources.

Withholding and Withdrawing Treatment

Based on the principle of informed consent, patients and their surrogate decision-makers have the option not only to consent to a specific treatment, but also to refuse treatment. Chapter 12, Section 2, discussed how advance directives can be used to document a person's wishes regarding refusal of treatment options. For example, patients exercise their right to refuse treatment when they opt not to begin a new course of chemotherapy when a cancer recurrence is diagnosed. Similarly, a patient with end-stage renal disease may decide to stop hemodialysis knowing that death will result within a few days or weeks.

In these examples, the patient has refused to initiate a treatment; however, situations occur where patients, surrogates, and/or health care professionals question the appropriateness of continuing a treatment. Sometimes these decisions are readily resolved. For example, when an infection is not responding to a specific antibiotic, the decision is made to stop the current drug and switch to a different antibiotic. However, other situations can occur in which the patient is not benefiting from a treatment, but the treatment is sustaining the patient's life. For example, a 75-year-old woman is placed on a ventilator and started on vasopressive drugs after a myocardial infarction. Despite these actions, the woman experiences repeated episodes of symptomatic hypotension. Her prognosis for recovery is doubtful based on her severely compromised cardiac function. At this point, three possible choices are identified: (1) continue treatment, (2) withhold further treatment, and (3) withdraw current treatment. First, a decision could be made to continue treatment and monitor her responses. Second, further treatment could be withheld, such as adding a second vasopressive drug. Third, a decision to withdraw treatment could be made. Whereas withdrawal could include stopping the current vasopressive drugs and beginning a different regime, withdrawal of treatment usually refers to stopping the current treatment, and not initiating further treatment. When treatment is withdrawn, the decision-makers have concluded that medical intervention is not beneficial. Thus, the decision is made to stop the intervention and not interfere further in the dying process, and to provide comfort measures.

These types of decisions can become complicated if individuals disagree on whether the treatment was beneficial by sustaining the person's life or harmful by prolonging the person's dying. How a person perceives withholding and withdrawing treatment can be influenced by values, religious ideologies, and knowledge of physiology, pathology, and/or pharmacology as well as current events, such as the case of Terry Wallis awakening after 19 years in a vegetative state (Glauber, 2003).

When a decision is made to withdraw treatment, such as withdrawing a ventilator, there is concern that the dying process could be uncomfortable, painful, and/or anxiety producing. To manage these symptoms, such as the patient's apparent suffering, a sedative or analgesic is given. The medication is given with the intent of relieving the anxiety, shortness of breath, or pain that the patient is experiencing, but a side effect of the medication may be respiratory depression or a response that could hasten death. Thus, the decision-maker must determine whether the intent for using these drugs is to decrease suffering or to hasten death. The doctrine of double effect is often used to justify the action of giving the medication. This doctrine forbids the achievement of good ends by wrong means, but permits actions with a double effect, both good and bad, under certain conditions:

1. The act performed is not itself morally evil.
2. The good effect does not result from the evil effect.
3. Only the good effect is intended.
4. There is a proportionate reason for causing the harm. (Shaw, 2002, p. 102)

Based on these conditions, the administration of an analgesic, such as morphine sulfate, when withdrawing a treatment is permissible because administering it is intended as a morally acceptable action that causes good by decreasing pain. A foreseeable negative effect of administering analgesics is respiratory depression; however, respiratory depression is not the intended outcome and is less likely to occur than the intended outcome of pain relief. Therefore, the use of an analgesic when withdrawing treatment can be a morally justifiable action based on the doctrine of double effect.

Euthanasia

Euthanasia comes from the Greek word *euthanatos*, which means "good death, but is an illegal act in the United States." (Battin, 1998). In euthanasia, one individual decides that another person's life is no longer worth living (often related to perceptions of the person's quality of life) and acts to cause the person's death. For example, an individual directly acts to end another person's life by administering an intravenous bolus of potassium chloride. A variety of descriptions have been ascribed to acts of euthanasia. *Voluntary euthanasia* occurs with the person's consent, such as when a person with a degenerative neuromuscular disease is unable to self-administer a lethal medication dose, and so asks another person to administer the medication. *Involuntary euthanasia* occurs despite the person's opposition, for example, a physician administers a lethal injection to a newborn with Down syndrome despite the parent's objections. *Nonvoluntary euthanasia* occurs when a person with advanced Alzheimer disease is unable to participate in the decision.

The Netherlands Experience

In February 2002, euthanasia by a physician became a legal option in the Netherlands. This legal action followed a period of 20 years in which euthanasia and assisted suicide were illegal but not prosecuted, based on Article 40 of the Dutch penal code, which "waives the liability to punishment for anyone who commits a crime while compelled to do so by *force majeure*, that is, by a psychological or moral force so strong that the perpetrator could not resist it. Physicians typically argued that they were compelled to commit euthanasia on moral grounds" (Welie, 2002, p. 42).

Based on this new legislation, Dutch physicians will no longer have to provide a moral justification for participating in an act of euthanasia. Instead, Dutch physicians are now required to demonstrate that the patient requested euthanasia and that the physician responded competently. Box 12-6 is a list of conditions that must be met for an act of euthanasia by a Dutch physician to be considered legal. It has been well documented, though, that Dutch physicians violated protocol and euthanized patients without their consent or knowledge. The Remmelink Report (1991), prepared by the Dutch government, found that 5981 patients were euthanized at their family's request or when their physician thought they should die, confirming the concern opponents of euthanasia have about the "slippery slope."

As other countries debate legalizing euthanasia, the role of other health care professionals, especially advanced practice nurses, will need to be outlined. In the Netherlands, euthanasia has been defined as a medical intervention; however, this does not mean that only a physician has the skills necessary to competently implement an act of euthanasia. Because euthanasia is often accomplished through a lethal dose of medication, the argument has been put forth that other health care providers, such as nurses and pharmacists, may also possess the necessary skills to competently perform euthanasia (Welie, 2002). Should the euthanasia movement gain momentum in the United States, this debate may challenge the American Nurses Association's (1994a) position that participation in acts of euthanasia is contrary to a nurse's moral and ethical "obligation to provide timely, humane, comprehensive and compassionate end-of-life care" (p. 1).

BOX 12-6

Dutch Euthanasia Conditions

Effective February 2002, for a Dutch physician "to be immune from punishment for performing euthanasia, a physician must:

1. Be convinced that the patient's request was voluntary, well considered, and lasting;

2. Be convinced that the patient's suffering was prospectless and unbearable;

3. Have informed the patient about his situation as well as about his prognosis;

4. Be convinced, together with the patient, that there was no reasonable alternative solution for his situation;

5. Have consulted at least one other independent physician who has seen the patient and has formed an opinion in writing about the requirements of due care described in (1) through (4);

6. Have terminated the patient's life with due medical care" (Welie, 2002, p. 43).

Source: Reprinted with permission.

Assisted Suicide

Assisted suicide occurs when an individual seeks and requests another person (often a loved one or health care professional) to provide the means to commit suicide. Providing the means for suicide could include providing a gun or access to a lethal overdose. End-of-Life Choices (formerly known as the Hemlock Society) provides its members with access to "the latest information, advice and tips on hastening death" (End-of-Life Choices, 2003). However, there is a lack of consensus on whether providing the knowledge and patient education about suicide options and resources constitutes providing the means for suicide.

In the book *Jean's Way*, Derek Humphry (1986) provided the following description of his wife's experience with assisted suicide:

She looked across at me and said, "Is this the day?" "Yes, my darling, it is, I replied." I had known for some time now. "All right," she declared, "I shall die at one o'clock. That's good. I am glad it's been decided." I was not surprised at her statement. For two years and four months, she had known she had cancer and almost a year previously we had made a pact about what to do when the end was close. In the four hours we had left, we . . . reflected on the happy years of our lives together. . . . We talked on until a few minutes before one o'clock when I left the room to make a hot drink. I prepared two mugs of coffee, both with milk, and into one mug I put a strong mixture of dissolved pain-killing and sleeping tablets which I knew would be lethal. When I returned to her room I handed this mug to her. "Is this it?" she asked. She knew what it contained. We gave one another a last embrace while we said farewell. She gulped the coffee, set down the mug on the bedside table barely in time before she began to pass out, murmuring, "Good-bye, darling." She fell into a deep sleep, breathing heavily. I watched over her until fifty minutes later her breathing stopped. (pp. 1–2)

In this description, Humphry illustrates the key elements of assisted suicide. The dying person initiates the event and asks for assistance. The assisting person agrees to provide assistance and carries out the steps necessary so that the dying person can carry out the final act (swallowing the pills, firing the gun, or sealing a bag over his or her head). It is important to remember that assisting a person with suicide is an illegal act, and the assisting person could be prosecuted for manslaughter or murder.

As in this case, many persons plan their suicide long before the need exists. Sometimes people wait too long and lose their ability (because of dementia or loss of physical strength or movement) to carry out their plan. When this happens, the person with whom the pact was made may experience distress if the dying person is left in a condition he or she never wanted to experience. Sometimes the *assisting* person may contemplate carrying out the plan without the person's autonomous involvement; however, doing so would be an act of euthanasia.

When discussing the moral permissibility of assisted suicide, proponents often make statements such as, "We treat animals better than humans. When an animal is suffering or unable to control bodily functions, we 'put a horse down' or 'put the pet to sleep.' Why do we treat suffering and dying animals more humanely than we do suffering or dying humans?"

Proponents of assisted suicide claim that it:

- Provides a compassionate end to life
- Is an autonomous decision
- Limits the suffering and pain that would be experienced from a protracted death
- Eliminates the person's fears of abandonment

In contrast, opponents of assisted suicide claim that it:

- Devalues life
- Illustrates a debasement of societal values
- Diminishes trust in the integrity and commitments of health care providers
- Weakens support for palliative care initiatives
- Violates the moral obligation of nonmaleficence (to do no harm)

Thus, assisted suicide involves ethical conflicts for health care professionals between honoring the autonomy of the patient and honoring the professional code that prohibits taking life. There is an assumption that a dying patient whose suffering cannot be relieved would want assistance in ending life rather than wait until death comes naturally. However, people who choose assisted suicide often do so because they fear dependency and loss of control or feel socially isolated.

Some people with disabilities fear that the assisted suicide movement will create pressure for them to accept suicide rather than use health care resources. The "Kevorkian experience" confirms that issues of terminal illness and disability can become conflated (Kirshner, Gill, & Cassel, 1997).

Oregon Death With Dignity Act

Oregon is the only state with legislation permitting physician-assisted suicide (nursing-assisted suicide is illegal) (Euthanasia.com, 2003). This is significant because a 1997 ruling by the U.S. Supreme Court held that "there is no federal constitutional right to physician-assisted suicide (PAS) but implied that individual states could nevertheless enact statutes permitting" PAS (Palmer, 2003, p. 2283). In addition, federal legislation passed in 1997 forbids financial reimbursement for PAS with federal monies, such as Medicaid and Medicare (Assisted Suicide Funding Restriction, 1997).

The general provisions of the Oregon Death with Dignity Act are clear in stating that the adult person must be a resident of the state of Oregon and have a terminal condition that has been confirmed by the person's attending as well as consulting physicians. To initiate the process, the person must inform the attending physician of his or her desire to die and complete the written Request for Medication to End My Life in a Humane and Dignified Manner form. After a mandatory 15-day waiting period, the person is required to verbally reaffirm the wish to die. At that time, if the attending physician is convinced that the person is making an informed and autonomous decision, he or she writes a prescription for a lethal dose. To avoid criminal or civil liability, the physician is required to submit documentation of the person's request and the physician's report to the State Registrar (Task Force to Improve the Care of Terminally-Ill Oregonians, 1998).

Although the citizens of Oregon have demonstrated continued support for this legislation, it has been challenged by a variety of groups and causes. For example, the U.S. Attorney General challenged the Oregon statute, and claimed that physicians who prescribe a lethal dose of medication are violating federal drug laws concerning controlled substances. The question arises of whether a lethal dose falls within the criteria that allow controlled substances to be prescribed for a medical purpose (Palmer, 2003). In addition, this law challenges the profession of pharmacy's refusal to distribute lethal doses of medication based on a commitment to do no harm.

Whereas the Oregon law specifically legislates the physician's role and responsibilities, a nurse practitioner is prohibited from prescribing medication to end life. In addition, the law clearly states that not every health care provider can administer a lethal injection. However, Oregon nurses might become involved in a variety of other ways. First, a patient might approach a nurse about a desire to die and ask questions about the process. Second, a nurse might be identified to serve as the designated health care facility witness for the Request of Medication form. Third, the patient might ask a nurse to be present when the medication is taken, or the nurse might unknowingly happen onto the scene (e.g. a home health or hospice nurse making a routine visit or a nurse at a long-term care facility might be asked to check on a resident after the resident does not appear for a meal). Therefore, nurses need to be aware of the current end-of-life options available in their state or province as well as be cognizant of differences between being present at and participating in the self-administration of the lethal dose. Participation is defined as "making the means of suicide available to a patient with knowledge of the patient's intention (e.g., administering pills, putting pills in a patient's hand, or holding pills while a patient takes them)" (Oregon Nurses Association, 1998). Nurses should develop skills in assisting patients to clarify their values regarding life, death, and suffering and document these discussions in the patient's record. In addition, nurses should prospectively consider their personal and professional values related to end-of-life choices so as to be prepared when approached for information and/or assistance with end-of-life choices. Finally, nurses need to be aware of how to implement a claim of conscientious objection if asked to engage in acts contrary to the nurse's moral code (see Chapter 16).

SUMMARY

In the decision-making process regarding end-of-life choices, the nurse must consider the patient's autonomy and the intentions guiding the decisions. Nurses need to be knowledgeable of current legislation and professional positions regarding various end-of-life choices, such as euthanasia and assisted suicide. Because nurses may be asked for information and/or assistance with end-of-life choices, nurses should prospectively consider their personal values and moral position regarding such choices. This self-awareness will assist them to respond compassionately to a patient's questions while protecting their own moral and legal status.

CLINICAL EXERCISES

1. Locate your clinical agency's policy and procedures for:

   - Withdrawal of life-sustaining treatment
   - Forgoing nutrition and hydration
   - Assisted suicide
   - Palliative care

2. After informing the nursing staff that you are discussing end-of-life choices this week in class, ask the nurse you are working with if a patient has ever asked him or her about end-of-life options. If the answer is yes:

   - What were the circumstances surrounding the request?
   - What questions did the patient ask?
   - What moral justifications were identified by the various individuals involved in the discussion?
   - What resources did the nurse consult or refer the patient to for further information?

3. A person's religious affiliation may influence his or her end-of-life choices. Use the Internet or meet with your agency's chaplain to identify whether various religions have formal positions regarding withholding or withdrawing life support or assisted suicide. For example, the United Methodist Church's (2004) Faithful Care for Dying Persons states, "There is no moral or religious obligation to use these [life-sustaining treatments] when they impose undue burdens or only extend the process of dying."

Discussion Questions

1. The ANA (1994b) definition of assisted suicide states that in such a situation "someone makes the means of death available." When a nurse provides a patient with information about assisted suicide options, methods, and/or resources, is the nurse making the means (knowledge) of death available and thus assisting in the patient's suicide? Explain your answer.
2. You are a nurse working in Oregon. How would you respond if asked by a patient to be present during the self-administration of a lethal dose of medication? What ethical principles support your position?
3. Ms. Song's surrogate has requested to have her feeding tube removed. During the intershift report, the day nurse is obviously distressed and says, "Do not patients have a right to be fed? I am so upset about this that I am not thinking straight! What should I do?" How would you reply?

SECTION 4: *Nursing of the Adult: Adult-Onset Genetic Issues*

In conducting a health history with an adult patient, the nurse is collecting genetic information when he or she asks whether anyone in the patient's family has high blood pressure, diabetes, cancer, or a mental illness. However, the possibility exists that neither the nurse nor the patient recognizes that the information disclosed is in fact genetic information that may have ramifications for both the patient and his or her family's insurability and confidentiality. Nurses who work with adult patients may be approached for information about genetic testing as well as emotional support while incorporating genetic information into health care and lifestyle decisions.

The goal of the Human Genome Project was to identify all the genes in the human body. With the accomplishment of this goal comes the added potential of being able to identify genetic disorders. As the availability for genetic testing moves out of the academic research arena and into the consumer market, nurses will be required to assist adults to make genetic testing decisions. Prenatal and preimplantation genetic issues are discussed in Chapter 13.

ETHICAL ISSUES OF PRESYMPTOMATIC DIAGNOSIS

Testing for adult-onset genetic disorders such as Huntington disease, familial cancers, polycystic kidney disease, or Alzheimer's disease engenders a variety of ethical issues because at present there is no cure for these conditions (Ensenauer, Michels, & Reinke, 2005). Because testing occurs before the incidence of any symptom, this type of testing is referred to as presymptomatic testing.

Presymptomatic genetic diagnosis identifies whether the person carries a known genetic marker. The ability to identify the marker often requires participation by other family members, especially those known to have the disease. The need for family participation is associated with several ethical issues.

First, do family members have a moral obligation to participate? In other words, does a family member have a duty to facilitate another family member's quest for genetic information? If we argue that such an obligation exists, then we must be willing to agree that the family member does not have a right to keep his or her medical information private from his or her family. However, arguing the opposite view—that there is no obligation to participate—minimizes the importance a shared genetic history holds among a family unit in addition to one of the fundamental roles of a family, to promote the well-being of its members. Thus, society continues to debate whether genetic information belongs to an individual or is shared by a family unit.

Second, participation in genetic studies requiring *pedigree* and *linkage analysis* has the potential for identifying multiple persons with the genetic marker who will also have the potential of manifesting the disease at some point in time even if they do not provide a blood sample (DiPietro, Giuli, & Spagnolo, 2004). For example, a grandfather has Huntington disease and the grandson desires genetic testing to determine whether he has the Huntington gene. Identifying the grandson's status will also diagnose his father's status because Huntington disease is an autosomal dominant disease, that is, one that is not gender specific, does not skip a generation, and carries a 50:50 probability that any child of the affected person will inherit the genetic marker (Jorde, Carey, Bamshad, & White, 2000). Thus, the possibility exists that if the grandson has genetic testing, the father by default will learn his Huntington disease status without providing informed consent or waiving his right to privacy.

Third, learning genetic information without the preparation that typically occurs during the informed consent process has the potential for creating harm to the nonconsenting individual. Continuing with the Huntington disease example, it might turn out that the father will experience depression or suicidal thoughts as a result of learning about a positive diagnosis. In addition, he might experience profound guilt after learning that he passed the gene on to his son. In contrast, the father might experience survivor's guilt if the family testing reveals that he and his son do not have the gene but aunts, uncles, and cousins do. The specificity of some genetic tests results is not always accurate. Thus, the possibility exists for an individual's results to indicate a low risk when in fact the risk is high or vice versa.

Fourth, presymptomatic screening for a disease for which there is no treatment or cure raises questions about what benefits are associated with learning such knowledge. Some individuals argue that possessing the information provides the individual with power to make better life decisions. For example, if the grandson learns that he does have the Huntington' disease marker, then he may choose to enter a career that does not require fine motor coordination (becoming a psychologist rather than a neurosurgeon), live in a one-story house, and/or make financial decisions that would favor an early retirement. Presymptomatic information also provides the opportunity for the individual to institute preventive measures, for example eating a low-fat diet to diminish the occurrence of cancer or heart disease. In addition, women who test positive for the breast cancer gene BRCA1 or BRCA2 may opt for a prophylactic mastectomy or total hysterectomy to prevent the occurrence of cancer by eliminating the site. Again, little is known about the long-term physical and psychosocial risks and benefits associated with these prophylactic surgeries. Presymptomatic diagnosis also provides an individual with the option to opt out of experiencing the disease through the act of suicide.

Fifth, awareness of a high risk for an adult-onset genetic disease has the potential for stigmatizing an individual and/or his or her children. For example, persons with a Huntington disease marker may not be allowed to become professional pilots even in the absence of any symptom. A person might be reluctant to enter into marriage with someone who potentially may become incapacitated by 50 years of age. Because of the potential for stigmatization, individuals may use an alias and pay for genetic testing directly without involving an insurance company.

Sixth, another harm that can occur during genetic testing is identification of paternity. When genetic testing reveals that the identified father is not the biological father, several ethical issues concerning rights and confidentiality arise. Does the health care professional have an obligation to disclose information concerning paternity if this information does not directly relate to the reason for testing, for example, if the genetic disorder is found on the Y chromosome? Does the mother have a right to privacy concerning her previous sexual encounters? Does the woman's spouse have a moral and/or legal right to this information? Similarly, does the child have a right to know his or her paternity (Ensenauer et al., 2005)? Because issues of paternity can create a multitude of harms to individuals as well as partners and families, how information related to paternity will be handled should be included in the informed consent process.

Actions That Promote Informed Consent

The decision to participate in genetic testing requires informed consent (see Section 2). When interacting with and/or educating the person and/or family, the nurse must be vigilant to present information in a nonbiased fashion as well as act to protect the individual's rights, which include the right not to participate.

Remaining Nondirective and Morally Neutral

Persons who provide genetic counseling (genetic counselors or geneticists) profess a commitment to providing information in a nondirective, morally neutral fashion (Evans, Bergum, Bamforth, & MacPhail, 2004). Hsai (1979) defined moral neutrality as "I judge it more advisable to give clients the genetic facts as objectively as possible and to refrain from giving the final recommendation of how these facts should be spliced into their personal equations" (as cited in Caplan, 1993, p. 151). In this definition, Hsai combines the objective data and autonomous client decision-making typically associated with nondirective counseling with the necessity of ignoring the professional's personal values, which is typically equated with being morally neutral. Although being nondirective and being moral neutral may have philosophical distinctions, these terms are used interchangeably by genetic counselors.

Genetic counselors and nurses might find their commitment to being nondirective or morally neutral challenged if a patient were to ask, "What do you think I should do?" One strategy for remaining nondirective and morally neutral is to refocus the patient onto his or her values and circumstances. For example, "How I would feel is not going to tell you how you would feel once you get back home. Given the options that are available to you, how do you think you would feel about each option once you are back home with the people whom you live with and love?"

One potential problem with remaining nondirective is that the patient is not given enough structure or guidance on how to make the important genetic decision. The possibility exists that the person will not know what to do with the information. The challenge of remaining nondirective is to not tell the patient what choice to make while guiding him or her through the decision process. Many institutions and special-interest groups (e.g., Huntington's Disease Society of America, Inc., 1994) have protocols designed to promote the patient's ability to make an informed decision in a supportive neutral environment.

Use of a Companion

Discussion Exercises 12-5

Mr. Lamb is 20 years old. He initiated the referral request after his mother died of Huntington's disease (HD). During the initial visit, Mr. Lamb comes alone. He states, "I recently moved to this city so I did not know who to ask to come with me." The HD protocol requires that a non—blood-related person be present as a companion.

1. What ethical issues are involved?
2. Because Mr. Lamb is unable to identify a support person to accompany him, would it be ethically permissible to not follow the protocol?

3. What suggestions would you make to resolve the ethical issues present in this case?
4. While talking with Mr. Lamb, you learn that he will be the first person tested in his family. Considering your commitment to being nondirective and morally neutral, how would you respond to this information?

One strategy proposed to promote informed consent while providing emotional support is to have a companion present. The companion attends all sessions (preconsultation, testing, and disclosure of results) and the informed consent process to provide the patient with another pair of ears about what information was communicated during each session. Although the intent behind using a companion is to promote the patient's objective understanding of the various issues related to presymptomatic diagnosis, the possibility does exist that the presence of a companion will be coercive. For example, the companion might say to the patient, "You have done all the prescreening tests, you really should not stop now."

Genetic testing protocols generally stipulate that the person serving as the companion should not be biologically related to the person considering testing. Therefore, a companion could be a spouse or friend, but not a sibling or parent. The rationale for not using a blood-related companion is again related to the need for objectivity and reducing the chance of coercion. If the companion were related by blood, the potential exists that he or she might learn information related to his or her genetic status and might encourage or discourage genetic testing because of the companion's preferences, thus threatening the autonomy of the person seeking genetic testing.

If a companion is used, the health care professional in charge of each session must verify that the patient desires the companion to be present and realizes that the companion will learn confidential and perhaps personal information simultaneously with the patient. Prior to assuming the role of companion, the person should be educated on his or her need to maintain confidentiality regarding the patient's genetic information.

Companions also need education about their supportive role, which includes identifying extreme depression and suicidal ideations so that resources can be accessed to assist the patient to cope with the genetic information learned. Thus, a companion has duties associated with decreasing harm and promoting good coping as well as promoting the patient's autonomous decision to engage in presymptomatic diagnosis.

SUMMARY

A decision to engage in presymptomatic genetic diagnosis requires that the individual consider harms and benefits as well as personal values. When working with individuals concerning presymptomatic genetic diagnosis, nurses need to remain nondirective and morally neutral while implementing actions to promote patient autonomy and maintain confidentiality.

CLINICAL EXERCISES

1. Review the medical record of your assigned patient to identify the types of genetic information included.
2. Identify whether your clinical agency has a policy and procedure regarding presymptomatic diagnosis of genetic conditions.

3. Identify the nearest genetic counseling center to your university or college. What services do they offer? Does the genetic counseling center's published or online information include any information regarding ethical and legal issues related to presymptomatic testing?

Discussion Questions

1. Six years ago, Mr. Nosal participated in a research study investigating a new genetic test. His results suggested the likelihood of premature death or disability. He is now applying for an individual life insurance policy. Does Mr. Nosal have an ethical obligation to disclose these research results to the insurance company?

2. Your family has an extensive history of breast and ovarian cancer. After participating in pretesting counseling, you consent to genetic testing. You are notified that you tested positive for both the BRCA1 and BRCA2 breast cancer genes. Using the decision analysis model of Chapter 5, identify what action based on your values is the best response for you concerning this information.

3. You are a nurse working in a neurology office. One day you answer the phone and are asked advice on the following situation: "My mother died of Huntington's disease last year. I have made the decision not to be tested, because I do not think I could keep a positive outlook if I tested positive for HD. My wife just found out she is pregnant and she is adamant that we have the baby tested for HD so we can abort if the test is positive. Agreeing to test our baby is the same as agreeing to test myself. What should I do?" How would you respond?

Special Topic: *Medical Directive Project*

The purpose of this project is to provide the student with a vehicle for self-reflection and analysis on the effect of culture and communication on end-of-life decision-making for himself or herself and another person. The project is designed to allow the student to first analyze his or her response to completing the Medical Directive Form (MDF). From this experience, the student will then design and implement a plan to use with someone else (older family member, someone with a chronic illness, patient, or family member) who the student will assist to complete the MDF.

In this process, there is an opportunity to analyze personal and cultural values and examine how values and culture influence and contribute to quality-of-life and important end-of-life decisions. In addition, this project will provide an opportunity for assessment and analysis of communication techniques as well as an opportunity to apply aspects of the decision-making model to end-of-life decision-making.

STEP 1.   Complete the full Medical Directive Form (MDF) based on your health and life situation.

STEP 2.   Using the decision analysis model graph presented in Chapter 5, complete the horizontal axis by identifying and prioritizing the values/outcomes that influenced how you answered the MDF in Step 1 (do not fill out the vertical axis).

STEP 3.   Reflect on your decisions as you filled out the answers to the MDF, and respond to the following questions:

    a. What did you learn about yourself?

    b. How have your personal values been shaped or influenced by professional and/or societal cultural values and/or your cultural group?

    c. How did you feel (both cognitively and emotionally) when completing Steps 1 and 2?

    d. Describe difficulties or areas of difficulty you had in filling out the MDF. (This could include such things as clarity of task, unclear terms or directions, or feeling that this was not relevant to you or that it was too repetitive).

    e. Identify areas that could be problematic for you when asking another person these questions.

STEP 4. After completing Steps 1 through 3, identify another person to complete the MDF. Provide a rationale for why you chose this person to be part of this project.

STEP 5. Develop a plan for assisting the selected person to complete the MDF.

    a. What difficulties do you anticipate from cultural and/or communication barriers?

    b. Explain how you will deal with these barriers as well as the problems you identified in Step 3E. What actions will you take to deal with these difficulties (e.g., an older adult who has visual difficulties, someone in pain)?

STEP 6. Implement your plan to assist the selected person to complete the MDF.

    a. Describe how and where you implemented your plan.

    b. How did you approach your identified person and gain agreement?

    c. Did anything unexpected happen?

STEP 7. Analyze this experience.

    a. Evaluate your plan for assisting this person to think through end-of-life decisions by completing the MDF.

    b. What are the selected person's evaluation/feelings regarding the MDF?

    c. How has the selected person's personal values been influenced or shaped by their cultural group and/or societal cultural values?

STEP 8. Summary of experience. What effect will what you have learned about the impact of culture and communication on end-of-life decision-making have on your future clinical practice? Provide pragmatic illustrations of how this new knowledge will be incorporated into your future nursing practice.

Special Topic: *It's Over, Debbie*

The call came in the middle of the night. As a gynecology resident rotating through a large, private hospital, I had come to detest telephone calls, because invariably I would be up for several hours and would not feel good the next day. However, duty called, so I answered the phone. A nurse informed me that a patient was having difficulty getting rest, could I please see her. She was on 3 North. That was the gynecologic-oncology unit, not my usual duty station. As I trudged along, bumping sleepily against walls and corners and not believing I was up again, I tried to imagine what I might find at the end of my walk. Maybe an elderly woman with an anxiety reaction, or perhaps something particularly horrible.

I grabbed the chart from the nurses station on my way to the patient's room, and the nurse gave me some hurried details: a 20-year-old girl named Debbie was dying of ovarian cancer. She was having unrelenting vomiting apparently as the result of an alcohol drip administered for sedation. Hmmm, I thought. Very sad. As I approached the room I could hear loud, labored breathing. I entered and saw an emaciated, dark-haired woman who appeared much older than 20. She was receiving nasal oxygen, had an IV, and was sitting in bed suffering from what was obviously severe air hunger. The chart noted her weight at 80 pounds. A second woman, also dark-haired but of middle age, stood at her right, holding her hand. Both looked up as I entered. The room seemed filled with the patient's desperate effort to survive. Her eyes were hollow, and she had suprasternal and intercostal retractions with her rapid inspirations. She had not eaten or slept in two days. She had not responded to chemotherapy and was being given supportive care only. It was a gallows scene, a cruel mockery of her youth and unfulfilled potential. Her only words to me were, "Let's get this over with."

I retreated with my thoughts to the nurses station. The patient was tired and needed rest. I could not give her health, but I could give her rest. I asked the nurse to draw 20 mg of morphine sulfate into a syringe. Enough, I thought, to do the job. I took the syringe into the room and told the two women I was going to give Debbie something that would let her rest and to say good-bye. Debbie looked at she syringe, then laid her head on the pillow with her eyes open, watching what was left of the world. I injected the morphine intravenously and watched to see if my calculations on its effects would be correct. Within seconds her breathing slowed to a normal rate, her eyes closed, and her features softened as she seemed restful at last. The older woman stroked the hair of the now-sleeping patient. I waited for the inevitable next effect of depressing the respiratory drive. With clocklike certainty, within four minutes the breathing rate slowed even more, then became irregular, then ceased. The dark-haired woman stood erect and seemed relieved.

It's over, Debbie.

Name Withheld by Request

Anonymous (1988). A piece of my mind: It's over, Debbie. *JAMA, 259(2)*, 272. Copyright © 1988, American Medical Association. All rights reserved.

Discussion Questions

1. What is the ethical issue(s) in this case?
2. What question(s) need to be resolved?
3. Identify two questions the resident could have asked to clarify Debbie's wishes and values.
4. Critique the role and actions of the nurse in this case.
5. If you were the nurse, what other options might you have suggested to the resident?
6. Was the outcome justifiable? Were the individuals involved satisified? Explain.

Resources

Aetna InteliHealth. (2004). Genetic testing: Decision guide: Colorectal cancer. Retrieved May 30, 2005, from http://www.intelihealth.com/IH/ihtIH/WSIHW000/32193/35150.html
An interactive test introducing ethical issues a person should consider before making a decision to engage in genetic testing.

American Academy of Family Physicians. (1999). Sample advance directive form. Retrieved September 2, 2003, from http://www.aafp.org/afp/990201ap/617.html

American Association of Retired Persons, the American Bar Association Commission on Legal Problems of the Elderly, and the American Medical Association. (1995). Shape your health care future with Health Care Advance Directives. Retrieved May 28, 2005, from http://www.abanet.org/lawinfo/fam1.html This site provides links to a variety of documents addressing end-of-life issues and estate planning

American Nurses Association. (1991). Position statement: Nursing and the Patient Self-Determination Act. Retrieved July 18, 2003, from http://nursingworld.org/readroom/position/ethics/etsdet.htm

American Nurses Association. (1991). Position statement: Guidelines for disclosure to a known third party about possible HIV infection. Retrieved May 30, 2005, from http://nursingworld.org/readroom/position/blood/blhiv.htm

American Nurses Association. (1992). Position statement: Nursing care and do-not-resuscitate decisions. Retrieved July 18, 2003, from http://nursingworld.org/readroom/position/ethics/etdnr.htm

American Nurses Association. (1992). Position statement: Foregoing nutrition and hydration. Retrieved May 30, 2005, from http://nursingworld.org/readroom/position/ethics/etnutr.htm

American Nurses Association. (1994). Position statement: Nurses' participation in capital punishment. Retrieved May 30, 2005, from http://nursingworld.org/readroom/position/ethics/etcptl.htm

American Nurses Association. (1991/2003). Position statement: Pain management and control of distressing symptoms in dying patients. Retrieved May 30, 2005, from http://nursingworld.org/readroom/position/ethics/etpain.htm

American Society of Transplant Surgeons. (2002). ASTS position statement on adult-to-adult living liver donation. Retrieved May 30, 2005, from http://www.asts.org/livingliverdonorupdated.cfm

Annas, G. J., Glantz, L. H., & Roche, P. A. (1995). The genetic privacy act and commentary. Retrieved May 30, 2005, from http://www.ornl.gov/TechResources/Human_Genome/resource/privacy/privacy1.html

Canadian Nurses Association. (1994). Policy statement: Joint statement on advance directives. Retrieved July 18, 2003, from http://www.cnanurses.ca/_frames/policies/policiesmainframe.htm

Canadian Nurses Association. (1996). Policy statement: Joint statement on resuscitative interventions. Retrieved July 18, 2003, from http://www.cna-nurses.ca/_frames/policies/policiesmainframe.htm

The Cleveland Clinic Department of Bioethics. (2002). Policy on do not resuscitate. Retrieved July 18, 2003, from http://www.clevelandclinic.org/bioethics/policies/dnr.html

Cook, A. F., Hoas, H., & Grayson, C. (2003). Asking for organs: Different needs and different values. *Journal of Clinical Ethics, 14*(1/2), 37–48.

DuBois, J. M., & Schmidt, T. (2003). Does the public support organ donation using higher brain-death criteria? *Journal of Clinical Ethics, 14*(1/2), 26–36.

End-of-Life Choices and Compassion in Dying [formerly the Hemlock Society]. Retrieved May 28, 2005, from www.endoflifechoices.org

Euthanasia.com. (n.d.). Retrieved May 28, 2005, from www.euthanasia.com/index.html

Faber-Langendoen, K., & Karlawish, J. H. T. (2000). Should assisted suicide be only physician assisted? *Annals of Internal Medicine, 132*(6), 482–487.

International Council of Nurses. (2000). Nurses' role in providing care to dying patients and their families. Retrieved May 30, 2005, from http://www.icn.ch/pscare00.htm

Institute of Medicine (1997). *Non-heart-beating organ transplantation: Medical and ethical issues in procurement.* Washington, DC: National Academy Press.

International Society of Nurses in Genetics. (2000). Position statement: Informed decision-making and consent: The role of nursing. Retrieved October 6, 2003, from http://www.globalreferrals.com/about/position_statements/consent.htm

International Society of Nurses in Genetics (2001). Position statement: Privacy and confidentiality of genetic information: The role of the nurse. Retrieved May 30, 2005, from http://www.isong.org/about/position_statements/privacy.htm

International Society of Nurses in Genetics (2002). Position statement: Genetic counseling for vulnerable populations: The role of nursing. Retrieved May 30, 2005, from http://www.isong.org/about/position_statements/vul_pop.html

International Society of Nurses in Genetics (2003). Position statement: Access to genomic health care: The role of the nurse. Retrieved May 30, 2005, from http://www.isong.org/about/position_statements/genetics_health care.html

King, P., & Jordan-Welch, M. (2003). Nurse-assisted suicide: Not an answer in end-of-life care. *Issues in Mental Health Nursing, 24*, 45–57.

Legal Counsel for the Elderly, American Association of Retired Persons. (n.d.). Individualized state advance directive forms can be obtained by writing to Legal Counsel for the Elderly, American Association of Retired Persons, P.O. Box 96474, Washington, D.C. 20090.

Les Turner ALS Foundation (n.d.). *Ventilation: The decision making process* [video; available to rent]. Retrieved May 30, 2005, from http://www.lesturnerals.org/

Lynn, J., Arkes, H. R., Stevens, M., Cohn, F., Koenig, B., Fox, E., et al. (2000). Rethinking fundamental assumptions: SUPPORT's implications for future reform. *Journal of the American Geriatrics Society, 48*(5), S214–S221.

McKenney, E., & Parker, B. (2003). Legal and ethical issues related to nonheart beating organ donation. *AORN Online, 77*(5), 973–976.

Murphy, P., Kreling, B., Kathryn, E., Stevens, M., Lynn, J., & Dulac, J. (2000). Description of the SUPPORT intervention. *Journal of the American Geriatrics Society, 48*(5), S154–S164.

National Cancer Institute. (n.d.). Legal and ethical issues. Retrieved May 30, 2005, from http://www.cancerdiagnosis.nci.nih.gov/specimens/legal.html#3a

National Center on Elder Abuse. (2003). Adult protective services: Ethical principles and best practice guidelines. Retrieved May 28, 2005, from http://www.elderabusecenter.org/pdf/publication/ethics.pdf

Sabatino, C. P. (n.d.). 10 legal myths about advance medical directives. Retrieved May 28, 2005, from http://www.abanet.org/aging/myths.html

State of New York Department of Health. (1995). Deciding about CPR. Do Not Resuscitate orders (DNR). A guide for patients and families. Retrieved May 30, 2005, from http://www.strems.org/dnr.html

University of Michigan. (2003). TransWeb: Questions about ethical issues in transplantation. Retrieved May 28, 2005, from http://www.transweb.org/qa/qa_txp/faq_ethics.html

U.S. Department of Energy Office of Science, Office of Biological and Environmental Research, Human Genome Program. (2004). Ethical, legal and social issues. Retrieved May 30, 2005, from http://www.ornl.gov/sci/techresources/Human_Genome/elsi/elsi.shtml

Williams, D. (2001). Living Wills Registry (Canada). Retrieved May 28, 2005, from http://www.sentex.net/~lwr/index.html

References

American Civil Liberties Union. (2000). State criminal statutes on HIV transmission. Retrieved May 28, 2005, from www.aclu.org/HIVAIDS/HIVAIDS.cfm?ID=9365&c=21

American Hospital Association. (1973, 1992). *The patient bill of rights.* Retrieved on December 6, 2005, from http://www.injuredworker.org/Library/Patient_Bill_of_Rights.htm

American Hospital Association. (2001). *The patient care partnership: Understanding expectations, rights and responsibilities.* Retrieved on December 6, 2005, from http://www.aha.org/aha/ptcommunication/partnership/index.html

American Nurses Association. (1991). Travel restrictions for persons with HIV/AIDS. Retrieved October 8, 2005, from http://nursingworld.org/readroom/position/blood/bltrav.htm

American Nurses Association. (1994a). Position statement: Active euthanasia. Retrieved September 3, 2003, from http://nursingworld.org/readroom/position/ethics/eteuth.htm

American Nurses Association. (1994b). Position statement: Assisted suicide. Retrieved September 3, 2003, from http://nursingworld.org/readroom/position/ethics/etsuic.htm

Anonymous. (1988). A piece of my mind. It's over, Debbie. *JAMA, 259*(2), 272.

Assisted Suicide Funding Restriction. (1997). 42 USC §§14401–14408.

Battin, M. P. (1998). Euthanasia: The way we do it, the way they do it. In J. F. Monagle & D. C. Thomasma (Eds.). *Health care ethics: Critical issues for the 21st century* (pp. 311–322). Gaithersburg, MD: Aspen.

Caplan, A. L. (1993). Neutrality is not morality: The ethics of genetic counseling. In D. M. Bartels, B. S. LeRoy, & A. L. Caplan (Eds.). *Prescribing our future: Ethical challenges in genetic counseling* (pp. 149–165). New York: Aldine de Gruyter.

Castledine, G. (2001). Euthanasia: What is the nursing and medical role? *British Journal of Nursing, 10(8),* 550.

Cruzan v Director, Missouri Dep't of Health. (1990). 110 S. Ct. 2841. Retrieved August 1, 2003, from http://biotech.law.lsu.edu/cases/consent/cruzan_sc.htm

DiPietro, M. L., Giuli, A., & Spagnolo, A. G. (2004). Ethical implications of predictive DNA testing for hereditary breast cancer. *Annals of Oncology, 15*(Supplement 1), i65 –i70.

End-of-Life Choices. (2003). Retrieved September 10, 2003, from http://www.hemlock.org/index.asp

Ensenauer, R. E., Michels, V. V., & Reinke, S. S. (2005). Genetic testing: Practical, ethical, and counseling considerations. *Mayo Foundation for Medical Education and Research,* 80(1), 63–73.

Euthanasia.com. (2003). Assisted suicide laws by state—July 1998. Retrieved September 3, 2003, from www.euthanasia.com/stlaws.html

Evans, M. Bergum, V., Bamforth, S., & MacPhail, S. (2004). Relational ethics and genetic counseling. *Nursing Ethics, 11*(5), 459–471.

Federal Patient Self Determination Act. (1990). 42 U.S.C. 1395 cc(a). Retrieved August 1, 2003, from http://www.fha.org/acrobat/Patient%20Self%20Determination%20Act%201990.pdf

Five wishes. (n.d.). Retrieved May 28, 2005, from www.agingwithdignity.org/5wishes.html

Glauber, B. (2003, July 13). Mom's faith borne out as son awakens after 19 years. *Chicago Tribune,* Section 1, pp. 1, 17.

Greenhouse, L. (1990, June 27). Right to reject life. *The New York Times,* p. A1.

History of CPR. (n.d.). Retrieved August 1, 2003, from http://www.ukdivers.net/history/cpr.htm

Humphry, D. (1986). *Jean's way.* New York: Harper & Row.

Huntington's Disease Society of America, Inc. (1994). *Guidelines for genetic testing for Huntington's disease.* Retrieved May 30, 2005, from http://www.hdfoundation.org/testread/hdsatest.htm

Illinois Public Health Communicable Diseases AIDS Confidentiality Act. (1997). 410 ILCS 305/9.

Jorde, L. B., Carey, J. C., Bamshad, M. J., & White, R. L. (2000). *Medical genetics* (2nd ed.). St. Louis: Mosby.

Lewis, R. (1994). *Human genetics: Concepts and applications.* Dubuque, IA: Wm. C. Brown Communications.

McCaffery, M., & Beebe, A. (1989). *Pain: Clinical manual for nursing practice.* St. Louis: Mosby–Year Book.

National Center on Elder Abuse. (2003). Frequently asked questions. Retrieved December 12, 2003, from http://www.elderabusecenter.org/default.cfm?p=faqs.cfm

Oregon Nurses Association. (1998). *Guidelines on the nurse's role related to the Death With Dignity Act.* Tualatin, OR: Author. Also retrieved September 10, 2003, from http://www.oregonrn.org/services-whitepapers-0001.php

Palmer, L. (2003). The legal and political future of physician-assisted suicide. *JAMA, 289*(17), 2283.

Pence, G. E. (1995). *Classic cases in medical ethics: Accounts of cases that have shaped medical ethics, with philosophical, legal, and historical backgrounds* (2nd ed.). New York: McGraw-Hill, Inc.

Remmelink Report. (1991). *Practice of euthanasia in the Netherlands.* Retrieved April 5, 2004, from www.euthanasia.com/hollchart.html

Rubin, S. B. (1998). *When doctors say no: The battleground of medical futility.* Bloomington, IN: Indiana University Press.

Shaw, A. B. (2002). Two challenges to the double effect doctrine: Euthanasia and abortion. *Journal of Medical Ethics, 28,* 102–104.

Steinberg, D. (2003). The antemortem use of heparin in non-heart-beating organ transplantation: A justification based on the paradigm of altruism. *Journal of Clinical Ethics, 14*(1/2), 18–25.

The Declaration of Independence of the Thirteen Colonies (July 4, 1776). Retrieved on September 8, 2003, from http://www.law.indiana.edu/uslawdocs/declaration.html

The Task Force to Improve the Care of Terminally-Ill Oregonians. (1998). *The Oregon Death With Dignity Act: A guidebook for health care providers.* Portland, OR: The Center for Ethics in Health Care, Oregon Health Sciences University.

Tilden, V. P. (2000). Advance directives. *American Journal of Nursing, 100(12),* 49, 51.

United Methodist Church. (2004). Faithful care for dying persons. Retrieved on December 9, 2005, from http://archives.umc.org/interior.asp?mid=1734

University of Washington School of Medicine. (2003). Learn CPR: History of CPR. Retrieved August 1, 2003, from http://depts.washington.edu/learncpr/book.html

Vazquez, E. (2001, November/December). Small town, big misperceptions. Positively aware. Retrieved September 15, 2003, from http://www.thebody.com/tpan/novdec_01/small_town.html

Welie, J. V. M. (2002). Why physicians? Reflections on The Netherlands' new euthanasia law. *Hastings Center Report, 32*(1), 42–44.

Wikepedia. (2005). Terri Schiavo. Retrieved May 30, 2005, from http://en.wikipedia.org/wiki/Terri_Schiavo

CHAPTER 13

Women's Health Nursing

Objectives

At the end of this chapter, the student should be able to:

1. Identify ethical issues relating to women's health care.
2. Discuss the ethical implications of new reproductive technologies.
3. Analyze complex ethical situations affecting women's health and caregiving roles.
4. Analyze the ethical issues in light of the nurse's obligation toward advocacy, truth-telling, confidentiality, and resource allocation.

KEY WORDS

- Abortion
- Assisted reproduction
- Caregiver burden
- Circumcision
- Contraception
- Genetic testing
- Maternal–fetal conflict
- Menopause
- Sexually transmitted infection (STI)
- Sterilization

SECTION 1: *Ethical Themes: Building From the Basic to the Complex*

In the last few decades of the twentieth century, issues relating to women's health were determined to be distinctly different from those relating to men's health even if one excluded obstetric and gynecological issues. The specialty of women's health has grown in the last 20 years, and new ethical issues have arisen. Reproductive and genetic technologies have allowed postmenopausal women to bear children. Couples can make decisions regarding unwanted genetic disorders prior to implantation of the fertilized ovum. More is known about menopause and health issues for that time in a woman's life. Women continue to outlive men and are frequently the caregivers for others in their families with chronic illnesses. This chapter reviews the ethical issues that arise in relation to women's health care across the lifespan. Although these are not exclusively reproductive issues, most of the ethical issues in women's health care are related to reproductive issues or the reproductive system. This chapter discussed the clinical ethical issues that students will most likely encounter in their clinical practice.

The basic ethical themes (confidentiality, truth telling, advocacy, and allocation of scarce resources) can become more complex in women's health nursing. This complexity may be related to society's values related to women as well as legal views on how to deal with issues that arise when the needs or rights of a woman are in conflict with those of her fetus or society.

CONFIDENTIALITY

In every aspect of health care, health information is kept confidential except under specific circumstances, in which (1) proper authorization is given to release information, (2) there are public health laws defining when and what information can be shared without consent, and (3) there is imminent harm to a third party.

Reproductive Care

When an adolescent girl seeks health care for contraception, pregnancy, or treatment of a sexually transmitted infection (STI), the health care provider (HCP) may treat her without parental consent or notification, depending on that state's statute. The HCP may urge the girl to tell her parents, but cannot disclose confidential information without the girl's written consent. Even though the HCP may believe that the girl is immature, troubled, or being exploited and needs parental assistance, he or she cannot disclose any information to the parents. If the HCP suspects abuse and/or neglect by the parent or legal guardian or a statutory rape has occurred, then he or she is obligated to break confidentiality and report the event as stipulated in that state's abuse and neglect statute.

Although this restriction may seem counterintuitive to family-centered care, the emerging autonomy of the adolescent girl must be respected. Although there is no evidence to support the idea that an adolescent girl would be able to make decisions related to some conditions (substance abuse, STI, pregnancy) but not others (urinary tract infection, asthma, acne), there is an assumption that she might refrain from seeking treatment for certain conditions (substance abuse, STI, pregnancy) if parental consent or notification was required. Also possibly counterintuitive is that adolescents may not consent to participate in research even for studies that involve treatments for which he or she can, by state statute, give consent (see Chapter 10). Nurses must stay apprised of relevant state statutes that affect their practice. The Alan Guttmacher Institute (2005) provides online tables showing relevant state laws on minors' access and rights to reproductive health care and rights as parents in all 50 states and the District of Columbia. Even though the law provides boundaries, the right course of action for the nurse may not be clear, as illustrated by the following case.

Case Study 13-1

Jennifer, age 15 years, attends the local high school. Her teachers notice that she has been gaining weight and refer her to the school nurse. With careful questioning, Ms. Klein, the school nurse, learns that Jennifer has been having consensual intercourse with several boys (all younger than 18 years of age) in her school and does not know when she had her last period. A pregnancy test is positive. Ms. Klein realizes that Jennifer should be tested for sexually transmitted infections, including HIV. According to state statute, Jennifer can be treated for pregnancy and STI without parental consent or notification. Ms. Klein would like to contact Jennifer's parents and discuss Jennifer's future health care needs with them. Jennifer does not want her parents notified, nor does not want anyone to know about the pregnancy. Ms. Klein explains to Jennifer that she should have tests to see how far advanced the pregnancy is and to make sure she has not contracted any infections from her partners. She further encourages her to be seen by a physician or midwife. She assures Jennifer that she will not tell anyone about the pregnancy, but soon it will be suspected because she will appear pregnant as the fetus grows. She strongly encourages Jennifer to confide in her parents because she will need to make plans about the pregnancy and birth if she continues the pregnancy.

Ms. Klein believes that it would be in Jennifer's best interests to include her parents in the decision-making, but she is constrained by state law from contacting them. If Jennifer breaks a finger in her physical education class, her parents would have to be notified for Jennifer to be treated, yet with pregnancy and possible STI, her parents cannot be informed without Jennifer's consent. Although Ms. Klein must keep Jennifer's information confidential, she has an ethical obligation to assist Jennifer to access appropriate health services.

TRUTH-TELLING

In the foregoing case, truth-telling was important. Ms. Klein told Jennifer that she would keep her information confidential. Her adherence to confidentiality is based on her belief that adolescents would be less likely to seek health care services if confidentiality was doubted. Sankar, Moran, Merz, and Jones (2003), in an extensive review of research on patient perspectives on medical confidentiality, reported that when people, especially adolescents, doubt that their confidentiality will be maintained, they are more likely to forgo medical care, withhold information, or provide incorrect information. Thus, a perception that a HCP is not being truthful can create a cycle of lack of trust and nontruthful disclosure between the patient and the HCP.

Ms. Klein may view her commitment to promote beneficence (first, preventing harm while also fostering good) for Jennifer and her fetus to be at moral odds with the ethical commitment to truthfulness. The probability is great that Jennifer is not aware of her legal rights regarding the confidentiality of her health records and/or student academic records. In some states, parents may legally obtain their child's school health records via the Family Educational Rights and Privacy Act (FERPA). Would it be ethical for Ms. Klein to manipulate Jennifer into disclosing her pregnancy ("for her own good") to her parents by the use of a nontruthful statement that FERPA would allow her parents access when in fact this is not true?

Toxicology Screening

Another quandary that arises in relation to truth telling involves the issue of toxicology screening for drugs in newborns. The National Institute on Drug Abuse estimates that 5% of pregnant women use illicit drugs during their pregnancy and nearly 19% use alcohol (2003). For women who deny drug use but whose infants display behaviors consistent with intrauterine drug exposure, urine toxicology tests on the newborn would confirm the exposure. Should maternal consent be obtained, or should the health care providers have the freedom to test the infant without the mother's consent?

Bundled within this truthfulness quandary regarding infant urine toxicology screening without maternal consent are questions of maternal–fetal conflict, maternal rights, deterrence to medical treatment, and the uneasy collaboration between health care delivery and the law. In an effort to advocate on behalf of the fetus, maternal rights may be violated when communication is avoided, incomplete, or deceptive. Women who are drug dependent may avoid interactions with the health care system even to the detriment of their fetus when the health care system becomes a vehicle for law enforcement. Is the fact that the fetus is at risk for developmental problems and even death through drug exposure a sufficient reason for violating the professional commitment to truthfulness? Should concern for the risk to the fetus outweigh the mother's right to privacy or her authority to consent to toxicology testing of her infant?

In the state of Illinois, each hospital establishes its own policies about which infants are tested for drug exposure. The hospital is mandated to report positive findings to the Public Health Department (Illinois Department of Public Health Division of Epidemiological Studies, 2001) for epidemiological purposes and the child welfare department, although most infants are not removed from their mother's custody based on the infant's positive toxicology. If the hospital sets its own policy, then nurses (both perinatal and neonatal) need to participate in the discussion and formation of policy. Before establishing a drug exposure testing policy, nurses need to consider the ethical underpinnings for the policy when answering a variety of questions. How should the value of truth telling be balanced with a woman's right to privacy and her right to know whether her infant is being tested for drugs? How should the woman's rights be balanced with the infant's interest to be free from harm? Should the nurse inform the mother if her infant will be tested for intrauterine exposure to illegal drugs? Is maternal consent required or is it sufficient that the mother merely be informed? Does a commitment to truth telling require that the mother be informed before the testing occurs? For more background on this topic, see Bornstein (2003), Burns (1997), Catlin (1997), Dailard and Nash (2000), and Tillett and Osborne (2001).

ADVOCACY

The area of women's health is replete with examples of opportunities for nurse advocacy. The primary role that nurses can play as advocates for women is in informed decision-making. Nurses can provide education, clarification, and referrals for more information on various women's health topics. Decisions about choice of contraception, termination of pregnancy, prenatal testing, circumcision of the newborn, hormone replacement therapy, genetic testing for breast and ovarian cancers, and domestic violence are all issues in women's health. In other areas of health care, it is not unusual for the nurse to want to advocate for the patient and the needs of other family members. What is unique in women's health is when the woman is pregnant, there are two patients within the one body (conjoined twins being another albeit rare example). There may be times, as in the example of intrauterine drug exposure, that the newborn needs an advocate apart from his or her mother. These and other issues are discussed in more detail in Section 2.

Postpartum Depression

Adjustment to birth of a child is a major life-altering experience. Usually with mixed feelings of great joy and some trepidation, women transition into their maternal roles. It is estimated that 1 woman in 10 experiences the "baby blues," a transient "letdown" as the impact of the transition affects her physically and emotionally (American Psychiatric Association, 2001). One view is that this is a normal response to a number of losses, such as loss of identity or social network or career interruption, or is due to feelings of guilt that the new mother does not identify with the ideal mother (Stanton, Lobel, Sears, & DeLuca, 2002). For some, however, the depression persists, especially for women with a previous psychiatric episode. The risk of recurrence for women who have had postpartum depression with psychiatric features increases with each pregnancy. Occasionally, women who have murdered their children have used postpartum depression or postpartum psychosis, a break with reality, as an insanity defense.

Andrea Yates was a 37-year-old mother of five children, of ages ranging from 6 months to 7 years. In June 2001 she drowned all five children in the bathtub. Prosecuted for murder, her defense was that she was suffering from severe postpartum depression and was insane at the time of the drownings. She was convicted of the murders and sentenced to life in prison. Her husband stated that he believed the health care system failed her and was responsible for the deaths of his children. Although Mrs. Yates was under treatment for postpartum depression, she reportedly had a psychiatric hospitalization shortened because of insurance restrictions and despite her husband's insistence that she was too sick to be discharged. Her story is relevant to the discussion about ethics in women's health for a number of reasons: (1) It reveals a lack of parity in insurance coverage for mental health treatment (an issue of resource allocation), (2) it challenges the prevailing cultural expectation that all mothers love and want their children, and (3) it demonstrates the use of criminal law to control the aberrant behavior of women.

The Mental Health Equitable Treatment Act was introduced into the Senate in 2001, but has yet to be passed. The bill requires parity in coverage, so that insurance companies cannot have limitations in mental health treatment that they do not impose in medical and surgical treatment. Just as medical conditions like diabetes, heart disease, and cancers are often influenced by the interaction between genes and the environment, so are mental health conditions. Discrimination in health care coverage is based on false beliefs such as mental illness is within the control of the person, it is a sign of low moral character, and the diagnosis cannot be objectively validated. Historically, women's medical complaints, if no pathology was discovered, were attributed to hysteria or hypochondriasis. The interaction between societal expectations of certain roles, like motherhood, and cultural messages of what constitutes a "good" mother, a "good" wife, and a "good" daughter creates unattainable models. Further assaulting a woman's self-esteem are labels of codependency or self-defeating personality disorder. Women who try to please others to the point of self-sacrifice are pathologized, even though the dominant cultural message is that good mothers, wives, and daughters meet their families' needs. Consistent with the "good mother" image is the myth that all women want children. Plato believed that female hysteria was caused "by a lonely womb that wanders through the body crying for a baby" (Tavris, 1992, p. 177).

Not all women want to have a baby, even those who have one or more children. Society expects a mother to bond with her children, and whereas most mothers do, some do not and may have feelings of guilt and inadequacy surrounding that role. When the ambivalence toward the infant is manifested in murder, the tendency is to believe that there must be a psychopathology because mothers are programmed to love their children. Another well-publicized case of a mother murdering her children is that of Susan Smith. Susan Smith, a 23-year-old, murdered her two small children by allowing them to drown when she rolled her car into a lake while they were asleep in the back seat. She was in the midst of a divorce from the children's father and had been rebuffed by her lover because he did not want to become further involved with a woman who had children (Pergament, 2004). Her defense was that she suffered from severe depression (her youngest child was 14 months old, so arguing postpartum depression may have been difficult), and the murders, to which she confessed, were part of a failed murder-suicide plan. She was convicted of two counts of murder.

These and other cases raise awareness of postpartum depression and its potentially devastating effects. Nurses have an ethical obligation to assess a woman after she has give birth for signs and symptoms of depression and to educate the woman as to resources and referrals. As with all specialties in nursing, careful documentation is essential.

ALLOCATION OF RESOURCES

Access to health care services like prenatal care, reproductive services, and drug treatment for pregnant women are allocation issues in women's health. There are broader societal issues raised by certain health care services available to women. As part of routine prenatal care, screening is done for Down syndrome, other atypical chromosomal conditions, and neural tube defects. A woman may or may not be aware that having these tests starts a trajectory of decisions should the tests reveal an abnormality. The rationale behind the testing is that a woman should know whether there is an abnormality with the pregnancy so she can decide whether she wants to continue it or so she can anticipate and prepare for needs she and her infant may have at birth and in the future. There is the assumption that a woman would want to know, and there have been malpractice cases brought against physicians who did not inform a woman that these tests were available.

Society tends to place a greater value on a "normal" infant than on an infant who is suspected or known to have disabilities. There are many reasons that enter into a decision not to continue a pregnancy of a fetus with probable disabilities, and it is likely that the mother considers her resources in making a decision—physical, psychological, social, and financial. She may not directly consider the effect on society, but societal attitudes toward people with disabilities can affect her decision-making. These are shaped by historical attitudes, competition for resources, and cultural values relating to the body, independence, and productivity. The disability rights movement is increasing societal awareness of the biases against and prejudices toward those with disabilities (Charlton, 1998; Fleischer & Zames, 2001; Longmore, 2003; Shapiro, 1994; Silvers, Wasserman, & Mahowald, 1998) and helping to change them.

Funding Decisions

What services are provided and which services are covered by various third-party payers (insurance company, Medicare, or Medicaid) are resource allocation decisions that reflect societal values and biases. For example, one of the authors (M.B.) was insured by a hospital-based health maintenance organization (HMO) that did not provide financial support for oral birth control pills but did cover the surgical termination of pregnancy. This reflects an inconsistency in policies regarding women's health. Supporting the use of oral contraceptives seems to be an easier and financially sounder action in comparison to the emotional and physical harms that can occur with decisions to surgically terminate a pregnancy.

Another resource allocation issue is created by the stance of a religion-affiliated health care system, such as the Catholic Church, on the use of the "morning-after pill," often referred to as emergency contraception. The Pontifical Academy for Life (2000) called the morning-after pill an abortifacient, and urged health care providers to morally object to its use. There are two medications that are used for emergency contraception: Plan B and Preven. A third type of emergency contraception uses a copper-releasing intrauterine device, which can be used up to 7 days after intercourse. The Ethical and Religious Directives for Catholic Health Care Services (United States Conference of Catholic Bishops, 2001) permit the use of medications that prevent ovulation or fertilization or decrease the capacity of sperm to fertilize the egg. Many states, such as Washington, Illinois, and California, require that women who were raped and are being treated in a hospital emergency department receive information about emergency contraception (Cooley, 2003). Catholics for a Free Choice, an advocacy group, conducted a survey that found that a little more than one-fourth (28%) of Catholic hospitals would provide emergency contraception to women who were raped, leaving three-fourths of Catholic hospitals in the United States that would not (Cooley, 2003). The Planned Parenthood Federation of America (2004) observed that there have been many mergers between Catholic and non-Catholic hospitals, and that half of the largest not-for-profit health care systems are operated by Catholic systems of care. In many areas of the country, the local hospital is Catholic, and rape victims may not be counseled about emergency contraception. Access to these services is becoming increasingly limited to many women, who may be unaware of them and might remain unaware if their only hospital is Catholic affiliated.

Gender Differences in Diagnosis and Treatment

It has been recognized that women experience and interpret symptoms differently than men. Historically, women were excluded from some types of clinical research, particularly women of child-bearing age in drug trials, because of concern for teratogenicity. Despite a National Institutes of Health (NIH) policy change to include women or justify their exclusion, it required a House of Representatives subcommittee investigation to expose the NIH's blatant disregard of their own policy (Sullinger, 2000). Through studies that focused on women's health, it is now known that coronary heart disease kills more women than any other disease, but women present with different signs and symptoms than men. There is a moral imperative for health care providers to be aware of the different presentations and to not dismiss women who are not showing "typical" signs and symptoms of heart disease.

Barsky, Peekna, and Borus (2001) reviewed the literature on somatic symptom reporting in women and men. They concluded that socialization beginning in childhood likely has an influence on how men and women differ in their recognition and reporting of somatic symptoms. Women have a higher prevalence of psychiatric diagnoses and higher rates of abuse. The researchers also found that there is a gender bias in research and clinical practice, in which women may be viewed as emotionally disturbed and their symptoms attributed to hysteria and so not further investigated. Nurses must be aware of the potential for the dismissal of symptoms reported by women and advocate for appropriate, unbiased evaluation.

The feminist movement of the late 1960s and 1970s may seem like ancient history to today's nurses, but it had an effect still felt on the current health care of women. Although women's roles have changed, so that women are now in the workforce in greater numbers, their child care and home responsibilities remain. Having the stresses of multiple roles and unrealistic expectations of being able to fulfill them all, women experience more psychiatric and psychosomatic disorders than men. There has also been a greater recognition of incest, sexual abuse, domestic violence, and posttraumatic stress disorder in women (Gold, 1998). There is ambivalence toward this recognition of the stresses and social ills that befall women. The psychiatric community, although identifying and treating women with these problems, also pathologizes women who respond to social inequities. In the 1800s, Dr. Samuel Cartwright diagnosed "drapetomania" in slaves—a "condition" defined as the uncontrollable urge to escape from slavery (Tavris, 1992, pp. 176–177). The problem, slavery, became the sickness of the slave, to be cured only by acceptance of his or her lot. This is an example of blaming the victim. The danger in recognizing society's pressures on women and the effect on their mental health is in accepting the medicalization of women's responses as pathological. Nurses must be aware of the influence of social inequities on women's lives and how the effect of those inequities manifest themselves in women's health.

Two psychiatric diagnoses represent the tension between blaming the victim and legitimizing psychiatric disturbances. The designation of late luteal-phase dysphoric disorder (LLPDD), characterized by transient debilitating depression during menstruation, was opposed by some as perpetuating myths that women were subject to madness during their menstrual cycle. Additional research in the disorder resulted in a refinement of the diagnostic criteria, and the name was changed to premenstrual dysphoric disorder. Another diagnosis, self-defeating personality disorder, characterizes a person as masochistic, someone who derives pleasure from being abused or dominated. Critics of this diagnosis pointed out that women may be socialized to be subservient, and that victims of abuse become too defeated to escape their abuser (Gold, 1998). Despite mounting protests against including the diagnosis in the *Diagnostic and Statistical Manual of Mental Disorders* (DSM), it was included. The editors of the DSM acknowledged that data from empirical studies were lacking, and the diagnosis was included based on a "rich clinical tradition" of psychiatrists' clinical experiences (Tavris, 1992, p. 182). An anonymous psychiatrist noted, "Yes, I have seen these women in my practice. It's the damnedest thing. They actually want to play the martyr" (Tavris, 1992, p. 182). The diagnosis was dropped from the fourth edition of the DSM.

Nurses may often be in positions to advocate for more appropriate, gender-sensitive policies for the individual woman as well as women in general. Conditions such as fibromyalgia and chronic fatigue syndrome, which predominantly affect women, defy easy diagnosis and classification. The etiologies are not known, and some bristle at the relegation of the disorders to a psychiatric disturbance, which harkens back to the assumption that unexplained symptoms are signs of hysteria. Because of the stigma and lack of parity between mental health treatment and medical-surgical treatment, there is resistance to identifying certain conditions as psychiatric conditions. There is also a trend toward complementary and alternative medicine (CAM) in seeking relief from conditions the medical establishment cannot effectively diagnose and/or treat.

SUMMARY

This section reviews the ethical themes of advocacy, truth-telling, confidentiality, and allocation of resources in relation to issues in women's health. It is important for nurses to understand the clinical relevance of various conditions and situations in women's health to identify and facilitate ethical decision-making in this specialty.

CLINICAL EXERCISES

1. If you are in a clinical rotation in a hospital, locate the hospital's policy on emergency contraception counseling for women who have been raped.
2. Investigate what your institution's policy is toward age of consent related to reproductive health services, such as treatment for sexually transmitted infection, birth control, pregnancy termination, and genetic counseling.

Discussion Questions

1. In a follow-up visit, Ms. Godfrey tells you that she thinks she is hearing voices telling her to smother her newborn. She asks you whether this is normal postpartum depression. What is your response to her, and what actions should you take? Give your ethical reasoning.
2. Ms. Jackson is being admitted to the labor room and smells of alcohol. She denies drinking anything but nonalcoholic drinks. She delivers within an hour after admission, and at birth, the infant is listless and requires resuscitation. Should the infant's urine be sent for toxicology? Defend your answer.

SECTION 2: *Informed Decision-Making*

As with all adults with decision-making capacity, adult women have the right to consent to or refuse medical treatment. Regardless of the person's gender, informed decision-making requires the understanding of the intended benefits and possible risks or complications of medical interventions. This chapter addresses situations unique to women.

As previously discussed, informed decision-making requires that information be given to the person making the decision in a manner that is understandable. Information should be complete, and the person should have an opportunity to ask questions for clarification. In medical decision-making, relevant information should include the condition that needs treatment, options for treatment, potential and known risks and anticipated benefits, alternatives to treatment, both immediate and long-term costs, and within what time frame a decision must be made. In some relationships, the husband or father may be the family decision-maker and the woman defers the decision to a male family member. In some cultures, women do not leave their home without a male chaperon; women are not examined by male health care providers. Although the expectation is that women should make autonomous decisions, it may be their preference, or custom, to defer to another. In other instances, women may desire autonomy but feel limited by their relationship, financial dependency, or lack of confidence in their ability to make decisions. The nurse can facilitate decision-making by being present when information is being shared, reinforcing and clarifying information, and referring the woman to other supportive services for assistance in decision-making.

BALANCING MATERNAL AND FETAL INTERESTS

Pregnancy can be a very physically stressful experience. There is an expectation that the pregnant woman will care for herself in a way that ensures her health and the health of her fetus. Some maternal behaviors may threaten the well-being of the fetus. As previously mentioned, the pregnant woman may ingest alcohol or drugs that could be teratogenic to the fetus, induce drug dependence in the fetus, or cause dangerous hemodynamic changes. Social response to these behaviors has been in the form of criminal prosecution for maternal behaviors that endanger the fetus. Although substance abuse has been approached as a disease and medically treatable condition, pregnant women who are substance abusers have been treated as criminals. Hospital staff at a South Carolina hospital noticed that there seemed to be an increase in cocaine use in pregnant women, so they adopted a policy of testing urine for cocaine and reporting positive results to the local police. Women with positive results were prosecuted for drugs offenses and/or endangering the fetus, depending on the stage of pregnancy. The urine testing was intended to force women into treatment. Ten women were arrested. They sued on the grounds that the urine test was an illegal search, and the U.S. Supreme Court, in its decision in *Ferguson v. City of Charleston* (2001), agreed with the women. Although roughly 5% of pregnant women abuse illegal substances, they are less likely to seek prenatal care (Bornstein, 2003). A facilitative approach, including comprehensive pregnancy and drug treatment, rather than a punitive approach has been shown to be more effective in promoting maternal and fetal health. The American Nurses Association (1997) opposes criminal prosecution of women who use drugs while pregnant.

When the pregnant woman's condition becomes life threatening and the standard of treatment is a blood transfusion, conflict exists if the woman refuses blood based on religious objection. Ordinarily, her refusal would be honored, although there would be an exhaustive attempt to ensure she was making an informed decision. When she is pregnant, though, the health care providers have an obligation to the fetus as well as the mother. If the mother dies, it is likely the fetus will die as well. Obstetricians also feel a moral duty to save the life of the pregnant woman when she has dependent children. It has become common practice to remove custody of children of Jehovah's Witnesses who are in need of life-saving blood transfusions for purposes of receiving treatment, then returning them to parental custody. The American Academy of Pediatrics Committee on Bioethics (1997) endorses court intervention when a child's life is threatened by parental refusal of treatment based on religious objection. To rescue the fetus, however, involves violating the woman's body. Sacks and Koppes (1994) noted that although careful monitoring and limiting of blood loss has become standard, there are still situations in which patients who refuse blood die. They suggested referring patients who are Jehovah's Witnesses to practitioners with similar views, but they remained troubled that the best interests of the fetus (and dependent children) are not served by this referral. Alternatively, they suggested having a mechanism within the institution so that a hearing can be quickly convened and conducted when lives are at stake. Nurses may also face the dilemma of advocating for the patient's wishes that may result in fetal and/or maternal death. The nurse must examine his or her beliefs and values, and if they are in conflict with the patient's, arrange for transfer of the patient's care to another nurse who can support the patient without reservation.

Pregnancy and HIV

According to the Centers for Disease Control and Prevention (2004), 91% of the cases of AIDS in children are attributed to perinatal transmission. The incidence decreased from 1000 to 2000 cases a year in the 1990s to 100 cases in 2001. The reason for the dramatic decrease is the improvement in HIV counseling and testing, use of zidovudine (AZT or ZDV) during pregnancy, treatment of the infected pregnant woman, treatment of the newborn after birth and delivery via Caesarean section (de Zulueta, 2002). Before testing, the pregnant woman must understand the risks of testing (discrimination, stigma, psychological stress) and the decisions that will need to be made if she tests positive. Pregnancy and delivery management are geared toward reducing perinatal transmission. The woman might be asked to take a combination of medications that have unpleasant side effects, and she must strictly adhere to the schedule. The recommended mode of delivery is Caesarean section, and the woman will be instructed not to breast-feed. At any point in the treatment plan, the woman may decide to stop taking medication, or she may refuse delivery via Caesarean section. Even though there is evidence to show that these measures should benefit the fetus, the woman has the right to make decisions that might not benefit the fetus. For example, suppose that a woman has been taking medication to prevent perinatal transmission of HIV, and with the onset of labor, a Caesarean section is recommended. Her physician advised her that this was the preferred method of delivery to prevent transmission, but she will not consent to the surgery. She states that she will take her chances that her baby will not contract HIV during vaginal delivery. Although current thinking is that Caesarean delivery provides some protection to the fetus, the woman has the right to refuse unwanted medical intervention, even if the decision does not appear to be in the best interests of the fetus.

Mandatory Bed Rest

Preterm labor is not uncommon, but occasionally, when preterm delivery is threatened, the pregnant woman is placed on complete bed rest. Some women may have jobs or other children to care for and cannot remain on bed rest. Is their behavior considered "noncompliant"? Some women find it very unnerving to remain on extended bed rest and decide to risk their pregnancy rather than risk their mental health. Should they be expected to endure the stresses of bed rest for the sake of fetal health? Again the woman's autonomy is in conflict with fetal interests. Bewley (2002) suggested that the relationship between a pregnant woman and her fetus is different, and that adhering to all the recommendations to avoid alcohol, tobacco, strenuous activities, have frequent check-ups, and submit to examinations is going above and beyond the call of duty. If a woman forgoes the opportunity to terminate a pregnancy, does she then have an ethical obligation to avoid harming the fetus? Current attitude is that the state has an interest in preventing harm to the fetus, and jurisdictions that recognize the fetus as a person may seek legal means to coerce the womens' behavior. But should the law be used to force a woman to remain on bed rest? The American College of Obstetricians and Gynecologists Committee on Ethics (2004) argued that the judicial intervention should rarely, if ever, be acceptable. Medical judgments are fallible, so pregnant women should be given information and advice and then be permitted to make their own decisions.

In the last 20 years, there have been cases of women forced to have Caesarean sections. The fetus may have been in distress or have been the first of multiple fetuses in breech position in a primiparous woman. The standard of care is that an emergency Caesarean section should be performed to deliver the fetus; the practitioner risks malpractice in not explaining the urgency and performing the surgery. In some cases, though, women refused the surgery. The health care professionals, unable to persuade the women to consent to surgery, obtained court orders to forcibly operate and deliver the fetuses. However, not all courts would rule against such women, and court-ordered Caesarean sections are rarely if ever done.

In contrast, some women desire a Caesarean section, believing that it is more convenient to schedule and allows them to avoid the discomfort and physical trauma to their bodies due to childbirth. The American College of Obstetricians and Gynecologists (2004) issued a statement that one method, vaginal delivery, has not been shown to be clearly superior to the other method, Caesarean section. It is speculated that their statement could invite more surgical deliveries when there is no medical indication but there is patient preference. Although the risks of Caesarean section are greater than those of vaginal delivery, should the woman's preference prevail over best medical judgment? Should Caesarean sections be performed only when medically necessary?

Pregnancy and Delivery

There are a number of other ethical issues surrounding pregnancy and delivery. Not all pregnancies are planned and welcomed, but there is an assumption that if the woman does not terminate the pregnancy, she has an obligation to avoid substances or activities that could harm the fetus. When women with chronic health problems desire to become pregnant, there is some planning about health maintenance that should occur. For example, a woman with a seizure disorder who has taken anticonvulsant medication since childhood may be concerned about the teratogenic effect of the medication on the developing fetus. She realizes the risk of seizures she would face if she stopped taking the anticonvulsants, yet the risk of birth defects is significant. She discusses these risks with her physicians and determines whether there are other options to her current medication and what the risks are with various medications. Ultimately she must decide whether she is willing to risk her health to prevent potential birth defects or believes the risk is too great and will either forgo pregnancy or continue her medication and risk affecting the fetus. In this case, the decision is the woman's, and she makes it after gathering and considering all the relevant information.

There was a trend toward criminalizing behaviors that result in fetal death, or, at a minimum, categorizing the behaviors as fetal abuse. The Unborn Victims of Violence Act (also known as Laci and Conner's Law) was passed April 1, 2004; it allows for the prosecution of anyone who harms or kills a fetus at any point in development, whether or not the perpetrator knew the woman was pregnant. The act does not provide for prosecution of medical personnel performing an abortion or if the mother harms the fetus. The law resulted from a case in California where a woman (Laci Peterson) who was 8½ months pregnant was murdered, but only her killing and not that of the fetus was prosecuted. The law did not recognize the fetus as a person, so the killing of the fetus could not be prosecuted. There is speculation that the supporters of this law were actually working to overturn *Roe v. Wade*, the U.S. Supreme Court case that legalized abortion in 1973. In recognizing the fetus as a legal person, the way might be paved to considering certain abortion procedures as killing a legal person.

The specific abortion procedure that is being targeted is so-called "partial birth abortion," or intact dilation and extraction. This procedure is performed in the second or third trimester of pregnancy. The fetus is partially delivered in breech position, with the head remaining in the birth canal. A craniotomy is performed to decompress the cranium and evacuate the cranial contents, then the head is delivered. Because the body but not the head is delivered, it is considered a partial birth, not a complete birth, so the infant is "born dead." When a fetus with undiagnosed hydrocephalus is being delivered in breech position, the procedure may need to be performed to save the life of the mother. Danforth's *Obstetrics and Gynecology* (2003) describes intact dilation and extraction as a procedure that is rarely performed in the United States. The American College of Obstetricians and Gynecologists (2003) opposed laws to ban the procedure and argued that it may be the best or most appropriate procedure in a particular circumstance to save the life or preserve the health of a woman, and only the doctor, in consultation with the patient, based upon the woman's particular circumstances, can make this decision.

CONTRACEPTION

Contraception is not exclusively a woman's concern, but the woman is the one who becomes pregnant, so when pregnancy is not intended, the woman must practice birth control or ensure that her partner uses a condom. In consultation with her health care provider, the woman makes an informed decision about whether to practice birth control and which method to use. Some religions prohibit the use of contraception other than abstinence. At the other extreme, some women use abortion as their method of choice. When the woman decides to use contraception, she needs information on the various methods presented in a nonjudgmental and confidential fashion. It may be critical for the woman to know how pregnancy occurs (ovulation, fertilization, implantation) so that she can select a contraceptive method that is consistent with her beliefs. For example, if she believes that human life and personhood begin at conception, she may want to prevent fertilization and use a barrier or hormonal method. If she believes that life does not begin until the fertilized egg is implanted, an intrauterine device that interferes with implantation may be an option. As noted in Chapter 11, Section 1, in most states adolescents can obtain contraceptives without parental consent or notification, but some states still require parental consent and/or notification.

Case Study 13-2

A woman is interested in selecting a birth control method, and visits a clinic for information. She sees a nurse practitioner, who takes a history, performs an examination, and describes the various options appropriate for this woman. Which of the following statements by the nurse practitioner best captures respect for the womens' autonomy?

  A. "You could select any of the methods I have described to you, but I recommend abstinence since you are not married."
  B. "You could use any of the methods I have described, but only these methods protect you from sexually infectious disease."
  C. "Before prescribing a method, I would like to meet with your partner to make sure he approves of the method."

Statement A interjects the nurse practitioner's values and attitudes toward premarital sexual relations. The nurse practitioner could discuss why she favors abstinence (100% effective against pregnancy and contraction of sexually infectious disease), but it is likely that the woman seeking birth control does not intend to practice abstinence.

Statement C implies that the woman should not select a method without her partner's approval. The nurse practitioner might suggest that the woman think about the acceptability or unacceptability of a method to her partner, and strategize with her if she selects a method her partner will reject. However, the woman is free to make her choice and have her decision kept confidential.

Statement B shows respect for the woman's right to make the decision, and repeats information that may help the woman distinguish the differences in the various methods. The ethical issues in these statements are those of autonomy and respect for the woman's right to make an informed decision consistent with her values and beliefs.

ABORTION

Abortion is legal, but is highly controversial and politicized. A political candidate's position on abortion is often a litmus test for his or her political ideology. Health care providers who perform pregnancy terminations have been murdered by antiabortion extremists; family planning clinics where terminations are conducted have been bombed. Even people who support a woman's right to choose to continue or end a pregnancy might find the use of abortion as a birth control method morally repugnant. Nurses who choose to work in women's health must provide care in a nonjudgmental fashion. Those nurses who feel compelled to influence a woman's decision about abortion to be consistent with the nurses' position should not work in this specialty. Although the individual nurse has the right to free speech in appropriate forums, such as holding a sign at a rally at the state legislature or expressing an opinion on a talk radio show, the intimate HCP–patient relationship is not the appropriate forum.

Although surgical abortion has been legal since 1973 (*Roe v. Wade*), medication has become available that provides a medically induced abortion. Mifepristone and methotrexate are two prescription drugs that cause abortion. There may be confusion between the "abortion pills," which cause the lining of the uterus to slough, and the "emergency contraception pill," also known as Plan B. Plan B works by preventing fertilization, ovulation, or implantation. Nurses working in the emergency room, clinics, or women's health centers need to clarify for women the different pills and different uses. The use of these medications is predicted to change the political and social landscape of pregnancy prevention and termination. Many more physicians, midwives, and nurse practitioners will be able to provide abortion services, and do so confidentially, without the public knowing who or where the services are being provided, thereby potentially averting the violence associated with attacks on abortion clinics.

One barrier to accessing medical abortion is that most providers charge more for medical abortion than surgical abortion. Henshaw and Finer (2003) attributed higher charge to the increased time in counseling and follow-up and possibly the cost of the drug. Because women have a legal right to terminate a suspected or real pregnancy, nurses have a professional responsibility to give accurate, timely information. Those nurses who conscientiously object to facilitating abortion should avoid working in emergency departments, ambulatory clinics serving women of child-bearing age, and the area of women's reproductive health.

As mentioned in Section 1, access to certain reproductive services is limited if the woman seeks them from a Catholic-affiliated hospital. These hospitals are prohibited by the Church from providing the service or information about it. For some women, their only health care facility may be Catholic affiliated, so they would have to travel outside their community to obtain certain services.

STERILIZATION

Another major decision in reproductive health is the decision to become sterilized. The informed consent process should include all the options available and a discussion of the permanence of the procedure. At some point in her child-bearing years, a woman may decide to adopt a permanent form of contraception, referred to as sterilization. When a couple has decided that they do not wish to have any further children (or any children at all), the man may decide to have a vasectomy or the woman may decide to have a tubal ligation. Both procedures are surgical procedures that usually can be performed on an outpatient basis. The vasectomy can be done under a local anesthetic; the tubal ligation requires general or spinal anesthesia, but can be done via laparoscopy. Sometimes women will ask for the procedure to be performed during a planned Caesarean section. Women should be aware that some hospitals with religious affiliations do not permit sterilization procedures to be performed. According to some religions, sterilization through oophorectomy, salpingectomy, or hysterectomy is permitted if the surgery is medically necessary to treat a condition such as hemorrhage after childbirth, placenta accreta, or cancer of the uterus.

In the past, physicians performing sterilization procedures required the consent of the patient and the patient's spouse. As recently as December 2004, a urological practice in Texas posted the consent for vasectomy on its website, and it required the consent of the spouse as well as the consent of the patient. It was also common that gynecologists would not sterilize a woman who was unmarried or a married woman who had never had a child. Such paternalism was characteristic in the past, but may persist today. Open and honest communication between partners is encouraged because sterilization is considered permanent, despite microsurgery to reverse the tubal ligation or vasectomy.

A new method of permanent birth control came on the U.S. market in 2002, known as transcervical sterilization. A tiny coil is inserted into each Fallopian tube through the cervix and uterus. Sterilization is accomplished through the scarring of the tube, thereby closing it off. A local anesthetic is used, and women who are not candidates for a tubal ligation may be candidates for this coil. Once the tubes are blocked, they cannot be reopened. During the informed consent process, it must be stressed that this method is not reversible.

The sterilization of women with developmental disabilities requires a more strenuous consent process. Considering the history of eugenics (discussed in Chapter 11) and the forced sterilization of women with disabilities, it has become more difficult to get authorization for sterilizing someone with an intellectual disability. However, the cultural legacy of the eugenics movement persists. In 1994, a woman was involuntarily sterilized at her mother's request, after 7 years of appeals. Cindy Wasiek, a 26-year-old woman with an intellectual disability and the functional ability reportedly of a 5-year-old, was sterilized because her mother feared she would be raped and become pregnant. Despite the fact that she had a guardian representing her interest not to be sterilized, Justice Souter refused to grant a routine stay (Block, 2000). As Block (2000) pointed out, sterilization would not protect Cindy Wasiek from being raped or from contracting a sexually transmitted infection. Block further contended that Cindy Wasiek was not sterilized for her safety, but to allay her mother's fears.

The American Association on Mental Retardation's (2002) Sexuality Policy Statement states that people with intellectual disability have the right to "protection from sexual harassment; physical, sexual, and emotional abuse; and involuntary sterilization" (p. 2). As advocates, nurses can participate in the assessment of the capacity of a woman with intellectual disabilities to make decisions pertaining to her sexuality. Developmentally appropriate sexuality education should focus on menstrual hygiene, socially appropriate expressions of affection, contraception, and sexual abuse avoidance training. Nurses who know the woman can participate in discussions with her and appropriate others to determine the need for contraception or sterilization. Informed decision-making by the woman with intellectual disabilities, supported by others of the woman's choosing, is critical in honoring her autonomy.

COMPLEMENTARY AND ALTERNATIVE MEDICINE (CAM)

The ethical issues in CAM revolve around informed decision-making. In 1993 the Office of Alternative Medicine was established within the NIH. A fact sheet is available that answers many questions about CAM and how to decide whether to use CAM therapy. Nurses might often be asked about the validity of a CAM treatment or for a recommendation for a practitioner of CAM. Many advanced practice nurses might incorporate CAM treatments into their repertoire. It is important for the woman (or any consumer of CAM) to have information with which to make a decision and to consult with her health care provider to ensure compatibility with any conventional treatment she is also receiving. Some insurers may cover certain treatments, such as chiropractic services or acupuncture, but the woman should check to see whether these treatments are covered by her plan.

MENOPAUSE

Menopause is the cessation of menstruation for at least 12 months. It is often preceded by perimenopause, with irregular periods and other symptoms of hot flashes, vaginal dryness, and sleep disturbances. After menopause, there is a greater risk of heart disease and osteoporosis, and, until recently, the literature supported the use of hormone replacement therapy (HRT) to prevent heart disease and osteoporosis and relieve unpleasant menopause symptoms. There was some suggestion that HRT could have positive effects on sexuality, memory loss, and depression associated with menopause, but the data are inconclusive. The Woman's Health Initiative issued findings of the Heart and Estrogen-Progestin Replacement Study Follow-Up and decided to stop the study of the popular and widely prescribed drug Prempro (Shelby, 2003). In February 2004, the NIH (2004) decided to stop the estrogen-alone trial of the study. Not only did the hormones fail to protect against heart disease, there was an increased risk of breast cancer, coronary heart disease, stroke and blood clots. There has also been a 220-fold increase in the risk of ovarian cancer for women taking HRT for 20 years or more (National Cancer Institute, 2002). The NIH decisions to stop the clinical trials dramatized the lack of evidence-based practice in the area of women's health. For more than 30 years, hormone replacement therapy was common, yet the data supporting its use and risks had never been systematically analyzed. The move toward evidence-based practice will provide information with which the woman can make an informed choice about the potential risks and benefits of hormone replacement therapy.

CAREGIVER BURDEN

Another allocation issue in women's health has to do with the caregiver role that is relegated most of the time to female family members. When the family member is older, 75% of the caregivers are women (National Alliance for Caregiving and AARP, 1997; U.S. Department of Health and Human Services, 1998). Many of these caregivers also work outside the home, which sometimes necessitates reducing paid work hours or taking unpaid leaves. Although many family members accept the caregiving role willingly, the role exacts a physical and psychological toll on the caregiver (Schulz & Beach, 1999; U.S. Department of Health and Human Services, 1998; Yee & Schulz, 2000). In pediatrics, there is the expectation that parents will meet the needs of their children, even if a child has extensive, pervasive, and unending needs, until he or she is independent, is placed outside the home in a residential facility, or dies. For unmarried adult children, such as a 21-year-old who is brain injured in a motor vehicle accident, often parents are expected to make the health care decisions and assume the follow-up care (the exception is when the 21-year-old has designated someone other than a parent to be the durable power of attorney for health care; see Chapter 12), even if the adult child has been living independently. Callahan (1988) questioned the limits of obligation a family has toward one of its members whose needs are so great. Must the family sacrifice its future for one needy member? Nurses are in the position of helping families to assess the needs of the ill or injured member, assess the strengths and limitations of the family, arrange for resources, anticipate the need for assistance and respite, and reevaluate the care plan. The care plan is primarily affected by the family's abilities and resources. An affluent family has many more resources than an impoverished family. Those with insurance through a managed care organization likely have many fewer resources and may not meet financial eligibility for government services.

SUMMARY

Informed decision-making in women's health presents new challenges because in many situations the woman balances her interests against the interests of her fetus when making health care decisions. Not only do her choices affect her health and well-being, but also the health and well-being of her fetus. Political forces impact the freedom with which women can exercise their autonomy in reproductive choices. Nurses working in women's health should recognize the variation in attitudes that women may have toward continuation or termination of pregnancy and be prepared to inform and support their decisions.

CLINICAL EXERCISES

1. Observe the informed consent process for some procedure in women's health, such as consent for a Caesarean section, hysterectomy, outpatient biopsy, or tubal ligation. How much detail was given? Do you believe the language was understandable to the patient? Was there opportunity for the patient to ask questions and have them answered? Who conducted the process? What was the nursing role?

Discussion Questions

1. Ms. Kwan has been taking hormone replacement therapy for 30 years. As you are taking her history, you learn that she is unaware of the recent findings of the Women's Health Initiative studies. What is your role in informing her? Give your ethical reasoning.

2. Ann Barr, 23 years old, presents to a family planning clinic for contraception. She explains that she was sexually abused as a child, and because of this, she has decided that she never wants to have children. She is seeking sterilization through tubal ligation. On questioning, she reveals that she is not sexually active, has undergone psychotherapy for several years, and believes that being sterilized will improve her mental health. The nurses in the clinic are split on whether it is ethical to acquiesce to her request. As a nurse in the clinic, you have been asked to ethically analyze this situation.

   a. Identify the ethical issues in this situation.
   b. Describe under what conditions it would be ethical to perform a tubal ligation on Ann.
   c. Describe why it would be unethical to perform a tubal ligation on Ann.
   d. Describe the nurse's role in facilitating Ann's decision.

3. Ms. Schmeckler, 35 years old, has been trying unsuccessfully to become pregnant. She weighs 265 pounds and tells you that she is thinking about having gastric bypass surgery to improve her chances of becoming pregnant.

   a. What are the ethical issues in this situation?
   b. What is your response to Ms. Schmeckler?
   c. What information do you need and what information does Ms. Schmeckler need?

4. You work in the antepartum unit, to which a woman is transferred because of a high census on the gynecological unit. The woman has had a prostaglandin infusion to abort her 20-week pregnancy. You have not cared for a woman undergoing an abortion and you have a moral objection to abortion.

   a. What are your obligations to this patient?
   b. How do you reconcile your personal beliefs with your professional duties?

SECTION 3: *Assisted Reproduction*

INFERTILITY

Although there is no universally accepted definition of infertility, the typical definition is the inability to conceive after at least 1 year of unprotected intercourse (Fidler & Bernstein, 1999). Epidemiologically, it is difficult to know the extent of infertility in the United States because unless a couple attempts to become pregnant (or does not practice contraception), their fertility is not known. However, it is estimated that 7% of married couples in the United States report difficulty in becoming pregnant, and 10% of women between 15 and 44 years of age report difficulty becoming pregnant or carrying a pregnancy to full term (Fidler & Bernstein, 1999). For women, infertility may be caused by dysfunction of the Fallopian tubes or ovaries or both. The most common causes of infertility are *Chlamydia* infection, advanced maternal age (older than 35 years), and, to a lesser extent, environmental exposure to pesticides, solvents, and other chemicals found in the workplace.

An infertility work-up includes invasive testing to image the reproductive system, examination following intercourse to examine sperm motility, and data collection by the couple on characteristics conducive to conception, such as cervical mucous viscosity and positions used for intercourse. The sexual relationship between the couple takes on a clinical atmosphere by making an intimate private act a planned technical event involving many individuals beyond the couple. However, the desire to have children often compels a couple to pursue a work-up and treatment. The ethical issues related to infertility are primarily in the realm of treatment.

ASSISTED REPRODUCTION

Assisted reproduction has many forms. Most commonly, the assistance takes the form of ensuring sperm is delivered to the egg, one technique being *in vitro fertilization* (IVF). With IVF, mature ova are harvested from the woman and fertilized in vitro (outside the body) rather than in vivo (in the body) with sperm. After a number of cell divisions, the fertilized ova are implanted into the woman. Since the late 1970s, when Louise Brown, the first "test tube" baby, was born, assisted reproduction techniques have expanded. Assisted reproduction technology (ART) can help infertile couples, single women without a male partner, postmenopausal women, and surrogate mothers. Ova can be the woman's own or from another woman, such as her mother, daughter, or sister or a completely unrelated stranger. One technique involves injecting ooplasm or mitochondrial DNA from a donor into fertilized ova to replace the deficient mitochondria. The offspring will have the DNA of three people, however. This technique has not been approved for use in the United States. Sperm can be donated from the woman's husband, unmarried partner, obtained from a sperm bank (issues involving the release of donor information are discussed later in this chapter), or retrieved from a man's body shortly after his death. Couples can obtain ova, sperm, or fertilized ova. The fertilized ova that are not used can be used at a later time, remain frozen indefinitely, donated to another woman, donated for research, or destroyed. It is estimated that there are 400,000 frozen embryos in cryopreservation in the United States (President's Council on Bioethics, 2004).

Before implantation of the fertilized ova into the woman, genetic testing can be done on a single cell when the fertilized ova are at the eight-cell stage to screen for a number of characteristics, such as gender, or genetic conditions, like cystic fibrosis. A technique called intracytoplasmic sperm injection is used both to insert one sperm into the ovum for fertilization and, after cells have multiplied, to withdraw one cell for genetic analysis.

Ethical issues abound. As with all technologies, informed consent is crucial. Nurses working in this specialty area can participate in the education of women who seek these services. With in vitro fertilization, risks to the woman of life-threatening hyperstimulation of the ovaries or later ovarian cancer should be fully explained. It is especially important for the healthy oocyte donor, whether acting altruistically or donating the eggs for a fee, to understand the risks. The fees for egg donation range from $1500 to $5000 (White, 2001). White (2001) reported that there have been ads offering as much as $50,000 for certain characteristics, although she could not document that the donor actually received that amount. Is it possible that the fee could act as an undue influence in the donor's decision?

There is little regulation of the ART industry. The new technologies have been driven by a marketplace competition between infertility programs to achieve higher success rates. Centers for Disease Control and Prevention (2002) data revealed that 34% of IVF procedures result in a clinical pregnancy; 19.9% resulted in a single fetus, 12.4% resulted in multiple gestation, and 2% ended in miscarriage. Live births occurred in 83% of the pregnancies, with 54% being single births and 29% multiples; the outcome in 16% of cases was miscarriage, abortion, or stillbirth (for less than 1% of cases, the outcome was not reported). Costs per cycle range from $6500 to $15,000 (Advanced Fertility Services, 2005). For multiple gestations greater than two fetuses, the likelihood for term delivery is decreased. The mother may be offered a selective reduction procedure in which one or more fetuses are injected with a lethal substance, killing it. The fetal tissue decomposes and is reabsorbed, increasing the survivability odds for the remaining fetus or fetuses. Thus, the woman is faced with a dilemma: Continue the multiple pregnancy and risk losing the pregnancy or ending the life of one fetus to promote the viability of another. For many women who have invested much money, time, and emotions into becoming pregnant, being asked to participate in selective termination is counterintuitive and emotionally draining.

Apart from the informed consent issues, there are broader societal issues related to allocation of resources. Should ART be available only to those who can pay for it? Should there be any limits to its use? Should an unmarried couple, a 60-year-old woman, or a lesbian couple use ART to become parents? Should insurance companies, including Medicaid, be mandated to cover the costs of ART? Although it is necessary to produce and implant a number of viable fertilized ova to increase the probability of a successful pregnancy, what should become of the unused embryos? Should they be kept frozen indefinitely? Should they be donated for research? Who owns them, that is, are they property or persons? Does the couple who "commissioned" their creation own them, or do the biological donors have any claims?

Once pregnancy occurs, there are additional broad social questions. Who are the parents of this child, the product of ART: the genetic parents, the biological mother who bore the child, or the people who have a legal contract for custody of the child? The answers may vary, depending on state law or the court that hears a specific case. Laws have not been written to address all the technological quandaries posed by ART.

Understanding and appreciating the deep desires some couples have to bear their own children (or have a surrogate mother bear a child) and the desperation and vulnerability that brings them to submit to multiple procedures is necessary for nurses to provide compassionate care. For nurses working in this area, it is useful to reflect on their own attitudes, beliefs, and biases. Ethical issues in assisted reproduction are very complex and worthy of careful examination and exploration by clinicians who have key roles in delivering the technology. Educating women about their options and facilitating their decision-making is a role for nurses.

ART may also be recommended for couples where one or both are HIV-positive. If only one partner is positive, ART can reduce the transmission between the partners. Opposition to the use of ART for couples with HIV is that the disease remains incurable and there is the risk of early death, so the child could be orphaned, and if the woman is HIV-positive, there is still the risk of transmission to the fetus.

Some critics of ART believe that women/couples should investigate adoption rather than undergo expensive, risky procedures. Many people desire children who have their DNA and thus have family characteristics. Others may specifically wish to avoid certain inherited disorders, so they seek IVF with prenatal genetic diagnosis. For those who consider adoption, they may want an infant with specific characteristics whose medical history is known and verifiable. If a baby meeting certain criteria is not available, many couples would forgo adoption and opt for IVF.

One of the recent issues in bioethics involving truth telling involves the disclosure to children, on reaching adulthood, of the identity of their biological fathers who were sperm donors. The Sperm Bank of California (n.d.) was the first in the nation to have an "identity-release" policy. With consent of the sperm donor, children conceived by the donors in this program can request the donor's full name, driver's license number, last known address and telephone number, and date and place of birth. Sperm donors have the prerogative of agreeing to have their identity released when the child reaches 18 or remaining anonymous. Under no circumstances, however, are sperm donors given any information about their offspring.

This policy was written in 1983, and so children conceived by these donors reached the age of 18 years in 2001. In December 2003, one California teenager came forward to learn her donor's identity, with her mother's approval. As a sperm donor, the biological father has no legal obligations to or claims on the children he fathered, but there are ethical questions. Should the donor provide genetic histories of blood relatives if asked? The child of the donor may want to have as much genetic history as possible if there is a question about inherited conditions. Although a donor may have consented to have his identity released, his family (wife, parents, siblings, children) may not wish their identities to be known. If any other offspring contact the donor and request to learn the identities of their half-siblings (the donor's own children or other sperm bank offspring), should the donor provide the information, or, as a minimum, act as a go-between? These issues are so new that the professional associations and consumer organizations have yet to respond with position statements. According to Dr. Sandra Carson of the American Society for Reproductive Medicine, "We do not have a lot of outcome data on anonymity versus non-anonymity. And until we do, we cannot say that one way is the right way'" (Muller, 2003).

The United Kingdom, New Zealand, and Japan are considering joining Sweden, Australia, the Netherlands, and other countries in permitting donor-conceived persons to identify their biological parents. Should children who are conceived through assisted reproduction be told how they were conceived? If the biological parent is different from the legal parent, should the child be told? Although the children would not have any legal claim on their biological parents, some donors may not wish to be identified, and the risk of being identified may discourage people from becoming donors. Is it strictly a parental prerogative to reveal this information to their children, or does a child have a right to know?

The European Society of Human Reproduction and Embryology (ESHRE) Task Force on Ethics and Law (2002) developed guidelines regarding ethical issues in gamete and embryo donation. The Task Force stated that children conceived through gamete or embryo donation have a right to all information that is provided by the donor. They also recommended a double-track system in which the donor can choose to be anonymous or identifiable and the recipient can select either an anonymous or an identifiable donor. The child conceived by the recipient can only learn the identity of the donor if both the donor and the recipient chose that option.

In addition to conception through sperm donation, oocyte donation is becoming increasingly popular. Between 1996 and 2001, assisted reproductive cycles with donated eggs increased 66%, and there was a 101% increase in live birth deliveries from 1996 to 2001 (Centers for Disease Control and Prevention, 2001, p. 60). In a qualitative study exploring parents' decision to disclose to their children that they were conceived through donor eggs, Hahn and Craft-Rosenberg (2002) reported that the majority of parents in their study intended to disclose. The parents who intended to disclose believed that it was in the child's best interests to know the truth and it would be harmful for the family to keep the information secret. The authors stressed the importance of the nursing role in preparing parents to disclose, if that is their choice, and preparing them for the child's possible responses. Having a plan for supporting a child who has a negative response is important.

Case Study 13-3

Angela and Bob (both nurses) have been married for 6 years and have been trying for 18 months without success to conceive a child. They actively searched the Internet and met with a fertility specialist to discuss options for creating a family. During a couples' infertility support group, Angela stated, "I really want to be a mother and have my own family. I do not really care if the baby has my DNA. However, I think the decision is going to come down to money. My insurance company is legally required to cover three attempts at ART, and adoption will cost at least $10,000. I am going to try ART solely because we cannot afford adoption. I feel badly that there are children out there looking for parents while we are seeking a child. Society's values seem to be inconsistent." For nurses working in fertility programs, would it be a conflict of interest for the nurses to advise parents on how they might get legal assistance in the adoption procedure? The clinic is a revenue-generating enterprise, yet is there an ethical obligation to identify the patient's goals of becoming a mother and assist the patient in reaching that goal?

FETAL SURGERY

There are a number of nonlethal conditions of the fetus that can be diagnosed in utero. Myelomeningocele (spina bifida) and sacrococcygeal teratoma are two examples. Surgical techniques that involve cutting open the uterus through the woman's abdomen, exposing the premature infant's back to repair the lesion, and returning the fetus to the uterus can be performed. Treatment through fetal surgery is highly controversial for a number of reasons: Is fetal surgery therapy or research? Have the procedures been validated? Are the risks known so that informed consent can be obtained? Should a technique be taught and practiced if it is considered experimental surgery?

Chervenak and McCullough (2002) recommended an ethical framework for fetal research (including fetal surgery) that recognizes the fetus as a patient, and they referred to the fetus and a previable fetal-subject. Next, there must be previous studies in animals that indicate the intervention is likely to be lifesaving or will reduce morbidity and the intervention has, on balance, acceptable risks to the mother and fetus. They also proposed that the physician-investigator who is knowledgeable about the procedure conduct the informed consent process and that the terms "treatment" or "therapy" should *not* be used in describing the procedure. Additionally, they believed that women who would electively abort or who would not consider abortion be excluded from the research. Their reasoning is that if a woman would electively abort, one can conclude that she is not viewing the fetus as a person and cannot adequately represent fetal interests in analyzing potential benefits and risks of surgery. If the woman would not consider abortion under any circumstances, she closes one option that the researchers want available to women if surgery has an adverse outcome. The researchers postulate that a woman must be vested in fetal well-being so that the decision to abort is based on fetal interests and not solely on maternal interests. The procedure should not be performed outside of the research context. Clinical equipoise should exist, meaning that it is not known whether fetal surgery is clearly a benefit.

SUMMARY

Assisted reproductive technologies, viewed as a blessing by many infertile couples, have also generated many complex ethical questions. The orchestration of conception and gestation challenges traditional views of pregnancy and identification of "parents." Questions of the limits of reproductive freedom are raised as the boundaries of technology continue to expand.

CLINICAL EXERCISES

1. Using the Internet, see how many fertility programs you can find in your community. How would you use this information to advise women interested in ART?
2. Look in your local newspaper classified ads for women seeking egg donors and women willing to donate eggs. How would you use this information to advise women interested in ART?

Discussion Questions

1. Should parents have certain qualifications in order to undergo ART? Defend your answer.
2. Ms. Eagle just learned that her fetus has spina bifida and she wants to find a surgeon who will operate in utero so the fetus will be "born normal." What information should you provide to her about fetal surgery?

SECTION 4: *Genetics in Women's Health*

GENETICS

Genetics in women's health involves reproductive decisions. The President's Council on Bioethics (2004) issued a report on reproductive issues and "new biotechnologies." Among the nine issues it identified were the following:

---

1. *Compassion for children with serious genetic diseases, and relief of the sorrows and burdens that they and those who love and care for them must bear. . . . Several expressions and avenues of human freedom, including the freedom of parents to make their own reproductive decisions or to use or refuse genetic screening, and the freedom of scientists to conduct research. As important, as well, is the necessity to protect the freedom of children from improper attempts to manipulate their lives through control of their genetic make-up or from unreasonable expectations that could accompany such manipulations. . . .*
2. *The promotion of justice and equality, including equitable access to the use and benefits of new technologies, equal respect and opportunity in a world that places great emphasis on genetic distinctions, and the prevention of discrimination against or contempt for genetic "defectiveness" or "inferiority." (p. 1).*

The report called for longitudinal studies of the effect of assisted reproductive technologies on the health of women and the health and development of children born through such technologies.

Prenatal Testing

There are a number of ways that genetic information about the fetus can be obtained prenatally. One way is through examining the mother's blood during pregnancy for certain indicators of genetic conditions. The maternal serum alpha-fetal protein can indicate Down syndrome or neural tube defect. The blood is drawn some time between weeks 15 and 20 of pregnancy. Two other tests, human chorionic gonadotropin (hCG) and estriol, can be done at the same time, with the three tests being referred to as the Triple Screen. Having the Triple Screen, however, starts the pregnant woman on a decision trajectory, and she should be aware of the purpose of the testing and future decisions that might have to be made.

If the Triple Screen indicates a likelihood that the fetus has a genetic condition, like Down syndrome, the next step is to perform an amniocentesis and/or ultrasound. An ultrasound may be sufficient to identify a birth defect such as a neural tube defect, but for chromosomal abnormalities, amniocentesis is preferred. Informed consent is obtained prior to the procedure. Risks such as miscarriage or the possibility that not all birth defects can be detected with amniocentesis should be fully disclosed. Should amniocentesis confirm the suspected genetic condition, the next decision the woman faces is whether to terminate the pregnancy. What many women may not realize is that there is an assumption that women will abort fetuses with birth defects. It is highly likely that women want to know and want the option, but it cannot be assumed that they will prefer to abort. Some women may want to be prepared in terms of pregnancy management, delivery options, newborn care, and future special needs. In the past, diagnostic procedures were not available unless the woman agreed to terminate the pregnancy if an abnormality was found. In the United Kingdom there is an expectation that women who conceive through IVF have a duty not to reproduce a child who could suffer "some form of demonstrable harm" through inheritance (McHale, 2002, p. 102). There is an assumption that all parents want a "healthy" baby, but there is evidence that some parents want children from their own DNA, even if the majority culture would disagree.

For example, Mr. and Mrs. Hahn have congenital deafness. They want a child, and they want the child to have the gene for deafness. Suppose through preimplantation genetic diagnosis (PGD) they can have the fertilized ova tested for the gene for deafness. If the gene is present, the ova are implanted; if the gene is not present, the ova are frozen, donated, or destroyed. The dominant culture views deafness as a disability, yet in the deaf culture, it is the norm. Should the genetic testing be performed with the expressed purpose of conceiving a child who is deaf? Genetic counseling is value-neutral (see Chapter 12, Section 4, for more details about genetic counseling); information is provided, and the couple makes a decision based on their own values.

Preimplantation genetic diagnosis is intended to provide information to aid the couple to make a decision. In the future there will be the ability to screen for more and more genes. Will society limit access to PGD to those couples at risk for having a child with a life-threatening or life-altering inherited condition? Should PGD be used for gender selection? Currently, PGD to identify gender is useful in identifying the risk of sex-linked disorders. If a couple wanted to use PGD to plan a family of all boys or all girls, is that ethical? As mentioned in Chapter 11, gender selection through ultrasound and infanticide of female infants has left India and China with a very lopsided male-dominated population. Is the decision strictly up to the couple, or should society interject and regulate the technology?

Genetic testing can also affect family relationships. Suppose a pregnant woman has a family history of Huntington disease (HD), an autosomal dominant neurodegenerative disorder that usually does not manifest until after age 40. She has not been tested, nor have her parents, but she has a paternal uncle with Huntington disease. She wants prenatal genetic testing on the fetus with the intention of terminating the pregnancy if the gene is present. If the gene is present, then it is highly probable that she inherited it from her father, and both she and her father have the HD gene. Because her father has not been tested, he may not want to know whether he has the gene. Depending on the family relationship (and his knowledge of the inheritance of the HD gene), if he learns of the results of the prenatal genetic diagnosis testing, he will learn of his own genetic inheritance. If the testing does not reveal the gene, it is still possible that both the pregnant woman and her father have the gene, but the gene did not get passed on to the fetus. Should the pregnant woman discuss with her father her intention to have the fetus tested? Should he have a say in whether she is tested? The Huntington Disease Society of America (1994) established guidelines that include extensive pre- and posttest counseling to assist the person to deal with the ramifications of testing.

Genetic Testing for Cancer

With more and more genetic tests becoming available, women will face choices about whether to submit to testing. By family history, the woman may be at risk for breast, ovarian, or colon cancer, and she can be tested to discover whether she carries the relevant gene. Although having the gene does not guarantee the person will develop the cancer, it does indicate the person is at a higher risk than the general population. For some women, that may be enough information to consider prophylactic measures such as increased surveillance, preventative medication like tamoxifen, or more drastic steps such as bilateral mastectomies, bilateral removal of the ovaries, or total hysterectomy. If the woman does not have the gene, it does not mean that she will remain cancer-free. There are other risks to being tested. Again, the ethical issues revolve around informed decision-making. Nurses should be aware of the implications of genetic testing for cancer risk. Although the exact effects are unknown, there is concern that genetic testing could lead to discrimination in employment and insurance. The psychological effects can be significant because a negative finding does not eliminate the risk and a positive finding does not ensure the disease will occur. Pasacreta, Jacobs, and Cataldo (2002) expressed concern that the psychological effects of testing could be worse than having a diagnosis of cancer confirmed. They encouraged nurses to be familiar with the indications for genetic testing for cancer, and if nurses work in a setting where testing is offered, it is critical that nurses have the education to support women who have testing.

Case Study 13-4

Ms. Harris has several female relatives who died from breast and ovarian cancers. She is now 50 years old and is convinced that she will eventually develop one or both types of cancer. She asks her gynecologist to test for the BRCA1/2 breast cancer genes. If she has either or both genes, she wants bilateral mastectomies and a total hysterectomy. Her physician does not want to remove healthy tissue, and recommends increased surveillance through tumor marker blood testing and breast ultrasounds. Ms. Harris said her quality of life is adversely affected by her constant and intense worrying. In addition, Ms. Harris has a 31-year-old daughter who wants the same testing and who says that she also would choose surgery rather than "wait for cancer to kill me."

SUMMARY

New technologies pose new ethical problems. How should the technologies be used? If a condition cannot be treated, is its discovery helpful or harmful? For those conditions that can be life-threatening, should prophylactic treatment such as surgery be promoted? Health care providers in women's health should stay current on the technologies and the best practices in their use. Staying current is critical, but even more critical is the influence professionals can have on attitudes toward genetic conditions. Routine prenatal testing for Down syndrome and neural tube defects assumes that women want to know in order to make a decision about continuation of the pregnancy. They may wish to know in order to plan for the needs of a child with such a condition, so those women may be interested in prenatal testing that does not pose a risk to the fetus.

CLINICAL EXERCISES

1. Investigate where a pregnant woman could go to have genetic testing in your community.

   a. Where is it done, what does it cost, and how does a patient get referred?
   b. What do you need to know to be able to inform patients of this service?
   c. What do you identify as the ethical issues in giving this information to patients?

2. Obtain a copy of a consent form that is used for genetic counseling.

   a. How does the content of the form differ from a consent form used for surgery?
   b. What is the ethical rationale for the differences?

Discussion Questions

1. In Case 13-4, how can the nurse assist Ms. Harris in her decision about genetic testing? What about Ms. Harris' daughter? What is the community standard for women who carry the BRCA1/2 genes?
2. Discuss the pros and cons of a woman learning whether she carries the BRCA1/2 genes. What are the benefits and risks of having the test?

Resources

American College of Obstetricians and Gynecologists (2003). Statement on "so-called" partial birth abortion law. ACOG News Release, October 3, 2003. Retrieved December 9, 2005, from http://www.acog.org/from_home/publications/press_releases/nr10-03-03.cfm

Family Educational Rights and Privacy Act (FERPA). (1974). 20 U.S.C. §1232g; 34 CFR Part 99.

National Institutes of Health. (1994). Inclusion of women in research. NIH guidelines on the inclusion of women and minorities as subjects in clinical research. Retrieved April 11, 2004, from http://grants2.nih.gov/grants/guide/notice-files/not94-100.html

Planned Parenthood Federation of America. (n.d.). Fact sheet. Laws requiring parental consent or notification for minors' abortions. Retrieved August 25, 2003, from www.plannedparent-hood.org/library/ABORTION/StateLaws.html

Stavis, P. F. (1991). Sexual activity and the law of consent. Retrieved August 25, 2003, from www.cqc.state.ny.us/counsels_corner/cc50.htm

Teenparents.org. (n.d.). Legal consent requirements for the medical treatment of minors. Retrieved August 25, 2003, from www.teenparents.org/consent.html

References

Advanced Fertility Services. (2005). Cost of IVF at Advanced Fertility Services. Retrieved May 15, 2005, from http://www.infertilityny.com/costs/index.html

Alan Guttmacher Institute. (2005). State policies in brief. Retrieved December 14, 2005, from http://www.guttmacher.org/statecenter/spibs/index.html

American Academy of Pediatrics Committee on Bioethics. (1997). Religious objections to medical care. *Pediatrics, 99*(2), 279–281.

American Association on Mental Retardation. (2002). Sexuality policy statement. Retrieved April 4, 2004, from www.aamr.org/Groups/si/SS/

American College of Obstetricians and Gynecologists Committee on Ethics. (2004). Ethics in obstetrics and gynecology. (2nd ed.). Retrieved April 4, 2004, from http://www.acog.org/from%5Fhome/publications/ethics/

American Nurses Association. (1997). Opposition to criminal prosecution of women for use of drugs while pregnant. Retrieved May 15, 2005, from http://nursingworld.org/readroom/position/drug/drpreg.htm

American Psychiatric Association. (2001). *Fact sheet: Postpartum depression*. Washington, DC: Author.

Barsky, A. J., Peekna, H. M., & Borus, J. F. (2001). Somatic symptom reporting in women and men. *Journal of General Internal Medicine, 16*(4), 266–275.

Bewley, S. (2002). Restricting the freedom of pregnant women. In D. L. Dickenson (Ed.). *Ethical issues in maternal-fetal medicine*. (pp. 131–146). New York: Cambridge University Press.

Block, P. (2000). Sexuality, fertility, and danger: Twentieth-century images of women with cognitive disabilities. *Sexuality and Disability, 18*(4), 239–254.

Bornstein, B. H. (2003). Pregnancy, drug testing, and the Fourth Amendment: Legal and behavioral implications. *Journal of Family Psychology, 17*(2), 220–228.

Burns, D. L. (1997). Positive toxicology screening in newborns: Ethical issues in the decision to legally intervene. *Pediatric Nursing, 23*(1), 53–75.

Callahan, D. (1988). Families as caregivers: The limits of morality. *Archives of Physical Medicine and Rehabilitation, 69*(5), 323–328.

Catlin, A. J. (1997). Commentary on Deborah L. Burns' article Positive toxicology screening in newborns: Ethical issues in the decision to legally intervene. *Pediatric Nursing, 23*(1), 76–78, 86.

Center for Disease Control. (2001). *2001 Assisted Reproductive Technology Success Rates. National Summary & Fertility Clinic Reports*. Washington, D.C.: U.S. Department of Health and Human Services.

Centers for Disease Control and Prevention. (2002). CDC reproductive health. 2001 assisted reproductive technology success rates. Retrieved May 15, 2005, from http://www.cdc.gov/reproductivehealth/ART02/PDF/ART2002.pdf

Centers for Disease Control and Prevention. (2004). Eliminating perinatal HIV transmission. Retrieved May 15, 2005, from http://www.cdc.gov/programs/hiv05.htm

Charlton, J. I. (1998). *Nothing about us without us: Disability, oppression and empowerment*. Berkeley, CA: University of California Press.

Chervenak, F. A., & McCullough, L. B. (2002). A comprehensive ethical framework for fetal research and its application to fetal surgery for spina bifida. *American Journal of Obstetrics and Gynecology, 187*(1), 10–14.

Cooley, M. (2003). Catholic hospitals refuse patients contraception. Women's *e*News. Retrieved May 15, 2005, from http://womensenews.org/article.cfm/dyn/aid/1209

Dailard, C., & Nash, E. (2000). State responses to substance abuse among pregnant women. The Guttmacher Report on Public Policy. Retrieved May 15, 2005, from http://www.guttmacher.org/pubs/tgr/03/6/gr030603.pdf

Danforth, D. N., & Scott, J. R. (2003). *Danforth's Obstetrics and Gynecology*. (9th ed.). Philadelphia: LWW.

De Zulueta, P. (2002). HIV in pregnancy: Ethical issues in screening and therapeutic research. In D. L. Dickenson (Ed.). *Ethical issues in maternal-fetal medicine*. (pp. 61–85). Cambridge: Cambridge University Press.

European Society of Human Reproduction and Embryology Task Force on Ethics and Law. (2002). Gamete and embryo donation. *Human Reproduction, 17*(5), 1407–1408.

Ferguson v. City of Charleston. (2001). 121 S. Ct. 1281.

Fidler, A. T., & Bernstein, J. (1999). Infertility: From a personal to a public health problem. *Public Health Report, 114*(6), 494–511.

Fleischer, D. Z., & Zames, F. (2001). *The disability rights movement: From charity to confrontation*. Philadelphia: Temple University Press.

Gold, J. H. (1998). Gender differences in psychiatric illness and treatments: A critical review. *Journal of Nervous and Mental Disease, 186*(12), 769–775.

Hahn, S. J., & Craft-Rosenberg, M. (2002). The disclosure decisions of parents who conceive children using donor eggs. *JOGNN, 31*, 283–293.

Henshaw, S. K., & Finer, L. B. (2003). The accessibility of abortion services in the United States, 2001. *Perspectives on Sexual and Reproduction Health, 35*(1), 16–24.

Huntington's Disease Society of America. Guidelines for Predictive Testing for HD (Huntington's Disease). (1994). Retrieved April 4, 2004, from http://www.circ.uab.edu/sergg/s95/guid.htm

Illinois Department of Public Health Division of Epidemiological Studies. (2001). Surveillance of Illinois infants prenatally exposed to controlled substances 1991–1999. Retrieved May 15, 2005, from http://www.idph.state.il.us/about/epi/pdf/Epi01-4.pdf

Longmore, P. K. (2003). *Why I burned my book and other essays on disability*. Philadelphia: Temple University Press.

McHale, J. (2002). Is there a duty not to reproduce? In D. L. Dickenson (Ed.). *Ethical issues in maternal-fetal medicine*. (pp. 101–112). Cambridge: Cambridge University Press.

Muller, J. (2003). Sperm search: California teen may become first to meet her sperm-donor father. Retrieved January 19, 2004, from http://abcnews.go.com/sections/wnt/DailyNews/sperm_donor021213.html

National Alliance for Caregiving and AARP. (1997). *Family caregiving in the U. S.: Findings from a national survey*. Washington, DC: Author.

National Cancer Institute. (2002). News center. Increased risk of ovarian cancer is linked to estrogen replacement therapy. Retrieved April 12, 2004, from http://www.cancer.gov/newscenter/Laceyovarian

National Institute on Drug Abuse. (2003). Pregnancy and drug use trends. Retrieved August 25, 2003, from www.drugabuse.gov/Infofax/pregnancytrends.html

National Institutes of Health. (2004). NIH news. NIH asks participants in Women's Health Initiative Estrogen-Alone Study to stop study pills, begin follow-up phase. Retrieved April 12, 2004, from http://www.nih.gov/news/pr/mar2004/nhlbi-02.htm

Pasacreta, J. V., Jacobs, L., & Cataldo, J. K. (2002). Genetic testing for breast and ovarian cancer risk: The psychosocial issues: For some women, anticipating the diagnosis is worse than receiving the diagnosis itself. *American Journal of Nursing, 102*(12), 40–47.

Pergament, R. (2004). Susan Smith: Child murderer or victim? Retrieved April 8, 2004, from http://www.crimelibrary.com/fillicide/smith/

Planned Parenthood Federation of America. (2004). Fact sheet. Obstructing access to emergency contraception in hospital emergency rooms. Retrieved December 17, 2004, from www.plannedparenthood.org/library/facts/obstructing_032102.html

Pontifical Academy for Life. (2000). Statement on the so-called "morning-after pill." Retrieved December 9, 2005, from http://www.vatican.va/roman_curia/pontifical_academies/acdlife/documents/rc_pa_acdlife_doc_20001031_pillola-giorno-dopo_en.html

Pregnancy and drug use trends. National Institute on Drug Abuse. Retrieved August 25, 2003, from www.drugabuse.gov/Infofax/pregnancytrends.html

President's Council on Bioethics. (2004). Reproduction and responsibility: The regulation of new biotechnologies (Prepublication version). Retrieved April 4, 2004, from www.bioethics.gov/reports/reproductionandresponsibility/exec_summary.html

Sacks, D. A., & Koppes, R. H. (1994). Caring for the female Jehovah's Witness: Balancing medicine, ethics and First Amendment. *American Journal of Obstetrics and Gynecology, 170*(2), 452–455.

Sankar, P., Moran, S., Merz, J. F., & Jones, N. L. (2003). Patient perspectives on medical confidentiality: A review of the literature. *Journal of General Internal Medicine, 18*, 659–669.

Schulz, R., & Beach, S. R. (1999). Caregiving as a risk factor for mortality: The Caregiver Health Effects Study. *Journal of the American Medical Association, 282*(23), 2215–2219.

Shapiro, J. P. (1994). *No pity: People with disabilities forging a new civil rights movement*. New York: Random House.

Shelby, K. (2003). Hormone replacement therapy: What we know now. *NurseWeek*, January 20, 2003, pp. 19–21.

Silvers, A., Wasserman, D., & Mahowald, M. B. (1998). *Disability, difference, discrimination: Perspectives on justice in bioethics and public policy*. New York: Rowman & Littlefield.

Sperm Bank of California. (n.d.). Available at www.thespermbankofca.org/aboutus/idrels.htm

Stanton, A. L., Lobel, M., Sears, S., & DeLuca, R. S. (2002). Psychosocial aspects of selected issues in women's reproductive health: Current status and future directions. *Journal of Consulting and Clinical Psychology, 70*(3), 751–770.

Sullinger, H. (2000). Women and heart disease: Identifying risk, overcoming barriers. *Topics in Emergency Medicine, 22*(1), 42–51.

Tarvis, C. (1992). *The mismeasure of woman: Why women are not the better sex, the inferior sex, or the opposite sex*. New York: Simon & Schuster.

Tillett, J., & Osborne, K. (2001). Substance abuse by pregnant women: Legal and ethical concerns. *Journal of Perinatal and Neonatal Nursing, 14*(4), 1–11.

United States Conference of Catholic Bishops. (2001). Ethical and religious directives for Catholic health care services. (4th ed.). Retrieved December 17, 2004, from http://www.usccb.org/bishops/directives.shtml

United States Conference of Catholic Bishops. (2001). Ethical and religious directives for Catholic health care services. (4th ed.). Retrieved December 17, 2004, from www.usccb.org/bishops/directives.shtml

U.S. Department of Health and Human Services. (1998). *Informal caregiving: Compassion in action*. Washington, DC: Author.

White, G. B. (2001). Young women wanted: The hopes and hazards of oocyte donation and what nurses can do. *AJN: American Journal of Nursing, 101*(6), 60–65.

Yee, J. L., & Schulz, L. R. (2000). Gender differences in psychiatric morbidity among family caregivers: A review and analysis. *The Gerontologist, 40*(2), 147–164.

CHAPTER 14

Mental Health Nursing

Objectives

At the end of this chapter, the student should be able to:

1. Identify the nurses' professional responsibility for truth-telling, advocacy, confidentiality, and resource allocation when caring for a person with a mental health disorder.
2. Discuss the nurse's professional obligation to simultaneously promote patient autonomy and prevent harm.
3. Discuss the ethical principles affecting the decision to implement an act of restraint with a patient.
4. Analyze personal and professional values and biases and cultural norms affecting ethical dilemmas in conflicts between patient autonomy and health care paternalism.
5. Discuss the professional nurse's obligation to provide care to difficult patients.
6. Identify strategies for fulfilling the nurse's commitment to respect persons when dealing with challenging patients.
7. Discuss the nurse's duty to protect third parties.

KEY WORDS

- *Anonymity*
- *Autonomy*
- *Best interests*
- *Challenging patient*
- *Chemical restraint*
- *Dangerous to self*

- *Deinstitutionalization*
- *Mental illness/Mental health disorder*
- *Noncompliance*
- *Paternalism*
- *Physical restraint*
- *Seclusion*

SECTION 1: *Ethical Themes: Building From the Basic to the Complex*

When dealing with person with mental health disorders (MHD), the nurse's actions and ethical obligations related to the basic ethical themes (confidentiality, truth-telling, advocacy, and allocation of scarce resources) may be affected by legislation as well as the social stigma associated with mental health disorders. The availability of social and financial resources for persons with MHD may affect how ethical issues are defined and resolved.

CONFIDENTIALITY

Confidentiality is the guarding of private information. *Anonymity* involves keeping a person's name and/or identify unknown to a third person, and thus is a more stringent standard than confidentiality. In the past, anonymity in public health care agencies was not possible because admissions to hospitals were often public record. In fact, many rural newspapers published hospital admissions in a column along with ambulance responses for services and police arrests or citations. Thus, high-profile persons (e.g., politicians or actors) might be admitted to an agency using fictitious names in an attempt to conceal their identities. However, this practice can raise issues related to continuity of care and billing when the patient's name does not match previous records or insurance policies.

Special Protections

The obligation to maintain patient confidentiality does not change when caring for persons with mental health problems. However, due to the social stigma frequently associated with a diagnosis of a mental illness, extra measures are often implemented to protect not only the confidentiality of persons with mental illnesses, but also their anonymity.

Illustrative Case 14-1

When a child is admitted to an in-patient child psychiatric unit, a list of names of persons who may call the child is prepared. Each of these persons is given a code word for identification purposes. When, say, the child's grandmother telephones or visits the in-patient child psychiatric unit, she must provide her name as well as the code word before the clerk can acknowledge the child's presence on the unit. The intention behind the use of a code word is to minimize the possibility that an unauthorized person would become privy to the knowledge that a specific child was receiving psychiatric care.

A second protection that agencies and independent therapists employ relates to the physical design of waiting areas and exits. A person's confidentiality/anonymity while seeking mental health services can be breached when they enter and/or exit buildings or offices.

Illustrative Case 14-2

Reverend Perkins made an appointment at the local mental health center after experiencing a panic attack. The mental health center maintains a large parking lot in front of the building that is used by patients as well as employees. Although each therapist has an individual office, all patients use a common waiting room. When exiting the therapist's office through the waiting room, Reverend Perkins recognizes and is greeted by Ms. Temple, the daughter of a parishioner of his church. A few days later, Reverend Perkins is approached by Ms. Temple's mother and asked, "Is everything OK?"

Several actions can be considered for improving the confidentiality of persons seeking mental health services. Ideally, receiving mental health services should not be stigmatizing, but for many they are. Separate waiting rooms could be used for each therapist, or appointment times could be staggered. Persons should be able to exit a therapist's office without going back through the waiting area. In addition, building entrances and parking lots could be configured to decrease the recognition of persons and their cars by other persons driving by the mental health agency. These strategies limit the likelihood that two persons seeking mental health services would encounter and recognize each other.

Threat to confidentiality can also occur during group therapy sessions (Cline, 2003). By coming to a group session, a person seeking mental health services reveals his or her identity. The use of pseudonyms may promote an element of anonymity for persons participating in a group, especially for persons (e.g., teachers, business leaders, or religious leaders) with names that may be easily recognized by others if mentioned outside of the group. A second threat to confidentiality is created by the expectation that participants will share personal information with the group; the possibility exists that a participant could accidentally or purposefully disclose information shared during the group meeting with a third party.

Illustrative Case 14-3

Mrs. Shaw joined a bereavement group after her husband's suicide. During one session, Mrs. Shaw disclosed that immediately following her husband's death she used illicit drugs to cope with her loss. Ms. Berstein, another member of the group, recognized Mrs. Shaw's name as being the same as her son's English teacher at the local high school. Several weeks later, Ms. Berstein's teenage son came home from school and reported, "Mrs. Shaw was really acting weird today in class." Ms. Berstein questioned her son: "Do you think she was high? She shared at the bereavement group that she's had a drug problem."

Discussion Exercises 14-1

Mrs. Patton has been contacting area health care facilities on a routine basis after the disappearance of her adult daughter, Angela, who has a history of mental illness. As the days progress, Mrs. Patton is becoming more distraught wondering whether her daughter is ill, wandering the streets, or dead. However, Angela Patton was brought to the hospital by the police 3 days ago after being found disoriented and wandering the streets.

1. Based on a commitment to patient confidentiality, how should you respond the next time Mrs. Patton contacts the hospital unit?
2. Do you believe that family members should have a right to know that their loved one is safe? If so, how would you go about advocating for the family's right to know? If not, what ethical commitments (besides confidentiality) should guide your interactions with the family members?

TRUTH-TELLING

Therapeutic relationships, especially those between a person receiving mental health services and a nurse, are based on trust. The professional nurse may be faced with an ethical dilemma concerning how honest to be with a patient with a mental illness. For example, a patient with impulse control problems may ask a senior nursing student during her psychiatric nursing rotation, "Are you afraid to be alone with me?" or a patient with a history of self-mutilation might state, "I bet you are not so perfect. You're so skinny. Do not tell me you have never purged or taken laxatives to stay thin!"

There is no one clear answer for how a nurse should respond to questions about his or her feelings, beliefs, and actions. The nurse's response will be influenced by the type of relationship he or she perceives exists with the patient and the nurse's interpretation of the motivations behind the patient's question. Nurses need to maintain professional boundaries when interacting with patients. When maintaining professional boundaries, the focus is on the patient, and thus the nurse does not discuss personal details or beliefs (Deering & Frederick, 2003). "Boundaries mark the parameter of the professional relationship" (Peternelj-Taylor & Yonge, 2003, p. 56). Failure to maintain professional boundaries may result in negative consequences for the patient's recovery (Diamond & Larsen, 2003). For example, if the nursing student did share with the patient her eating disorder history, the patient might conclude, "How can this nursing student ever help me? She had just about the same problem as I do!" On the other hand, if the patient believed that the student nurse was not responding honestly, then the patient may lose trust in the student nurse's ability to assist in the patient's recovery.

The nurse should also consider potential harm to self when deliberating on how honestly to answer a question. For example, a nurse should never disclose personal information such as that he or she lives alone or his or her address or daily routine to any patient, especially to a patient with a history of impulse control issues or stalking behavior. Similarly, a nurse should never disclose information to a patient that the nurse would not want to become public knowledge. For example, a nurse should not disclose intentions to change employment to a patient unless the nurse has already submitted a formal resignation.

Finally, nurses may also be confronted by a patient asking, "If I tell you, will you keep it a secret?" Nurses do not work in isolation. They are part of the health care team; therefore, any promise to keep a patient's secret could be detrimental to the health care team's effectiveness and ultimately the patient's ability to make therapeutic changes. When asked to keep a secret, a nurse must answer the patient directly about the nurse's obligations to promote good for the patient and commitments to other health care team members. In addition, the nurse may have a legal obligation to disclose specific information, such as abuse or fraud. The nurse may have an ethical obligation to warn a third party of the possibility of imminent harm (see Section 4). Thus, when faced with a request to maintain secrecy, the nurse will need to respond compassionately, yet directly. For example, the nurse might say, "I cannot promise that I will not share the information you might tell me with other members of your health care team if they need to know. As a nurse, I have the legal obligation to report actions such as abuse and neglect of children or elders. I can promise you that I will not disclose information to people who are not involved in your treatment and thus do not have a need to know." In addition, the nurse should attempt to ascertain why the patient perceives the need for secrecy.

Discussion Exercises 14-2

A patient in an in-patient psychiatric unit refused to take his or her prescribed medications. The staff cornered the patient in his room. After the door was closed, members of the health care team held the patient down while a nurse administered an intramuscular injection of medication.

1. What ethical justification can be provided to support and negate this practice?
2. Are health care professionals lying when they tell patients during the admission process "You have the right to refuse treatment, including medications"?
3. Virginia Henderson makes a moral claim by defining nursing as follows:

   The unique function of the nurse is to assist the individual, sick or well, in the performance of those activities contributing to health or its recovery (or to a peaceful death) that he would perform unaided if he had the necessary strength, will or knowledge. And to do this in such a way as to help him gain independence as rapidly as possible. (As cited in Marinner-Tomey, 2002, p. 101)

Do the actions in this case fulfill the moral obligations of a nurse as set forth by Henderson? Explain your answer.

Nurses in every clinical setting experience challenges to their professional boundaries; thus, it behooves professional nursing organizations and health care agencies to provide resources the individual nurse can access when facing ethical issues related to boundary crossings and/or violations. These resources could include, but are not limited to, self-awareness questionnaires [e.g., Pilette, Berck, & Achber's (1995) Nursing Boundary Index], self-monitoring inventories [e.g., the Relationship Security Risk Warning Signs Self-Assessment Checklist (Love, 2001)], individual and/or group peer debriefing sessions, clinical supervision, proactive guidelines for clinical practice, and continuing education about professional relationships and the potential for abuse of power that can occur in any therapeutic relationship (Peternelj-Talyor & Yonge, 2003).

ADVOCACY

Western medicine recognizes the patient's right to autonomy, which includes the right to make informed decisions to accept or reject medical intervention.

Autonomy: The Right to Make a Bad Decision

In nonpsychiatric settings, nurses often are required to accept what he or she considers to be a bad plan based on the patient's right to self-determination. For example, a patient with cancer may decide not to have chemotherapy despite the fact that the treatment has a 95% success rate for curing that form of cancer. Thus, the patient makes an informed refusal of treatment knowing that there is a high probability that he or she may die without treatment.

A competent patient's right to refuse treatment continues even if he or she is receiving mental health services, as long as there is no evidence of significant immediate harm to self or others.

Illustrative Case 14-4

Mr. Lubicky is in an acute psychotic state and refusing to eat. He is 6 feet tall and weighs 100 pounds. His serum albumin is 1.7 mg/dl. Based on these and other findings, the health care team concludes that Mr. Lubicky is severely malnourished and is causing significant harm to himself. Because of the health care team's moral obligation to prevent harm, Mr. Lubicky is started on feedings via a nasogastric tube. His son legally challenges the health care team's actions. A judge rules in favor of Mr. Lubicky's right to refuse to eat because the health care team did not follow applicable state law. The judge rules that the health care team violated Mr. Lubicky's rights by force feeding him for 72 hours without initiating legal proceedings to legally challenge his competence.

Thus, every nurse must be aware of the applicable laws and court cases that affect clinical decisions regarding a patient's right to refuse treatment.

Discussion Exercises 14-3

Ms. Horner is admitted to a geropsychiatric unit for depression. She is receiving total parenteral nutrition (TPN) because of her difficulty in tolerating oral food. She is refusing all medications except for the TPN. The gastrointestinal (GI) specialist suggests that she would benefit from having a gastrostomy tube (G-tube) placed; however, Ms. Horner refuses. Although she is depressed, Ms. Horner is alert, oriented to person, place, and time, and makes all of her own decisions. The GI specialist believes that TPN is not a long-term solution to her nutritional issues and that not placing a G-tube may shorten Ms. Horner's life.

1. Based on what criteria should decisions about Ms. Horner's decisional capacity be made?
2. If Ms. Horner were found to lack decisional capacity and you were assigned to serve as her surrogate decision-maker, what factors and values should guide how you make decisions for her? How would you identify these factors and values if you had no prior relationship with her?

No-Suicide Contracts

An attempt to commit suicide is a commonly accepted reason for overriding a patient's autonomy to act. After a thorough assessment, a no-suicide contract is sometimes implemented to minimize the likelihood that a patient will attempt suicide. No-suicide contracts are often initiated in community settings or verbally via suicide hotlines when the health care professional concludes that the risk for suicide is low. In a no-suicide contract, the patient may promise, "No matter what happens, I will not kill myself, accidentally or on purpose, at any time" (Drye, Goulding, & Goulding, 1973, p. 172; as cited in Farrow & O'Brien, 2003, p. 200). Alternatively, the patient may agree to contact the therapist if the patient experiences increased suicidal ideations.

The use of no-suicide contracts is not without ethical challenges. First, the health care professional must determine that the person has the decisional capacity necessary to make an informed decision. If the person has decisional capacity, then the health care professional has an obligation to provide him or her with information necessary to make an informed decision about the various options available. Second, the possibility exists that the decision to enter into a no-suicide contract may not be voluntary. A person with suicidal ideations may be informed, "If you do not sign the no-suicide contract, then I'll have no choice but to have you involuntarily committed because you are at risk of imminent harm." Finally, there is limited empirical evidence to suggest that no-suicide contracts do result in lower suicide rates, and thus they may not be a beneficial intervention (Farrow & O'Brien, 2003).

RESOURCE ALLOCATION

After World War II, advocates for persons with mental illnesses called attention to the unethical treatment many persons with mental illness received in state psychiatric hospitals. The National Mental Health Act was passed in 1946, and the National Institute of Mental Health was created in 1949 to promote the care of persons with mental illness (Huggins, Anderson, & Odom, 2003).

Deinstitutionalization of Mental Health Services

The advent of antipsychotic drugs (such as chlorpromazine) in the 1950s made it possible for many persons with mental illnesses to control their disease/symptoms without the need for institutionalization. Unfortunately, their leaving the structured environment of a mental institution resulted in decreased compliance with antipsychotic drug regimes for many persons with mental illnesses living in the community, which frequently resulted in the *revolving door syndrome*, in which the patient is admitted for treatment, stabilized, relapses, and is readmitted (Conn, 2003).

In 1963, the federal government enacted legislation that created community mental health centers. This legislation allowed states to shift much of the financial burden for mental health care away from the individual states to the federal government. Persons with mental illnesses were released from institution-based care and moved into the community for housing and community-based outpatient services (Conn, 2003). The *deinstitutionalization* of mental health services reflects the ethical commitment to autonomy by providing services in the least restrictive setting possible. Although intentions were good, the need for services outweighed the resources available then and now and resulted in many persons with mental illnesses receiving less than optimal and, at times, no care. Thus, ethically, one must question whether the least restrictive setting is equivalent to the most therapeutic setting.

As a result of the community's inability to absorb the thousands of persons with mental illness who were deinstitutionalized (discharged from state hospitals), many of these persons became homeless. It is estimated that one-third of all homeless persons have a mental health disorder (Rickelman, 2003). Life on the streets is not easy for anyone. Unfortunately, the combination of homelessness, MHD, poor nutrition, and behavior that challenges social norms has resulted in many homeless persons with MHD being reinstitutionalized in prisons after displaying violent behaviors. Thus, the penal system seems to be coming the twenty-first-century equivalent of the asylum or state mental hospital.

The U.S. experience with deinstitutionalizing persons with mental illnesses provides several ethical lessons. When making any change, decision-makers have an ethical obligation to ensure that it occurs at the highest level possible. In retrospect, politicians and health care professionals had good intentions, but sufficient resources were not allocated to ensure that these were met. For example, the system was unable to provide sufficient housing, community-based mental health services, and social supports necessary to maintain the deinstitutionalized person's welfare and treatment goals.

This deinstitutionalization process illustrates how an individual's needs can be overlooked when making decisions based on the greatest good for the greatest number. Theoretically, deinstitutionalization should have been cheaper overall than maintaining institutionalized care, which should have resulted in more financial resources being available to meet the mental health (and other needs) of all patients. However, lack of coordinated services and communication breakdowns undermined the success of a community-based mental health system for many individuals. For example, without a mailing address, homeless persons might be unable to apply for or receive financial assistance or community-based programs. Although deinstitutionalization was a beneficial change for many persons with mental illness, many individuals were harmed by deinstitutionalization. For example, many persons with mental illness were unable to independently maintain their medication regimen without a structured environment. Therefore, when instituting a global change, health care professionals have an obligation to consider and advocate for the individual's needs as well as the group's shared needs.

Medications Rather Than Psychotherapy Due to Reimbursement Issues

Ideally, health care (including mental health care) should be a clinical decision based on the state of the science and not a business decision. Unfortunately in the era of health management organizations (HMOs) and insurance plans, this ideal may not be reality.

Every insurance policy or HMO plan stipulates the type, frequency, and limits to care that will be applied to every participant in the plan. These stipulations can be so specific as to address exactly which drug will or will not be covered by the drug plan. For example, the insurance or HMO drug policy may stipulate that only formulary medications will be covered, or drug A but not drug B within a specific drug category. Thus, a person who experiences side effects from the dye used in a generic drug or drug A may be prohibited based on the insurance/HMO plan from purchasing drug B at the reduced co-pay cost (i.e., $20) and thus be required to pay the full cost of drug B, which could be hundreds of dollars a month.

Another way insurance or HMO plans may create an allocation-of-resource dilemma is by not paying for long-term psychotherapy or for an agency not affiliated with the plan. Patients with limited financial resources who might benefit from individual or group therapy may be unable to access these individualized services. Thus, health care providers with prescriptive power may opt for pharmaceutical intervention, which is covered, rather than fighting the system to obtain a waiver for psychotherapy services.

Illustrative Case 14-5

Scott is 7 years old and was recently diagnosed with attention-deficit/hyperactivity disorder after failing his second-grade state-level exams. His primary care physician suggests a treatment plan that includes stimulant medication (methylphenidate) concurrently with psychosocial interventions, including behavior and cognitive therapy. When the nurse attempts to schedule Scott for the behavior and cognitive therapy, she discovers that no agency within a 5-mile radius from Scott's home accepts the insurance plan that covers him. When confronted with these facts, Scott's mother is faced with the dilemma of accepting the services that are readily available or negotiating with the insurance/HMO and an accessible agency to work out a plan for treatment. Situations like this can test the advocacy skills and tenacity of the insured individual or surrogate as well as the health care team members. When advocating for individualized services, the person/health care provider may need to demonstrate that what appears to be the more expensive therapy will in the long run save the insurance company/HMO money by preventing hospitalization or other costly interventions. Thus, nurses (individually and collectively) need to work to ensure parity of insurance coverage between physical and psychological needs.

SUMMARY

The ethical commitments for the nurse working with a patient with a MHD are not changed; however, state or federal law or insurance reimbursement policies may influence how these commitments are operationalized. The nurse must be skilled in capacity assessment so that persons with MHD are allowed to remain autonomous decision-makers despite their condition. Nurses, both individually and as a profession, need to advocate for the rights of persons with MHD to obtain quality health care in the least restrictive condition possible.

CLINICAL EXERCISES

1. When you are in the clinical setting, observe the actions the agency and/or health care professionals take to maintain patient confidentiality. For example:

- Signage for an in-patient psychiatric unit
- Visibility to third parties of clients or significant others when entering the unit/agency
- Manner in which the phones answered
- Directions and/or assurances of confidentiality given to patients before they begin group therapy

2. Discuss with a staff nurse how he or she has responded to personal questions asked by a client.
3. Go to the National Alliance for the Mentally Ill (NAMI) website (www.nami.org/Hometemplate.cfm) and select Inform Yourself/About Public Policy. Select either Court Watch or Current Policy News & Alerts. Read one of the reports. What ethical rationales, ethical commitments, ethical violations, or ethical issues can you identify?
4. Locate your state's mental health code. Identify the process that must be followed to obtain a court-appointed guardian for a person with a mental illness.

Discussion Questions

1. Many community self-help groups (such as Alcoholics Anonymous) maintain a closed meeting as a means for protecting the privacy of the participants from inquisitive outsiders. In the past, nursing students were assigned to attend community self-help group meetings as a means for learning about group process and interactions. Analyze this practice from either the utilitarian or deontological perspective (see Chapter 1). Would the theory justify the implementation of this educational strategy?
2. How should a nurse respond to a psychotic patient who expresses delusional statements? What is the ethical justification for this communication technique?

SECTION 2: *Autonomy Versus Paternalism*

Patient autonomy is a fundamental moral expectation in the Western health care delivery system. For the concept of autonomy to be actualized, the patient must have the decisional capacity necessary to make an informed decision to consent to or refuse treatment (as discussed in Chapter 12). However, a person's ability to make autonomous decisions may be compromised by the presence of an MHD. Ethical dilemmas can occur when a patient with an MHD makes a decision that a health care professional does not believe is in the patient's best interest, thus necessitating an assessment of the patient's decisional capacity. This may be perceived as a challenge to the patient's autonomy and viewed as an exertion of power on behalf of the health care provider. However paternalistic it might appear, the health care provider has an obligation to evaluate the patient's decision-making capacity when the patient's decisions could result in harm to him or her.

A foundational premise behind the concept of *autonomy* is that the person desires and is able to discern what actions are in his or her best interests. For example, a person should desire to be safe and should be able to recognize and implement actions to enhance the potential for safety, such as choosing a well-lighted route for traveling at night, making sure a car has gas and a functional spare tire, and/or carrying a cellular phone. However, the possibility exists that a person with an MHD may not be able to recognize actions that are harmful or not in his or her *best interests* or may have a non-mainstream view of what actions or outcomes are in his or her best interests.

Illustrative Case 14-6

Ms. Flood lives on the street and has been diagnosed with schizophrenia with paranoid features. Because of her disease, she believes that everyone is attempting to steal her personal belongings and physically harm her. Because of this fear, Ms. Flood refuses to avail herself of community-sponsored health clinics, soup kitchens, or warming shelters even when encouraged to do so. When the outside temperature drops below 0°F, the question must be raised whether Ms. Flood's refusal to seek shelter and health care services for exposure-related symptoms is in her best interests. When considering her options, Ms. Flood prioritized safeguarding her possessions, which are instrumental to her ability to survive on the streets, over sleeping overnight in a warming shelter. Thus, the ethical dilemma involves questions associated with short- and long-term consequences. If, on evaluation, Ms. Flood is found to have the capacity to make this decision, she has the freedom to risk harm and remain outdoors.

Paternalism is a common societal response for protecting another (usually someone the person perceives to have less knowledge and experience and/or fewer problem-solving skills) from harm. Paternalism is derived from the word *parent*. Throughout a child's infancy, childhood, and teenage years (and sometimes into adulthood), a parent acts to prevent harm to the child even if the child desires or prefers to undertake risky behavior. Each of us has probably at one time or another been told by a parent or other adult, "Just because (insert your best friend's name) wants to jump off a bridge does not mean you should jump," or "It's your bedtime. Tomorrow is a school day. I do not care if you want to watch TV or do not feel tired. You are going to bed now."

When determining what is in a person's best interests, one needs to consider which of the available options has the greatest potential to create benefit to that person and promote the possibility of achieving his or life goals. The best-interest standard reflects a utilitarian perspective with the emphasis on consequences and greatest utility. When evaluating the various options, the decision-maker should consider, but not be limited to, the person's life goals and values, as well as the potential for pain and suffering (Beauchamp & Childress, 2001). As illustrated, parents and their children may have competing goals for the child's life (living a good life as promoted by sufficient sleep to facilitate a good education versus living a good life by being entertained). Similarly, a person with an MHD that affects decision-making capacity may define what is in his or her best interests differently than a person with a healthier mental status. Thus, determining how to promote the autonomy of a patient with an MHD while minimizing paternalistic care and decisions is an important skill for any nurse working with persons with such illnesses or limited decision-making capacities associated with drug or alcohol use, neurological injuries, or limited cognitive abilities.

Providing Treatment Against the Patient's Will

Autonomous persons are free to make decisions on whether to seek or refuse medical treatment and to make decisions that others (including family or health care providers) believe are not in their best interests, or in other words, decisions that are perceived as harmful or wrong. An ethical quandary can occur when a person with an MHD refuses treatment for the disorder or refuses to listen to a health care professional's explanation of the person's condition or treatment options. Is the person unable to realize the need for mental health treatment and refusing solely because of the disorder itself?

Based on the Preamble of the Constitution of the United States, the government has a *parens patriae* interest in promoting the welfare and liberty of the country and its citizens and future generations. Thus, the government has an interest in protecting individuals who are believed to be a "danger to self" and because of the disorder cannot make informed decisions regarding treatment that could be beneficial in ameliorating their disorder. The concept of "dangerous to self" is ambiguous and is defined differently in various state laws or court decisions; thus, it behooves each professional nurse to know and understand the definitions and state laws that are applicable to his or her work setting. Most definitions of "danger to self" include references to threats to or attempts of suicide and/or violent behavior or immediate threats to others.

A variety of civil legislation as well as court decisions direct the practice of emergency or involuntary admissions related to MHD. Because of these, health care professionals often view this process as a legal issue, and might not consider the ethical ramifications related to paternalistically inhibiting a person's autonomy and physical freedom. One must always remember that just because an action is legal, the action may not be ethical, and vice versa.

Whenever limitations are placed on a person's freedoms by a health care institution, the restrictions should always meet the criteria of being the *least restrictive possible*. This entails "the objective of maintaining the greatest degree of freedom, self-determination, autonomy, dignity, and integrity of mind, body, and spirit for the individual while he or she participates in treatment or receives services" (President's Commission on Mental Health, 1978, p. 14; as cited in Farrance & Kinglsley, 1990, p. 37). An example of least restrictive conditions related to involuntary treatment is admitting a patient to mandatory outpatient treatment rather than an in-patient treatment unit.

Mandating Treatment

Beneficence is a primary rationale used to justify mandated treatment for a person with MHD; however, situations exist where one must question whether mandated treatment does in fact promote the person's life goals. First, in Western society, a court may rule that a person with an untreated MHD lacks the ability to participate in his or her legal counsel and therefore cannot be prosecuted. For example, Mr. Turner has a dissociative identity disorder and has three documented distinct identities. While in a dissociative fugue, Mr. Turner engaged in a robbery during which a police officer was killed. The county prosecutor charges Mr. Turner with murder and seeks the death penalty. Based on his current level of mental health, everyone agrees that Mr. Turner cannot be tried for this crime. The county prosecutor is working within the legal system to obtain a court order mandating treatment for Mr. Turner so that he can one day be tried for this crime.

The county prosecutor's actions may cause an ethical dilemma for Mr. Turner's health care team. Health care providers have a moral commitment to assist Mr. Turner to obtain the highest level quality of life possible. This commitment does not seem consistent with the probability that if he is found guilty, his life will be ended via a lethal injection. Thus, the health care team may question whether participating in mental health treatment is ultimately in Mr. Turner's best long-term interest.

A second scenario that health care professionals may experience related to mandated treatment occurs when a patient who lacks decisional capacity as a result of his or her MHD is required to participate in mandated therapy with the goal that the person will regain decisional capacity. Once the person regains decisional capacity, he or she will be allowed to refuse further treatment with a foreseeable outcome that the patient will again lack decisional capacity. For example, Ms. Prinz has schizophrenia. She previously told the staff at the local health clinic that she does not like how she feels when she is taking her required medication and believes that her life is better when she is not taking it. She is brought to the emergency room by the police after she threatened pedestrians with a wooden board on a major city street. Under threat of prosecution, she participates in mandated treatment. After a few weeks, Ms. Prinz is believed to have her schizophrenia under control and demonstrates decisional capacity. During a counseling session with the psychiatric nurse, Ms. Prinz states, "When I am taking this medicine, I do not feel like myself. It is like there is stranger inside my skin. I know you will not agree with me, but I do not want to live like this. I want to feel like myself even if that means I may experience periods of violence again."

In this situation, the nurse may experience a conflict between the patient's autonomous right to define what represents a quality life and the nurse practitioner's definition of quality. One option the nurse should discuss with Ms. Prinz at this time is the option of completing a psychiatric advance directive. In such a directive, the person expresses in writing his or her autonomous directions regarding psychiatric treatment in the event that a psychiatric relapse occurs. It "can include the patient's preferences for psychotropic medication, ECT, hospital preference, selection of a psychiatrist/psychotherapist, attorney and any other preferences" (American Psychiatric Nurses Association, 2003, p. 3). Thus, completing a psychiatric advance directive may prevent Ms. Prinz from being subjected to another episode of treatment. The Illinois Psychiatric Advance Directive is shown in Box 14-1.

USE OF RESTRAINTS

The practice of restraining a person is implemented throughout society as a means for promoting safety. For example, toddlers are placed in playpens while their mothers cook dinner, and travelers in airports are confined to the terminals and not allowed to roam throughout the baggage area or tarmac. The practice of restraints has also been implemented as punishment. Teenagers are grounded after violating curfew, and criminals are contained in prisons. In health care situations, the practice of restraining a patient is only ethically justifiable based on a commitment to nonmaleficence or doing no harm. Unfortunately, the possibility exists for the practice of restraints to be

(Text continues on p. 327)

BOX 14-1

Illinois Psychiatric Advance Directive

DECLARATION FOR MENTAL HEALTH TREATMENT

I _____, being an adult of sound mind, willfully and voluntarily make this declaration for mental health treatment to be followed if it is determined by 2 physicians or the court that my ability to receive and evaluate information effectively or communicate decisions is impaired to such an extent that I lack the capacity to refuse or consent to mental health treatment. "Mental health treatment" means electroconvulsive treatment, treatment of mental illness with psychotropic medication, and admission to and retention in a health care facility for a period up to 17 days.

I understand that I may become incapable of giving or withholding informed consent for mental health treatment due to the symptoms of a diagnosed mental disorder. These symptoms may include:

_____

_____

PSYCHOTROPIC MEDICATIONS

If I become incapable of giving or withholding informed consent for mental health treatment, my wishes regarding psychotropic medications are as follows:

_____ I consent to the administration of the following medications:

_____

_____ I do not consent to the administration of the following medications:

_____

Conditions or limitations:_____

_____

_____

ELECTROCONVULSIVE TREATMENT

If I become incapable of giving or withholding informed consent for mental health treatment, my wishes regarding electroconvulsive treatment are as follows:

_____ I consent to the administration of electroconvulsive treatment.

_____ I do not consent to the administration of electroconvulsive treatment.

Conditions or limitations: _____

_____

_____

(Continued)

BOX 14-1 (CONTINUED)

ADMISSION TO AND RETENTION IN FACILITY

If I become incapable of giving or withholding informed consent for mental health treatment, my wishes regarding admission to and retention in a health care facility for mental health treatment are as follows:

_____ I consent to being admitted to a health care facility for mental health treatment.

_____ I do not consent to being admitted to a health care facility for mental health treatment.

This directive cannot, by law, provide consent to retain me in a facility for more than 17 days.

Conditions or limitations:_____

_____

_____

SELECTION OF PHYSICIAN
(OPTIONAL)

If it becomes necessary to determine if I have become incapable of giving or withholding informed consent for mental health treatment, I choose Dr. _____ of _____ to be one of the 2 physicians who will determine whether I am incapable. If that physician is unavailable, that physician's designee shall determine whether I am incapable.

ADDITIONAL REFERENCES OR INSTRUCTIONS

_____

_____

Conditions or limitations: _____

_____

ATTORNEY-IN-FACT

I hereby appoint:

NAME _____

ADDRESS _____

TELEPHONE # _____

to act as my attorney-in-fact to make decisions regarding my mental health treatment if I become incapable of giving or withholding informed consent for that treatment.

(Continued)

BOX 14-1 (CONTINUED)

If the person named above refuses or is unable to act on my behalf, or if I revoke that person's authority to act as my attorney-in-fact, I authorize the following person to act as my attorney-in-fact:

NAME _____

ADDRESS _____

TELEPHONE # _____

My attorney-in-fact is authorized to make decisions that are consistent with the wishes I have expressed in this declaration or, if not expressed, as are otherwise known to my attorney-in-fact. If my wishes are not expressed and are not otherwise known by my attorney-in-fact, my attorney-in-fact is to act in what he or she believes to be my best interest.

_____
(Signature of Principal/Date)

AFFIRMATION OF WITNESSES

We affirm that the principal is personally known to us, that the principal signed or acknowledged the principal's signature on this declaration for mental health treatment in our presence, that the principal appears to be of sound mind and not under duress, fraud or undue influence, that neither of us is:

A person appointed as an attorney in fact by this document;

The principal's attending physician or mental health service provider or a relative of the physician or provider;

The owner, operator, or relative of an owner or operator of a facility in which the principal is a patient or resident; or

A person related to the principal by blood, marriage or adoption.

Witnessed By:

_____
(Signature of Witness/Date) (Printed Name of Witness)

_____
(Signature of Witness/Date) (Printed Name of Witness)

ACCEPTANCE OF APPOINTMENT AS ATTORNEY-IN-FACT

I accept this appointment and agree to serve as attorney-in-fact to make decisions about mental health treatment for the principal. I understand that I have a duty to act consistent with the desires of the principal as expressed in this appointment. I understand that this document gives me authority to make decisions about mental health treatment only while the principal is incapable as determined by a court or two physicians. I understand that the

(Continued)

> ## BOX 14-1 (CONTINUED)
>
> principal may revoke this declaration in whole or in part at any time and in any manner when the principal is not incapable.
>
> _____
>
> (Signature of Attorney-in-fact/Date) (Printed Name)
>
> _____
>
> (Signature of Attorney-in-fact/Date) (Printed Name of Witness)
>
> *Source:* Illinois Mental Health Treatment Preference Declaration Act (1998). 755 ILCS 43/75. Retrieved April 22, 2005, from www.ilga.gov/legislation/ilcs/ilcs2.asp?ChapterID=60

abused, leading to the perception that the patient is being considered wrong rather than in danger of harming self or others, and thus is being punished. The practice of restraining a patient is the epitome of a paternalistic action because it limits the patient's ability to act voluntarily or be in control of his or her destiny, in other words, act autonomously.

Physical Restraints

A variety of *physical restraints* are used in health care institutions, including soft and hard limb restraints, vest restraints, mitten restraints, and belt restraints. Physical restraints are used as a last resort to limit the potential that the patient will cause physical harm to himself or herself.

Illustrative Case 14-7

Ms. Byrd has been in a catatonic state after surviving a traumatic experience. Because her catatonic state has impaired her ability to eat, a feeding tube was placed (after obtaining consent from the appropriate surrogate decision-maker). Because she has excess motor activity without purpose, the decision is made to place her hands in mitten restraints so she does not grab and pull out the feeding tube. Mittens were selected over soft arm restraints because they are less restrictive. However, if even with the mitten restraints on, Ms. Byrd exhibited the ability to tug on the feeding tube, the nurse may need to use soft arm restraints instead.

Illustrative Case 14-8

Mr. Carr is HIV+, is in a manic state, and has not slept for more than 48 hours. When approached by a nurse, he says, "Keep away from me or I'll bite you!" He then picks up and throws a brown paper sack filled with soda cans at the nurse. Because of the need to protect the staff as well as Mr. Carr, he is placed in hard limb restraints and his significant other is notified. Within minutes of being restrained, he is asleep. The use of physical restraints may have provided the structure he needed but could not provide for himself. With his significant other, his legal surrogate, present, it was no longer necessary for the health care provider to act paternalistically; the surrogate could employ substituted judgment and exercise autonomy on Mr. Carr's behalf.

Seclusion

The practice of *seclusion* occurs in mental health settings and rarely in other clinical settings. The practice of secluding a patient often in a "safe" room, which may include padded walls and floor, is used to limit harm to the patient by decreasing/limiting environmental stimuli (as was illustrated by the case of Mr. Carr). However, because of childhood experiences with timeouts, being sent to our rooms, or being grounded, many persons in Western society perceive seclusion as punishment and not a viable intervention for assisting someone to gain control over emotions, thoughts, and actions. As with all types of restraints, other actions, such as communication, diversion, limit setting, and promoting a calm milieu reflecting an atmosphere of collaboration, should be attempted prior to implementing an act of seclusion (American Psychiatric Nurses Association [APNA], 2000). As part of their commitment to preventing the need for using physical restraints in the psychiatric setting, the American Psychiatric Nurses Association (2000) outlined a standard according to which physical restraints and seclusion should not be used concurrently.

Chemical Restraints

Chemical restraints are a greater threat to patient autonomy than physical restraints or seclusion because the patient's cognitive abilities are affected, which threatens the patient's ability to make an informed decision and/or participate in discussions and decisions related to the plan of care. Because the length of time a person loses his or her autonomy due to chemical restraints is contingent on the pharmokinetics of the medication as well as the person's metabolism, they should be used only when all other, less restrictive efforts have failed.

Chemical restraints (also referred to as medications for treatment) are often administered during intense moments when the patient is especially vulnerable. The patient may be physically outnumbered by health care professions and held down while an intramuscular injection invades his or her patient's physical space and integrity (Parker, 1995).

Illustrative Case 14-9

Scott is 12 years old and has been diagnosed with a conduct disorder. When he was admitted to the in-patient unit, Scott and his parents participated in the creation of a plan of care indicating a multistep approach if his behavior became aggressive and impulsive. Initial attempts to redirect Scott's behavior and minimize overstimulation have failed. Scott is standing in the middle of the common area swinging a pool cue and cursing. Scott's physician has ordered intramuscular lorazepam in the event that Scott's actions put him or others at risk. Surrounded by various members of the health care team and told by the nurse that he will be receiving a "shot" to "help him cope," Scott begs the nurse not to administer the medication and promises to put down the pool cue and not to hurt anyone.

Scott's request creates a new dilemma for the nurse:

Giving the child an injection against his will violates his own body and prevents autonomy. Not giving the injection involves the issue of veracity because the nurse has told the client what will happen if he is unable to control his behavior. Backing out of the decision to give the injection or giving different consequences for the same behavior can be extremely confusing for children. (Parker, 1995, p. 27)

This request from Scott requires the nurse to evaluate whether giving or not giving the injection will result in the greatest good related to preventing harm to Scott as well as to other patients and staff on the unit. The nurse must consider the possible short- and long-term consequences associated with not giving the injection. The nurse must consider which action would promote beneficence related to Scott's ability to achieve previously identified health care goals and his ability to act autonomously, in addition to preventing harm to the tentative trust that has been established between Scott and the health care team. How the nurse prioritizes these competing principles will depend on his or her values, experience, and clinical expertise and the unit's culture related to this type of decision.

Let us assume for this discussion that the nurse does administer the injection to Scott. Following the administration of the medication, the nurse must ensure that Scott is in a safe and quiet environment. Depending on the dose and Scott's response to the medication, he may at the least become calm and at the most somnolent. Because of these changes in his mental status, he may lose his ability to actively engage in plans about his care or express his wishes. The loss of autonomy due to the use of a chemical restraint invokes the principle of double effect because the loss of autonomy is a recognized but unintended result of the chemical restraint. While Scott is unable to participate in decision-making, the nurse must make every effort to advocate for his welfare and create a milieu that will foster his ability to function voluntarily.

NURSING OBLIGATIONS

When any form of restraint is being considered or has been implemented, the nurse must be cognizant of the possibility that the patient's behavior may be related to a physiological or organic problem rather than an emotional or psychological problem. Thus, the nurse has the moral responsibility to conduct a thorough and ongoing assessment including the patient's physical and emotional status, responses to intervention, and potential for new or further harm. Because of the moral commitment to patient advocacy and patient autonomy, the nurse has the obligation to remove or minimize the level of restraint as soon as is safely possible. Additionally, before implementing an act of restraint, one requires an order from a physician or licensed independent practitioner (LIP). The patient must also be assessed by a physician or LIP within 1 hour of being restrained (or as directed by agency policy or appropriate regulatory body) (APNA, 2000).

Any nurse who has the potential to implement restraints must be adequately trained on the use of every approved restraint device. Nurses have a moral and legal obligation to use only devices approved for use by the institution. This obligation supports nursing's commitment to promoting safety because unapproved restraint devices (such as using a bed sheet as a waist restraint) may result in harm to the patient or others. Nurses, both individually and collectively (as unit staff or an entire agency), need to consider personal and institutional biases, cultural factors, values, or perceptions that affect their actions related to patient autonomy and the use of restraints. For example, are children with certain physical characteristics, medical history, or social ranking more likely to be chemically restrained than other children without these characteristics? In addition, nurses need to be aware of how the patient's age, maturation, previous experiences with the health care system, medical and psychological history (including abuse), and the actions and side effects of any prescribed or illicit drugs may affect the patient's response to a nurse's attempts to limit or restrict the patient's autonomy (APNA, 2000).

SUMMARY

Nurses have a moral obligation to advocate for their patients while at all times protecting their civil rights. Nurses need to be aware of applicable laws and court rulings that affect a patient's rights to refuse mental health services. Whenever a decision to restrict a patient's freedom/autonomy is made, the nurse must act to ensure that the least restrictive conditions are implemented and the restrictions are lifted as soon as possible.

CLINICAL EXERCISES

1. Does your institution or agency have a restraint policy? If so, does this policy reflect physical, chemical, and social/environmental restraints? Does the institution/agency have a restraint policy specific for persons with mental illness or for psychiatric care areas?
2. Ask the staff nurse whether he or she has had to restrain a patient against the patient's will. What actions were attempted prior to the act of restraint? In your opinion, what was the nurse's ethical justification for restraining the patient against the patient's will?
3. Does your institution or agency have a policy regarding mandatory treatment for psychiatric illnesses? Talk with a staff nurse about his or her experience with admitting a patient for mandatory treatment against the patient's will.
4. In consultation with your clinical instructor, determine whether a current patient is receiving mandatory treatment. Was any additional documentation required during the admission process and subsequently because of the mandatory order to treat?
5. Does your institution or agency have a policy on seeking/identifying a legal guardian for a person with mental illness who lacks decisional capacity? If so, what actions are included to protect the patient's autonomy and limit paternalism?

Discussion Questions

1. In many institutions, security officers are present when a patient is being "taken down." What ethical principles can be used to justify this practice? What ethical principles can be used to refute this practice?

2. Refer to Illustrative Case 14-9 regarding the administration of a chemical to restrain Scott. What decision would you make if you were Scott's nurse? Explain the ethical rationale supporting your decision. Write a nurse's note to record this situation and the actions you implemented.

3. Divide the clinical group in half and debate the practice of mandating psychiatric treatment so that a criminal will be mentally competent for execution.

SECTION 3: *Caring for the Challenging Patient*

Nurses have a responsibility to provide compassionate nursing care "unrestricted by considerations of social or economic status, personal attributes, or the nature of the health problem" [American Nurses Association (2001b) Code of Ethics for Nurses, Provision 1]. However, nurses (in every clinical setting, not just mental health settings) may find that fulfilling this ethical obligation is stressful when the patient is perceived as "difficult" or "challenging." This section considers factors influencing such perceptions and offers suggestions for how a nurse can use ethical principles to facilitate work with difficult patients.

At the end of a clinical day, nursing students frequently conclude, "Today was a great clinical experience. My patient was *so nice.*" By being nice, the patient promoted the student's perception of being competent and in control of the nursing plan of care activities. Thus, this *nice* patient and the student were able to work together to meet mutual goals. Fortunately, most patients and their significant others are kind, friendly people who are interested in helping a nursing student to learn and develop skills. As a means for promoting a positive learning environment, staff nurses and clinical instructors may consider the patient's and/or significant other's personality and mood before assigning a nursing student to work with the patient.

However, every nursing student will some day experience working with a patient that he or she perceives as not being nice, but rather mean, disinterested, noncompliant, and/or lacking the ability to control his or her emotions, thoughts, and/or behavior. At the end of this clinical experience, the nursing student may say, "Clinical today was awful. My patient was so difficult. He would not cooperate with anything. He refused his medications. He even refused to explain why he would not attend group sessions." Thus, a patient is considered *challenging* because he or she denies "both the authority and therapeutic value of the nursing staff, not as a result of the 'difficult' behaviour" (Breeze & Repper, 1998, p. 1301). In this section, the concept of *challenging* will be considered in relation to patients; however, it could apply to any person (colleague, physician, supervisor, etc.) who creates a situation in which the nurse perceives a loss of control and competency in guiding the situation to a positive outcome. When a nurse is required to assist a challenging or difficult patient, every aspect of the nurse's psychiatric and mental health skills are called into play to assist such a patient regardless of the specific clinical setting.

Noncompliance

The perception that someone is challenging may be related to a variety of factors. A nurse might perceive a patient as being challenging when he or she does not comply with the outlined treatment plan. For example, Mr. Faux is a 55-year-old man with a long history of depression. His physician has prescribed an antidepressant and professional counseling. Mr. Faux is brought to the emergency department after a failed suicide attempt. On admission, his toxicology screen is negative for any antidepressant. When asked why he had not taken the antidepressant, he replies, "I did not like how it made me feel. I did not feel like myself and I was not able to perform sexually." His response illustrates that for some patients noncompliance simply means that their goals are different from those identified by the health care professional.

When the patient and nurse have competing goals for treatment, a communication breakdown can result and the patient's autonomy can be in conflict with the health care team's paternalism. The nurse must work with the patient to ascertain the patient's goals and desires. Refer back to the scenario involving Mr. Faux. The health care team's goal is to treat his depression. Whereas Mr. Faux may agree with this goal, he has other goals (maintaining sexual intimacy and "feeling like myself") that have a higher priority for him. The nurse should assist Mr. Faux to clarify his goals, and facilitate communication with the health care team to arrive at a therapeutic dosage to treat his depression with minimal undesirable effects.

Unfortunately, the possibility exists that a patient may make an autonomous decision to implement a course of action that the nurse and other health care team members believe is unsafe or not in the patient's best interest. However, as long as the patient maintains legal competency, Western society holds that an autonomous individual has the right to make even a *bad* decision. Thus, a medical nurse might encounter a patient with a deep vein thrombosis who refuses to use the urinal and repeatedly walks to the bathroom to urinate. The psychiatric nurse may encounter a patient who has stopped taking medication (such as valproic acid) because of the unpleasant side effects of weight gain and increased incidents of suicide attempts or an adult with decisional incapacity who engages in self-mutilation (cutting) but is not attempting suicide.

Inadequate Resources for Dealing With a Challenging Patient

A challenging patient situation might occur when the resources needed to meet the patient's needs are unavailable. For example, inappropriate staffing patterns can lead a patient to the conclusion that a nurse is incompetent. When the nurse/patient ratio is not appropriate, the nurse may be unable to prioritize and organize his or her plan of care, but rather finds himself or herself "putting out fires" and jumping from crisis to crisis without an organized plan. Thus, because he or she has too many responsibilities, the nurse might be unable to gain control over the therapeutic milieu.

Another example of inappropriate resources leading to the perception of a challenging patient may occur when the patient is being treated in the wrong setting. For example, a rural day clinic may not have the diagnostic or treatment resources required to competently treat a critically ill psychiatric patient compared to the resources available at an in-patient psychiatric unit at an academic medical center with 24-hour services.

The skills of the individual practitioner represent another potential source of inappropriate resources for providing competent care for the challenging patient. When the nurse (or other health care personnel) has limited experience, his or her ability to be therapeutic may be limited by lack of knowledge related to the disease, treatment plan, and/or organizational structure and resources. For example, a new nurse with limited clinical experience working on an in-patient psychiatric unit may lack the expert clinical judgment necessary to recognize that a patient who defecates on his meal tray may do so as a form of attention-seeking behavior. This new nurse may not possess the sophisticated communication skills necessary to assist the patient to behave in a socially appropriate manner within established boundaries. In addition, practitioners with limited experiences may not have the expertise necessary to view a patient's plan of care holistically rather than episodically. Thus, nurse managers must be cognizant of the skills mix of the available nursing staff when making assignments, both unit scheduling and nurse-patient.

UNMET EXPECTATIONS

A patient might be perceived as being challenging if the nurse believes that the patient's expectations are unrealistic or wrong. Some patients with high emotional needs may expect that the nurse will provide undivided attention, which is unrealistic when the nurse has been assigned to care for multiple patients. An example of a patient's expectations being wrong can occur when a police officer is voluntarily being treated in a drug and alcohol rehabilitation unit. When admitted to the unit, the police officer may initially refuse to relinquish his weapon, stating "I am required by law to be armed at all times." This statement illustrates the police officer's wrong expectation because all weapons (including those carried by the agency's security officers) must be secured for the safety of all persons (employees and patients) on the unit. A patient may also be labeled as challenging when his or her values and/or religious beliefs vary drastically from the mainstream religious practices of the community. For example, animal sacrifice may be a common practice by immigrants from the Caribbean who practice the Santeria religion (Ontario Consultants on Religious Tolerance, 2003). However, expectations of being able to practice animal sacrifice in a conservative evangelical Christian community may engender a clash of values and the perception of being challenging if the patient and significant others are adamant about continuing their faith practices in the hospital.

Discussion Exercises 14-4

You are the charge nurse of a unit that includes unlicensed assistive personnel (UAP) and an ethnically diverse group of people. A male patient is admitted to the unit at 1:30 P.M. He says that he is a member of the KKK and the National Socialist White Americans' Party. He states that he does not want a "Jew" or "Negro" taking care of him. He wants a "White" nurse to care for him. At 2:15 P.M., you look at the evening work schedule and notice that the three RNs scheduled to work are Mary Kohn (an Orthodox Jew), Susan Jones (a Haitian who immigrated to the United States at the age of 15) and Jane Su (a Chinese American).

1. Do you believe that this patient is a challenging patient? If so, what factors are affecting the patient's and nursing staff's decision-making?

2. Use the decision analysis model presented in Chapter 5 to guide your decision-making as the charge nurse about how you will staff the evening shift.

- Identify three prioritized values that are or should be guiding your decision-making.
- Identify three potential action alternatives you could implement to resolve this ethical issue regarding how to staff the evening shift.
- Based on your probability calculations, which action would you implement?

3. The charge nurse has decided that you are the best nurse to care for this patient. Considering your ethnicity, personal values, and professional skills, how will you approach this patient to identify his plan of care for the shift?

Rights Versus Privileges

The possibility exists that a patient may be perceived as being challenging if the patient or his significant other forcefully and/or repeatedly uses rights language to make claims on the nurse and/or health care institution or disregard the rights of others. A right is a justifiable claim a person can make regardless of time or location based on law or widely recognized standards, such as those proposed by the Joint Commission on Accreditation of Healthcare Organizations (JCAHO) or the American Hospital Association (AHA). In 2003, the AHA proposed a Patient Care Partnership: Understanding Expectations, Rights and Responsibilities, which replaced their Patient Bill of Rights (American Hospital Association, 1973/1992). The Patient Care Partnership emphasized the concept that with rights comes responsibilities; thus, a patient cannot make claims based on rights without also acting to facilitate the health care team's ability to fulfill that right. Specifically, the AHA (2003) stated that a hospitalized patient has a right to be involved in his or her care. However, this right to be involved comes with an expectation that the patient will communicate values and goals related to health care and spiritual beliefs. In addition, the health care personnel also have associated responsibilities to fulfill as a means of protecting the patient's rights. Thus, the health care team and institution have an obligation to incorporate the patient's values and spiritual beliefs into the patient's plan of care.

The existence of a right creates duties for others to fulfill. Negative rights require people not to act. For example, the right to life is a negative right that requires others not to act in a manner that may shorten another person's life. This right not to be harmed is the ethical basis for the use of restraints or seclusion when a patient in a psychiatric setting is unable to control his or her behavior. In contrast, positive rights require people to implement an action to promote the occurrence of the right. For example, if the United States was to recognize the positive right to health care, then the country would be required to develop a payment system to make access to health care possible for everyone.

Whereas Western society widely recognizes that patients have rights associated with health care, there is less consensus regarding whether health care professionals, including nurses, have special rights related to their professional role (B. Bandman, 1978, 1981; E. Bandman, 1981; Wiseman, 2001). Thus, the American Nurses Association

> ## BOX 14-2
>
> ### The 2001 American Nurses Association Bill of Rights for Registered Nurses
>
> **1.** Nurses have the right to practice in a manner that fulfills their obligations to society and to those who receive nursing care.
>
> **2.** Nurses have the right to practice in environments that allow them to act in accordance with professional standards and legally authorized scopes of practice.
>
> **3.** Nurses have the right to a work environment that supports and facilitates ethical practice, in accordance with the Code of Ethics for Nurses and its interpretive statements.
>
> **4.** Nurses have the right to freely and openly advocate for themselves and their patients, without fear of retribution.
>
> **5.** Nurses have the right to fair compensations for their work, consistent with their knowledge, experience, and professional responsibilities.
>
> **6.** Nurses have the right to a work environment that is safe for themselves and their patients.
>
> **7.** Nurses have the right to negotiate the conditions of their employment, either as individuals or collectively, in all practice settings.
>
> Reprinted with permission from the American Nurses Association (2001). *Bill of rights for registered nurses.* Washington, DC: Author. Also available at http://nursingworld.org/tan/novdec02/rights.htm

(2001a) proposed a Bill of Rights for Registered Nurses (Box 14-2) to indicate how the public and health care organizations can support the professional nurse's ability to provide quality patient care. Nurses have the same human rights as every citizen, including the right to be free from harm, constitutional rights to free speech, and the right to dignity and respect as a person. In addition, nurses have special privileges related to their role. However, privileges are revocable and not absolute. For example, nurses have privileges that are bestowed by a patient based on the patient's rights; thus, nurses have the privilege (not the right) to administer medications or assist a patient in the activities of daily living based on the patient's right to informed consent. Similarly, patients in psychiatric settings have privileges related to participation in, for example, recreational activities or shopping.

APPLICATION OF ETHICAL PRINCIPLES TO FACILITATE WORKING WITH CHALLENGING PATIENTS

Respect for Persons

The ANA (2001b) Code of Ethics for Nurses mandates that nurses have an ethical commitment to respect persons: "The nurse, in all professional relationships, practices with compassion and respect for the inherent dignity, worth and uniqueness of every individual, unrestricted by considerations of social or economic status, personal attributes, or the nature of health problems" (Provision 1). Based on this standard, the professional nurse is obligated to fulfill his or her professional obligations to assigned patients except for the rare occasion when the nurse must engage in conscientious objection (see Chapter 16, Section 2). Fulfilling these professional obligations requires the nurse to work to correct factors that contribute to power struggles and/or inability to meet desired goals. When desired goals cannot be met, the nurse must communicate with the patient, provide supporting rationale, and problem solve with the patient and other members of the health care team to identify available alternatives.

One method for demonstrating respect for the challenging patient is to spend time with him or her. Nurses must actively work against the temptation to ignore or limit time with challenging patients because patients might consider the amount of time the nurse spends with them as a measure of how much the nurse cares about him or her. In addition, the quality as well as the quantity of time the nurse spends with any patient may affect the nurse's ability to hear and understand the patient's values and goals (Breeze & Repper, 1998).

Advocacy

According to Provision 2.1 of the ANA (2001b) Code of Ethics for Nurses,

> *Nursing holds a fundamental commitment to the uniqueness of the individual patient; therefore, any plan of care must reflect that uniqueness. The nurse strives to provide patients with opportunities to participate in planning care, assures that patients find the plans acceptable and supports the implementation of the plan. Addressing patient interests requires recognition of the patient's place in the family or other networks of relationships. When the patient's wishes are in conflict with others, the nurse seeks to help resolve the conflict. Where conflict persists, the nurse's commitment remains to the identified patient.* (Reprinted with permission from nursesbooks.org.)

In this provision, the ANA sets forth a high level of expectation for the profesional nurse. The nurse is required to focus on and promote the challenging patient's interests while working to correct existing goal and value conflicts.

One way to promote the patient's interests is to empower the patient to participate in decision-making, which promotes patient autonomy and diminishes paternalism. An empowered patient is more likely to verbalize goals and values, which may diminish overt acts of power against the patient, such as involuntary admission or restricting his or her movement (Breeze & Repper, 1998).

Another way a nurse can promote the patient's interests and power is to believe and communicate honestly with the patient . When a patient feels his or her position has been heard and understood, he or she will feel more autonomous and in control of his or her life and decisions. However, a nurse must not blindly trust a patient, but must use good nursing judgment to discern what is in the patient's best interests. For example, a nurse assigned to a patient with suicidal ideations will need to consider multiple data sources before agreeing that the patient no longer needs constant monitoring despite the patient's promise not to hurt himself or herself (Breeze & Repper, 1998). Because knowledge is power, both the patient's and the nurse's power base will be increased through truthful dialogue.

Competent Practitioners

According to Provision 3.3 of the ANA (2001b) Code of Ethics for Nurses, "Nursing administrators are responsible for assuring that the knowledge and skills of each nurse in the workplace are assessed prior to the assignment of responsibilities requiring preparation beyond basic academic programs." Individual nurses must work with nursing administrators to ensure that for each shift the nursing unit is staffed with competent practitioners. In some institutions, nurses are allowed to pick shifts and rotations based on seniority; therefore, the possibility exists that less desired shifts or days, such as holidays, may be staffed with less experienced staff. Although each staff member has demonstrated basic competencies for the particular environment, a challenging patient often requires the intervention of a seasoned practitioner who is secure in his or her skills and competency. Thus, expert practitioners may have an ethical obligation to work the less desired shifts as a means of supporting and mentoring novice practitioners. In addition, administrators should offer continuing education on decision-making, negotiating, and limit setting as a means for assisting new nurses to improve their confidence and interpersonal skills.

SUMMARY

Professional nurses will interact with a variety of persons (patients, family members, and other health care professionals) whom the nurse perceives as being challenging. When interacting with challenging persons, the nurse must be able to recognize conflicting goals and unmet expectations and then work to improve communication and resources with the hope that collaboration and understanding will be fostered.

CLINICAL EXERCISES

1. Ask the staff nurse you are working with to describe a patient that he or she has worked with that he or she perceived as being challenging.
2. Does your clinical institution have a policy for dealing with challenging persons (whether patients, visitors, or employees)? If not, does the nurse you are working with believe such a policy is needed?

Discussion Questions

Consider the challenging patient who the staff nurse described to you in Clinical Exercise 1.

1. What factors affected the staff nurse and your perception of why the patient was "challenging"? Do the factors reflect moral absolutes, a difference in culture, or a difference in expectation of outcomes or cost/benefit analysis?
2. What actions could be suggested to resolve or prevent the factors that resulted in the perception of the patient being challenging?

3. "Some may say that there are no difficult patients, only difficult situations" (Maupin, 1995, p. 11). What do you believe? Explain your answer.
4. At what point would you or would you not believe that a person may be denied access to health care services for "noncompliant" behavior? What is the ethical justification for your position?
5. A patient diagnosed with paranoid schizophrenia and insulin-dependent diabetes refuses to take insulin because she thinks the insulin is poisoning her.

    a. Do you believe that this patient is a challenging patient? If so, what factors are affecting the patient's and nursing staff's decision-making?

    b. What ethical principles should guide the nurse's problem-solving with this patient?

SECTION 4: *Confidentiality Versus the Duty to Protect Third Parties*

Traditionally, the information disclosed by a patient to his or her therapist is viewed as being confidential, similar to the relationship held between a parishioner and a priest. However, the 1976 legal decision in *Tarasoff v. Regents of the University of California* has forced mental health workers (including nurses) to rethink this commitment to confidentiality in light of a competing duty to protect a third party from imminent harm.

CONFIDENTIALITY

The ethical obligation to protect confidential patient information is well recognized. In fact in this book, confidentiality is identified as one of the four fundamental ethical themes that a professional nurse encounters in every clinical setting. By protecting confidential patient information, the professional nurse builds the foundation for a trusting nurse–patient relationship. Although establishing a trusting relationship is important to every nurse–patient relationship, the success of mental health treatment is contingent on the patient's ability to trust and feel accepted by the mental health workers involved in his or her care. However, the ethical culture of mental health care changed dramatically after the 1976 *Tarasoff* ruling.

TARASOFF V. REGENTS OF THE UNIVERSITY OF CALIFORNIA

Prosenjit Poddar was an international student from India who was studying at the University of California at Berkeley. He met and spent time with Tatiana (Tanya) Tarasoff during the fall of 1968. On December 31, 1968, Tarasoff told Poddar that she was not interested in dating. During the spring of 1969, Poddar became extremely depressed. He continued to profess love for Tarasoff while also describing to a friend his intention to kill her by means of an explosive. In the summer of 1969, Tarasoff traveled to Brazil and Poddar began psychotherapy. On August 18, during his ninth therapy session, Poddar confessed to Dr. Lawrence Moore his intention to kill a woman on her return from Brazil. Although Poddar would not specify the woman's name, Dr. Moore knew, based on information discussed during previous sessions, that Poddar was referring to Tarasoff.

On August 20, 1969, Dr. Moore attempted to initiate a 72-hour emergency detention order because he believed that Poddar was experiencing a paranoid schizophrenic reaction and was a threat to himself and others. The campus police took Poddar into custody. Despite warnings from Dr. Moore to the contrary, the police released Poddar after concluding that he was thinking rationally and that therefore no threat of harm existed.

Poddar stopped seeing Dr. Moore sometime after this detention event. Tarasoff returned from Brazil in October. Shortly thereafter, Poddar learned about an affair Tarasoff had while in Brazil. On October 27, 1969, Poddar went to Tarasoff's home, but was told by her mother to leave because Tanya was not home. Later, Poddar returned with a kitchen knife and a pellet gun. Tanya was home alone. He shot her with the pellet gun and chased her into the yard, where he stabbed her to death. Immediately after killing Tarasoff, Poddar notified police and requested to be arrested.

Poddar pled not guilty by reason of insanity. During the trial, Dr. Moore's aborted attempt to involuntarily detain Poddar became public knowledge. Poddar was found guilty of second-degree murder. The conviction was overturned during appeal based on a technicality related to the judge's failure to appropriately instruct the jury about diminished mental capacity. Rather than retry the case 5 years after the fact, the state prosecutor dropped the case after Poddar agreed to return to India and never return to the United States.

Tarasoff's parents subsequently filed a wrongful death claim against the University of California at Berkeley and the various psychotherapists involved in Poddar's treatment. The Alameda County Superior Court dismissed the case, and the parents appealed. The California Supreme Court dismissed three of four claims and concluded that:

- The therapists were not liable for not originally detaining Poddar.
- Dr. Powelson (the hospital director of psychiatry) was not liable for punitive damages related to attempts to conceal actions on or following August 20.

Thus, the Tarasoffs had only one viable claim, that Dr. Moore failed to warn Tanya Tarasoff (or anyone else in the position of protecting her) of Poddar's threat (Buckner & Firestone, 2000). The court concluded,

---

Obviously, we do not require that the therapist, in making that determination, render a perfect performance; the therapist need only exercise that reasonable degree of skill, knowledge and care ordinarily possessed and exercised by members of that professional specialty under similar circumstances. . . . The protective privilege ends where the public peril begins. (Tarasoff II, 551 P.2d at 345 & 347)

PRIVILEGE

Confidentiality is not synonymous with *privilege*, "which denotes an individual's right to keep private from legal settings information revealed in the context of specific fiduciary relationships (e.g., physician–patient, priest–penitent, or attorney–client)"

(Pinals & Gutheil, 2001, p. 113). The legal concept of privilege between a therapist (in this case a social worker) and a client was supported in *Jaffee v. Redmond*, in which the court of appeals "qualified its recognition of the privilege by stating that it would not apply if 'in the interests of justice, the evidentiary need for the disclosure of the contents of a patient's counseling sessions outweighs that patient's privacy interests'." (Supreme Court of the United States, 1996). A similar standard requires an attorney to disclose knowledge of a client's intentions to commit a crime (Sterns, 2001). Because the concept of privilege is not an absolute, the nurse must make decisions about disclosure based on the interests and harms present in each individual case.

DUTY TO PROTECT

The *duty to protect* requires the health care professional to take action to personally inform a third party and law enforcement (or others with the skills to protect the third person) that the third person is in imminent and significant threat of harm. The *Tarasoff* case established that a "psychotherapist has a duty to use reasonable cause to protect third parties from becoming victims of a psychotherapist's patient" (Stern, 2001, p. 2). This duty to protect is based on the premise that the therapist's priority is to the third party rather than the patient.

Right to Be Free From Harm

This duty to protect is in response to the belief that citizens in Western society have an inherent right to be free from harm as typified by the reference in the Preamble to the Constitution of the United States to an entitlement to life, liberty, and the pursuit of happiness. The right to be free from harm may be considered a negative right. A negative right stipulates that a person must refrain from exposing another person to a specific action (in this case harm). Typically when a person refrains from doing something, the person is required not to act, in other words, to do nothing. However, the duty to protect requires the health care professional to carry out a specific action, which implies that the right to be free from harm is also a positive right (Beauchamp & Childress, 2001).

Requirements for Duty to Protect

To carry out this duty, the psychotherapist must believe that the third party is at risk of serious danger due to an action that might be carried out by the patient. However, the possibility exists that a psychotherapist could place more credence on a patient's comments than the patient really intends. Everyone at some point of time, perhaps in anger, has proclaimed, "I want to kill him!" even if her or she had no true intention or plan for caring out this threat. Thus, the therapist must use all available assessment and communication skills to ascertain the veracity and intentions related to the patient's comments.

The patient must also identify a specific person or collection of persons by name. In some cases, like the *Tarasoff* case, the patient may only be able to infer the identity of the third party (in this case, the woman who will be returning from Brazil), but the duty to warn exists if the therapist has reason to believe he or she knows the identity of the person (Stern, 2001).

When the decision to protect a third party is made, the therapist could implement several actions including personally warning the identified party and encouraging the third party to take action to protect himself or herself and notifying the local law enforcement agency. The therapist should also act to prevent the patient from carrying out the harm. This might include voluntary or involuntary commitment to a psychiatric facility or around-the-clock supervision or monitoring of the patient (Stern, 2001).

STRATEGIES

One key way for a nurse or other health care provider to avoid the need to breach confidentiality is to enlist the patient's assistance. Through education and therapeutic communication, the nurse could educate the patient on the importance of preventing harm to others by disclosing pertinent information, such as positive HIV status or suicidal ideations. Confidentiality is not broken if the patient either discloses the information or provides permission for the health care professional to disclose (Pinals & Gutheil, 2001).

When questioning the need to disclose confidential patient information for the purpose of protecting a third person, the nurse should consider the following questions before making a decision:

1. *Who will suffer if this information is not revealed?*
2. *How will the patient suffer if the information is revealed or is not revealed?*
3. *Is there any potential gain to anyone in revealing the information?*
4. *What kind of relationship do I have with this patient and how can that be used or strengthened in the way I approach this dilemma? (Pinals & Gutheil, 2001, p. 118)*

If, after considering these questions, the nurse believes that there is a duty to protect a third party, then he or she must consider how to convey the necessary warning while disclosing the least amount of personal information possible (Pinals & Gutheil, 2001). For example, the psychiatrist might have said to Ms. Tarasoff, "It is my professional responsibility to warn you that Mr. Poddar has stated his intent to kill you. While I cannot disclose any further information, I urge you to take the precautions necessary to protect yourself."

Nurses as well as all health care professionals need to be cognizant of current state and national laws related to mandatory reporting (e.g., abuse and communicable diseases) and parental notification limitations and requirements with regard to mature minors (e.g., reproductive decisions or psychiatric care) (Pinals & Gutheil, 2001). On admission or during the initial treatment session, the patient should be notified in writing of the exception to confidentiality deriving from the duty to protect third parties. The patient should sign the notice to acknowledge his or her informed decision to proceed with the relationship (Stern, 2001).

Nurses need to be active participants in their clinical setting in developing protocols related to the use of communication technology and transmission of confidential information. These protocols should address the use of cell phones, fax machines, and e-mail for transmitting and/or discussing private patient information (Pinals & Gutheil, 2001).

SUMMARY

Nurses have a moral obligation to promote the welfare of individual patients as well as society. At times, the nurse may experience an ethical conflict when the need to protect others in society requires him or her to violate other ethical obligations, such as confidentiality, to an individual patient. Nurses need to be aware of mandatory reporting requirements that can affect their practice. Enlisting the patient's cooperation and using therapeutic communication skills are instrumental when faced with a duty to warn others.

CLINICAL EXERCISES

1. Determine whether the psychiatric facility has a policy on duty to protect third parties or a confidentiality policy that is different from the policy used in other specialty areas.
2. Ask your staff nurse if she or he has ever been involved in a situation involving the duty to warn a third party. If so, ask her or him how "public peril" was defined, who was notified, and what role she or he had in this situation.

Discussion Questions

1. One argument against the duty to protect is that this practice will deter other people from seeking treatment. What ethical theory or principle supports this argument?
2. Divide the students into two groups to engage in a debate regarding the following claim by Martinez (2001):

   The *Tarasoff* case is often cited with regard to the duty to warn and the risk of HIV infection. . . . However, the risk of harm in the HIV case is not as clear. . . . There is arguably some obligation on the partners to protect themselves. . . . Moreover, the transmission of HIV through sexual contact is not as certain as a gunshot wound from a gun. (p. 1)

3. Identify at least two situations that you believe illustrate that the interests of justice outweigh the patient's privacy interests and thus would require the need to disclose the contents of a patient's counseling sessions.
4. A patient on your unit makes the following statement during the morning community meeting: "When I get out of here, I will go back to the office and I will show them who I am. They will get what they deserve."

   - How do you assess this patient's thought process?
   - When you completed this patient's admission data, you noticed that he works at the same company as your brother-in-law. What actions should you take to ensure patient confidentiality?
   - Do you have a duty to protect his co-workers?

Resources

Association of Child and Adolescent Psychiatric Nurses Division of International Society of Psychiatric-Mental Health Nurses. (1999). A position on the rights of children in treatment settings. Retrieved April 16, 2005, from www.ispn-psych.org/html/position_statements.html

Austin, W., Bergum, V., & Goldberg, L. (2003). Unable to answer the call of our patients: Mental health nurse's experience of moral distress. *Nursing Inquiry, 10*(3), 177–183.

Backler, P., & Cutler, D. L. (2002). *Ethics in community mental health care: Commonplace concerns.* Boston: Kluwer Academic.

Bazelon, D. L. (2003). Advance psychiatric directives. Retrieved April 16, 2005, from www.bazelon. org/issues/advancedirectives/index.htm

International Society of Psychiatric-Mental Health Nurses. (1999). Position statement: The use of restraint and seclusion. Retrieved April 16, 2005, from www.ispn-psych.org/html/position_statements.html

International Societ of Psychiatric-Mental Health Nurses. (2001). Position statement: Response to clinical psychologists prescribing psychotropic medications. Retrieved April 16, 2005, from www.ispn-psych.org/html/position_statements.html

Maupin, C. R. (1995). The potential for noncaring when dealing with difficult patients: Strategies for moral decision-making. *Journal of Cardiovascular Nursing, 9*(3), 11–22.

Miller, I. (1998). The National Coalition of Mental Health Professionals and Consumers: Eleven unethical managed care practices every patient should know about (with emphasis on mental health care). Retrieved April 16, 2005, from www.nomanagedcare.org/eleven.html

Quinn, D. K., Geppert, C. M., & Maggiore, W. A. (2002). The Emergency Medical Treatment and Active Labor Act of 1985 and the practice of psychiatry. *Psychiatric Services, 53*(10), 1301–1307.

Roberts, L. W., & Dyer, A. R. (2004). *Concise guide to ethics in mental health care.* Arlington, VA: American Psychiatric Publishing.

Scheurich, N. (2004). Moral attitudes and mental disorders. *Hastings Center Report, 32*(2), 14–21.

Simon, J. R., Dwyer, J., & Goldfrank, L. R. (1999). The difficult patient. *Emergency Medicine Clinics of North America, 17*(2), 353–370.

Telson, H., Glickstein, R., & Trujillo, M. (1999). Report of the Bellevue Hospital Center Outpatient Commitment Pilot Program. Retrieved July 6, 2004, from www.psychlaws.org/Medical-Resources/Bellevue%20Report%202%20web.htm

The Federal Psychotherapist-Patient Privilege (*Jaffee v. Redmond*, 518 U.S. 1), History, Documents and Opinions. (n.d). Retrieved July 23, 2004, from www.jaffee-redmond.org/

U.S. Department of Health and Human Services, Substance Abuse and Mental Health Services Administration. (n.d.). Special report: Annotated bibliography for managed behavioral health care 1989–1999. Retrieved April 16, 2005, from www.mentalhealth.org/publications/allpubs/SMA00-3424/SMA00-3424ch9.asp

VandeCreek, L., & Knapp, S. (2001). *Tarasoff and beyond: Legal and clinical considerations in the treatment of life-endangering patients.* Sarasota, FL: Professional Resource Press.

References

American Hospital Association. (1973/1992). Patient bill of rights. Retrieved April 16, 2005, from www.injuredworker.org/Library/Patient_Bill_of_Rights.htm

American Hospital Association. (2003). The patient care partnership: Understanding expectations, rights and responsibilities. Retrieved April 16, 2005, from www.aha.org/aha/ptcommunication/partnership/index.html

American Nurses Association. (2001a). *Bill of Rights for Registered Nurses.* Washington, DC: Author. Retrieved on April 22, 2005 from http://nursingworld.org/tan/novdec02/rights.htm

American Nurses Association. (2001b). *Code of ethics for nurses with interpretive statements.* Washington, DC: Author.

American Psychiatric Nurses Association. (2000). Position statement on the use of seclusion and restraint. Retrieved April 16, 2005, from www.apna.org/resources/positionpapers.html

American Psychiatric Nurses Association. (2003). Mandatory outpatient treatment (MOT). Retrieved May 21, 2005, from www.apna.org/resources/positionpapers.html

Bandman, B. (1978). The human rights of patients, nurses, and other health professionals. In E. L. Bandman & B. Bandman (Eds.). *Bioethics and human rights* (pp. 321–331). Boston: Little, Brown.

Bandman, B. (1981). Do nurses have rights? No. *American Journal of Nursing, 78*(1), 84–86.

Bandman, E. (1981). Do nurses have rights? Yes. *American Journal of Nursing, 78*(1), 84–86.

Beauchamp, T. L., & Childress, J. F. (2001). *Principles of biomedical ethics* (5th ed.). New York: Oxford University Press.

Breeze, J. A., & Repper, J. (1998). Struggling for control: The care experiences of 'difficult' patients in mental health services. *Journal of Advanced Nursing, 28*(6), 1301–1311.

Buckner, F., & Firestone, M. (2000). "Where the public peril begins": 25 years after *Tarasoff*. *Journal of Legal Medicine, 21*(2). Retrieved April 16, 2005, from http://cyber.law.harvard.edu/torts01/syllabus/readings/buckner.html

Cline, J. L. (2003). Working with individuals. In W. K. Mohr (Ed.). *Johnson's psychiatric-mental health nursing* (5th ed.) (pp. 135–150). Philadelphia: Lippincott Williams & Wilkins.

Conn, V. (2003). Working with families. In W. K. Mohr (Ed.). *Johnson's psychiatric-mental health nursing* (5th ed.) (pp. 169–189). Philadelphia: Lippincott Williams & Wilkins.

Deering, C., & Frederick, J. (2003). Therapeutic relationships and communication. In W. K. Mohr (Ed.). *Johnson's psychiatric-mental health nursing* (5th ed.) (pp. 53–75). Philadelphia: Lippincott Williams & Wilkins.

Diamond, R. S., & Larsen, G. (2003). Legal and ethical aspects of psychiatric-mental health nursing. In W. K. Mohr (Ed.). *Johnson's psychiatric-mental health nursing* (5th ed.) (pp. 113–131). Philadelphia: Lippincott Williams & Wilkins.

Drye, R. C., Goulding, R. L., & Goulding, M. E. (1973). No-suicide decisions: Patient monitoring of suicidal risk. *American Journal of Psychiatry, 130*, 171–174.

Farrance, C. A., & Kingsley, B. J. (1990). Least restrictive conditions. *Nursing Connections, 3*(3), 37–41.

Farrow, T. L., & O'Brien, A. J. (2003). 'No-suicide contracts' and informed consent: An analysis of ethical issues. *Nursing Ethics, 10*(2), 199–207.

Huggins, M., Anderson, J. A., & Odom, S. E.(2003). Community mental health, support, and rehabilitation. In W. K. Mohr (Ed.). *Johnson's psychiatric-mental health nursing* (5th ed.) (pp. 291–310). Philadelphia: Lippincott Williams & Wilkins.

Illinois Mental Health Treatment Preference Declaration Act. (1998). 755 ILCS 43/75 Retrieved April 22, 2005 from www.ilga.gov/legislation/ilcs/ilcs2.asp?ChapterID=60

Love, C. C. (2001). Staff-patient erotic boundary violations: Part one—Staff factors. *On the Edge: The Official Newsletter of the International Association of Forensic Nurses, 7*(3), 4–7.

Marinner-Tomey, A. (2002). Virginia Henderson: Definition of nursing. In A. Marinner-Tomey & M. R. Alligood (Eds.). *Nursing theorists and their work* (5th ed.) (pp. 98–111). St. Louis, MO: Mosby.

Martinez, W. (2001). January 2001 internal house staff conference: Duty to warn. Retrieved April 16, 2005, from http://www.med.utah.edu/ethics/Casearch-2001.htm

Ontario Consultants on Religious Tolerance. (2003). Santeria, A syncretistic Caribbean religion. Retrieved April 16, 2005, from www.religioustolerance.org/santeri.htm

Parker, J. G. (1995). Chemical restraints and children: Autonomy or veracity? *Perspectives in Psychiatric Care, 31*(2), 25–29.

Peternelj-Talyor, C. A., & Yonge, O. (2003). Exploring boundaries in the nurse–client relationship: Professional roles and responsibilities. *Perspectives in Psychiatric Care, 39*(2), 55–66.

Pilette, P. C., Berck, C. B., & Achber, L. C. (1995). Therapeutic management of helping boundaries. *Journal of Psychosocial Nursing and Mental Health Services, 33*(1), 40–47.

Pinals, D. A., & Gutheil, T. G. (2001). Sanctity, secrecy, and silence: Dilemmas in clinical confidentiality. *Psychiatric Annals, 31*(2), 113–118.

President's Commission on Mental Health. (1978). *Report to the President.* Washington, DC: U.S. Government Printing Office.

Rickelman, B. L. (2003). The client who displays angry, aggressive, or violent behavior. In W. K. Mohr (Ed.). *Johnson's psychiatric-mental health nursing* (5th ed.) (pp. 555–573). Philadelphia: Lippincott Williams & Wilkins.

Supreme Court of the United States. (1996, June 13). *Carrie Jaffee, Special Administrator for Ricky Allen, Sr., Deceased, Petitioner v. Mary Lu Redmond et al.* On writ of certiorari to the United States Court of Appeals for the Seventh Circuit. No. 95-266. Retrieved April 16, 2005, from http://apsa.org/pubinfo/jr-opin.htm

Stern, E. (2001). *Tarasoff* cases weight patient's confidentiality rights with society's protection needs. *MassPsy.com, 12*(6). Retrieved April 16, 2005, from www.masspsy.com/columns/0407ne_stern.htm

Tarasoff v. Regents of California. 131 Cal. Rep. 14, 1976.

Tarasoff II, 551 P.2d at 345 & 347.

Wiseman, R. (2001). The ANA develops Bill of Rights for Registered Nurses: Know your rights in the workplace. *American Journal of Nursing, 101*(1), 55–56.

CHAPTER 15

Community and Public Health Nursing

Objectives

At the end of this chapter, the student should be able to:

1. Identify situations in community/public health nursing in which autonomy and paternalism are in conflict.
2. Identify resources that assist in resolving ethical issues in community/public health nursing.
3. Recognize situations in which cultural differences could pose ethical problems.
4. Identify resources that assist in providing nursing care when issues of cultural differences arise in health care practices.
5. Analyze ethical issues in public health relevant to nursing.
6. Describe broader social justices issues for nurses to address through political activism.
7. Assume the advocacy role for clients.

KEY WORDS

- *Abandonment*
- *Communitarianism*
- *Culture*
- *Decisional capacity*
- *Female genital mutilation*

- *Health disparities*
- *Index patient*
- *Medical neglect*
- *Moderate paternalism*

The clinical education of many nurses who are practicing today was primarily based in the hospital. In the last decade, however, there has been a shift toward reducing hospital admissions, reducing in-patient lengths of stay, and expanding the sites of health care delivery to a variety of settings. Nurses deliver care in facilities such as nursing homes, residential facilities, halfway houses, ambulatory care centers, school-based clinics, surgicenters, parish houses, correctional facilities, and patient homes, among other sites. Even such technologies as ventilators, dialysis, and chemotherapy can be provided in the patient's home. The shift from hospitals to the community poses different ethical issues, which are the focus of this chapter.

Public health activities began as early as 494 BC, with the Roman Office of Aedile being the earliest known regional health department (Basta, 1992). It focused on sanitation, ventilation, and environmental effects on public health. Public health measures such as quarantine were instituted as early as 1377 in response to the bubonic plague. Care of the sick was usually provided by female family members in the home. The Sisters of Charity, founded in 1633 by St. Vincent de Paul and a precursor to public health nursing, were the first to perform home visits to minister to the sick. After Florence Nightingale's work during the Crimean War in the mid-nineteenth century, developments in nursing education and epidemiology helped to shape professional nursing. Like Nightingale, other nurses have been activists for public health. In the 1890s Lillian Wald founded the Henry Street Settlement in New York City, where nurses lived and worked with poor immigrant communities. She is credited with being the first person to use the phrase "public health nurse." As the first president of the National Organization for Public Health Nursing, Wald pushed to standardize both the practice and education of public health nursing through education and certification. Recognizing the need for a university education for nurses, she lobbied for baccalaureate education as the entry level.

The American Nurses Association's membership unit was restructured in the 1980s, and the section on public health nursing was renamed community health nursing to include all nursing practices outside hospitals. Public health nurses, however, preferred to keep their identity, so the term public health/community health is often seen. Although the labels of community health and public health nursing may be used interchangeably, there is a philosophical commitment to public health and the health of populations that distinguishes public health nursing from other types of community health nursing.

SECTION 1: *Ethical Themes: Building From the Basic to the Complex*

ADVOCACY

Often community and public health nursing (C/PHN) is initiated after an in-patient hospital stay or an out-patient office visit. Accessing health care and navigating the confusing bureaucracy of home health can be very challenging to clients (the preferred name for patients outside of the hospital). Rules and regulations about the type of care, scope of practice, procedures, treatments, supplies, equipment, and medication can be enormously confusing and frustrating to the client and family, and the nurse can often help to enlist others to help secure services for clients.

There may be situations, however, in which for various reasons clients are unable to advocate for themselves, and the nurse can fulfill the advocacy role as needed. Knowing the rules, regulations, and the system may still not be sufficient for the nurse to manage all advocacy situations that arise. For example, Ms. Baker and Ms. Taub, elderly sisters, live in a two-flat, dilapidated building. Ms. Baker, 80, has congestive heart failure and uses oxygen continuously through a portable tank. Her sister, 84, lives upstairs and is unable to perform any activities of daily living (feeding, dressing, bathing, toileting) unassisted and has several large decubiti ulcers over her heels, hips, and sacrum. Ms. Baker is the caregiver of her sister, but has difficulty providing the care because of her own physical limitations. With Ms. Baker's recent hospitalization, Ms. Taub was left without any caregiver. Despite arrangements made by the home health nurse for a home health aide, Ms. Taub was left alone except for the daily visits of the aide. Both sisters refuse to consider nursing home placement and desire to remain in their homes. The nurse believes that continuing home health services, which are inadequate for meeting all of the sisters' needs, is perpetuating an unsafe situation. Perhaps if the home health agency discontinued services, the sisters would be forced to accept placement, ideally, together. The nurse is concerned that stopping services would be abandoning the sisters. *Abondonment* occurs when the provider ends the relationship with the client without proper notification (Ladd, Pasquerella, & Smith, 2002). Would discontinuing services that are meeting some but not all of their needs in order to compel the elderly sisters to accept other services that will likely meet many if not most of their needs be abandonment? Purposely limiting the sisters' options can be construed as violating their autonomy; advocating for them would seem to require that the nurse facilitate their autonomy. Notifying the sisters that their home health services will be terminated permits them to explore all their options and make an informed decision. Discontinuing services is not abandonment because, with adequate notification, usually in the form of a certified letter, the agency can inform the clients that they will no longer provide services after a specific date.

The nurse has the goal of finding a place where the sisters can be together and receive care that addresses their health needs within their limited resources. The sisters, however, may have the goal of remaining together in their home until their deaths, even if doing so may hasten their deaths. Is the nurse advocating for the sisters by being paternalistic and forcing them to move, or would the nurse be advocating for the sisters by respecting their wishes, mobilizing whatever resources are available to keep them in their home, and continuing home health services? Whatever the ultimate decisions, the nurse should document (1) the risks to the clients if they remain in their home, (2) her conversations advising them of their risks and alternatives, and (3) notifications to their physician and the nurse's home health agency supervisor.

The nurse's feelings that he or she is indirectly causing harm by perpetuating the home situation can be a source of palpable distress. Realizing that competent clients have the right to make decisions, even decisions that may result in harms, may be little consolation. One activity the nurse can engage in is to advocate for improved services for the elderly who want to remain in the community. Another level of advocacy that is critical in community health nursing involves working with others within the nurse's agency, community, professional associations, and relevant state and federal agencies to affect policies and resource allocation decisions.

Discussion Exercises 15-1

Based on current service/billing guidelines, the home health agency is required to "provide all supplies required by the client for his care." This phrase has been interpreted to mean that the agency must provide all supplies for every medical condition even if this condition is not related to the reason for services. Mr. Phillips is admitted to the home health care agency because of a stage 4 pressure ulcer. When completing the admission database, the nurse learns that 20 years ago Mr. Phillips received a colostomy. Mr. Phillips is independent in his colostomy care. The nurse recognizes that the home health agency does not carry the brand of ostomy supplies that Mr. Phillips normally uses. In addition, the nurse realizes that if the agency provides the ostomy supplies, then it will lose money by accepting Mr. Phillips as a patient.

1. Mr. Phillips is financially able and willing to purchase the ostomy supplies independently. Does the nurse have to disclose the option that the agency can provide ostomy supplies to him?
2. If Mr. Phillips' finances were limited and he was unable to use the brand of ostomy supplies provided by the home health agency, should the nurse advocate with the agency to provide his usual brand of supplies?
3. Should the agency refuse to accept Mr. Phillips as a client solely based on the fact that it would be providing services at a financial deficit if he wants it to provide his ostomy supplies?

There may be other situations in which the nurse is concerned about abandoning the client. By virtue of being the only health care provider in the home, nurses have an ethical problem when the relief nurse does not arrive. In the hospital setting, there is a new shift of nurses to cover all the patients, although at times not with the desirable level of staffing. In the home, if the next shift's nurse does not appear, the current nurse in the home may believe it is unsafe to leave until a replacement arrives. Yet with the multiple commitments nurses have, is it reasonable to expect the nurse to remain in the home if he or she is also expected to pick up children from a babysitter or keep a previous appointment? For example, Mr. Franklin, age 85, requires assistance in the activities of daily living (ADLs), including a shower and transfer into bed in the evening, and he has overnight jejunostomy feedings. He has few visitors or phone calls and enjoys talking with the home health nurse. He often delays his care to prolong her stay. Despite her explanation that she needs to leave his home by 9 P.M., he continues to postpone his evening care. Can she ethically leave without performing the nursing care? He is at risk for dehydration without the overnight feeding, and he is not capable of managing the feedings on his own. Because of therapies and other treatments during the day and his intolerance for activity when feeding, the feedings must be done overnight.

What option does the nurse have? She can discuss with him her need to leave on time and suggest that he arrange for another nurse to relieve her and complete his care and accommodate his preferred schedule. If there is no one available or willing to visit that late in the evening, the nurse could investigate other agencies. Looking into the reason behind his delaying his care, the nurse might learn that he is lonely and particularly enjoys her company. Addressing his psychosocial needs may facilitate the evening care. If, despite addressing other needs, the nurse still is unable to complete his care by 9 P.M., she may require that he make a contract with her that authorizes her to have him transported to a local emergency department rather than leave him at risk of dehydration. Is that a paternalistic approach? The nurse feels obligated to provide care that, if not given, could result in serious harm to the client, and she offers him a choice, albeit a limited one, of allowing his care to be completed or going to an acute care facility with 24-hour staffing.

Power Differential in Home Health Nursing

In the previous example, the nurse attempts to balance the client's needs with her commitments; she wants to honor his autonomy and prevent harm (nonmaleficence) by applying paternalism that she believes is appropriate to the situation. Negotiating an outcome that is agreeable to both client and nurse is one way to honor the client's autonomy. However, there is a power differential in this relationship. The nurse is a "guest" in the client's home and has been allowed to enter based on an agreement for services she will provide. If there is a lack of agreement on the services, then the nurse should clarify the goals of the nurse–client relationship. The power in the relationship lies with the client and the client's desire to continue the relationship. In the example of Mr. Franklin, the nurse advises him of the consequences of not having his care completed by the time she must leave and her concern of the possible harm he could sustain. Mr. Franklin is placing the nurse in the difficult situation of choosing to leave on time and not completing his care or staying and missing important time with her children. Is the nurse exerting her power, however, in the implied threat that she will have him removed from his home rather than risk harm to him through dehydration? If Mr. Franklin has decisional capacity, is it not his decision to risk dehydration and remain in his home? Perhaps he does not believe the nurse will call an ambulance if she is ready to leave and he has not started his overnight feedings. With the advice and support of her supervisor, the nurse should proceed with the plan of care she has negotiated with Mr. Franklin, reassess his needs in light of the agency policies and ability to meet his needs, and document all discussions with Mr. Franklin, his physician, and her supervisor.

CONFIDENTIALITY

Suppose that Mr. Franklin has a daughter who lives in a distant state, and she calls one evening. Mr. Franklin asks the nurse to answer the phone. When the daughter identifies herself, she asks for information about her father. Without Mr. Franklin's permission to share information, the nurse cannot give any confidential information to his daughter. In another situation, though, it may be necessary to share confidential information with others.

Mr. Vox is a 29-year-old man who had his annual tuberculosis (TB) test at work and was informed it was positive. He is notified by the occupational health nurse that he needs follow-up. On confirmation of active TB, he is referred to the public health department for treatment. Should his immediate family (his parents), with whom he resides, be contacted for testing? Do any of his co-workers need to be informed? What about other people he may have had more intimate contact with? Does Mr. Vox's right to keep his medical information confidential supersede the right of others not to be harmed? According to the Centers for Disease Control and Prevention (2003), the "index patient," in this case the person with TB, is asked to identify persons with whom he or she has had close contact, such as people with whom he or she lives or works. The public health nurse then notifies and informs them they could have been exposed to TB and should be tested, but the nurse does not divulge the identity of the index patient. It is possible, though, that the identity could be surmised, and the index patient should be counseled that the breach of confidentiality could occur. For example, if Mr. Vox works in close quarters with others, he may be advised to be away from work for 2 to 3 weeks after starting medication. His co-workers might presume that he was the person who exposed them if he is away from work for several weeks.

Suppose that Mr. Vox has a thorough medical work-up that also reveals he is HIV-positive and has gonorrhea. The modes of transmission are different for HIV and gonorrhea than for tuberculosis. Who should be notified of their exposure? Each state may have its own laws regarding partner notification; the differences among states reflect the tension between one person's autonomy and another's person right not to be harmed.

One might assume from an ethical point of view that all sexual partners or persons who shared needles with Mr. Vox should be notified so they can seek medical evaluation and treatment. However, the law protects Mr. Vox's confidential medical information to an extent. He will be asked to reveal his sexual partners, who will be notified that they may have contracted gonorrhea. He may also reveal names of persons with whom he has shared needles or syringes for intravenous (IV) drug use because they are at risk for contracting HIV. Depending on the state in which Mr. Vox resides, the nurse may not be able to inform his sexual or IV drug partners that they have been exposed to HIV; only his spouse, if he is married, can be given the information. This information, based on the principle of nonmaleficence would be shared with his spouse only if he is unwilling to inform her of his HIV status. The states, in permitting authorized disclosure of confidential medical information, hold the principle of non-maleficence higher than an individual's autonomy. The diagnosis of HIV remains stigmatizing, even though treatment has improved longevity and quality of life. Other sexually transmitted infections, like gonorrhea or syphilis, although embarrassing, do not have the same stigma as HIV, and are completely curable through antibiotic therapy. Nurses should be aware of the current law in their state regarding notification for communicable diseases.

The community health nurse may also find himself or herself confronted by a client and/or a client's family asking that extra actions be instituted to protect the client's confidentiality. For example, Ms. Dodd is 96 years old and very proud of her ability to live independently. She was hospitalized for uncontrolled atrial fibrillation. Prior to being discharged from the hospital, her primary care physician notifies her, "You will need to have your INR level evaluated every other day until you are on a routine warfarin dose. However, you will not be able to drive for at least 4 weeks. Therefore I am going to arrange for a home health nurse to come to your house to draw your blood." Ms. Dodd replies, "If it has to be, but I do not want the neighbors to know I am sick. Does the nurse have to come in a uniform? What kind of vehicle will she drive?"

While Ms. Dodd's concerns for her privacy are important, the nurse may not be able to comply with her requests for a variety of reasons. The use of a uniform or company vehicle serves to identify the nurse to Ms. Dodd and thus protect her safety. Wearing the uniform of a community health nurse and driving a company car may augment the nurse's safety. Community health nurses have reported that "looking like a nurse" makes them recognizable to persons in the community, which can be especially important when they are visiting clients who live in neighborhoods with high incidents of violence. Because of this recognition, community persons may monitor, promote, and/or protect the nurse's movement through the neighborhood. Thus, it may not be in the nurse's best interest to conceal his or her occupation.

Neighbors may ask the nurse questions as he or she enters or exits the building. For example, a neighbor might say, "I see that you have been coming every day this week. Is Ms. Dodd doing worse?" Or, "I know Ms. Dodd cannot hear me if I telephone. Is she doing OK? Is there anything I could do for her?" Although it is tempting to engage in conversation with persons who appear concerned about the client's welfare, the community nurse (just like the hospital-based nurse) must divert all questions to the client and/or seek approval from the client before answering specific questions raised by neighbors.

TRUTH-TELLING

As in other areas of nursing practice, telling the truth is foundational to ethical behavior. There are a few exceptions, however. Mrs. Robinson, who is 76 years old, lives in an assisted living facility. She has been diagnosed with Alzheimer disease and experiences short-term memory loss. The home health nurse visits daily to ensure that she completes her activities of daily living (ADLs); she also administers Mrs. Robinson's medication. Frequently Mrs. Robinson asks where her husband is. He died suddenly a few weeks ago, and although her family informed her, she does not remember. The home health nurse explains in a very sensitive and compassionate way that Mr. Robinson died. Mrs. Robinson becomes very upset and distraught each time she is told her husband died, as though it was the first time she was hearing it. In consultation with her family, the nurse decides that it is better to deceive Mrs. Robinson into believing her husband is away rather than cause her the distress each time she is told of her husband's death. The nurse discusses with the family what is plausible to tell Mrs. Robinson when she asks about her husband.

Another example of truth-telling involves the treatment plan. Mrs. Robinson has difficulty walking and standing because of extensive osteoarthritis. She resists doing exercises recommended by the physical therapist. Her family has told her that if she performs her exercises daily, she will be accepted for joint replacement surgery. The nurse is aware that she is not a candidate for surgery, but Mrs. Robinson believes she is and will do her exercises with this encouragement. The exercises are not harming her and may improve her functional status. Is it ethical for the nurse to join the family in telling this lie to Mrs. Robinson? There is a direct benefit to Mrs. Robinson if she believes the lie, but what is the harm if she discovers it is a lie and the nurse has been taking part in it? In every situation, the nurse should assess the potential benefits and harms and decide the course of action to take. In this situation, some may believe that it is acceptable to lie to Mrs. Robinson to enlist her cooperation to improve her functional status. Others may believe it is unacceptable to lie even in this situation, and would find other strategies to enlist Mrs. Robinson's cooperation.

ALLOCATION OF RESOURCES

Most counties in the United States and provinces in Canada have public health departments. Smaller counties may merge resources with other counties, and the state and local municipalities make allocation decisions. In evaluating epidemiological data for their area, the public health departments prioritize their efforts. Data showing, for example, increased teen pregnancy rates, motor vehicle accidents, or increased deaths from pulmonary conditions may reveal areas that could be affected by targeted education. Counties could lobby for funds to conduct sex education programs and awareness campaigns to reduce driving under the influence or tobacco use. Although all of these efforts are laudable, it may not be possible to fund them at a meaningful level. The allocation decision is an ethical decision that must be justified to the taxpayers. Aroskar, Moldow, and Good (2004) observed that the effects of policies are rarely discussed in the nursing literature. They conducted a study with multiple focus groups of practicing nurses, many of whom were community health nurses. The nurses had a mean age of 51 years and more than 20 years of experience, which the authors cited as a limitation because it indicated that younger nurses were not represented in the groups. The authors reported four themes of ethical concern that affected community health nursing, although these themes crossed all practice arenas.

The first theme was the emphasis on cost containment. Reimbursement mechanisms in terms of diagnostic-related groups and managed care adversely affected the quality of care for clients. What the payer will pay for becomes the criterion for what the client receives, rather than what the client needs. The prospective payment system that recently became effective in home health requires a home health agency to meet all the needs of the client, including medication and supplies, while receiving a fixed payment for the diagnostic category. The second theme is closely related. The nurses expressed concern regarding the effect of quality of care as a result of decreased use of professional nurses. The replacement of RNs with unlicensed assistive personnel and the lack of sufficient RN staffing were viewed as major ethical issues in community health. The third theme also is related to RN staffing; inadequate discharge planning and teaching mean that clients and families are ill-prepared to manage at home, and, as a result, are readmitted to an inpatient facility. This is especially significant when a client is terminally ill but has not executed an advance directive or made a plan for home care. The lack of access to clinics was also cited as a major ethical problem for home health nurses and accounted for the inappropriate use of the emergency department.

The fourth theme reflected a dissatisfaction of the nurses in this study about the way in which nursing has changed. The nurses felt disenfranchised from the policy-making and allocation decisions that had a direct effect on their practices. None regretted choosing nursing as their career, but they feared that fewer qualified people would choose nursing. Box 15-1 lists the authors' recommendations.

Aroskar et al. (2004) maintained that it is an ethical obligation for nurses to be involved in politics and policy-making. They can do this as individuals or through their professional associations. Bringing the reality of health care delivery through the "nursing voice" (Aroskar et al., p. 275) to politicians and policy-makers is vital to the quality of client care.

SUMMARY

The nature of the relationship between nurse and client is altered when care is delivered in the community setting. Power shifts from the health care provider to the client. Issues of confidentiality, truth-telling, and allocation of resources remain, and take on new significance in the home and/or community settings.

BOX 15-1

The Nursing Voice in Health Care Policy

- Involve nurses who provide direct patient care.

- Give attention to the long-term care crisis, pain management, and appropriate end-of-life care.

- Educate patients and families to help them to navigate the health care system and to promote and maintain health.

- Provide payment for medications as preventive measures in appropriate circumstances.

- Develop consumer incentives to participate in and take more responsibility for self-care.

- Provide funding to recruit and retain nurses.

Adapted from Aroskar, M., Moldow, D. G., & Good, C. M. (2004). Nurses' voices: Policy, practice and ethics. *Nursing Ethics, 11*(3), 274.

CLINICAL EXERCISES

1. Does your home health/public health agency have a confidentiality policy regarding highly sensitive information?
2. Talk with the nurse you are working with about his or her experiences with being recognized as a nurse out in the community. Has this recognition had positive or negative consequences for the nurse and/or client?

Discussion Questions

1. An outbreak of pertussis (whooping cough) occurs in an upper-middle-class suburb. Numerous teenagers who for religious reasons have not been vaccinated develop whooping cough. Several of these teenagers are in a work-study program in the high school–based day care center. The child care center accepts children as young as 6 weeks old who have not yet been vaccinated against pertussis. The public health nurse conducts a public education awareness session during which she is asked the following questions. What ethical commitments should the nurse consider when determining if or how to answer these questions?

   - "I am a mother of 7-week-old in day care. Do I not have a right to know if my child is being cared for by someone not vaccinated for whooping cough?"
   - "I want to move my child to another day care away from the school. However, one director told me that they were not accepting nonimmunized children who have a high likelihood of being exposed to the whooping cough for the next 2 months. Can a day care discriminate against my child just because she is not old enough to have received the vaccine?"
   - "Shouldn't there be some website we as parents can go to learn where the whooping cough has occurred and what locations these persons have

been at? Why doesn't the health department just quarantine the nonimmunized teenagers or better yet force them to be immunized if they want to go to public schools!"

SECTION 2: *Autonomy Versus Paternalism*

Previous chapters focused on the importance of the autonomy of the health care recipient in making informed decisions. In community and public health nursing, autonomy remains highly valued and respected, but can pose various challenges. In home health, for example, a client who is diabetic might reuse the disposable syringes and needles because she pays a portion of the costs for equipment and supplies. The nurse believes that the client is risking contamination of the insulin and encourages her to discard the used supplies. The client refuses, however, so the nurse consults with a colleague in infectious disease to determine the best way to clean the supplies. Although the nurse believes reusing the equipment poses a risk of infection, she respects the client's decision to accept the risk after verifying that the client is making an informed decision.

There may be situations in which the needs of a community trump an individual's autonomy. The ethical theory of *communitarianism* is often cited as being the prevailing framework in public health. Communitarianism is a social theory that places "communal values, the common good, social goals, traditional practices and cooperative virtues" (Beauchamp & Childress, 2001, p. 362) above individualism. For example, for the welfare of all citizens in the United States, children are required to be immunized for certain communicable diseases prior to entering public school. There are risks associated with immunizations, and parents are mandated to have their children immunized. There are exceptions to this mandate, such as when the immunization is contraindicated for a specific child or if parents have religious objection to vaccinations (state statutes describe what is required to obtain exemption for school entry). Another example of communitarianism taking precedent over autonomy occurs with so-called direct-observation therapy (DOT). In DOT persons with a communicable disease such as tuberculosis are observed as they ingest oral medication; if they do not agree to the DOT, they may, as a last resort and only through a court order, be involuntarily isolated. Their autonomy and freedom would be sacrificed to prevent the spread of a communicable disease.

Paternalism involves making judgments about the best interests of others. Conflict can arise, however, when the nurse and the health care provider do not agree on what constitutes best interests as well as whose best interests should be considered. For example, Mrs. Miller, a 73-year-old woman and retired veterinary assistant, lives alone. She has congestive heart failure and osteoporosis and had a splenectomy a number of years ago. She uses a walker and limits her movement to the bathroom, kitchen, and bedroom. Most of the day she sits in a recliner and watches television. She has a number of cats and allows them unrestricted movement throughout her house. Her limited mobility and energy interfere with her housekeeping. Home health nursing services were ordered to monitor Mrs. Miller's cardiac status after a recent hospitalization, so the home health nurse plans to visit daily during the first week after discharge. The home health nurse is alarmed by the lack of cleanliness throughout the house and believes Mrs. Miller is at increased risk of infection because of her splenectomy. The nurse explores with Mrs. Miller the possibility of her hiring someone to clean and cook for her. Mrs. Miller, who states she cannot afford that on her limited income and is not concerned about the cleanliness of her home, states, "If I have not gotten sick by now then I doubt that I will."

Is this an ethical issue? Does the lack of cleanliness endanger Mrs. Miller's health? Home health nurses may encounter many situations different from what they would find in a health care facility. The client, in this case Mrs. Miller, may clean (or not clean) her house as she chooses. She might find it distressing to forgo a prescription or food in lieu of hiring a housekeeper, and she would not consider giving away her cats. It is her choice to decide how she will spend her money and how clean she will keep her house. The community health nurse, respecting Mrs. Miller's autonomy, could explore other options. Perhaps there are family or friends who could assist her with some housekeeping duties. There may be help available from the Department on Aging or a community agency. With Mrs. Miller's permission, the nurse can investigate options, present them to her client, and assist in the implementation of the option selected, while preserving Mrs. Miller's autonomy.

Suppose instead of the issue being the state of cleanliness of the house, it was Mrs. Miller's inability to perform activities of daily living, so that her health was affected. Suppose that she frequently fell and at times was unable to get up. She would be left alone on the floor for hours, sometimes more than a day. When the community health nurse discovers her, Mrs. Miller refuses to go to the emergency department, and states that she cannot afford a medical alert system. The nurse is concerned that Mrs. Miller is unsafe in her own home. Again, the nurse respects Mrs. Miller's autonomy, but believes it is in Mrs. Miller's best interests that the unsafe conditions be changed. The nurse is being paternalistic in believing that she knows what is best for Mrs. Miller over what Mrs. Miller considers what is best for her. Thus the dilemma for the nurse is how to improve the safety of the home environment and continue to respect Mrs. Miller's autonomy.

DECISIONAL CAPACITY

When a client makes a decision that would appear to jeopardize his or her health or welfare, the nurse might question the client's ability to make decisions. In Mrs. Miller's case, the nurse may wonder whether she has the capacity to make an informed decision. Ruling out any physiological reason for decreased capacity, the nurse can evaluate Mrs. Miller's ability to make decisions using one of a number of decision-making frameworks (e.g., Grisso & Appelbaum, 1998). Once she is satisfied that Mrs. Miller has the capacity to make decisions about her health and welfare, the nurse must then accept her decision to remain in her home and forgo a medical alert system. The nurse may investigate other options for Mrs. Miller to improve the safety in her home. Autonomy wins out over paternalism.

In another scenario, suppose Mrs. Miller lives in an apartment, and she is forgetful. She left a pan on her stove that started a small fire. She is jeopardizing not only her safety, but also the safety of others in her apartment building. Does the safety of others override Mrs. Miller's autonomy? Does the nurse have a duty to warn others (the landlord, any of Mrs. Miller's closest relatives or friends)? Using her best clinical judgment, the nurse must decide whether this situation warrants violating Mrs. Miller's autonomy and confidentiality. The nurse returns to her agency and informs her supervisor of the situation, and they follow the agency policy for intervening in this type of situation.

PARENTAL AUTONOMY

In another situation, say the community health nurse visits a child with cerebral palsy who was discharged after a brief hospitalization for seizures. During the hospitalization, blood was drawn, and the results determined that the child had a subtherapeutic level of anticonvulsants. The nurse assesses the home situation and finds that the parents do not have a system for remembering when to medicate their child or how much medication to give him. The nurse suggests a calendar and a timer with an alarm, and reviews the importance of maintaining a therapeutic level of anticonvulsant to prevent seizures. In a week, the child is seen in the emergency department for seizures related to subtherapeutic anticonvulsant levels. The community health nurse revisits the family and discusses the medication plan. The parents state that they forget to reset the timer, so some doses might be missed. Given that the parents can repeat what they were told about the importance of regularly medicating their child and have demonstrated the ability to give the child the appropriate dose, it appears that they are electing not to medicate their child as recommended. Does the parents' behavior constitute medical neglect? Or is it in the parents' purview to medicate the child whenever they remember? As discussed in Chapter 11, *parental autonomy*, while not absolute, gives parents a wide berth in making decisions for their children.

The community health nurse views the child as the client; the child's needs are being unmet, and his health is jeopardized by the subtherapeutic anticonvulsant levels. Ruling out physiological reasons for the subtherapeutic levels, what should the nurse conclude? The parents are responsible for the well-being of their child and admit that they do not medicate him as recommended. Does their behavior constitute *medical neglect*, which is the denial of medically indicated care? Some may argue that it is medical neglect because the child required two hospital visits for seizures. Others may say that the parents have the prerogative to accept or reject medical treatment for their child. The community health nurse may want to consult her supervisor, the agency policies, and state statutes mandating reporting of suspected or documented abuse and/or neglect. In the instances of children, the elderly, and other vulnerable people, it may be appropriate for the nurse to be paternalistic.

Other issues involving family can pose ethical problems for the nurse. Mr. Herman, a 35-year-old man, has been discharged from the hospital after treatment for an opportunistic infection associated with AIDS. He has not told his family what his diagnosis is. His mother and pregnant sister will be assisting in his care. He is incontinent and frequently expectorates sputum. In the hospital, standard precautions are followed, but in his home, it is unlikely, especially if the family does not know his diagnosis, that any special procedures will be followed to limit their exposure to his bodily fluids. The nurse respects the client's decision and keeps his information confidential, but discusses with the client the need to follow certain infection control procedures to prevent others from being exposed. After consulting with the client, the nurse instructs the family on standard precautions to protect both him and them from exposure.

FAMILY PATERNALISM

Nurses, acting in the best interests of the client, are sometimes asked by families to provide treatment that the client is refusing. This case illustrates a dilemma a hospice nurse may face. Mrs. Lane is a 70-year-old woman who was diagnosed with breast cancer that has metastasized to bone. To provide pain relief, she requires a dose of oral morphine that causes her to sleep all the time. She wants to be awake as much as possible, and has decided not to take enough medication to completely manage her pain. Other pain medications and pain management techniques have failed to provide comfort. Her family asks the hospice nurse to make Mrs. Lane take a higher dose of pain medication or provide her with a higher concentration of morphine without telling her the strength. They find it unbearable to watch her writhe in pain. The nurse wishes to respect Mrs. Lane's preference to avoid sedation. Again, the resourcefulness of the nurse may provide a solution to the ethical dilemma. With consultation from a pharmacist or pain management team, the nurse may find a medication or combination of medications that provides better pain relief without sedation, thereby satisfying both Mrs. Lane and her family and preserving Mrs. Lane's autonomy.

Again, valuing autonomy is weighed against other values, such as comfort, truth-telling, and family cohesion. In this example, the hospice nurse was able to provide comfort while fully disclosing the methods and getting the client's consent and having the approval of the family. It is not always possible to honor all the values at once. Suppose the hospice nurse is unable to obtain an order from the physician for her proposed pain management strategy. The physician may be unfamiliar with the combination of medications, and instead prescribes a continuous midazolam (Versed) infusion, an *amnesiac* that will not alter Mrs. Lane's pain medication, but will interfere with her ability to recall events. The physician advises the nurse to instruct Mrs. Lane that her doctor wants her to have a medication that will make her more comfortable, but the nurse is not to tell Mrs. Lane about the amnesiac effect. The nurse is now faced with two ethical problems—the first is nondisclosure to the client about medication and the second is the decision on whether to follow the physician's order. The nurse should be able to discuss her concerns with the physician and arrive at a plan that is acceptable to the nurse, physician, family, and, above all, the client. Resources such as the nursing supervisor, an ethics committee, or an ethics consultant may assist the nurse to resolve the ethical problems. The nurse may feel powerless to oppose the medical plan and not wish to compromise her integrity by deceiving the client. A request for ethics review may provoke the physician and family into reexamining their decisions in light of the increased scrutiny.

SUMMARY

Paternalism takes on a new meaning when applied to a population versus an individual client. Restricting the autonomy of a person or group of people for the protection of others requires paternalism that is enforced by law, for example, public health initiatives requiring immunizations, restriction on sales of alcohol and tobacco, and speed limits are mandated. Communities frequently condone paternalism based on a commitment to benefit the greatest number. However, the nurse must be vigilant in maintaining his or her commitment to the individual client when serving in the community or public health setting.

CLINICAL EXERCISES

1. Discuss with the nurses in your assigned agency how they assess decisional capacity.
   a. What resources do they have available to them?
   b. What criteria do they use to decide when to perform the assessment?
   c. Are they more likely to challenge a client's capacity when the client disagrees with the plan of care?

2. Investigate the agency policy toward clients who disregard medical advice.

    a. On what basis is the decision made to continue or discontinue services?
    b. How does the agency ensure the client is making an informed decision?

Discussion Questions

1. On a well-baby home visit, the public health nurse (PHN) discovers that none of the other children, ages 2, 3, and 5 years, have ever been immunized. There has been a recent outbreak of measles in their town. The mother states that because they were all breast-fed, they do not need immunizations. Understanding that immunizations before school age are not mandatory but highly recommended, what should the PHN tell the mother?

    a. What are the ethical issues?
    b. What is the PHN's obligation to the nonimmunized children?
    c. What is the PHN's obligation to the rest of the community?

2. Mrs. Yan is 70 years old and diagnosed with Alzheimer disease. Her 72-year-old husband is her caregiver. The home health nurse has observed bruising on Mrs. Yan's wrists and asks Mr. Yan about them. He responds that to keep Mrs. Yan from wandering when he goes out, he ties her in a chair.

    a. What are the ethical issues?
    b. Does this type of physical restraint constitute elder abuse?
    c. If Mrs. Yan were to wander away from the house, would Mr. Yan be negligent in his care?
    d. What are the nurse's ethical obligations if Mrs. Yan were to say, "That man keeps trying to hurt me. I am afraid; please take me with you."

SECTION 3: *Cultural Competency*

Although cultural competency is expected in every nursing specialty, it warrants special attention in community and public health nursing. When health care is delivered in the hospital, there is an attempt to accommodate patients who have requests related to their culture. Such requests might include providing kosher food and permitting the wearing of a scapular or religious object to the operating room. The patients, however, are usually expected to conform to the hospital rules and routine. In community and public health nursing, the nurse is the one who accommodates the client. The nurse may refrain from visiting the home of a client who is an Orthodox Jew on a Saturday. Knowing certain rituals and unacceptable behaviors, the nurse would greet a client or compliment a child according to the norms of the culture. The nurse also should know as much as possible about the health beliefs of a specific culture and validate those beliefs with clients of that culture. Although the term "culture" is being applied very broadly, the nurse should avoid thinking stereotypically about groups. Not all members of a culture subscribe to all its rituals, beliefs, and customs. It is worthwhile, though, for nurses to be aware of the health beliefs and practices in order to begin a dialogue with the clients about their personal health beliefs and practices.

Culture is a "collection of beliefs, values, and behaviors that permit a group of people to interact effectively with their environment" (Jones, 1992, p. 282). Attitudes toward health and health care are shaped by one's culture. Beyond knowing, in general, various cultures' health beliefs and practices, nurses need to be culturally competent so that they can respectfully interact with and provide services for clients from different cultures. From an agency standpoint, nurses can assess whether their agency delivers services that are culturally and linguistically appropriate by referring to the U.S. Department of Health Office of Minority Health (2001) national standards as a guide. Campinha-Bacote (2003) offered a model of cultural competence that evolves from a desire to become competent, to an introspective review of one's biases and prejudices, to the acquisition of knowledge and skills, and to opportunities to engage with people of other cultures. She coined the acronym ASKED, which stands for Awareness, Skill, Knowledge, Encounters, and Desire. Even culturally competent nurses encounter ethical problems in practice.

In previous sections, autonomy has been identified as an important principle. Truth-telling is based on the principle of autonomy, in that one needs to have truthful information in order to make decisions and thus be self-determining. Autonomy is a Western notion, though. Some cultures have a person other than the client, such as the head of the household or another family member, make decisions.

For example, Mrs. Cass, a 70-year-old widow, has been diagnosed with cancer of the colon with metastasis to the liver. Her prognosis is poor for survival beyond 2 to 3 months. She has a large, extended family. She has two brothers who are in the medical field, although they are not physicians. One brother speaks to the physician and requests that Mrs. Cass not be told her diagnosis and prognosis. He says that it would be too difficult for her to deal with the information and it would be better if she were not told. The physician agrees, and Mrs. Cass is discharged home with home health nursing. The nurses are informed that the family does not want the diagnosis and prognosis revealed to the client. Although the medical literature promotes truth-telling even when clients do not want to know their prognosis (Neff, Lyckholm, & Smith, 2002), there is an acknowledgment that some clients prefer to have their families make decisions about what and how much they should be told (Candib, 2002; Lapine, Wang-Cheng, Goldstein, Nooney, Lamb, & Derse, 2001; Mazanec & Tyler, 2004). Rather than viewing autonomy as a primary ethical commitment, some clients and/or their families may believe that a family should protect the individual from harm, including bad news and the associated decisions. Rather than taking an individualistic perspective, some clients view the family as the unit and believe that the interests of the family supersede those of the client. This perspective emphasizes the need for cultural competency on the part of the health care providers who serve these groups.

The idea of keeping a terminal diagnosis from the client is morally distressing for many nurses, and they need to fully understand what is behind the family's request. The nurses may be able to facilitate communication of this difficult discussion between the client and family by assessing the client and family's values and beliefs about health care and health care decision-making. With the family, the nurse can learn how their culture prepares for death. Issues such as addressing unfinished business, saying good-bye, and making decisions regarding comfort measures may or may not be important, but should be reviewed with the family, and if appropriate in this culture, with the client. It is possible, however, that the client lacks experience in making major decisions or prefers to have family members whose advice he or she trusts make the decisions. As in the foregoing case, Mrs. Cass deferred to her husband for major health care decisions and, on his death, relied on her brothers to make the decisions. A nurse who insists that Mrs. Cass hear her diagnosis and prognosis and make her own decisions risks being disrespectful to Mrs. Cass and her family. Although it is uncomfortable for nurses, it may be consistent with their culture and long-existing family dynamics and it could be more disruptive to Mrs. Cass and the family to disregard their wishes.

CULTURAL/RELIGIOUS PRACTICES

The religious beliefs of some families influence their health care choices. Jacob is a 15-year-old who was sent to the nurse's office at school because he is complaining of an intense frontal headache and has a yellowish-green nasal discharge. His parents belong to a faith community that does not accept medical treatment, but instead believe in healing through prayer. After an examination, the school nurse suspects that he has a sinus infection and recommends that a physician evaluate him. She has seen cellulitis and a brain abscess develop from an untreated sinus infection. She notifies his mother, who politely thanks the nurse for her concern but explains that his congregation is praying for him and he will be healed through prayer. Is this a matter of freedom of religion or could this constitute medical neglect? In cases in which the treatment is known to be efficacious and the risk of nontreatment is extremely high for death or morbidity, the courts have stepped in and allowed children to be treated against their parents' wishes. Conversely, some practices that are culturally based are illegal.

The use of *peyote*, a hallucinogen, in some Native American medicoreligious rituals is legal (Shultes & Hoffman, 1992). *Moxibustion*, the heating of the skin at acupuncture points by burning dried leaves, is an alternative therapy (Ergil, 2001). *Cupping and bleeding* of the skin over certain points on the body is part of Chinese medicine (Ergil, 2001). Although a nurse might have concerns that these therapies could be harmful, they are legal, and when performed by a competent practitioner, they should be safe. Nurses working in palliative or home hospice nursing may encounter clients who smoke marijuana for medicinal purposes when undergoing chemotherapy. In a few states, medical marijuana is legal, but it is illegal in most states. What is the nurse's role? Should the nurse "look the other way" if marijuana is relieving the client's symptoms? Is the nurse or the nurse's agency complicit in the illegal activity if it is not reported to appropriate authorities? Does it matter whether the client's family is growing the marijuana or buying it from a local drug dealer? What if the family asks the nurse for assistance in obtaining marijuana; how should the nurse respond?

The nurse needs to be aware of those activities that legally must be reported. Depending on state laws, suspected or actual child abuse and/or neglect or abuse of a person age 65 years or older must be reported to the proper authorities. It may not always be clear, however, what is a cultural practice and what is abuse/neglect. Mrs. Patel is 86 years old, has deteriorating health and cognitive function, and has stopped eating. She is Jain, a very old religion practiced by Southeast Asian Indians. Her family believes that she has stopped eating because she believes it is time for her to die. Her family respects her decision and does not attempt to feed her. Her physician wants to insert a percutaneous endoscopic gastrostomy tube and give her enteral feedings. Is it elder abuse if they do not agree to insertion of the tube? Should they attempt to force feed her? Should the home health nurse respect the family's wishes or report them?

Other ethical issues can arise that are not life-and-death scenarios. As discussed in Chapter 11 some cultures practice both male and female circumcision. Female circumcision, also referred to as *female genital mutilation*, can be done to varying degrees, ranging from removal of the clitoral hood to infibulation—removal of the labia minora and majora, with the remaining tissue sewn together, almost completely covering the perineum. It may be illegal for a girl younger than the age of majority (18 or 21 years, depending on state law) to undergo female circumcision, even if it is customary in their culture. A newly immigrated family brings their daughter to the health department for routine immunizations. Her mother asks where to find a physician or a midwife to perform a circumcision on her daughter, who is 10 years old. The nurse in the clinic informs her that it is illegal in their state; the mother says she will find someone in her community to do it, but she was hoping that it could be done with anesthesia and under sterile conditions. How does the nurse reconcile respect for the family, cultural sensitivity, and the duty to prevent harm? Should the dominant culture prevail and prevent female genital mutilation, or should it be a matter of parental choice? Having the procedure done in a health care facility may prevent more harm than if it is done under nonsterile conditions and without anesthesia. The family believes it is an important rite of passage and that it is the parents' decision. What should the nurse do?

Discussion Exercises 15-2

You are employed in a family clinic in an area of town with a fast-growing population of immigrants from Somalia. In recent months, several Somali women and female children have been treated for complications caused by the practice of female circumcision. The clinic organizes a meeting with several leaders from the Somali community and their wives to discuss this practice. One of the wives states, "Circumcision is one way that we teach our girls to remain pure. We do not tolerate sexual promiscuity like you Americans do." One of the nurse practitioners responds, "I was at a conference last month and I heard about how another community approaches female circumcision. In this plan, the girl is brought to the clinic and the physician, using sterile technique, performs a 1-cm cut. This cut is small enough that the natural anatomy is protected, but the symbolic nature of the circumcision is maintained. I am wondering if we might be able to create a similar plan."

1. Would you support an agreement for symbolic female circumcision to be done in a medical setting? Explain.
2. What could go wrong with this plan that the clinic workers and community leaders should think about in advance?

In another example in which religion dictates certain rules, a male nurse makes a home visit to a female infant who had an elevated bilirubin at discharge. He intends to draw blood through a heel stick from the infant. He will also examine her. On entering the home, he becomes aware that the family is Muslim. The infant appears very jaundiced, and her mother says she is listless and not sucking very well. The nurse is aware that Muslims prefer that a health care examiner be the same gender as the patient and that a woman be present when a female patient is being examined (Athar, n.d.). The nurse is concerned that a delay in obtaining the blood sample could delay treatment.

What should the nurse do? The nurse wants to respect the family's wishes, and he also wants to prevent any harm to the infant that might be caused by delaying care. He could explain his concerns to the parents and ask their permission to draw the blood from the infant in their presence. If they refuse, he could contact his supervisor to see how quickly a female nurse could be sent to the home. As a last resort, he could instruct the family to take the infant to their pediatrician or local pediatric clinic to have blood drawn.

Not all cultural differences are based on religion or ethnicity. Sometimes there is a difference in the value some people place on health care. Although they accept health care through an emergency department or acute and rehabilitation hospitals, once they are discharged they cease to perform health maintenance activities. Some of their behaviors might be detrimental to their health. Mr. Vasquez, a 25-year-old, has a spinal cord injury that requires him to use a wheelchair for mobility. The nurse makes a post-hospitalization visit to monitor a sacral decubiti he treated. Mr. Vasquez lives in a third-floor walk-up in a dilapidated apartment building. Although he is on a list for a first-floor apartment in public housing, he may have to wait more than a year. Supplies for his bowel and bladder program get stolen because the deliveryman leaves them on the first floor by the mailboxes. His mother wants him to move in with her in her home, but he refuses. The nurse suspects he is abusing illicit intravenous drugs. His neighborhood is known for gang activity, and the nurse has seen gang members leaving his apartment. He has new areas of skin breakdown, and he is not doing intermittent catheterization, but will occasionally credé his bladder. He is not continent. He missed his follow-up appointments and does not plan to return to the physician. The nurse is concerned that he is seriously jeopardizing his health. The nurse may not be able to change his environment, but can make some changes in how his supplies are delivered. She also can try to interest Mr. Vasquez in wheelchair sports, and, perhaps, in a peer-mentor program for men with spinal cord injury. Using various strategies to engage Mr. Vasquez in his care shows respect for his autonomy, possibly prevents complications in his forgoing health maintenance, and, in the end, promotes good health.

SUMMARY

Many beliefs, attitudes, and practices clients have regarding health care, illness, dependency, death, and dying stem from their culture. It is important for nurses to be knowledgeable and open to education about the client, family, and community cultures. Being respectful of and sensitive to culture and cultural differences is the first step to building a therapeutic relationship.

CLINICAL EXERCISES

1. Identify resources in your agency for learning more about different cultures and their health care beliefs and practices.
2. Identify the mechanism within your agency for resolving conflicts when client's cultural practices pose threats to their health.
3. Does your agency have a policy regarding cultural sensitivity or religious freedom?

Discussion Questions

1. In the example discussed earlier, do you believe the nurse should inform Mrs. Cass of her diagnosis and prognosis? Give your rationale in defense of your position.
2. What would you advise the mother who wants her 10-year-old daughter to be circumcised under sterile conditions? Justify your answer.
3. What incentives do nurses have or what incentives are needed to encourage them to consider cultural and subcultural variables in their work with patients?

SECTION 4: *Ethics in Public Health*

The federal government has broad powers over many aspects of its citizens' lives. The local, state, and federal governments mandate certain laws for the benefit of its citizens' health. Mandatory immunizations, seat belt laws, helmet laws, and laws related to food handling in restaurants are examples of *moderate paternalism* (Arisaka, n.d.). These laws are paternalistic because they infringe on personal liberties for the betterment of the general public. Public health departments provide many services, but usually have to prioritize their initiatives because of limited resources. Based on the leadership of the public health departments and the political climate, certain activities get funded. There may be a concern about an increase in cases of sexually transmitted infections or in the rate of teen pregnancy. Or there may be a public outcry about mental health services when a mother is accused of killing her infant because of postpartum depression. A community can focus on specific issues and target activities to address those issues. Decisions about what activities get funded are political and are not always based on statistical data or clinical significance to a large portion of the population, but instead might be based on persuasion and political ramifications. For example, during the Kennedy administration, funding for the prevention of premature births increased because of the premature birth and subsequent death of Patrick, the president's second son.

HEALTH PROMOTION AND DISEASE PREVENTION

Callahan and Jennings (2002) identified four areas of public health ethics: health promotion and disease prevention, risk reduction, epidemiological and other public health research, and structural and socioeconomic disparities. Health promotion and disease prevention are public health goals, but how those goals are reached creates ethical issues. Issues surrounding alcohol use offer examples relating to individual liberty and responsibility. Adults older than 21 years of age (in some states, 18 years) can legally ingest alcohol. There are rules that limit personal freedom, such as driving while under the influence, because drivers under the influence have a higher probability of having an accident. The rationale supporting drunk driving legislation is to reduce traffic accidents. Alcohol is also a contributing factor to violence and accidents in the home. Abuse of alcohol can lead to addiction and chronic disease. Yet, drinking alcohol is a personal liberty. A public health department may, in concert with state and federal agencies, launch a public awareness campaign, such as promoting the slogan "Friends do not let friends drive drunk." The aim is to reduce drunk driving and thereby reduce accidents associated with it.

Similarly, there have been national campaigns regarding tobacco use, safe sex, domestic violence, and obesity. All activities involve choice, although tobacco and alcohol use and overeating may be considered compulsive disorders. For health promotion and disease prevention, there must be some limits to personal freedom, and behavior change through persuasive peer pressure. How far the government can go to promote good health by limiting personal freedom is an ethical issue. Public health nurses can work toward health promotion and disease prevention not only on an individual and family level, but also with communities in terms of programs offered, such as smoking cessation, safe sex, and healthy eating.

Another area is risk reduction. How far should the government be allowed to go to reduce risk? In the state of Illinois, helmet laws for motorcyclists have been passed and repealed. Drivers want the freedom to wear or not wear a helmet, and have lobbied legislators to repeal helmet laws. The Centers for Disease Control and Prevention (2004) estimate that direct medical costs for motorcyclists is greater than $8 billion/year. They have funded an initiative to persuade states without helmet laws to mandate helmet use. Public health nurses can be involved in educating communities about the dangers of unhelmeted motorcycle riding. They also can assess risks in their community and plan educational programs to increase awareness.

Another example of risk reduction is the practice of contact tracing and notification. Public health departments have mandated reporting of certain sexually transmitted infections and will notify the index patient's sexual partners that they have been exposed to such an infection. They protect the confidentiality of the index patient, although it may be possible for a partner to discern who the index patient is if the patient has only one sexual partner. The confidentiality of the index patient is potentially breached to reduce the risk of untreated infection in others. Public health nurses may be involved in interviewing the index patient and contacting sexual partners.

A third category is public health research. The United States has a blighted history of public health research, including the Tuskegee syphilis study (see Chapter 10) and human radiation experiments in which certain communities were exposed to radiation without their consent (U.S. Department of Energy, 2004). In the Tuskegee syphilis study, it was a public health nurse who was central in the continued deception of the men who were left untreated after penicillin was available for treatment. There is a history of abuse to be overcome. With evidence-based practice, it is very important that public health interventions be based on data. Yet there is difficulty in doing population-based research. Consider the following ethical issues that may arise during various types of population-based research:

- People with HIV/AIDS may not wish to participate in studies where they cannot remain anonymous, yet longitudinal studies require follow-up and tracking. There is concern about confidentiality.
- People may be reluctant to participate in genetics studies for fear of discrimination in insurance or employment if they are discovered to have a certain genetic trait, like the gene for breast cancer. Although data are supposed to be de-identified, potential research participants may not wish to risk a breach of confidentiality.
- In large interventional studies involving communities, community representatives should be included in the planning and implementation of the study. It is a subject of debate whether individual consent needs to be obtained from each person in the community.

For example, the National Cancer Institute studied interventional strategies for decreasing smoking in 11 matched pairs of communities. One community of each matched pair was randomized to the experimental group while the other community became the control. The people in the communities were surveyed annually by phone or mail about their smoking habits and were blind to their designated group (COMMIT Research Group, 1995a, 1995b). Brody (1998) raised the question of whether individual informed consent is needed when recruiting communities. Identifiers were recorded for people in this study because they were recontacted annually. He questioned whether the people in the study should be informed that they are in a study, that they will be randomized to an experimental or control group, and they will be recontacted annually.

Community research, especially on topics such as HIV transmission or infant feeding, is often conducted abroad. As discussed in Chapter 10, research conducted abroad must meet the standards of the home country of the researcher as well as comply with standards of the country in which the study is being done. Western traditions of insisting on a signature to indicate agreement to participate, or even asking for consent from an individual, are atypical in some countries.

Some international projects are not "research" but require attention to culture and ethics. In public health there has been a great deal of emphasis on the global impact of AIDS and on AIDS prevention. Peer-leader programs have been shown to be effective, but some countries do not have the expertise or resources for implementing such a program. In the spirit of social justice, international projects were undertaken by nurses to collaborate with nurse leaders from other countries (Norr, McElmurry, Slutas, Christiansen, Marks, & Misner, 2001).

Health disparities—differences in incidence, prevalence, morbidity, and/or mortality based on race, ethnicity, and socioeconomic level—represent the last category of public health ethics identified by Callahan and Jennings (2002). The U.S. Department of Health and Human Services Office of Minority Health (2004) cited six areas where significant health disparities exist. For example, the African-American infant mortality rate is 14.1 per 1000 live births, compared to the national average infant mortality rate of 6.9 per 1000 live births. Cervical cancer rates in Vietnamese women are five times higher than in white women. African Americans have a 29% higher death rate from cardiovascular disease (40% higher from strokes) than do whites. Hispanics/ Latinos, Mexican Americans, African Americans, Native Americans, and Alaskan natives have diabetes at rates from 1.9 to 2.6 times greater than that of whites. The last two areas in which health disparities exist are with regard to immunization rates and HIV/AIDS incidence. Both childhood and adult immunizations are the focus of Centers for Disease Control and Prevention (CDC) goals. Although it is improving, the rate of childhood immunization is still not 100%. This may never be possible because parents may opt not to vaccinate based on religious objection. Immunization of older adults (65 years and older) for influenza and the organism that causes pneumonia is targeted at 60%. HIV/AIDS is the leading cause of death for African-American men 35 to 44 years of age. The CDC have a number of programs targeted at specific ethnic groups. They have the goal of reducing health disparities by 2010 through the education of health care providers and recipients so as to reduce risk factors and through early identification of signs and symptoms of disease. Will this be enough? There may be other causal factors such as economics and availability that also have ethical implications.

With events of September 11, 2001, the worst terrorist attacks on U.S. soil, resources for public health were affected by the shift toward emergency preparedness and response to another potential attack. Public health departments and health care facilities reviewed their plans for disaster, which included intentional attack by an explosive device or through chemical or biological warfare. Other events, such as potential epidemics due to West Nile virus or severe acute respiratory syndrome (SARS) and natural disasters such as the hurricanes that struck the southeastern and Gulf Coast states in 2004 and 2005, tax public health department resources. Allocation decisions are made in response to the most critical needs. Nurses are at the forefront in identifying and addressing immediate needs, especially as first responders to disasters or other health threats.

SUMMARY

Public health initiatives stem from a communitarian approach to improving the health and lives of communities. It is necessary to balance personal liberties with the communal good. Allocation of resources revolves around need, power, and politics. Nurses take part in allocation decisions in various ways: participating in research, educating clients, families, and communities, and lobbying (individually and as part of a nursing organization) politicians and policy-makers. For there to be social justice, clients' voices must be heard and addressed.

CLINICAL EXERCISES

1. Find your agency's disaster plan. Discuss with the staff nurses whether the plan was altered after September 11, 2001, and if so, how. Did the terrorist attacks affect how resources have been allocated in this agency?

Discussion Questions

1. The school nurse is preparing an educational intervention to reduce injuries from unhelmeted motorcycle riding because helmets are not mandatory in her state. She will present a program entitled "Donors on Wheels" in which she will give the statistics on brain death and organ donation in the 16- to 19-year-old group and ask the students to indicate on their driver's licenses that they wish to become organ donors if they have decided not to wear a helmet.

   a. What are the ethical issues with her approach?
   b. How does this compare with the tactics of showing a cancerous lung to students who smoke?

2. Nurses in an outpatient rehabilitation clinic draft a position paper opposing gun violence and endorsing a political candidate because they like his position on gun control. The director of nursing informs the nurses that they cannot use the agency's name in their endorsement because a member of the agency's board of directors opposes gun control.

   a. What are the ethical issues?
   b. How should the nurses respond to their director of nursing?
   c. Should the nursing profession or health care agencies be allowed to mandate that nurses/employees follow current public health initiatives in their personal life? For example, should the profession or agencies mandate that

nurses must wear helmets when on a motorcycle, make attempts to stop smoking, and so on?

3. Read the American Nurses Association (ANA) (1997) position statement on Opposition to Criminal Prosecution of Women for Use of Drugs While Pregnant.

a. What are the public health issues?
b. What ethical issues are present in this practice?
c. Do you agree with the ANA position? Explain the ethical reasoning supporting your decision.

4. Your nursing student association is considering becoming involved in a community project. Identify and prioritize at least four ethical principles/concepts that you believe the association should consider when making their decision.

Resources

American Nurses Association. (1993). Position statement. AIDS/HIV disease and socio-culturally diverse populations. Retrieved October 1, 2004, from http://nursingworld.org/readroom/position/blood/bldvrs.htm

American Nurses Association. (1991). Position statement: Cultural diversity in nursing practice. Retrieved December 6, 2005, from http://nursingworld.org/readroom/position/ethics/prtetcldv.htm

Common Sense for Drug Policy. (2005). Drug war facts: Medical marijuana. Retrieved December 6, 2005, from http://www.drugwarfacts.org/medicalm.htm

Loyola University Chicago Stritch School of Medicine and The Neisswanger Institute for Bioethics and Health Policy. (2004). Resources in cultural competency. Retrieved December, 6, 2005, from http://www.meddean.luc.edu/depts.bioethics/resources/cultural

Referencses

American Nurses Association. (1997). Opposition to criminal prosecution of women for use of drugs while pregnant. Retrieved May 15, 2005, from http://nursingworld.org/readroom/position/drug/drpreg.htm

Arisaka, Y. (n.d.). Ethics. Arisaka. Liberty limiting principles (LLP). Retrieved October 11, 2005, from www.arisaka.org/ethics02LLP.html

Aroskar, M. A., Moldow, D. G., & Good, C. M. (2004). Nurses' voices: Policy, practice and ethics. *Nursing Ethics, 11*(3), 266–276.

Athar, S. (n.d.). Information for health care providers when dealing with a Muslim patient. Retrieved October 11, 2005, from www.islam-usa.com/e40.html

Basta, S. M. (1992). The historical context. In M. J. Clark (Ed.). *Nursing in the community* (p. 20). Norwalk, CT: Appleton & Lange.

Beauchamp, T. L., & Childress, J. F. (2001). *Principles of biomedical ethics* (5th ed.). New York: Oxford University Press.

Brody, B. A. (1998). *The ethics of biomedical research: An international perspective.* New York: Oxford University Press.

Callahan, D., & Jennings, B. (2002). Ethics and public health: Forging a strong relationship. *American Journal of Public Health, 92*(2), 169–176.

Campinha-Bacote, J. (2003). Many faces: Addressing diversity in health care. *Journal of Issues in Nursing, 8*(1). Available at http://nursingworld.org/ojin/topic20/tpc20_2.htm

Candib, L. M. (2002). Truth telling and advance planning at the end of life: Problems with autonomy in a multicultural world. *Families, Systems & Health, 20*(3), 213–228.

Centers for Disease Control and Prevention. (2003). TB control and confidentiality. Retrieved September 1, 2004, from www.phppo.cdc.gov/PHTN/tbmodules/modules6-9/m7/7-19.htm

Centers for Disease Control and Prevention. (2004). National Center for Injury and Prevention and Control. Projects in prevention: The mortality attributable to unhelmeted head injuries. Retrieved September 20, 2004, from www.cdc.gov/ncipc/profiles/icrcs/ucsf_projects.htm

COMMIT Research Group. (1995a). Community intervention trial for smoking cessation (COMMIT): I. Cohort results from a four-year community intervention. *American Journal of Public Health, 85*(2), 183–192.

COMMIT Research Group. (1995b). Community intervention trial for smoking cessation (COMMIT): II. Changes in adult cigarette smoking prevalence. *American Journal of Public Health, 85*(2), 193–200.

Ergil, K. V. (2001). Chinese medicine. In M. S. Micozzi (Ed.). *Fundamentals of complementary and alternative medicine* (2nd ed.) (pp. 303–344). New York: Churchill Livingstone. ·

Grisso, T., & Appelbaum, P. (1998). *Assessing competence to consent to treatment: A guide for physicians and other health professionals.* New York: Oxford University Press.

Jones, M. J. (1992). Cultural influences on community health. In M. J. Clark (Ed.). *Nursing in the Community* (pp. 280–341). Norwalk, CT: Appleton & Lange.

Ladd, R. E., Pasquerella, L., & Smith, S. (2002). Ethical issues in home health care. *Newsletter on Philosophy & Medicine, 2*(1), 196–197.

Lapine, A., Wang-Cheng, R., Goldstein, M., Nooney, A., Lamb, G., & Derse, A. R. (2001). When cultures clash: Physician, patient, and family wishes in truth disclosure for dying patients. *Journal of Palliative Medicine, 4*(4), 475–480.

Mazanec, P., & Tyler, M. K. (2004). Cultural considerations in end-of-life care: How ethnicity, age, and spirituality affect decisions when death is imminent. *Home Healthcare Nurse, 22*(5), 317–324.

Neff, P., Lyckholm, L., & Smith, T. (2002). Truth or consequences: What to do when the patient does not want to know. *Journal of Clinical Oncology, 20*(13), 3035–3037.

Norr, K. F., McElmurry, B. J., Slutas, F. M., Christiansen, C. D., Marks, B. A., & Misner, S. J. (2001). Mobilizing Lithuanian health professionals as community peer leaders for AIDS prevention: An international primary health care collaboration. *Nursing & Health Care Perspectives, 22*(3), 140–145.

Shultes, R. D., & Hoffman, A. (1992). Plants of the gods: Their sacred, healing, and hallucinogenic powers. Retrieved September 21, 2004, from www.peyote.org

U. S. Department of Health and Human Services Office of Minority Health. (2001). National standards for culturally and linguistically appropriate services in health care. Retrieved October 1, 2004, from www.omhrc.gov/omh/programs/2pgprograms/finalreport.pdf

U. S. Department of Health and Human Services Office of Minority Health. (2004). *Eliminating racial and ethnic disparities.* Retrieved September 27, 2004, from http://www.cdc.gov/omh/Aboutus/disparities.htm

U.S. Department of Energy. (n.d.). Openness: Human radiation experiments. Retrieved September 20, 2004, from www.eh.doe.gov/ohre/index.html

Ethical Issues Impacting the Professional Nurse's Values

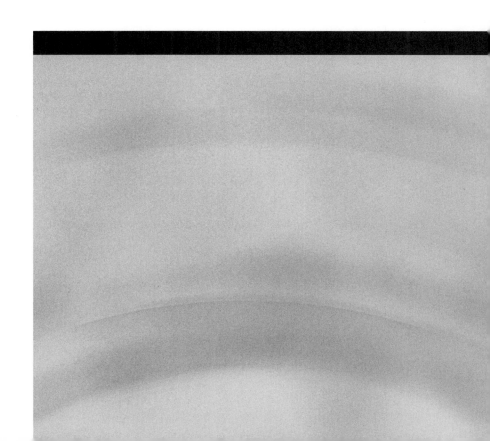

CHAPTER 16

Professional Ethical Issues Facing the Individual Nurse

Objectives

At the end of this chapter, the student should be able to:

1. Discuss the pros and cons associated with mutual recognition licensure models.
2. Identify the professional nurse's ethical obligations in response to an identified clinical error.
3. Identify the rights and obligations related to workplace violence.
4. Debate the nurse's right to privacy regarding the nurse's personal health and concurrent obligation to protect patients.
5. Outline actions a nurse should implement to protect personal information in the workplace.
6. Debate whether routine mandatory testing of nurses for drugs is ethically permissible.
7. Discriminate between an appeal to conscience and an appeal to the principle of nonmaleficence.
8. Discuss laws protecting conscientious objection.
9. Analyze cases that include claims of conscientious objection.
10. Discriminate among incompetent, unethical, illegal, and impaired practice.
11. Name the modifiable variables that can result in a nurse's incompetent or impaired practice.
12. Discuss strategies for identifying, assisting, and finally reintegrating the impaired nurse back into a practice setting.
13. Identify strategies for maintaining competent practice throughout a nursing career.
14. Apply legislative standards and ethical principles in considering how to respond when a colleague displays incompetent or impaired practice.

15. Identify the requirements of whistle-blowing.

16. Differentiate between illegal and unethical practice.

17. Discuss resources and strategies needed and/or available before and after making a whistle-blowing decision.

KEY WORDS

- *Appeal to conscience*
- *Appeal to nonmaleficence*
- *Conscience*
- *Conscientious objection*
- *Controlled-drug misuse*
- *Culture of silence*
- *Illegal practice*
- *Impaired practice*
- *Incompetent practice*
- *Integrity*

- *Interstate compact*
- *Mutual recognition model*
- *Reciprocity*
- *Right*
- *Substance abuse*
- *Unethical practice*
- *Unsafe practice*
- *Whistle-blowing*
- *Workplace violence*

SECTION 1: *Ethical Themes: Building From the Basic to the Complex*

When considering professional issues facing the individual nurse, the focus of the four ethical themes discussed earlier in this book switches from the patient to the individual nurse. Thus, this section considers the nurse's moral commitment to promote confidentiality, truth-telling, advocacy, and allocation of resources as these apply to the individual nurse.

CONFIDENTIALITY

Confidentiality requires that personal data be protected and shared only on a need-to-know basis, but how does this concept pertain to the individual nurse's personal data? Such data are kept confidential by actions implemented by the nurse and safeguards implemented by others.

Self-Regulation of Confidential Information

One common practice used by nurses to protect their personal data is setting professional boundaries, which limit the type of information shared in a professional relationship. However, the type of information shared may vary based on the type of relationship. For example, a nurse may share how she coped emotionally with infertility treatment as a way to establish an empathetic link with a patient, but not disclose the reasons for her infertility. In addition, a nurse might disclose a current medical problem to a supervisor to justify a need to leave work early the next day, but choose not to disclose her medical condition to colleagues because they have no need to know why she is leaving early.

Another way nurses keep personal information confidential is by protecting personal passwords, codes, and identifying information, such as social security, employee, and credit card numbers. For example, during clinical rotations students may be required to access narcotic medications with their faculty or a staff nurse. On busy days, the temptation is great for the faculty member to give the student the faculty's identification number and/or password. However, doing so could create numerous potential problems because knowing the faculty's identification number could provide a student with access to the faculty's personnel record, student records, or restricted computer databases depending on how the university and/or agency has linked them.

Nurses who conduct personal business by cell phone during their lunch break could also be broadcasting their information to anyone walking by the doorway to the nurse's lounge, thus threatening the integrity of their credit accounts if credit card numbers are read out loud. Similarly, nurses frequently mark out their credit card numbers when submitting credit receipts to apply for reimbursement after attending a continuing education program.

Regulation of Employee Information

Employers have an obligation to protect employee information. At first glance, this seems obvious. The Health Insurance Portability and Accountability Act (HIPAA) required that everyone receive confidentiality notices from health care providers and pharmacies on how their accounts and files will be protected. However, other threats to privacy can occur routinely in the workplace. For example, many nursing units have an employee Rolodex (or computer database) with phone numbers that is often accessible to any unit employee or person entering the unit's nurses lounge or office. This practice can threaten the privacy of a nurse with an unlisted phone number or provide a disgruntled employee or family member with access to harass the nurse by phone.

Another way nursing leadership or colleagues might inadvertently breach a nurse's confidentiality can occur when the nurse calls in sick. A routine response to learning that someone is ill is to ask what is wrong; the nurse is not obligated to disclose a diagnosis to the charge nurse when calling in sick. The charge nurse's question could be justified if he or she is attempting to find out how long the nurse anticipates being off work so that alternate staffing could be arranged. Depending on the agency's policy, the nurse may be required to disclose his or her medical history and obtain clearance from the employee health service to return back to work after an illness.

Nursing leadership has a duty to protect a nurse's confidentiality related to employee performance evaluations. Only nurses who are assigned as preceptors or have staff education responsibilities should be privy to a nurse's professional development plan unless the nurse divulges this information to colleagues. In the same vein, a nurse's chemical addiction history must be protected when he or she is returning to work after successfully completing a rehabilitation program. Often, the nurse and agency will agree that the nurse will return to new unit and/or shift as a means for protecting the nurse's history from other nurses. Thus, nursing leaders must design mechanisms for monitoring the nurse's behavior without arousing the curiosity of the other nursing team members. When creating these mechanisms, the nursing leader will need to identify who has a need to know about the nurse's addiction. For example, does the shift charge nurse need to know? Does this "need to know" change if the charge role is held by one designated person versus being rotated among four different persons?

Another threat to employee confidentiality can occur via routine monitoring reports. Often nursing leaders will post a staff roster highlighting the names of the persons who have not complied with the expected standard, such as annual tuberculosis testing. Thus, the staff nurse may feel forced to explain, "I am PPD positive" or "I received BCG before my stint in the Peace Corps, therefore, I cannot have a TB test." To many this may seem a benign threat, but the possibility exists for an uninformed person to treat the nurse differently based on an inaccurate assumption that the nurse has tuberculosis.

Finally, a nurse's confidentiality can be violated by colleagues with good intentions. For example, a nurse receives a needle-stick injury while decannulating the Port-a-Cath of a patient with HIV. In an attempt to create peer support and/or to prevent similar harm to other nurses, the charge nurse might announce the occurrence during a staff meeting. Thus, the injured nurse's colleagues might ask her about her HIV test results out of concern and not consider that for a variety of reasons she might not want to discuss them. In addition, news frequently travels fast through a health care agency; thus, the potential exists for the nurse's significant other, who is also an employee, to learn about the injury through the grapevine.

Thus, nurses have an obligation to protect not only their personal and professional data, but also those of their peers. In addition, nursing administrators and agencies have an obligation to institute practices that protect employee data while providing the necessary resources for the nurse to be successful and safe in his or her job. Thus, every employee must always consider whether he or she needs to know some information before seeking it about a professional colleague.

TRUTH-TELLING

Disclosure of Mistakes

Chapter 7 discussed the nurse's obligation to fulfill the ethical requirements of veracity as well as reasons that have been used to justify nontruthful disclosures. One reason proposed for not telling the truth was to prevent harm to self. Health care providers may consider following this rationale after an adverse event has occurred, such as a medication error. Based on this rationale, the nurse fears that disclosing the medication error could cause professional, legal, and/or personal harm to him or her. For example, the nurse might think, "If the patient finds out about this error, I might get sued," or, "I am still on probation, if my unit leader finds out about this mistake, I will lose my job." Often these fears prove to be unfounded. For example, hospitals with full-disclosure policies experience lower malpractice costs (Banja, 2001).

Another rationale that may be used to justify not disclosing an error is that of preventing further harm to the other person. For example, a nurse might hypothesize, "The patient was not really harmed by receiving the medication late, and telling him will only make him worry and undermine his faith in his health care team; therefore, not telling him about this error is the kindest thing I can do." Whereas the temptation to conceal errors can be great, nurses and other health care professionals have a moral obligation to disclose not only a harm-causing error, but also errors that do not produce a harm. Failure to disclose an error negates the patient's ability to make informed autonomous decisions:

Patients have the right not to be maltreated; but if they are, they have the right to consider some form of redress for the harm they suffered—which can only happen if they are informed of the error. The health provider or institution that fails to inform harms the patient twice: first, by failing to deliver care that met the professional standard (i.e., that involved negligence), and second, by failing to alert the harmed party to the error and so accommodate his or her right to redress. By failing to disclose, then, the health provider is conspicuously placing his or her self-interests above the patient's. (Banja, 2001, p. 2)

Acknowledging and reporting an error is an act of moral courage (Banja, 2001) by which the nurse safeguards the patient's rights while protecting his or her own. Thus, when truthfully acknowledging an error, the nurse is forced to "accept her own humanity and the humanity of the patient" (Husted & Husted, 2001, pp. 64–65).

Since the publication of the Institute of Medicine's (2000) report *To Err is Human: Building a Safer Health System*, much effort has been exerted to identify mechanisms to prevent errors, including reporting structures, system review, and education.

Reporting Systems

The reporting of medical errors can occur both internal and external to the agency. For example, many agencies report errors or "unusual occurrences" via a standardized form that requests information on what happened, who was involved, who witnessed the incident, and who was notified (Figure 16-1). Nursing leadership has the discretion of using these unusual occurrence forms to fulfill a variety of ethical commitments. First, the nurse leader has an ethical commitment to benefit the nurse employees; thus, unusual occurrence information could be used to justify a continuing education series on, for example, intravenous delivery systems. Second, the nurse leader has an ethical commitment to protect patients from harm; thus, repeated evidence of errors despite educational interventions by a single nurse may require disciplinary action. Third, the nurse leader can use the unusual occurrence information to look for patterns that might relate to system issues. Consider Figure 16-1. During a 1-week period, the nurse leader on the neurosurgical unit noted three separate incidents in which a patient received an intravenous (IV) dose of mannitol early. When talking with the staff nurses, the nurse leader found that mannitol was supplied by the pharmacy in a multidose bag. Thus, a nurses would set the pump to deliver 250 cc from a 1000-cc bag. When the 250 cc was delivered, the IV pump would stop. However, errors occurred when the pump alarmed and the IV piggyback restarted along with the primary IV solution when a nurse not assigned to the patient responded to the alarm.

UNUSUAL OCCURRENCE FORM

_____✓_____ PATIENT _____ VISITOR _____ OTHER (check one)

Date of incident: _____February 10, 2006_____ Time of incident: _____9:30_____ A.M. _____ P.M. ___✓___

Location of incident: __Neuro Surgical Unit_____

                                                 (Unit/Area)

Attending physician: __Jones_____

Witness: _____None_____ Phone No.: _____

Witness: _____ Phone No.: _____

TYPE OF INCIDENT: Medication Error

INCIDENT FACTS/DATA (Should be consistent with what is written in the medical record)

> Patient status postcraniotomy. Has triple-lumen catheter, continuous IV fluids, and mannitol IV piggyback every 6 hours. Staff nurse requested that student perform patient's blood draw for ordered laboratory tests. Nursing student stopped IV pump prior to blood draw. IV pump was connected to 1000-cc normal-saline bag and a 500-cc mannitol IV piggyback bag (pharmacy supplies mannitol as a multidose bag). Student turned IV pump back on, following the blood draw, with primary IV, then infusing. At 10:45 PM, the staff nurse noted that the mannitol IV piggyback bag was infusing, not the primary IV fluids. Staff nurse stopped the infusion of mannitol, and the IV pump was reprogrammed to infuse the primary IV fluids at the ordered rate. The patient's vital signs and neurological assessment remain unchanged. Dr. Jones notified of event. 12 midnight dose of mannitol to be held per Dr. Jones' order.

Preparer's Signature:

Sally Smith, Nursing Student   Date: February 10, 2006   Time: 11:30 PM
Jane Brown, RN

Figure 16-1
Unusual occurrence form.

Based on this information, the nurse leader and staff nurses strategized on mechanisms for preventing future errors. Potential strategies included the use of single-dose mannitol IV bags, disconnecting the multidose IV piggyback from the primary tubing after the dose was administered, adding a burretrol, and/or placing a warning sticker on the IV pump. Because three nurses were willing to report their actions, future patients and nurses were spared from experiencing the same error.

Some agencies have also initiated an anonymous "Oops, I almost made a mistake" hotline. These hotlines are intended to identify system issues that create the potential for errors without placing employees at disciplinary risk. In addition, the Medical Errors Reporting Program, a national voluntary reporting structure for medication errors, receives 1000 reports annually. The confidential information is used by pharmaceutical companies, the Food and Drug Administration, and other regulatory agencies to improve standards, labeling, and manufacturing designs (Cohen, 2000).

Thus, truthful disclosure of errors is evidence of an ethical commitment to promoting informed decision-making, autonomy, and nonmaleficence. A nurse who is honest and forthcoming about actual and potential errors exemplifies the profession's commitment to quality nursing care as stipulated in Provision 3.4 of the American Nurses Association (ANA) (2001) Code of Ethics for Nurses:

Nurses should be active participants in the development of policies and review mechanisms designed to promote patient safety, reduce the likelihood of errors. . . . When errors do occur, nurses are expected to follow institutional guidelines in reporting errors committed or observed to the appropriate supervisory personnel and for assuring responsible disclosure of errors to patients. Under no circumstances should the nurse participate in, or condone through silence, either an attempt to hide an error or a punitive response that serves only to fix blame rather than correct the conditions that led to the error. (Reprinted with permission from American Nurses Association, *Code of ethics for nurses with interpretive statements,* © 2001 nursesbooks.org, American Nurses Association, Washington, D.C.)

Disclosure of a Nurse's Personal Health Status

One of the first lessons that a beginning nursing student learns is that in a helping therapeutic relationship "it is inappropriate for the nurse to share her own needs and problems with the client" (Sundeen, Stuart, Rankin, & Cohen, 1998, p. 187). The rationale supporting this claim is that in a therapeutic relationship all actions and conversation should focus on meeting the patient's health goals. However, the nurse's ability to fulfill this expectation becomes difficult when the nurse's personal problem has the potential of causing harm to the patient. Answering this question becomes more complex when the nurse has to consider who needs to know this information. Therefore, this quandary involves both issues of confidentiality and truthfulness.

Disclosure to Protect the Nurse
Nurses can be exposed to a variety of contagious infections in their professional roles. Because of this potential exposure, a variety of isolation techniques and personal protective gear is implemented on a daily basis in every health care setting. Personal

protective gear includes gowns, gloves, and eye goggles. In spite of these protections, agencies may develop policies limiting who can and cannot enter a room. For example, the isolation plan for a patient with herpes zoster ("shingles") may include excluding anyone who is pregnant or has not had or been vaccinated for varicella ("chickenpox") from entering the room. This limitation may put a health care provider in an awkward position of having to disclose a pregnancy or past medical history.

Although disclosing one's immunization status may be viewed as fairly benign and perhaps considered a topic for general conversation (especially when the virus is going around the local grade school), nurses may be reluctant to disclose pregnancy for a variety of reasons.

Some nurses may evade disclosing personal information by volunteering for other patient assignments, such as "I would like more experience working with a patient with pancreatitis, why don't I take Mr. Jones and you take Ms. Smith?" Nurses may also evade the disclosure of personal information to peers by telling white lies or making up information. For example, instead of disclosing her pregnancy, a nurse might claim to not have had varicella or the varicella vaccine as a way to avoid being assigned to care for the patient with herpes zoster. A utilitarian would argue that the nurse was justified in lying about her immunization status because the end justifies the means. The nurse should not be in contact with the patient. The patient's health care goals were not compromised by the lie and the nurse's personal life remained confidential; thus, telling the lie seems to have created more benefit than harm. However, a deontologist would counter that truthfulness is always a good action and should always be promoted. In addition, a nurse has a duty to respect her peers, and lying to them does not fulfill this duty; if the deception is recognized, long-term harm may occur to the peer relationship.

Disclosure to Protect the Patient

A nurse may also find himself or herself in a situation in which he or she must consider whether to disclose personal health information as means for protecting the patient. Sometimes this is easy to decide. Mr. Smith is immunocompromised after a bone marrow transplant. His primary care nurse may disclose that "I think I am coming down with a cold; therefore, I have decided not to work with you today. While I will miss working with you, I believe that this decision is in your best interests." For many persons, admitting to an upper respiratory infection is of little consequence because the symptoms are generally visible to the public. However, this is not always the case with other infections.

After an incident in which a dentist transmitted HIV to several patients, questions were raised about whether a health care professional should disclose his or her HIV, hepatitis, or other blood-borne pathogen status to patients, and, if so, to which patients. The ethical issue centers on the nurse's need to balance doing no harm to the patient and not causing harm to himself or herself (e.g., threat to the nurse's financial situation if his or her job was lost due to the disclosure of HIV status). Another way this ethical issue can be described is as a conflict between the patient's right to informed consent and autonomy and the nurse's right to privacy. Despite the progress science has made with treating HIV, a social stigma still remains attached to the infection, which has the potential to harm a nurse's personal and profession goals if disclosed (Singh, 2001). Whereas nurses are required to treat all patient information confidentially, there is not an expectation that a patient will or should treat the nurse's personal information in such a manner. In other words, patients are free to discuss information about any health care provider with any other person (Fost, 2000).

This ethical question becomes more complex when one realizes that a potential for a double standard exists. A patient is expected to disclose his or her infectious disease to health care professionals to allow them to implement the necessary and appropriate actions needed to provide effective treatment for the patient and protect themselves from his or her infection. However, patients are often not given the opportunity to make a comparable decision. In other words, a patient cannot make an informed decision about how to protect himself or herself if the patient is not aware of the health care provider's infectious status. Patients select their health care providers based on a variety of subjective and objective criteria (Fost, 2000; Singh, 2001). It is not unreasonable for a pregnant woman to select a nurse midwife who has tested seronegative for HIV if the woman has a history of tearing that requires vaginal sutures. Similarly, a nurse midwife would want to know the woman's HIV status so that appropriate precautions could be taken throughout the labor and birth process. This reciprocal and generalizable expectation is a nice illustration of the principle of universality, which was introduced in Chapter 1.

Whereas a patient may select a health care provider based on specific criteria, such as HIV status, it is not ethical for a nurse to refuse to provide care to a patient with HIV (assuming protective gear is available). This expectation is included in the first provision of the ANA (2001) Code of Ethics for Nurses: "The nurse, in all professional relationships, practices with compassion and respect for the inherent dignity, worth and uniqueness of every individual, unrestricted by consideration of social or economic status, personal attributes, or the nature of health problems." (ANA, 2001. Used with permission.) This expectation is also addressed in the ANA (1994a) position statement on Risk Versus Responsibility in Providing Nursing Care:

The general principle of practice is that nurses are morally obligated to care for all clients. However, in certain cases the risks of harm may outweigh a nurse's responsibility to care for a given client. For example, a nurse who is immunosuppressed may be justified in refusing to care for clients with certain infectious processes. Risk, therefore, must be assessed by each individual nurse. Accepting personal risk which exceeds the limits of duty is not morally obligatory; it is a moral option. (p. 2)
(Reprinted with permission from nursesbooks.org)

Current Requirements
The Center for Disease Control and Prevention's (CDC) (1991) recommendations stipulate that:

HCWs [health care workers] who are infected with HIV or HBV [hepatitis B virus] (and are HBeAg [hepatitis Be antigen] positive) should not perform exposure-prone procedures unless they have sought counsel from an expert review panel and been advised under what circumstances, if any, they may continue to perform these procedures. Such circumstances would include notifying prospective patients of the HCW's seropositivity before they undergo exposure-prone invasive procedures. (p. 5)

The CDC (1991) recommendations also stipulate that:

HCWs who perform exposure-prone procedures should know their HIV antibody status. HCWs who perform exposure-prone procedures and who do not have serologic evidence of immunity to HBV from vaccination or from previous infection should know their HBsAg [hepatitis B surface antigen] status and, if that is positive, should also know their HBeAg status. (p. 5)

Many health care professionals are reluctant to be tested (Fost, 2000). These individuals believe that "If I do not know my status then I can honestly say I do not know and I do not have to face the dilemma of whether to lie or not." Although this line of reasoning may sidestep questions related to veracity, refusal to be tested and/or treated can create potential harm not only to the health care provider, but also his or her significant others and perhaps patients.

The Americans with Disability Act (1990) offers protections for health care providers who are unable to carry out their usual job duties due to the potential transmission of an infectious disease. Employers are required to assist the health care worker to retrain if necessary for a job that does not involve the risky activities (Fost, 2000). For example, a surgeon could become a radiologist and a trauma nurse could assume the emergency department triage position.

Many institutions have policies and procedures related to employees with various infectious diseases. Each nurse must comply with the institution's policy and procedure. Complying with the policy may require the nurse to trust his or her private information with the designated person(s); however, following the institution's policy should protect the nurse if questions are raised about the nurse's status.

ADVOCACY

Workplace Violence

Nurses are often concerned about their safety when commuting to work because of the need to work odd hours and possibly travel through neighborhoods with high crime rates. They have also become increasingly aware that working in a health care facility does not guarantee their safety (Henderson, 2003; Love, Morrison, & AAN Expert Panel on Violence, 2003). In fact, in 1999 the Australian Institute of Criminology ranked nurses as the next to the highest in incidence of workplace violence claims, surpassing prison workers and police officers (Jones & Lyneham, 2000).

Workplace violence can encompass a variety of abuses, including physical, sexual, emotional, and verbal. In addition, physical abuse can range from a threat of physical harm to shoving to the use of weapons. One nurse described work place violence as:

Anything that makes you feel unsafe, fearful or anything that does not allow you to perform your job through intimidation, repression, fear of repercussions or not

*respectful of you as a person in your own right as a nurse, be it from medical col-
leagues, clients, management, relatives etc. Where your concerns are pushed aside
and they make you feel inadequate. (Jones & Lyneham, 2000, p. 28)*

Thus, workplace violence can be blatantly obvious to all present or insidious and
secretive.

The escalation in workplace violence has been linked to a variety of factors,
including the following:

- *Increased waiting times and frustrations;*
- *Increased use of weapons (in society);*
- *Inadequate systems of security (in health care facilities);*
- *Culture of silence;*
- *Inadequate support for emergent mental health needs;*
- *Lack of reporting (to both law enforcement and administrators);*
- *Lack of institutional concern and systems of support; and*
- *Demands of triage nursing. (Jones & Lyneham, 2000, p. 27)*

Additionally, nurses who work alone, with medications, with people with emotional or
substance abuse problems, and in clinical areas undergoing institutional reform may
be more likely to experience workplace violence (International Labour Office, International Council of Nurses, World Health Organization, & Public Service International, 2002).

Nurses, like all persons, have a moral right to be safe and free from harm. When
a moral right exists, others as well as that individual have an ethical obligation to
advocate to protect the individual from harm. The easiest way for a person to respect
a nurse's right to be safe is to refrain from committing a harmful act, such as a physical or verbal assault. However, this failure to act, although praiseworthy, may not be
sufficient to protect the nurse's right to be free from harm. Thus, nursing and agency
administrators as well as security personnel have an ethical obligation to engage in
positive actions that increase the safety of the nurse's work environment. Actions that
have been implemented by many health care institutions include requiring that all
employees wear their agency identification while in the building, locking specific
units, such as the newborn nursery and psychiatric units, and ensuring the around-
the-clock presence of security guards in the emergency department.

In addition, agencies may implement policies that assist in monitoring and/or
limiting the number and/or location of visitors. For example, agencies may limit the
number of entries after 5 P.M. or on weekends and holidays, require all visitors to sign
in and wear visitor tags, and not allow family members arriving after posted visiting
hours to walk through without first being cleared by the charge nurse and/or having
an escort.

The increasing incidence of workplace violence is forcing nurses, individually and
collectively, to be active advocates for promoting the nurses' right to work in a safe

and supportive environment. Effective advocacy requires that nurses break the culture of silence that has often surrounded workplace violence, especially when the violence is between a nurse and someone with greater perceived positional power, such as a nursing administrator or physician. Thus, nurses have an ethical obligation to report acts of workplace violence.

Other actions an individual nurse could take to promote his or her safety include knowing current policy and procedures related to workplace violence and filing a grievance, when appropriate; requesting continuing education on cultural sensitivity, interpersonal communication skills, assertiveness, and/or self-defense training; developing stress management and crisis management skills; and promoting a workplace culture that is open and supportive (International Labour Office et al., 2002).

Nursing administrators have additional advocacy responsibilities. Nursing administrators need to advocate for workplace safety by creating appropriate staffing ratios and addressing system issues that could escalate into violent situations if not addressed, including the physical environment (noise, lighting, and environmental comfort) and workplace access, space, waiting areas, and security systems (International Labour Office et al., 2002). When incidents or workplace violence occurs, nursing administrators must work to counter a nurse's possible feelings of responsibility by providing resources for debriefing and counseling, emergency medical care if needed, and assistance with police and/or legal reports. Finally, staff nurses and nursing administrators have an ethical obligation to support their colleagues during their time of recovery and confidence rebuilding (International Labour Office et al.).

Creating a safe workplace is an ethical obligation shared by every employee, administrator, and visitor. Nurses have an ethical duty to protect their personal interests, which includes their physical, emotional, and sexual safety. Workplace violence represents an arena in which the nurse's primary responsibility may be to himself or herself. Once the nurse's safety is assured, he or she can then work to assure the safety of others in the environment. Although nurses may choose to engage in altruistic actions, there is no ethical mandate for a nurse to risk his or her safety for others in the workplace.

ALLOCATION OF RESOURCES

Interstate Licensure

The licensing of professional nurses demonstrates the commitment of the nursing profession and the individual states to nonmaleficence. Through the National Council Licensure Examination (NCLEX), the nursing profession and the individual states attempt to protect the public from nurses unable to demonstrate a minimum level of competency. The current nursing licensure process does not evaluate the graduate nurse's psychomotor skills or ability to apply nursing knowledge in a real clinical setting; this evaluation remains the responsibility of the nursing education system.

The power of individual states to license nurses and other health care providers is based on the Tenth Amendment to the U.S. Constitution (Hall, 1996), which asserts, "The powers not delegated to the United States by the Constitution, nor prohibited by it to the States, are reserved to the States respectively, or to the people." Despite the fact that the NCLEX is a national exam given in all states and territories, a nurse's license is granted by the state in which the exam was taken, based on the assumption that this is the state in which the nurse will work; however, this is not always the case. Nurses frequently move for career or educational opportunities and/or to be closer to family or friends or be in specific geographic locales.

When a nurse desires to engage in nursing activities (either as a paid employee or volunteer), he or she must possess a nursing license for the state in which the nursing activities will be performed. If the nurse holds a nursing license granted by another state, he or she must apply for licensing reciprocity, according to which the new state will recognize the original nursing license as evidence of the nurse's competency and grant a new nursing license without requiring the nurse to retake the NCLEX, which would be required if the nurse had never passed it or has an expired license.

The reciprocity process allows other states to review a nurse's licensure status and ascertain whether he or she is in good professional standing in his or her original state. For example, the new state could inquire into whether the nurse had ever had a judgment awarded in a malpractice suit or had practice limitations due to a history of substance abuse. Because many registered nurses hold a nursing license in more than one state, one can easily realize the amount of work the reciprocity process can create (Hellquist & Spector, 2004). Reciprocity demonstrates how individual states act to maintain a safe level of nursing practice; however, this system is not without problems.

One frequently experienced problem is that the reciprocity process takes time, and states do not guarantee a decision within a specific amount of time. Thus, the possibility exists that a nurse could relocate, but not have been granted a new nursing license. The failure to obtain a nursing license in a timely fashion could cause a variety of harms for the individual nurse as well as the institution where the nurse wishes to affiliate. For example, the nurse may suffer financial harms if he or she is prohibited from starting a new job or is forced to work as an unlicensed assistive personnel until the new nursing license is granted. In addition, the institution's goals may be delayed or thwarted if a new employee cannot work. Finally, the failure to obtain a timely nursing license through reciprocity can create potential harm to patients in the new state if the healthcare agency is unable to provide safe staffing ratios.

Based on these concerns, The National Council of State Boards of Nursing proposed a "mutual recognition model" that would operate similar to the current U.S. driver's license system (Kulig, 2001). The mutual recognition model "allows a nurse who holds a license in one state to practice in others without additional licenses" (Kulig, 2001, p. 51). This model is especially attractive as more nurses engage in electronically delivered nursing care (Muller & Flarey, 2004) or are employed as traveling nurses, which requires them to frequently cross state borders. Twenty-one states have agreed to this mutual recognition model by entering into an interstate compact agreement (Box 16-1).

Although the mutual recognition model provides many benefits, this plan is not without criticism. First, the creation of any large database for reporting information pertinent to a nurse's license raises questions about how to protect a nurse's confidentiality (Ray, 1999). Second, disciplinary actions are usually filed in the nurse's state of residence, but the possibility exists for actions to be filed in both the residency as well as the remote-practice state, which could compound the nurse's legal costs (Ray, 1999). Third, the practice state may rescind a nurse's ability to practice in that state, but cannot revoke the nurse's nursing license granted by the residency state. Fourth, in the event of a nursing strike, the mutual recognition model may facilitate an institution's efforts to hire nonunionized nurses (Kulig, 2001), which can be perceived

---

BOX 16-1

States Implementing the Nurse Licensure Compact

State	Implementation Date
Arizona	7/1/2002
Arkansas	7/1/2000
Delaware	7/1/2000
Idaho	7/1/2001
Iowa	7/1/2000
Maine	7/1/2001
Maryland	7/1/1999
Mississippi	7/1/2001
Nebraska	1/1/2001
New Hampshire	To be determined
New Jersey	To be determined
New Mexico	1/1/2004
North Carolina	7/1/2000
North Dakota	1/1/2004
South Carolina	To be determined
South Dakota	1/1/2001
Tennessee	7/1/2003
Texas	1/1/2000
Utah	1/1/2000
Virginia	1/1/2005
Wisconsin	1/1/2000

Source: Reprinted with permission from National Council of State Boards of Nursing. (2005). Nurse licensure compacts: Compact implementation. Retrieved December 7, 2005, from http://www.ncsbn.org/nlc/rnlpvncompact_mutual_recognition_state.asp

---

as a threat to nursing unions and professional solidarity. Fifth, because each state has its own nurse practice act, the interstate model does not define nursing practice (Muller & Flarey, 2004). Finally, this model does not include advanced practice nurses (Kulig, 2001).

In addition to these interstate issues, the mutual recognition model raises questions about whether the United States should have a mutual recognition model with other countries such as Canada, England, the Philippines, or Ireland. International graduate nursing students are prime examples of nurses who could benefit from such a model; however, this idea also raises the previously discussed concerns regarding confidentiality and discipline.

SUMMARY

Professional nurses can encounter a variety of ethical situations in which their commitment to the patient can be in conflict with the their personal and/or professional goals. Nurses need to be aware of current institutional as well as state and federal laws when deciding how to act. As with many ethical issues, prospective thinking and peer support can facilitate a nurse's decision-making when confronted with an ethical issue involving his or her professional role.

CLINICAL EXERCISES

1. Does your clinical agency or university have a violence prevention program or policy addressing workplace violence, verbal or physical abuse, and sexual harassment?
2. Identify your agency's policy on employee disclosure of personal health information.
3. Whitley, Jacobson, and Gawrys (1996) suggested the following clinical exercise: How aware are you of the resources and potential liabilities in your clinical environment? How quickly could you get to an exit from your assigned patient care location? How would you obtain assistance if needed? Are there any objects present that could be used as a weapon? What objects are available to protect you if someone were to approach you with a weapon? How would you describe the milieu of the clinical area (sedate, tense, chaotic, etc.)? What factors could result in a rapid change in the clinical area's milieu?
4. Ask a nurse at your clinical site about his or her experiences with seeking a nursing license in a different state than the one on which he or she took the NCLEX. How long did the process take? What type of documentation did he or she need to provide? Was he or she asked any personal information (e.g., some states require information about child support)?

Discussion Questions

1. You are completing the application to take the NCLEX. You need to identify the state in which you want to take the exam. Should you select a neighboring state that is part of the mutual recognition program rather than your home state that does not belong? Why or why not?
2. Describe how you would respond (Whom would you notify? How would you document the event? What actions would you take? etc.) to the following discoveries:

   a. When administering your 12 noon medications, you notice that the 9 A.M. antibiotic IV piggyback did not infuse.

b. When transcribing orders, you notice that the physician ordered "100 units of SQ regular insulin before each meal"; however, during the admission interview, the patient clearly stated "I take 10 units of SQ regular insulin before each meal."

c. You are administering medications for a group of patients on a cardiac step-down unit. After administering medications to the patient in Room 201 Bed B, you realize that the medication Kardexes for Room 201 Bed A and Room 201 Bed B were interchanged. Although you gave the two correct medications, the doses were not correct (e.g., the patient received 150 mg rather than 200 mg of Drug A and 500 mg rather than 325 mg of Drug B).

d. You are hepatitis B virus–positive and are completing a rotation on a pediatric psychiatric unit. Your 6-year-old patient begins to act out and bites your forearm deep enough to cause bleeding. What ethical questions does this situation raise? What actions should you take? What resources are available to assist you in your decision-making?

e. Before the United States were to enter into a mutual recognition model with another country, such as the Philippines, what ethical and social justice issues would need to be addressed first?

3. Based on the criteria suggested by Anderson (2002), evaluate your clinical agency's or university's violence policy for the following:

- How is violence defined?
- What are the goals of the policy?
- What employee actions are expected?
- What training and preventive measures are outlined?
- What risk factors are identified?
- What actions for dealing with violence are included?
- How clear is the reporting structure?
- What legal and counseling resources are identified?

4. Several years ago, you were enrolled in an anger management program, as directed by the court, after a family dispute. Today, you recognize the mother of your pediatric patient as another participant in the anger management program. The mother approaches the charge nurse and says, "I do not want that student working with my son. I know for a fact that the student has an anger problem." What factors will you need to consider before responding to the charge nurse's question about this mother's concerns?

5. Identify the ethical rationale supporting and negating the routine mandatory testing of all nurses for HIV and hepatitis B virus.

SECTION 2: *Professional Nurse Issue: Conscientious Objection*

Conscientious objection is frequently discussed in relationship to the professional nurse's participation in pregnancy termination, a timely and sometimes controversial women's health issue. However, questions about conscientious objection can occur with a variety of other issues that involve values.

Conscientious objection is a term that is frequently used by some professionals but is poorly understood by other professionals, including nurses. Conscientious objection is based on an appeal to conscience when a person believes that if a given action were implemented, then he or she would experience harm. Conscience is a form of self-reflection or judgment about whether actions are (1) obligatory or prohibited, (2) right or wrong, or (3) good or bad. Conscience is based on one's personal standards and calls attention to the (potential) loss of one's integrity and wholeness (Beauchamp & Childress, 2001).

Integrity can be described in two ways. First, *moral integrity* reflects a commitment to moral principles over time. Persons lacking moral integrity are often referred to as being hypocritical or insincere. The second type of integrity is *personal integrity*, which reflects a commitment to one's personal goals. People with personal integrity may not have moral integrity (Beauchamp & Childress, 2001). For example, Jesse James, the infamous outlaw of the U.S. West in the 1880s, displayed personal integrity. He worked hard to achieve his goals of acquiring personal wealth; however, most would agree that he lacked moral integrity! Unfortunately, recent corporate scandals, like that involving Enron, are providing more examples of persons who lack moral integrity.

APPEAL TO CONSCIENCE

Conscientious objection comes into play when a nurse refuses to participate in an action based on religious beliefs or the equivalent moral conviction if the nurse is not religious. For example, a nurse who is an active member of an Orthodox Jewish temple and is employed at a nursing home may refuse to discontinue an elderly patient's feeding tube with the intent of allowing the patient to die. This nurse's conscientious objection is based on the belief that life, regardless of the quality, should be promoted and protected. Typically when confronted with an appeal to one's conscience, a nurse would state something like, "I would not be able to live with myself if I participated in this action." Thus, a nurse engaging in conscientious objection is attempting to act consistently with his or her values and moral beliefs to avoid violating his or her belief system and harming his or her psychological state (Brushwood, 1993).

Conscientious Objection Laws

The three types of laws exist to protect a person engaging in conscientious objection (Brushwood, 1993). First, *employment laws* are based on professional codes, such as the ANA (2001) Code of Ethics for Nurses. Second, *religious discrimination laws* stipulate that a person cannot be discriminated against based on his or her religious practice. Finally, *conscience clauses* are included in specific legislation. For example, Illinois has a Right of Conscience Act (Amendment to the Illinois Right of Conscience Act, 1997), which states:

> *It is the public policy of the State of Illinois to respect and protect the right of conscience of all persons who refuse to obtain, receive or accept, or who are engaged in, the delivery of, arrangement for, or payment of health care services and medical care whether acting individually, corporately, or in association with other persons; and to prohibit all forms of discrimination, disqualification, coercion, disability or imposition of liability upon such persons or entities by reason of their refusing to act contrary to their conscience or conscientious convictions in refusing to obtain, receive, accept, deliver, pay for, or arrange for the payment of health care services and medical care. (Section 2)*

The definition of conscience included in this law is as follows:

> *Conscience: means a sincerely held set of moral convictions arising from belief in and relation to God, or which, though not so derived, arises from a place in the life of its possessor parallel to that filled by God among adherents to religious faiths. (Section 3e)*

Thus, an Illinois nurse using the Illinois Right of Conscience Act as rationale for refusing to act must be able to identify a religious value or its equivalent that was at risk during the situation in question. However, the Act does not require the person to identify a specific commandment or tenet that requires the refusal.

Discussion Exercises 16-1

Ann Niemeczura has been an operating room scrub nurse for 10 years and has willingly participated in pregnancy termination. Last week, Ann witnessed a termination that made her change her position on assisting at such procedures. After being notified by Ann about the change in her stance, her supervisor questions whether Ann can qualify as a conscientious objector after having been a willing participating for 10 years.

1. Provide and explain your professional opinion on whether Ann can now claim to be a conscientious objector.
2. What actions do you believe Ann must or should take professionally now that she has made this claim?

APPEAL TO NONMALEFICENCE

What recourse does a nurse have when he or she believes that he or she should not participate in an action, but the reason for not participating has nothing to do with a religious belief or its equivalent? When a nurse refuses to participate in an action because the action would cause harm to another, the nurse is making an appeal to nonmaleficence. For example, a nurse might refuse to administer a preoperative sedative to a patient with mild dementia who is agitated and yelling, "I do not want surgery!" This refusal would be based on the nurse's belief that administering the injection would be a violation of the patient's right to refuse treatment. Refusals to participate based on an appeal to nonmaleficence are always supported by the nurse's professional knowledge and judgment (Brushwood, 1993).

Discussion Exercises 16-2

You are employed as a nurse in a state penitentiary. The state's first execution by lethal injection is scheduled to occur next week. After consulting the ANA (1994c) Position statement: Nurses' Participation in Capital Punishment, answer the following questions.

1. Although the lethal injection itself is administered by a non–health care provider, the policy states that the prisoner's intravenous access is to be started in the prison infirmary by the nurse on duty. Assuming you are scheduled to work the day of the execution, explain and justify your intentions regarding starting the intravenous access.
2. The policy also states that the nurse on duty will prepare the body to send to the medical examiner/morgue. Assuming you are scheduled to work the day of the execution, explain and justify your intentions on preparing the body after execution.

ACTIONS TO REMOVE THE NEED TO CONSCIENTIOUSLY OBJECT

What can a nurse do to remove the need to conscientiously object? First, the nurse needs to actively identify and evaluate his or her morals and values. For example, does the nurse believe that food and hydration are a basic right that every person should receive?

Second, the nurse needs to think prospectively about what could threaten these values. One way to do this would be to know an institution's mission statements before seeking employment there. In addition, the nurse should be aware of relevant clinical situations. For example, a certified registered nurse anesthetist (CRNA) described her experience when moonlighting in a surgical center. She was confronted with the assignment to provide anesthesia for a pregnant patient scheduled for a therapeutic dilation and curettage (D & C), which would terminate her pregnancy. The CRNA realized that she never asked whether the center performed terminations, and as a devout Catholic found herself with a dilemma.

Third, use terms correctly; do not refer to conscience when your refusal is based on applying the principle of nonmaleficence to another person. For example, a nurse should not claim, "I have a conscientious objection to administering KCl by IV push to this patient" when the objection is based on her knowledge of pharmacology, not on a religious or equivalent belief, and thus in fact is based on an appeal to nonmaleficence. Finally, live out your values consistently.

SUMMARY

Conscientious objection based on nonmaleficence happens often and reflects the nurse's knowledge base. Conscientious objection based on an appeal to conscience is a rare occurrence that most nurses will never have to experience.

CLINICAL EXERCISES

Does your clinical agency have a policy on "conscientious objection" or "refusal to participate." Use the policy to examine the following issues. If the clinical agency does not have a policy, work individually or as a group to draft a sample policy that addresses the following issues.

1. How does your clinical agency define the term *conscientious objection*?
2. Does the agency outline a process to be followed when a nurse is a conscientious objector? If so, what steps are to be taken?
3. What safeguards are included to protect the nurse, the patient, and/or the agency when claims of conscientious objection occur?
4. Identify whether any professional specialty organizations have a position statement on conscientious objection. For example, see the ANA (1995) position statement regarding the nurse's right to accept or reject an assignment.
5. Investigate what type of law your state has related to conscientious objection.

   a. Is it (1) an employment law, (2) a religious discrimination law, or (3) a conscience clause?
   b. How does your state define conscientious objection?

6. Discuss with a religious or spiritual advisor (the agency's or yours) his or her religion's or culture's stance on the moral permissibility of participating in:

   - Abortions
   - Withdrawal of life support
   - Assisted suicide
   - Obligation to provide food and hydration
   - Assisted reproduction
   - Birth control
   - Organ transplantation, including the use of fetal tissue for transplantation
   - State-sanctioned execution
   - Administration of blood or blood products

Discussion Questions

1. Brushwood (1993) stated that "A conscientiously refusing professional usually will say something like 'I cannot do that, because I could not live with myself if I were to do it'" (p. 204). Name one professional situation in which you could not participate because if you did, you "could not live with yourself." What value is at stake?
2. Provide an example of an appeal to nonmaleficence that you or another nurse has made professionally.
3. A nurse you know from your fitness center tells you, "My hospital is requiring all nurses working in the emergency department to be vaccinated against smallpox. Is there any way I can refuse to be vaccinated without getting in trouble or fired?" What advice would you give to this nurse? Explain your rationale.

4. What reasons might explain why so few nursing organizations have official position statements on conscientious objection?

SECTION 3: *Professional Nurse Issue: Whistle-Blowing*

Whistle-blowing is a serious action that should be engaged in only after all internal resources have been exhausted and careful consideration has been given to the personal and professional ramifications that will follow the whistle-blowing event. This section builds on the previous discussion of conscientious objection. Nurses often have objections based on an appeal to nonmaleficence. Usually these objections are dealt with effectively by educating the involved individuals about the potential harms to specific individuals, institutions, and/or society. However, despite this, unethical or harmful situations may sometimes continue, which may force the nurse to consider "should I blow the whistle?"

The knowledge most people have about whistle-blowing may be based on what they learned through movies like Julia Roberts' *Erin Brockovich*. Although most nationally publicized whistle-blowing events are related to big businesses, such as Enron, nurses are also confronted with such issues. One famous whistle-blowing case involving a nurse occurred in 1996 when Barry Adams was fired after challenging Youville Hospital's staffing procedures (Frank, 2000).

Whistle-blowing is not the same as reporting a problem, tattling, or filing a complaint. Questions about whether to blow the whistle represent a classic moral dilemma (consequentialism vs. deontology). In this dilemma, the nurse is unsure whether the consequences (to the involved individuals, agency, and self) that might occur if the whistle is blown outweigh the nurse's duty to protect patients and the public from harm (Canadian Nurses Association, 1999). Making the decision based on the consequences would be employing a consequentialist approach; deciding which action to take based on the goodness or rightness of the action would be using a deontological approach.

Whistle-blowing questions arise when a nurse recognizes a lack of commitment to doing what is right by an individual, group, or agency. This lack of commitment to doing what is right may include illegal, incompetent, or unethical behaviors, for example:

- Illegal behaviors: abusive behavior, falsifying records, billing fraud
- Incompetent behaviors: health care professionals who fail meet the standard of practice, impaired practitioners, employees assuming responsibilities beyond their training or education
- Unethical behaviors: unsafe staffing patterns, breaches in maintaining confidentiality of patient records, conflicts of interest, failure to obtain informed consent before enrolling a subject into a clinical research study

When a nurse recognizes actions that fail to meet current ethical, legal, or professional standards, the nurse has a moral obligation to act. Provision 3.5 of the ANA (2001) Code of Ethics for Nurses stipulates:

When the nurse is aware of inappropriate or questionable practice in the provision or denial of health care, concern should be expressed to the person carrying out the questionable practice. Attention should be called to the possible detrimental affect upon the patient's well being or best interests as well as the integrity of nursing practice. When factors in the health care delivery system or health care organization threaten the welfare of the patient, similar action should be directed to the responsible administrator. If indicated, the problem should be reported to an appropriate higher authority within the institution or agency, or to an appropriate external authority. (ANA, 2001. Used with permission.)

Discussion Exercises 16-3

During your surgical rotation, you are assigned to a unit that is staffed with only one RN during the night shift. Before beginning the day shift, you come in early one morning to review your patient's chart. While walking down the hallway, you notice the night RN discarding liquid from a syringe into a paper cup on top of the medication cart. Later, you notice the same nurse drinking from the same paper cup as she pushes the medication cart back to the nurse's station. After your shift, during a post-conference discussion with your clinical group, one student says, "I just do not understand how my patient could receive a pain shot every three hours all night long and still rate his pain as 9/10 on the pain scale." Several other students confirm that their patients had the same experience last night, but that their patients all seemed to achieve better pain control during the day shift with the same medications.

1. Based on your colleagues' discussion, should you share your observations with your clinical group? Why or why not?
2. What is the chain of command for reporting potential ethical or legal breaches in clinical practice at your clinical agency?

Health care organizations typically have a structured reporting hierarchy for reporting an issue in which the alleged wrongdoer is informed of the problem through the possibility of notifying his or her immediate supervisor. For example, if a nurse observes a transporter verbally abusing a patient with expressive aphasia, the nurse first intervenes to stop the verbal abuse. Then after ensuring the patient's safety, the nurse counsels the transporter regarding professional behavior and demeanor when working with patients. After consulting the agency's organizational hierarchy, the nurse may also notify the transportation supervisor as well as the nursing manager. In an ideal world, once a problem or an ethical concern is noted, the responsible party would act immediately to resolve the problem. Unfortunately, this ideal is not always fulfilled. Therefore, if no actions are taken to rectify the ongoing behavior, the nurse may need to continue to report instances of patient abuse through the organization's structure.

Whistle-blowing occurs when the nurse has exhausted all internal resources and options available to assist in resolving the ongoing problem and goes beyond the agency's internal reporting structure to notify an external resource about the problem. This external resource might be a news agency, a political group, the state nursing organization, or an accrediting body, such as the Joint Commission on Accreditation of

Health Care (JCAHO) (Sloan, 2002). Thus, whistle-blowing requires the nurse to publicly accuse someone of wrongdoing and disagree with how the problem has been handled, which has the potential of painting the nurse as a disloyal employee or colleague (Canadian Nurses Association, 1999).

A nurse must not engage in an act of whistle-blowing hastily or without careful thought and supporting documentation. Feliu (1983) provided advice for actions to take prior to blowing the whistle:

---

1. Verify facts, document claims.
2. Begin to make your concerns known within the organization.
3. Exhaust all internal remedies.
4. Get a lawyer. (p. 1387)

Documenting claims includes creating a written account of the event, including who was involved, witnesses, dates, time, and location. The nurse should always retain a copy of any written documentation. When submitting the documentation, the nurse must be diligent in following the agency's policy and procedure for filing a grievance or complaint as well as documenting each step (Sloan, 2002).

Discussion Exercises 16-4

Charlotte Cecilio is beginning her first job as a registered nurse on a skilled unit in a retirement facility in a small, rural community. During her first month after orientation, she is the only RN working the 11 P.M. to 7 A.M. shift when a hospice patient requires larger amounts of narcotic pain medication to control his pain. Charlotte uses the last of the patient's narcotic supply at 3 A.M. The pharmacy with the contract to provide the facility's medications is closed from 10 P.M. until 9 A.M. Because no other patient is currently receiving narcotics, Charlotte is unable to administer any pain medication for the rest of the shift. During the change-of-shift report, Charlotte describes the problem to the day shift nurse, stating "I did not know what to do. There is no way to get more drugs during the night shift." The morning nurse whispers, "There is a stash of drugs that the nurses keep for situations like you have described. None of the nurses wants patients to endure pain because of the inability to get medication during the night." The day shift nurse then advises Charlotte to keep quiet about the "stash" because the medications are left over from previous patients.

1. What ethical, legal, and/or professional issues are involved in this case?
2. What actions should Charlotte take initially based on this conversation?
3. Should Charlotte discuss this situation with anyone? If so, whom? If not, why not?
4. Charlotte decides to discuss this situation with her former clinical instructor. After hearing the story, the instructor replies, "If it is happening at your facility, how do I know that nurses are not keeping personal stashes

of narcotics here at the university hospital?" What ethical principles or commitments are affecting this instructor's remark?

5. Is Charlotte's consulting her former professor about a clinical issue an act of whistle-blowing? Why or why not?

6. What actions or resources would Charlotte need to exhaust before considering whether she should "blow the whistle" on this surgical unit?

7. Is there any whistle-blowing legislation that Charlotte should consider while deliberating on how to respond to this situation?

WHISTLE-BLOWING LEGISLATION

Concurrent with verifying the facts and documenting the event, the nurse should also review pertinent laws, such as those covering mandatory reporting of abuse and whistle-blowing. Unfortunately, the United States does not have a comprehensive whistle-blower protection law. Instead, a variety of federal laws and agencies provide protections for specific types of problems in specific employment settings (Table 16-1). In addition, 13 states have whistle-blower protection legislation (California, Florida, Kentucky, Maryland, Massachusetts, Minnesota, New Jersey, New York, Ohio, Oregon, Texas, West Virginia, Wisconsin) and other states have introduced such legislation (ANA, 2002). Anyone contemplating an act of whistle-blowing should contact an experienced attorney prior to making any accusations.

FALLOUT FROM ACTS OF WHISTLE-BLOWING

Despite their good intentions and precautions, persons who engage in acts of whistle-blowing usually suffer a variety of negative consequences. These consequences can include being fired from their job, being blackballed within the profession from gaining future employment, and suffering post-traumatic stress disorder, finance loss, and divorce. Unfortunately, the investigation of allegations or wrongdoing in the health care arena can often last for years and wear on the whistle-blower's resolve. For example, Barry Adams stated that whistle-blowing "is a position no one should be in. . . . It has consumed my life for two years" (Fletcher, Sorrell, & Silva, 1998, p. 1). Thus, a nurse must be aware that engaging in whistle-blowing can change his or her life forever.

In light of the prolonged nature of procedures involving whistle-blowing, the Office of Research Integrity (2001) proposed a "Whistleblower's Bill of Rights" that should apply to all whistle-blowers. A whistle-blower has the right to:

1. *Communication*
2. *Protection from retaliation*
3. *Fair procedures*
4. *Procedures free from partiality*
5. *Information*
6. *Timely processes*
7. *Vindication (pp. 1–2)*

When a right exists, such as those just listed, associated obligations exist for the individual possessing the right as well as for those with the power to influence that person's

Table 16-1	Whistle-Blowing Legislation and Resources	
Legislation or Resource	Applies to:	Protections Provided
First and Fourteenth Amendments to the U.S. Constitution	U.S. citizens	Free speech and guarantee of due process and equal protection of laws
The 1863 Federal False Claims Act, as amended in 1986	Any individual who testifies, investigates, reports, or participates in a *qui tam* lawsuit	On behalf of the federal government, individuals can sue employers for fraud against federally funded programs, such as Medicare; individuals can receive a portion of any monies collected; protects from wrongful loss of employment or demotion and harassment
Civil Service Reform Act of 1978	Federal employees	Protects employees who identify mismanagement of monies or legal or regulatory violations
National Labor Relations Act	Nongovernment employees	Offers protections when employees work to correct illegal or unsafe practices
Individual union contracts	Union employees	Varies by contract
Whistleblower Protection Act of 1989	Federal employees who engage in whistle-blowing	Invalidates previous decisions that limit the employee's chances of winning a legal suit; protects the employee merit system and promotes the employee's right to work or get paid during appeals
Corporate and Criminal Fraud Accountability Act of 2002 (Sarbanes-Oxley Act)	Persons employed at publicly traded companies, including contractors and subcontractors	Protects employees from being fired, demoted, or harassed after reporting securities fraud to a supervisor or the government
Section 11(c) of the Occupational Safety and Health Act	Private and governmental employees	Protects workers after they make claims or testify about safety and health issues in the workplace

Adapted from Brownsey, D. (2001). Nurses and their right to whistle blow. *AORN Online, 73*(3), 693–697; Gallagher, R. M., & Kany, K. (2000). Does JCAHO see the truth? *American Journal of Nursing, 100*(4), 74; Nolan, K. J. (2003). Federal False Claims Act. Retrieved April 29, 2003, from http://www.whistleblowerfirm.com/federalfalseclaimsact.html; Quyen-Nguyen, B. (2001). Blowing the whistle: Nurses' rights and responsibilities when employers' conduct is unethical. *American Journal of Nursing, 101*(7), 79; U.S. Constitution; Whistleblower Protection Act. (1989). 5 U.S.C. Secs. 1201 et seq. Retrieved July 25, 2003, from http://cwx.prenhall.com/bookbind/pubbooks/dye4/medialib/docs/whistle.htm and http://peregrinos.us/jtexplanstate1989excerpts.htm#4512

ability to claim it. The involved individuals (including the whistle-blower) have an obligation to promote these rights by being truthful and acting in a manner that does not undermine or delay the resolution of the complaint.

SUMMARY

Whistle-blowing is a serious action and should be undertaken only when all internal resources and options have been exhausted. A nurse must consider the personal and professional risks as well as the patient care and/or social issues involved prior to engaging in whistle-blowing.

CLINICAL EXERCISES

1. Investigate what types of whistle-blower laws exist in your state. You may need to contact your state nurses association for assistance.
2. Find your clinical agency's protocol for reporting illegal, unethical, or unprofessional conduct. Identify the chain of command a nurse should follow in that agency. Does the agency have any required forms or documentation processes? If so, what?
3. Identify your college or university's policy on reporting illegal, unethical, or unprofessional conduct. Describe the key points.
4. Does your student malpractice insurance cover claims related to illegal, unethical, or unprofessional conduct? If so, how? If not, how else might students be protected?

Discussion Questions

1. When a nurse has exhausted all internal resources and avenues and has decided to "blow the whistle," what agency or person should the nurse contact first? Explain.
2. When pursuing all internal resources and avenues in an attempt to resolve a clinical situation and prevent the need for whistle-blowing, should the nurse be concerned about maintaining confidentiality? Explain.

SECTION 4: *Professional Nursing Issue: Professional Misconduct—Incompetent and Impaired Practice*

U.S. society holds the profession of nursing in high esteem (Jones, 2005). Many instruments (such as licensing exams and annual competency reviews) have been put in place to ensure that every nurse meets a minimal level of performance. Unfortunately, these safeguards cannot guarantee that every nurse will always meet this minimal level of performance. When a professional nurse becomes aware of professional misconduct related to incompetent or impaired practice of another health care provider, the nurse has an obligation to protect the public from potential harm and to assist the erring health care professional to receive appropriate educational or treatment interventions.

Most students entering the health professions express a desire to help people and create a better and healthier society and/or world. These desires are based on an explicit commitment to nonmaleficence, beneficence, advocacy, and justice. Undoubtedly, each of us has at one time or another stated, "I just want to be the best nurse possible!" Most of the time, we are able to act on these desires and provide competent, individualized holistic care to our individual patients, groups, and/or communities.

However, for some nurses or health care professionals this is not always the case. The purpose of this section is to identify and discuss the professional nurse's role, obligation, and rights when he or she is unable to provide competent high-quality nursing care or witnesses another health care professional's inability to provide safe care to patients, groups, and/or communities.

Provision 3.5 of the American Nurses Association (2001) Code of Ethics for Nurses states:

The nurse's primary commitment is to the health, well being, and safety of the patient across the life span and in all settings in which health care needs are addressed. As an advocate for the patient, the nurse must be alert to and take appropriate action regarding any instances of incompetent, unethical, illegal, or impaired practice by any member of the health care team or the health care system or any action on the part of others that places the rights or best interests of the patient in jeopardy. (p. 14). (ANA, 2001. Used with permission.)

Despite these basic commitments to patient safety, there has been a long history of denial about the magnitude of the problems of impaired nurses. Actions must be taken to break this "conspiracy of silence" that pervades the professional nursing culture. This conspiracy of silence may be due to a nurse's lack of knowledge regarding the signs and symptoms associated with incompetent or impaired practice (Table 16-2) or reluctance to cause problems or upset the status quo. Rather than admitting that a colleague is not performing competently, a nurse may act as an enabler by covering up the colleague's inactions such as by augmenting the colleague's charting or covertly assisting to make sure the colleague's work is completed (Box 16-2) (Serghis, 1999). This conspiracy of silence is often perpetuated when supervisors opt to terminate the nurse's employment rather than deal with the cause(s) for the lack of quality nursing care (Shewey, 1997). The conspiracy of silence is an attempt to minimize the short-term harm to the nurse's professional career and perhaps the agency's current patients. Nevertheless, such a culture increases the risk of potential and actual long-term harms to the nurse, other patients and agencies, and the nursing profession.

INCOMPETENT PRACTICE

A nurse is considered to be competent when he or she possesses "sufficiency of means or ability" (Thomson, 1997, p. 16). Incompetency is a pattern of behavior and not generally a single isolated mistake (Thomson, 1997). A nurse's inability to meet the competency expectations may be related to lack of knowledge or experience or to lapses in judgment.

Nurses may fail to meet the expected levels of competency because they have not been exposed to or understood key pathophysiological, pharmacological, or nursing knowledge. Nurses cannot use information that they do not possess. Thus it behooves nursing supervisors, preceptors, and faculty to validate the knowledge of nurses and nursing students and provide them the opportunities to practice certain skills.

BOX 16-2

Enabling Behaviors

Have I:

Excused or ignored behaviors in a peer that may be suggestive of impairment and justified those behaviors as "just having a bad day" or "stress?"

Never told the supervisor about possible behaviors indicative of impairment that I observed because I was afraid of being wrong and did not want anyone to get angry with me?

Accepted responsibility for my colleague's unfinished work and at times attempted to counsel and solve their problems?

Believed that nurses do not use drugs or alcohol to the point of practice impairment and that substance use can be stopped at any time unless the person is morally weak?

Like to use drugs or alcohol myself to relax or enjoy with friends? I do not want anyone to look at me. In fact, I have used a few discontinued drugs from work myself. Doesn't everyone?

Exonerated a peer's irresponsible actions by covering for attendance or tardiness? Have I cosigned wastes I have not truly witnessed or corrected the narcotic count to account for a discrepancy?

Defended a colleague when it was suggested there may be a problem with impairment?

Source: Reprinted from Smith, L. L., Taylor, B. B., & Hughes, T. L. (1998). Effective peer responses to impaired nursing practice. *Nursing Clinics of North America, 33*(1), 107, © 1998, with permission from Elsevier.

Illustrative Case 16-1

Nursing student Lola Ricci is doing a clinical rotation in the intensive care unit and is working with a new staff preceptor. The physician wrote orders for blood gases to be obtained from the arterial bloodline (A line). The staff preceptor asks Lola if she has ever drawn blood. Lola responds, "I did it once a few weeks ago."

Both Lola and the staff preceptor must now determine whether Lola (1) is competent to perform the task independently, (2) is competent to perform the task with supervision, or (c) is not able to perform the task and should observe the staff preceptor. Thus, Lola's knowledge and experience must be evaluated. Lola continues, "We had problems with the line when I drew the blood before; I would like to try again, but I'll need your assistance."

At this point, the staff preceptor could verbally assess Lola's knowledge of the procedure and/or refer Lola to the policy and procedure for drawing blood from an arterial line. After assessing Lola's knowledge, the staff preceptor states, "Ok, you can do it, but I will be there to help you."

Lola and the staff preceptor enter the room and explain the procedure to the patient and his family. The family opts to remain in the room during the procedure. While Lola is drawing the blood, the staff preceptor makes suggestions to facilitate Lola's skills and dexterity, for example, "Always turn the stopcock this way," or, "Stop and think about what the next step should be." On hearing these remarks, the family exclaims, "Should this student be doing this? I do not want a student practicing on my loved one!"

Table 16-2	**Behaviors Indicative of Substance Abuse**	
Behavior	Alcohol	Drugs
Preference in assignment	Less demanding Independent role Isolated Does not volunteer for difficult/additional assignments	Areas with high-volume use of drug of choice Patients with decreased awareness Lack of supervision Often volunteers for 3-11 or 11-7 shift
Absenteeism	Above average rate of absenteeism Apt to call at last minute to extend time off Use of sick time at beginning of shift Calls in sick after shift has begun	Exhibits "workaholic" syndrome
Time on unit	Late arrival Early departure	Arrives early Stays late Skips lunch and breaks
Charting and reports	Handwriting noticeably affected Failure to file incident reports on errors Discrepancies between oral and written reports Diminished quality of notes	Discrepancies between patients' and nurses' reports, especially with regard to pain, meds, etc. Errors in narcotic count Handwriting noticeably affected Failure to file incident reports on errors Discrepancies between oral and written reports Diminished quality of notes
Psychosocial behaviors	Most often observed in 40- to 45-year age group (now changing to younger age group) Financial problems Excessive use of coffee/cigarettes Prone to auto accidents Wide mood swings Difficulty in all types of relationships Irritable with staff and patients Defensive and suspicious Projects blame on others	Most often in late 20s (now changing to an older age group) Preoccupied with obtaining and using drugs Wide mood swings Difficulty in all types of relationships Irritable with staff and patients Defensive and suspicious Projects blame on others

Source: Reprinted from Lowell, J., & Massey, K. (1997). Sounds of silence. *Nursing Management, 28*(5), 40j.

At this point the staff preceptor and the student need to review the criteria for competency and use them to address the family's concerns. Because the student is being monitored by an experienced staff nurse and the policy and procedure for blood draws from an arterial line is being followed, no breach of nursing standards is occurring. The patient is not being put in a compromised or unsafe situation; thus, the family's fears about Lola being an incompetent practitioner are unfounded. However, the staff preceptor and/or the student's clinical instructor should emphasize to the family the teaching mission of the facility and reassure them that the students are closely supervised.

Discussion Exercises 16-5

Melinda Adams has been a registered nurse for 15 years and is employed at a 1000-bed hospital on an adult medical unit. During her professional nursing career, she has worked on an adult medical-surgical unit and a cardiac step-down unit. She recently passed the Academy of Medical-Surgical Nurses Medical-Surgical Nursing Certification Exam. When she arrived at work, the nursing supervisor informed her that her unit was closed because of low census and she had been reassigned to the pediatric unit for the rest of the week. Nurse Adams' immediate response is, "I have not taken care of a child since I was a junior in college. I am not qualified to work on the pediatric unit."

1. Do you believe that this nurse has failed to meet her ethical requirement to maintain competency? Why or why not?
2. Do you believe that Nurse Adams should agree to float to the pediatric unit? Explain.

UNETHICAL PRACTICE

A nurse's practice is deemed unethical when his or her actions fail to meet the ethical standards established by the profession through codes and societal standards. A wide variety of examples of unethical practice have been discussed throughout this book, including lying or cheating, failure to respect a patient's autonomy, failure to act to prevent harm to others, and inequitable use of scarce resources. As presented previously in this chapter, a nurse has a moral responsibility to act to stop and prevent future incidences of unethical practice. In extreme situations, the nurse might be required to engage in whistle-blowing if the institutional structure is unable or unwilling to act to prevent future episodes of unethical practice.

ILLEGAL PRACTICE

A nurse's practice is illegal when his or her actions violate local, state, or national laws. Many examples of illegal practice are situation specific, for example, failure to comply with abortion laws or fetal tissue regulations. However, other examples of illegal practice cut across specialty areas, such as sexual misconduct, posing as a nurse, and diverting controlled drugs for self-use or sale to others (Tranbarger, 1997; Zook, 2001). Whenever a nurse becomes aware of an illegal practice, he or she must immediately follow the agency's policy and procedure for reporting illegal behavior.

IMPAIRED PRACTICE

Professional impairment is present when the nurse "is unable to meet the requirements of the professional code of ethics and standards of practice because cognitive, interpersonal, or psychomotor skills are affected by conditions of the individual in interaction with the environment" (Shewey, 1997, p. 15). Thus, a nurse's practice could be impaired by alcohol or drug abuse as well as mental illness (Beckstead, 2002).

Substance Abuse (Alcohol or Drugs)

Although the incidence of substance abuse is similar for nurses and the general population (Beckstead, 2002), if, as believed, approximately 8% of U.S. nurses have a problem with alcohol or drugs, this is a significant enough number to represent a threat of impaired clinical practice (Aldersberg, 1997/2002).

Substance abuse has been associated with a combination of biological (genetic as well as neurobiological) factors, personality and behavioral characteristics, and social and environmental factors (Griffith, 1999). In evaluating the causes of substance abuse among nurses, one cannot ignore their ready access to controlled substances. In fact, frequent workplace access to controlled substances as well as ineffective control and/or monitoring are environmental factors that make a nurse's misuse of controlled or prescription drugs possible (Dwyer, Holloran, & Walsh, 2002).

In communicating potential examples of substance abuse, one should always simply report the facts as they occurred and focus on the actions, refraining from providing interpretation or commentary. For example, one might report simply that the narcotic record reflects that 10 mg of morphine sulfate was removed; the patient's medication record reflects that 4 mg of morphine sulfate was administered at 2 P.M., which leaves the remaining 6 mg of morphine sulfate unaccounted for (Shewey, 1997).

Mental Health Disorder

A nurse's ability to practice safely can also be impaired by a variety of mental conditions, such as, but not limited to, depression, bereavement, emotional breakdowns, schizophrenia, and bipolar disorder (Carlowe, 1997). Unfortunately, nurses with mental health disorders may experience difficulties in controlling them due to the stresses related to changes in sleep routine and diet, forgetting to take medications during long shifts, or anniversaries of previous illness episodes (Carlowe, 1997). Thus, the nurse with a history of mental health disorder needs to consider whether the nursing supervisor or other management personnel fits within the need-to-know category. For example, the supervisor may be able to assist the nurse to monitor his or her condition and/or provide assistance to limit work-related stressors, such as limiting the frequency the nurse rotates between shifts. However, the decision to disclose a history of mental health disorder should not be made hastily because the nurse must also consider the potential harms to his or her career that might occur because of preconceived opinions held by the supervisor or other administrators.

Burnout

Another cause of impaired practice is burnout (Carpenter, 1994). Burnout occurs after continued exposure to work-related stress. When experiencing burnout, the nurse exhibits signs of mental, emotional, and physical exhaustion (Pines & Aronson, 1981).

A nurse's ability to meet the standards of practice can be compromised by the depersonalization and apathy that come with burnout. (Stordeur, D'Hoore, & Vandenberghe, 2001). For example, a nurse experiencing burnout might fail to meet current standards of care by failing to provide patient treatments or medications as scheduled. Incompetent practice due to burnout is often evident during the change-of-shift report, when a nurse might state, for example, "There was just too much for me to do today, I could not get to all the dressing changes, not that it would have made a difference for Mrs. Jones' prognosis anyway."

Cognitive Threats

A nurse's practice can be impaired by threats that limit his or her cognitive abilities and threaten his or her abilities to recognize, evaluate, and act on pertinent data. One frequent cognitive threat that nurses experience is lack of sleep. This can result from rotating shifts and competing responsibilities or activities that prevent the nurse from getting sufficient rest. For example, a nursing student may experience sleep deprivation as a result of staying up until 2 A.M. to prepare for the next day's clinical rotation, or a nurse might be kept awake during the night by a sick child. A nurse can also experience difficulties in sleeping during the day due to outside neighborhood noises or changes in sleep patterns.

Generally, nurses are cognizant of the fact that they are sleepy and demonstrate extra caution and diligence with psychomotor tasks or drug administration. However, a nurse might note, "I read my charting from last night and it did not make much sense. In one chart, I wrote 'he patient is sitting in a dress at the side of the chair' when I meant to write 'the patient is sitting in a chair in no distress.'" Although the misinformation conveyed in this illustration likely would not cause any harm to the patient, the possibility exists for harm to occur when a nurse fails to meet the standards of clear documentation.

Similarly, a nurse's ability to think critically and accurately can be threatened by low blood sugar levels due to not eating. Thus, nurses, especially those with diabetes or hypoglycemia, need to be particularly diligent to make sure that they fulfill their nutritional needs so as to guarantee their professional competency.

> ### Illustrative Case 16-2
>
> At 9 P.M., Nurse Bonnie Juarez sits down in the staff lounge to do some charting while taking a short break. Noticing Bonnie's home-baked treat, Nurse Jacqueline Olson says, "I am so hungry I can hardly think straight. I would sure would like one of those goodies." Realizing that Jacqueline has made similar requests over the last few shifts, Bonnie replies, "I am sorry, but maybe you do not know that I am a diabetic. I have found that when I do a 12-hour shift I need a snack to maintain my blood sugar until I can get home and fix supper. Why don't you tell the charge nurse that you are going to go down to the cafeteria for a quick supper break now?"
>
> Nurse Juarez is displaying a commitment to preventing threats to her cognitive abilities. In addition to encouraging her colleague to take a supper break now, Nurse Juarez should work with the unit leadership to ensure that every nurse has the opportunity to have a meal break during shifts.

Finally, a nurse's cognitive abilities can be compromised by fear of failure and threats to his or her self-esteem. Everyone can remember an academic clinical moment when fear prevented him or her from answering correctly or completing a psychomotor skill. Sometimes this fear can get out of control and create a cycle of fear, poor performance, and more fear of failures. Every nurse, especially those with managerial responsibilities, need to be observant for signs that a colleague's nursing care and judgments are being influenced negatively by fears and misperceptions. Actions to prevent cognitive impairments due to fear include noting examples of good nursing care as they occur, offering emotional support following a mistake or difficult situation, validating that the nurse's perception of the incident or situation is realistic, and facilitating the use of appropriate resources to augment skills or knowledge base as a means of regaining confidence.

REPORTING PROFESSIONAL MISCONDUCT

Most states via their respective nurse practice acts have clear guidelines for the reporting of professional misconduct. However, when dealing with the impaired nurse, most states favor treatment over disciplinary punishment (Griffith, 1999).

Provision 3.6 of the ANA (2001) Code of Ethics for Nurses states:

Nurses must be vigilant to protect the patient, the public, and the profession from potential harm when a colleague's practice, in any setting, appears to be impaired. The nurse extends compassion and caring to colleagues who are in recovery from illness or when illness interferes with job performance. In a situation where a nurse suspects another's practice may be impaired, the nurse's duty is to take action designed both to protect patients and to assure that the impaired individual receives assistance in regaining optimal function. Such action should usually begin with consulting supervisory personnel and may also include confronting the individual in a supportive manner and with the assistance of others or helping the individual to access appropriate resources. . . . Nurses in all roles should advocate for colleagues whose job performance may be impaired to ensure that they receive appropriate assistance, treatment and access to fair institutional and legal processes. This includes supporting the return to practice of the individual who has sought assistance and is ready to resume professional duties. (ANA, 2001. Used with permission.)

Although differences might exist in the specific procedures of individual states or agencies, a standard approach to intervening with impaired nurses follows the following steps. When the impaired practice has been identified, a confidential verification of the facts must occur. It is imperative that the suspected nurse's confidentiality be maintained. Thus, when investigating a complaint, a manager must be careful not to disclose facts or assumptions to the nurse's colleagues and associates. After the impaired practice has been substantiated, the impaired nurse must be confronted directly, yet confidentially. After being confronted, the nurse has two options. Ideally, he or she will admit to the impairment and voluntarily seek treatment. The type of treatment will depend on the cause of the impairment. For example, diabetics would need to work with their endocrinologist, and a person with mental health problems would need to seek appropriate intervention and treatment. However, a nurse with a substance abuse problem would need to enroll in a treatment program and potentially continue long term in a 12-step program. When the nurse has successfully completed treatment and the cause of the impairment removed or successfully controlled, then he or she will need to work with the nursing leadership to return to practice. Every institution needs to have a clear policy for guiding the nurse's re-entry into the clinical setting. Often the nurse's return is stipulated in a contract that may include evidence of ongoing peer support or random drug testing (Griffith, 1999; Hocking, 1999; Lowell & Massey, 1997; Shewey, 1997). The American Nurses Association (1994b) supports the use of random drug testing when there is a history of impaired practice related to substance abuse.

However, if the nurse refuses voluntarily to seek treatment or fails to complete it the agency has no recourse but to follow its impaired-practice policy and procedure, report the incidence to the state board of nursing, and terminate the nurse's employment. When notified, the state will investigate and conduct a hearing if necessary. If the complaint of impaired practice is supported, the nurse may face revocation of his or her license (Lowell & Massey, 1997).

Legal Protections

Nurses whose practice has been impaired by chemical substance abuse or mental illness have some legal protections regarding their job. The Federal Family and Medical Leave Act of 1993 includes provisions for up to 12 weeks of unpaid time off in the event that a nurse is experiencing a serious health condition, which includes treatment for substance abuse.

In addition, the Americans with Disabilities Act offers guidance regarding employment decisions. Nurses with impaired practice secondary to mental illness and possibly substance abuse may be eligible for protections if actions are initiated to terminate their employment. In addition, the Act may offer some legal assistance for those nurses whose impairment is related to the demands of rotating shifts or mandatory overtime.

STRATEGIES

Nurses both individually and collectively have a moral obligation to create work environments that are conducive to and promote the practice of safe, competent care. Specific actions that can be recommended to assist impaired nurses include the following:

- Develop ways for documenting and communicating the efficacy of substance abuse rehabilitation programs.
- Develop strategies for changing attitudes about chemical substance abuse without moralizing.
- Increase the availability and visibility of institutional employee assistance programs.
- Create an institutional culture in which employees feel free to share concerns about substance abuse and mental health disorder (Beckstead, 2002).
- Implement educational strategies that facilitate positive rather than palliative coping mechanisms (such as drugs and alcohol) for dealing with

the stresses associated with the professional role (Bell, McDonough, Ellison, & Fitzhugh, 1999; Trinkoff & Storr, 1998).
- Target educational efforts in specialties where higher incidences of substance abuse may occur, such as emergency departments and critical care and psychiatric units (Trinkoff & Storr, 1998).

SUMMARY

Nursing is a demanding profession with a variety of physical and mental stressors. Most nurses are successful in meeting the profession's expectations for practice. Unfortunately, some nurses experience difficulties in providing competent and safe care. A nurse who believes he or she observes professional misconduct should consult the agency's policy and procedure manual, the state's nurse practice act, and the ANA (2001) Code of Ethics for Nurses for guidance in how to intervene to prevent harm to patients as well as to provide aid to the impaired nurse.

CLINICAL EXERCISES

1. Check with your state board of nursing and/or state nurses association to determine whether your state has a law mandating that nurses and other health care providers with known impaired practice be reported to the department of professional regulations. If your state does have a mandatory reporting law, (a) what is the penalty if a registered nurse fails to report an impaired colleague and (b) does the law provide protection to the impaired practitioner who is in a voluntary intervention program?
2. Does your state's nurse practice act include any disciplinary actions for nurses found to be (a) chemically impaired or (b) diverting controlled substances? If so, what disciplinary actions are described?
3. Locate your college's policy on chemical impairment. Is there an identified resource person or group that an impaired student could contact for assistance? If so, who?
4. Locate your agency's policy on chemical impairment. Is there an identified resource person or group that an impaired nurse could contact for assistance? If so, who?
5. Find your agency's policy and procedure for inventorying controlled substances. If possible, observe the inventory-taking process. What procedure is followed if a discrepancy in the controlled substance inventory is found?

Discussion Questions

1. What sanctions do you believe are ethically justifiable for a nursing student whose clinical performance is impaired due to:

   a. Lack of sleep?
   b. Being "hung over"?
   c. Lack of knowledge secondary to failure to prepare?

  d. Lack of knowledge secondary to inability to understand pertinent patho-physiology and/or pharmacology concepts?

2. Because intervention and treatment is preferable to punishment for nurses experiencing impairment (Badzek, Mitchell, Marra, & Bower, 1998), what resources do you believe should be available for students with the impairments listed in Discussion Question 1? Provide your rationale.

3. The ANA (2001) Code of Ethics for Nurses states that a nurse has the ethical obligation to maintain competency (Provision 5). Explain what criteria you believe should be used to determine whether a nurse is competent to practice.

Resources

Agency for Healthcare Research and Quality. (2000). Patient fact sheet. 20 tips to help prevent medical errors. Retrieved May 14, 2005, from www.ahcpr.gov/consumer/20tips.htm

Ahern, K., & McDonald, S. (2002). The beliefs of nurses who were involved in a whistle blowing event. *Journal of Advanced Nursing, 38*(3), 3003–3009.

American Nurses Association. (1984). *Addictions and psychological dysfunctions in nursing.* Kansas City, MO: Author.

American Nurses Association. (1992). Position statement: HIV infected nurse, ethical obligations and disclosure. Retrieved May 14, 2005, from www.nursingworld.org/readroom/position/blood/blhvrn.htm

American Nurses Association. (1994). Workplace violence: Can you close the door on it? Retrieved May 14, 2005, from www.nursingworld.org/osh/wp5.htm

American Nurses Association. (1994). Position statement: Drug testing for health care workers. Retrieved May 14, 2005, from www.nursingworld.org/readroom/position/drug/drtest.htm

American Nurses Association. (2001). Position statement: Opposition to mandatory overtime. Retrieved May 14, 2005, from www.nursingworld.org/readroom/position/workplac/revmot2.htm

Bletcher, M. B. (2002). What color is your whistle? Reporting incidents of wrongdoing in your workplace is always a risky business—but for minority nurses who blow the whistle, the stakes are even higher. *Minority Nurse, 2002*(Spring), 50–55.

Braithwaite, C. (1995). *Conscientious objection to various compulsions under British Law.* York, England: Sessions.

Council of Special Mutual Help Groups. (n.d.). List of members. [Eleven groups providing recovery assistance and/or networking opportunities to a wide range of health care professionals.] Retrieved May 14, 2005, from www.crml.uab.edu/~jah/members.html

Francione, G. L., & Charlton, A. E. (2001). Animal rights law: Students' rights and conscientious objection to harming animals: Your constitutional rights. Retrieved May 14, 2005, from www.animal-law.org/srco

Haddad, A. (1996). Acute care decisions. Ethics in action . . . conscientious objection. *RN, 59*(9), 70–71.

Institute of Medicine. (2000). *To err is human: Building a safer health system.* Washington, DC: National Academy Press.

International Labour Office, International Council of Nurses, World Health Organization, & Public Service International. (2002). *Framework guidelines for addressing workplace violence in the health sector.* Geneva: Authors. Also retrieved May 14, 2005, from http://icn.ch/guide_violence.pdf

Joint Commission on Accreditation of Healthcare Organizations. (2003). Reporting of medical/health care errors: A position statement of the Joint Commission on Accreditation of Healthcare Organizations. Retrieved May 14, 2005, from www.jcaho.org/accredited+organizations/patient+safety/medical+errors+disclosure/hc_errors.htm

National Whistleblower Center. (n.d.). *News from the center.* [A nonprofit educational advocacy organization that works for the enforcement of environmental laws, nuclear safety, civil rights, and government and industry accountability through the support and representation of employee whistleblowers.] Retrieved May 14, 2005, from www.whistleblowers.org

Nelson, K. D. (1998). "By reason of religious training and belief. . . ." A history of conscientious objection and religion during the Vietnam War. Retrieved May 14, 2005, from http://members.macconnect.com/users/k/knelson/co/co.html

Nolan Law Firm. (2004). Qui Tam lawsuit representation. [Whistle-blower resources website with links to federal laws and resources with an emphasis on the 1986 Federal False Claims Act.] Retrieved May 14, 2005, from www.whistleblowerfirm.com

Nurse Licensure Compact Administrators. (2004). Frequently asked questions regarding the National Council of State Boards of Nursing (NCSBN) nurse license compact (NLC). Retrieved May 14, 2005, from www.ncsbn.org/pdfs/FrequentlyAskedQuestions.pdf

Occupational Safety and Health Administration. (2003). Guidelines for preventing workplace violence for health-care and social-service workers. Washington DC: U.S. Department of Labor. Also retrieved May 14, 2005, from www.osha.gov/Publications/osha3148.pdf

Pierce, C. S. (2001). Implications of chemically impaired students in clinical settings. *Journal of Nursing Education, 40*(9), 422–425.

Public Concern at Work. (n.d). Making whistleblowing work. [Website with links to international organizations that assist potential whistle-blowers and links to policies and publications.] Retrieved May 14, 2005, from www.pcaw.co.uk/index.html

Quality Interagency Coordination Task Force. (2000). Doing what counts for patient safety: Federal actions to reduce medical errors and their impact: Report of the Quality Interagency Coordination Task Force (QuIC) to the President. Retrieved May 14, 2005, from www.quic.gov/report/

Recovery Works. (2001). Your addictions resource center. [Website with recovery links regarding drug, sexual, alcohol, gambling, grief, work, food, and Internet addictions.] Retrieved May 14, 2005, from www.addictions.org/recoveryworks/

Salmon, D. A., & Siegel, A. W. (2001). Religious and philosophical exemptions from vaccination requirements and lessons learned from conscientious objectors from conscription. *Public Health Reports, 116,* 289–295.

Spier, B. E., Matthews, J. T., Jack, L., Lever, J., & McHaffie, E. J. (2000). Impaired student performance in the clinical setting: A constructive approach. *Nurse Educator, 25*(1), 38–42.

St. Vincent Hospital. (1995). Memorandum of understanding for circumcision procedure. Santa Fe, NM: Author. Retrieved May 14, 2005, from www.cirp.org/nrc/Memorandum_of_Understandin.html

U.S. Department of Labor. (2005). The Family and Medical Leave Act of 1993, Section 825.114(d). Retrieved May 14, 2005, from www.dol.gov/elaws/esa/fmla/fmlamenu.asp

Whistleblowers. (2004). Blowing-the-whistle. Retrieved October 12, 2005, from www.whistleblowing.com/index.html

Wilmot, S. (2000). Nurses and whistle blowing: The ethical issues. *Journal of Advanced Nursing, 32*(5), 1051–1057.

References

Adlersberg, M. (1997/2003). *Chemical dependency—Helping a nurse return to work.* Retrieved May 14, 2005, from www.rnabc.bc.ca/registrants/nursing_practice/articles/chemdep1.htm

Amendment to the Illinois Right of Conscience Act. (1997). P.A. 90-246, eff. 1-1-98.

American Nurses Association. (1994a). *Risk versus responsibility in providing nursing care.* Washington, DC: Author. Also available at www.nursingworld.org/readroom/position/ethics/etrisk.htm

American Nurses Association. (1994b). *Drug testing for health care workers.* Washington, DC: Author. Also available at www.nursingworld.org/readroom/position/drug/drtest.htm

American Nurses Association. (1994c). Ethics and human rights position statement: Nurses' participation in capital punishment. Retrieved on December 9, 2005, from http://www.nursingworld.org/readroom/position/ethics/etcptl.htm

American Nurses Association. (1995). The right to accept or reject an assignment. Retrieved October 12, 2005, from www.nursingworld.org/readroom/position/workplac/wkassign.htm

American Nurses Association. (2001). *The code of ethics for nurses with interpretive statements.* Washington, DC: Author.

American Nurses Association. (2002). 2002 Legislation: Whistleblower protection. December, 2002. Available at www.nursingworld.org/gova/state/2002/whistle.htm

Americans with Disabilities Act. (1990). Public Law 336 of the 101st Congress, enacted July 26. Retrieved May 14, 2005, from www.usdoj.gov/crt/ada/pubs/ada.txt

Anderson, C. (2002). Workplace violence: Are some nurses more vulnerable? *Issues in Mental Health Nursing, 23,* 351–366.

Badzek, L. A., Mitchell, K., Marra, S. E., & Bower, M. M. (1998). Administrative ethics and confidentiality/privacy issues. *Online Journal of Issues in Nursing* (December 31). Retrieved May 14, 2005, from www.nursingworld.org/ojin/topic8/topic8_2.htm

Banja, J. (2001). Ethics news & views: Moral courage in medicine: Disclosing medical error. Retrieved May 14, 2005, from http://ethics.emory.edu/news/archives/000188.html#more

Beauchamp, T. L., & Childress, J. F. (2001). *Principles of biomedical ethics* (5th ed.). Oxford: Oxford University Press.

Beckstead, J. W. (2002). Modeling attitudinal antecedents of nurses' decisions to report impaired colleagues. *Western Journal of Nursing Research, 24*(5), 537–551.

Bell, D. M., McDonough, J. P., Ellison, J. S., & Fitzhugh, E. C. (1999). Controlled drug misuse by certified registered nurse anesthetists. *AANA Journal, 67*(2), 133–140.

Brownsey, D. (2001). Nurses and their right to whistle blow. *AORN Online, 73*(3), 693–697.

Brushwood, D. B. (1993). Conscientious objection and abortifacient drugs. *Clinical Therapeutics, 15*(1), 204–212.

Canadian Nurses Association. (1999). Ethics in practice: I see and am silent/I see and speak out: The ethical dilemma of whistle blowing. Retrieved May 14, 2005, from http://cnaaiic.ca/cna/documents/pdf/publications/Ethics_Pract_See_Silent_November_1999_e.pdf

Carlowe, J. (1997). Mental health: The secret history. *Nursing Times, 93*(33), 32–34.

Carpenter, M. A. (1994). The impaired nurse. *MEDSURG Nursing, 3(2), 139–141.*

Centers for Disease Control and Prevention. (1991). Recommendations for preventing transmission of human immunodeficiency virus and hepatitis B virus to patients during exposure-prone invasive procedures. Retrieved July 3, 2003, from www.cdc.gov/mmwr/preview/mmwrhtml/00014845.htm

Cohen, M. R. (2000). Editorials: Why error reporting systems should be voluntary. *BMJ, 320,* 728–729.

Dwyer, D., Holloran, P., & Walsh, K. (2002). "Why did not I know?" The reality of impaired nurses. *Connecticut Nursing News, 75*(1), 20–22.

Feliu, A. G. (1983). Thinking of blowing the whistle? *American Journal of Nursing, 83,* 1541–1542.

Fletcher, J. J., Sorrell, J. M., & Silva, M. C. (1998). Whistle blowing as a failure of organizational ethics. *Online Journal of Issues in Nursing* (December 31). Retrieved March 24, 2003, from www.nursingworld.org/ojin/topic8/topic8_3.htm

Fost, N. (2000). Patient access to information on clinicians infected with blood-borne pathogens. *JAMA, 284*(15), 1975–1976.

Frank, G. (2000). Two nurses and a doctor: Health care workers allege retaliation for blowing the whistle on understaffing. *Journal of Emergency Nursing, 26*(6), 598–600.

Gallagher, R. M., & Kany, K. (2000). Does JCAHO see the truth? *American Journal of Nursing, 100*(4), 74.

Griffith, J. (1999). Substance abuse disorders in nurses. *Nursing Forum, 34*(4), 19–28.

Hall, J. K. (1996). *Nursing ethics and law.* Philadelphia: WB Saunders.

Hellquest, K., & Spector, N. (2004). A primer: The National Council of State Boards of Nursing nurse licensure compact. *JONA's Healthcare, Law, Ethics, & Regulation, 6(4),* 86–89.

Henderson, A. D. (2003). Nurses and workplace violence: Nurses' experiences of verbal and physical abuse at work. *Canadian Journal of Nursing Leadership, 16*(4), 82–98.

Hocking J. (1999). Testing times. *Nursing Standard. 13(26),* 18–19.

Husted, G. L., & Husted, J. H. (2001). *Ethical decision making in nursing and healthcare* (3rd ed.). New York: Springer.

International Labour Office, International Council of Nurses, World Health Organization, & Public Service International (2002). *Framework guidelines for addressing workplace violence in the health sector.* Geneva: Authors.

Jones, J., & Lyneham, J. (2000). Violence: Part of the job for Australian nurses? *Australian Journal of Advanced Nursing, 18(2),* 27–32.

Jones, J. M. (2005). Nurses remain atop honesty and ethics list. Retrieved on December 7, 2005, from http://poll.gallup.com/content/default.aspx?ci=20254&pg=1

Kulig, N. (2001). Interstate licensure: Nursing beyond your state's borders. *Nursing, 31*(2), 51.

Love, C. C., Morrison, E., & AAN Expert Panel on Violence. (2003) American Academy of Nursing expert panel on violence policy recommendations on workplace violence (adopted 2002). *Issues in Mental Health Nursing, 24,* 599–604.

Miles, D. (2003). Protecting the whistleblower: The Sarbanes-Oxley Act expands OSHA's investigative authority to include discrimination associated with corporate fraud cases. *Job Safety & Health Quarterly, 14*(2). Retrieved July 25, 2003, from www.osha.gov/Publications/JSHQ/winter2003html/whistleblowers.htm

Muller, L., & Flarey, D. L. (2004). Interstate practice. *Lippincott's Case Management: Managing the Process of Patient Care, 9*(3), 117–120.

National Council of State Boards of Nursing. (2005). Nurse licensure compacts: Compact implementation. Retrieved May 14, 2005, from www.ncsbn.org/nlc/rnlpvncompact_mutual_recognition_state.asp

Nolan, K. J. (2003). Federal False Claims Act. Retrieved April 29, 2003, from www.whistleblowerfirm.com/federalfalseclaimsact.html

Office of Research Integrity. (2001). Responsible whistle blowing: A whistleblower's bill of rights. Retrieved May 14, 2005, from http://ori.hhs.gov/misconduct/Whistleblower_Rights.shtml

Pines, A., & Aronson, E. (1981). *Burnout: From tedium to personal growth.* New York: Free Press, Inc.

Quyen-Nguyen, B. (2001). Blowing the whistle: Nurses' rights and responsibilities when employers' conduct is unethical. *American Journal of Nursing, 101*(7), 79.

Ray, M. M. (1999). Crossing state lines: Are interstate licenses in nursing's future? *AWHONN Lifelines, 3*(1), 21–22.

Serghis, D. (1999). Caring for the carers: Nurses with drug and alcohol problems. *Australian Nursing Journal, 6*(11), 18–20.

Shewey, H. M. (1997). Identification and assistance for chemically dependent nurses working in long-term care. *Geriatric Nursing. 18*(3), 115–118.

Singh, D. (2001). Health care workers with AIDS: The patient's right to know. *Medicine and Law, 20,* 49–62.

Sloan, A. (2002). Whistle blowing: Proceed with caution. *RN, 65*(1), 67–69.

Smith, L. L., Taylor, B. B., & Hughes, T. L. (1998). Effective peer responses to impaired nursing practice. *Nursing Clinics of North America, 33*(1), 105–118.

Stordeur, S., D'Hoore, W., & Vandenberghe, C. (2001). Leadership, organizational stress, and emotional exhaustion among hospital nursing staff. *Journal of Advanced Nursing, 35*(4), 533–542.

Sundeen, S. J., Stuart, G. W., Rankin, E. A. D., & Cohen, S. A. (1998). *Nurse–client interaction: Implementing the nursing process.* St. Louis, MO: Mosby.

Thomson, S. (1997). Incompetent criteria. *Nursing Standard, 11*(39), 16.

Tranbarger, R. E. (1997). A nurse executive's nightmare: The rogue nurse. *Nursing Management, 28*(2), 33–36.

Trinkoff, A. M., & Storr, C. L. (1998). Substance use among nurses: Differences between specialties. *American Journal of Public Health, 88*(4), 581–585.

Whistleblower Protection Act. (1989). 5 U.S.C. Secs. 1201 et seq. Retrieved July 25, 2003, from http://cwx.prenhall.com/bookbind/pubbooks/dye4/medialib/docs/whistle.htm and http://peregrinos.us/jtexplanstate1989excerpts.htm#4512

Whitley, G. G., Jacobson, G. A., &. Gawrys, M. T. (1996). The impact of violence in the health care setting upon nursing education. *Journal of Nursing Education. 35*(5), 211–218.

Zook, R. (2001). Sexual misconduct by health care providers. *Journal of Psychosocial Nursing, 39*(6), 41–47.

CHAPTER 17

Professional Ethical Issues Facing the Nurse—Manager

Objectives

At the end of this chapter, the student should be able to:

1. Discuss the nurses' professional responsibility for truth-telling, advocacy, confidentiality, resource allocation, and empowerment.
2. Describe mechanisms that can assist nurses to maintain confidentiality and identify professional harms that could be created by breaches in confidentiality.
3. Explain how an absence of resources can create an ethical issue.
4. Discuss how staffing mix can affect patient care.
5. Identify the ethical issues that can arise as a result of the nursing shortage.
6. Identify the management structure within the institution, and describe how managers can advocate for patients and staff and the ethical conflicts that can arise.
7. Describe the ethical issues related to nurses' empowerment and political activity.

KEY WORDS

- *Advocacy*
- *Autonomy/self-determination*
- *Charge nurse*
- *Collective bargaining*
- *Competence*
- *Confidentiality*
- *Discrimination*
- *Empowerment*
- *Grievance*

- *Harassment*
- *Mandatory overtime*
- *Moral distress*
- *Resource allocation*
- *Shared governance*
- *Staffing mix*
- *Staffing ratio*
- *Paternalism*
- *Truth-telling*

SECTION 1: *Ethical Themes: Building From the Basic to the Complex*

In considering professional nursing issues, the focus of the four ethical themes of confidentiality, truth-telling, advocacy, and allocation of resources moves from the patient or individual nurse to a broader orientation in which the interests of individuals need to be balanced against the needs of the profession. Thus, this section considers how the nurse, as part of the nursing profession, should act to promote these key concepts.

Professional issues are numerous and diverse, and some of them affect the nurse's performance, attitude, and perception more than others. The following examples should promote a greater understanding of how the key concepts are integrated into daily professional nursing practice. Nurses frequently make decisions about how to handle confidential information from peer situations and institutional decisions. Nurses are also responsible for truth-telling, not only when making care decisions, but also during professional interactions with physicians and other employees of the institution at which they work. Nurses become advocates not only for the patients entrusted to their care, but also for the institution and the profession. Finally, nurses' roles are often governed by resource allocation because this frequently affects staffing decisions and patient safety and advocacy. The key concepts will be discussed as they relate to professional nursing issues.

CONFIDENTIALITY

Maintaining *professional confidentiality* carries the same importance as maintaining *patient confidentiality*. Professional relationships form the foundation for proficient health care, and breaches in confidentiality can adversely affect the relationships between health care providers within an institution (e.g., nurses and physicians) and between institutional departments (e.g., nursing and pharmacy) as well as with other institutions (hospitals and long-term care facilities).

Interagency Communications

Health care agencies are often in competition with one another for resources, patients, and nurses, which creates an ongoing challenge. As costs escalate and reimbursement decreases and as smaller institutions are incorporated into larger health care systems, the competition for resources, patients, and nurses increases. When competition increases, communications may change. When this happens, inappropriate or misleading information may be exchanged to safeguard the institution against competition. Although patient privacy and confidentiality are enforced by federal regulations, such as the Health Information Portability and Accountability Act (HIPAA) of 1996, there are no specific guidelines for the regulation of information that is shared between institutions, such as staff wages, staff ratios, new services, or adverse events.

Hospitals competing with each other for nurses may not share the hourly wages or bonuses they offer to new nurses. This lack of communication might become a hindrance to a hospital that is trying to hire experienced nurses if, for example, the wages and benefits it offers are not competitive in the marketplace. Before making a decision about where to work, a nurses who is seeking employment will have to interview at each institution to learn this information. Although competition and the free market are foundations of the Western economy, the keeping of this information confidential becomes frustrating to nurses and increases the competition among hospitals. Newspapers and journals frequently advertise open nursing positions, but the advertisements seldom include wages, benefits, or bonuses. Although nurses usually do not select their jobs based on salary alone, they should be privy to this sort of financial information so they can utilize it to bargain among hospitals for higher wages. For example, a nurse who interviews at hospital A and receives hospital A's salary information can then go to hospital B and ask hospital B for wages higher than hospital A offered. The nurse may also return to hospital A with a counter proposal based on information obtained at hospital B. This bargaining eventually affects resource allocation within the institutions, and it may lead to an inequity of wages between similarly prepared nurses. Although nurses have the right to bargain for wages in this manner, similarly prepared nurses who do not exert that right may be compensated at a lower rate than the nurses who did bargain. Confidentiality can also affect competing agencies in areas other than resource allocation and inequity of wages.

An example of an interagency breach of confidentiality is a discussion between two nurse–managers who are friends and are employed at competing hospitals. At lunch, they begin to discuss general staff problems. This leads to a more specific discussion that includes problems about a specific nurse, who is named. A few months later, this nurse applies for a position at the competing hospital. As a result of the information shared by the nurse–managers at their earlier lunch meeting, the nurse is denied the position. The breach in confidentiality regarding the nurse's performance has affected the nurse's ability to become employed at the competing institution. The former nurse–manager's indiscrete remark might also be perceived as slander, making her legally liable for the consequences of her remarks for that staff nurse's career.

Similar confidentiality breaches that occur within an institution may alter relationships within it. Two nurse–managers within the same institution begin to discuss a personnel issue in a casual manner, and again a specific nurse is named. The nurse then requests and is denied a transfer to one of the manager's units based on information discussed earlier by the managers. The confidentiality breach has affected the nurse's mobility within the institution.

Personal Issues

Although nurses work together closely to provide safe patient care, not all nurses become friends with their peers. Adversarial relationships between nurses could easily lead to public discussions about private information. Such discussions can create distrustful relationships among staff, can affect the milieu of the unit, and can ultimately affect patient care. Nurses occasionally form small groups, or cliques, of individuals who develop friendships to the exclusion of other nurses. These small groups may be prone to gossiping about other nurses from their unit or from other units in the hospital. For example, Joshua Hill, a recent graduate, confides in another nurse that he failed the National Council Licensure Examination (NCLEX) twice before he finally passed it. The other nurse tells co-workers, and they complain to the nurse–manager that they are too short-staffed to take the time to extend the new nurse's orientation. No one wants to be his preceptor. This makes for an uncomfortable situation for the new nurse, who regrets disclosing the NCLEX story and decides to find work at a different hospital.

In the long run, the nurses on this unit remain short-staffed because they alienated the new nurse. Could the nurse–manager have averted the situation by advising the new nurse to keep the NCLEX story private? Having a competency-based orientation that is individualized would make the new nurse's NCLEX exam scores irrelevant, and such an orientation would identify and address deficient areas in the new nurse's skill base.

Another example that illustrates the damaging effects of breaches in confidentiality involves Juanita Pierz, a nurse who has just been hired at hospital A. Juanita had previous problems with alcohol impairment but received treatment and is now in recovery. Julie Chism remembers Juanita from another hospital, and tells co-workers that Juanita is a drunk and is undependable. The other nurses formulate an opinion of Juanita before getting to know her. Regardless of Juanita's competence, this misuse of confidential information has already created an aura of skepticism, and possibly mistrust, at hospital A. As a result of the adversarial environment created by Julie's sharing this information, Juanita's tenure at this new job may be limited. Nurses often may not recognize how damaging breaches in confidentiality can become, not only to the person involved, but to the nursing unit and to the patients. Nurses' support of other nurses is essential for creating a nonhostile working environment.

Managers also have a responsibility to maintain the confidentiality of information regarding employees, other managers, and hospital personnel. Managers have access to confidential information from interviews, personnel reports, and evaluations. Employees expect this information to remain confidential. A manager's misuse of this information can create an environment of distrust within the unit or hospital. For example, unless a pregnant employee gives her nurse–manager permission to tell others about the pregnancy, a nurse–manager who tells other nurses about the pregnancy is violating the nurse's confidentiality.

Nurses have also been known to reveal information that their managers asked them to keep confidential. For example, when one of the authors (D.J.) was a nurse–manager, she received a compensation pool of money each year to distribute as merit increases. Although the formula the hospital used to develop the pool was 3% for each nurse, the manager was given the discretion to award more money to those nurses who deserved larger merit bonuses. Thus, the distribution of the money varied from 3% in some instances to higher merit bonuses to outstanding nurses and slightly lower merit bonuses to others who were not so outstanding. Each time the merit increase was discussed with the individual nurses, they were requested they keep the information confidential. However, each time, within moments of the merit distributions, all the nurses knew everyone else's merit amounts, and the complaints began. Those nurses who received less were dissatisfied. According to the principle of justice, however, distribution of goods should be fair in light of what may be owed to a person. Although this principle allows for equal treatment of equal people, it also permits unequal people to be treated unequally (Beauchamp & Childress, 2001). Justice allowed those nurses who excelled to obtain greater merit increases than those who performed at a lower level. Therefore, how would the outstanding nurses have reacted if they had received the same merit amount as the other nurses? Someone would have been unhappy either way, which is why all the nurses were asked to keep their merit bonuses confidential. The nurses' practice of discussing their merit raises always created a period of disharmony within the unit. Eventually, the milieu returned to normal, but relationships among nurses were permanently affected.

A final area for consideration regarding confidentiality is any situation that involves a grievance, harassment, or discrimination. These situations can all lead to confidential information becoming legally open for discussion among certain institutional personnel.

A *grievance* is a process whereby an employee can protest an action taken against him or her. Usually a grievance is filed when the employee believes that he or she has been unjustly or unfairly treated or has been falsely accused of wrong doing. A grievance can be filed through a *collective bargaining* unit or through an employee advocate. A grievance can be directed toward another employee or toward a manager. For example, two nurses who are equally qualified were being considered for a charge nurse position. The nurse who was not chosen filed a grievance claiming that the manager chose unfairly based on a friendship with the other nurse. Whether or not the allegations are true, the grievance will need to be investigated to resolve the issue. The investigation into why one nurse was chosen over the other may reveal confidential information that could harm either or both of the nurses.

In addition to grievances, another issue that may confront employees is harassment. *Harassment* includes any situation where another person repeatedly confronts an employee. Sexual harassment is often reported to be the most common type of harassment, although harassment for other reasons is certainly possible. For example, a phlebotomy technician at a hospital is harassing a nurse. This technician follows the nurse around the hospital and to her car, and has left notes on her car. The nurse reports the incident through the proper channels, such as through security and to her manager, and only tells her closest friends about the incident. One of the nurse's friends tells others about the harassment complaint, though, and then friends of the technician begin to also harass the nurse about filing the complaint. This breach in confidentiality has now led to additional harassment for the nurse, and it could result in harm to the nurse.

A final mechanism that can lead to the compromise of confidentiality is discrimination. *Discrimination* occurs when an unjust distinction is made based on race, sex, ethnicity, or sexual orientation. For example, two nurses have interviewed for a position in an emergency department in an urban medical center. One nurse is a man and the other a woman. The female nurse has 10 years and the male nurse just 2 years of emergency department experience. The male nurse is offered the position over the female nurse. When the female nurse asks a friend about the decision, she is informed that, although she was more qualified for the position, the presence of a man in the emergency department would create a stronger image for the hospital and would diversify the staff. This breach of confidential information has alleged a discriminatory practice at the hospital. As in this example, any breach of confidentiality has the potential to cause harm or create adverse situations for all of the individuals involved.

TRUTH-TELLING

The importance and difficulties of *truth-telling* were discussed in Chapter 7. Interactions between health care providers are based on truthful information. Just as being untruthful or lying to patients can result in harm to patients, failure to disclose information or lying to peers can hamper professional relationships. Truth-telling is a professional expectation that should be upheld by all nurses.

Nurses' Responsibilities

Nurses have a responsibility to be honest and straightforward with patients, physicians, staff, and the institution. Because truth-telling is based on respect, autonomy, nonmaleficence, and beneficence, values that are all desired in nurses, they have a duty to uphold these principles. Nurses' honesty and forthrightness may make the difference between a good and a poor patient outcome. For example, during shift report, Jon Packo tells Sophia Stack that a particular patient received acetaminophen for a headache. The patient again requests the medication for a headache, so Sophia checks the patient's chart to see what time Jon gave the last dose. However, Sophia does not see the previously reported dose charted in the patient's medication record. Instead of contacting Jon, who administered the earlier dose, to clarify what time it was given, Sophia administers the medication again. Sophia later sees that Jon had documented in the narrative notes that the earlier dose of medication was given just before change of shift. Sophia then decides not to document the dose she administered because it would require completing a risk report and she might be disciplined for the medication error even though no harm came to the patient. Although the patient was not harmed by the extra dose of medication or by the omission in documentation, Sophia is omitting essential information from the patient's medical record to protect herself. This act is a violation of truth-telling, and it undermines respect for both the patient and the professional role. Would the nurse's expectation to truth-tell have changed if the patient had suffered adverse effects from the extra dose of medication?

Another example of a breach in truth-telling involves information a nurse provides to a physician. A nurse is caring for a disoriented patient who is having difficulty sleeping. The nurse contacts the patient's physician and states, "The patient is requesting medication for sleep." The physician orders sleep medication for the patient, which the nurse administers. The patient falls asleep. Although the nurse's intention was to benefit and maybe even prevent harm to the patient, the nurse was not completely honest with the physician in communicating the need for sleep medication.

Nurses can also be dishonest with other nurses. For example, Shawn Turner asks Liz Kiley to switch a day on the schedule. Liz does not wish to make the switch, but instead tells Shawn that she has to take care of a sick aunt who lives 80 miles away, and so she cannot make the change. On the day in question, Shawn sees Liz at the local mall. Shawn now feels deceived by Liz, and the trust between them has been betrayed. This may affect their future working relationship.

Finally, nurses are responsible for being honest with the institution that employs them. For example, a nurse requests a particular day off to attend a concert but ends up being scheduled to work that day. Instead of attempting to find coverage by another nurse or talking to the manager, the nurse takes no further action and calls in sick that day. Although the unit is able to cover the nurse's absence, patients could have been adversely affected by the nurse's dishonesty.

Although no harm occurred to the patients, or to anyone else, involved in these situations, they all exhibited a degree of dishonesty. These small "white lies" undermine the integrity of the nurses involved, and they could potentially lead to greater degrees of dishonesty and harm in the future.

Administrative Responsibility

Just as staff nurses have a responsibility to tell the truth to patients, physicians, and peers, administrators are required to be truthful with nurses. Nurse administrators are expected to be truthful when hiring new employees, during the interview process, when placing information in an employee's file, and when nurses are not performing within the institution's guidelines. Administrative responsibilities when hiring new employees include being truthful about the role responsibilities, about the required training, and about the job's scheduling and wages. For example, a nurse–manager is interviewing a very skilled nurse and really wants to impress the nurse so that the nurse will consider accepting the position. In wooing the candidate, the nurse–manager could promise the nurse that he or she will receive extensive training, no rotation to evening or night shifts, and a high salary. However, once the nurse accepts the position and begins to work, the manager notifies the nurse that due to staffing shortages, his or her training will be significantly shortened and he or she will have to rotate shifts for a few months. If the manager was untruthful during the interview, the nurse will feel betrayed and will become distrustful of the manager. This could result in an adversarial relationship between the nurse and the manager that could affect the entire unit and patient care.

Another example of a manager's responsibility involves a nurse being reported for a breach in institutional policy. A truthful manager should address the issue with the nurse and inform him or her whether there will be a notation placed in the nurse's file. If the manager addresses the issue with the nurse and informs him or her that the information will remain between the nurse and the manager, but then places a notation in the nurse's file, the manager is violating the requirement for truthfulness.

A final example relates to a nurse who consistently performs below hospital and nursing standards. Other nurses' report and document the poor performance, and their nurse–manager informs them that the issues will be addressed. Because the manager does not want to dismiss the poorly performing nurse, the manager files the information away and never discusses it with the nurse. This situation could result in patient harm, but the manager chooses to ignore the other nurses' documented complaints. This choice could create a negative or adversarial relationship between the manager and the nurses who documented their concerns, which they wanted to be heard and validated; they might feel betrayed when their concerns are dismissed as unimportant. In attempting to avoid creating a negative relationship with the one poorly performing nurse, the manager actually ends up creating an adversarial relationship with all the other nurses on the unit.

Just as administrators have a responsibility to be truthful with nurses, nurses have a reciprocal responsibility to be truthful with administrators. During the interview process, managers trust that nurse-candidates are honest and forthright. A dishonest nurse may not fully disclose information during the interview or may falsely characterize information to attain the position. For example, nurses might exaggerate their skill levels and claim to have greater capabilities than they actually possess. Or they might be dishonest about why they left their last position, and say that they were sexually harassed when actually they were dismissed for poor performance. As a final example, a nurse might conceal pertinent personal information from administrators during the interview process, such as the fact that his or her license is suspended in another state.

A final issue that pertains to truthfulness involves inaccurate letters of recommendation. A nurse–manager could give a poorly performing employee a highly positive recommendation letter for another position, which shifts the burden of the problem employee to another, unknowing institution. Vague recommendations or letters without full disclosure can deceive managers. A manager being asked for a recommendation could avoid this ethical dilemma by only confirming a former employee's dates of employment and not commenting on the employee's performance. A letter of that type usually conveys the manager's reluctance to recommend the employee without forcing the manager to risk libeling the employee. Conversely, managers may write dishonest recommendations to eliminate problem employees from their current positions. This type of dishonesty could potentially harm patients or could place nurses in adversarial situations. Truth-telling is an important nursing responsibility, and dishonesty in any capacity could affect not only patient care, but also professional interactions and relationships that are built on trust and honesty. Truthfulness, in conjunction with confidentiality, facilitates the creation of a respectful working environment for nurses and helps to foster professional relationships.

ADVOCACY

Advocacy most often refers to the activities of health care providers in promoting and protecting patients' rights. For professionals, advocacy includes the support of causes or principles that forward the mission of the profession. There are several professional issues that health care providers can advocate for. Lack-of-resource issues revolve around the lack of competent nurses in the workforce. Such a shortage of adept nurses interferes with a health care institutions' ability to safely provide patient care. Therefore, nurses who demand appropriate staffing levels and mix are advocating not only for the profession, but for the patients as well.

Nurses expect to have a voice in major decisions that affect their nursing roles. Participating in shared governance is one means for nurses to attain this goal. In addition, they may participate in collective bargaining, and may even go on strike to improve working conditions and the patient-care situation. Nurses who wish to have a greater influence may become politically active at the local, state, or national level. Finally, by listening to and representing nurses' concerns within their institution or agency, nurse–managers can play a pivotal role in advocating for all nurses.

Competent Staff

To provide safe and effective patient care, the nursing staff must be competent in caring for a particular category of patients. Nurses who question an unsafe or inappropriate patient assignment and managers who refuse to accept unqualified supplemental staff are performing as advocates. However, if a nurse–manager or charge nurse accepts supplemental staff who cannot safely provide patient care, then management is not advocating for the nurses or the patients. In addition, if a nurse accepts a patient assignment for which he or she is unqualified, the nurse is not functioning as an advocate. For example, if an adult critical care nurse accepts an assignment in a pediatric critical care unit for which he or she is unqualified, that nurse is not advocating for the patient, for the institution, and/or for the profession. By accepting a patient assignment that is beyond his or her scope of knowledge and experience, that nurse is putting himself or herself at high risk for causing harm to the patient. It is the nurse's responsibility to object to that patient assignment and request that he or she only be assigned to patients for which he or she is qualified to safely care. However, if the pediatric unit manager mandated the assignment over the objections of a nurse who felt ill prepared to care for pediatric patients, then management would be the ones not advocating for patient safety or for the professional needs of the nurse. As this example illustrates, both the bedside nurses and management need to work as advocates to guarantee that safe nursing practices are in place to ensure the delivery of safe patient care.

ALLOCATION OF RESOURCES

Allocation of resources is commonly viewed in terms of the use of equipment or other resources within the institution, but nurses are also accountable for other forms of resource allocation. One important issue is that of "time theft." In many institutions, nurses manually complete their time sheets or time cards using the honor system. Nurses can add additional time by signing in early or signing out late, or more commonly by not indicating their breaks or their lunch times on the sheet. Nurses who are accountable to time clocks can also "steal time" by taking extra long lunches and then leaving late because they did not catch up on their work during their shift, or by clocking out late because they were visiting with other nurses.

Another type of theft involves patient equipment and supplies. There are two types of theft involving patient supplies; one concerns charging patients inappropriately, the other concerns a loss of revenue for the institution. In the former, nurses borrow supplies or medications from other patients in the interest of providing timely and expedient care to their patients. However, "borrowing" from one patient for another patient becomes "stealing" if the nurse does not replace the supplies/medications that he/or she took from the first patient or if the nurse does not go back and charge the supplies/medications to the appropriate patient. Patients can also be inappropriately charged when nurses do not give them "credit" for medications they refused to take.

Institutions can also lose revenue in a variety of ways. Failure to record patients' charges equates to lost revenue for the institution. Hospital staff taking food from patient meal trays, taking extra meal trays for themselves, or eating items from the patient nourishment center costs the institution money. Nurses may also be guilty of taking stock medications for personal use, such as taking acetaminophen for a headache. The occasional use by a nurse of stock medication is not usually an ethical concern on a unit, but any other diversion of medication, such as taking narcotics, tranquilizers, sedatives, or other controlled substances, is absolutely forbidden. Finally, nurses often inadvertently go home with items in their pockets such as tape, pens, alcohol pads, and syringes, although they probably bring these items back the next day. If they were stocking their home office with reams of computer paper or obtaining their children's school supplies from material from the unit, then they would be stealing.

SUMMARY

There are many challenges in the health care arena. Nurses will be frequently confronted with professional ethical situations that relate to confidentiality, truth-telling, advocacy, and resource allocation, as well as other issues. By reviewing some of these situations and discussing how to foresee, and possibly prevent, adversarial situations, nurses can promote a concerted effort to provide superior patient care and safety. Nurses are in a position to positively affect the future of health care, both as individuals and as collective units, by exhibiting ethical practice within institutional settings.

CLINICAL EXERCISES

1. Observe nurses working on the nursing unit and determine the number of instances in which nurses borrow items from one patient to treat another

patient. Can you identify any ethical justification for this disparity in resource allocation?
2. Observe the nursing unit for any actual or potential professional breaches in confidentiality. Do nurses talk adversely about others in their absence? Do these breaches cause adverse working relationships?
3. Observe the level of peer support on the unit. How can the absence of support alter working relationships?

Discussion Questions

1. A nurse is interviewing for a job on a medical unit. She is recently divorced and is the single mother for three young children. She left her last two positions because she was unable to rotate shifts due to lack of flexible child care. The manager intends to offer her a position on the day shift, but may assign her to another shift if needed. She does not tell the nurse about the expectation that she will need to work evenings or nights occasionally. Discuss how much information should be disclosed during the interview. What are the possible ethical consequences of failure by either party to disclose information?
2. Nurse Anita Eybel overhears Nurse Barbara Hodges on the telephone and learns that Nurse Hodge's mother-in-law is an inpatient on the mental health/psychiatric unit. Nurse Eybel tells others on the unit. Discuss the ethical ramifications of Nurse Eybel's actions.
3. You have been working with a nurse for the last 10 months on a busy surgical unit. The nurse often leaves tasks undone, her patient rooms are messy, and you have received patient complaints about her care. This nurse has just asked you to write a recommendation letter for her for a new position at another institution.

   a. As her manager, will you write the letter?
   b. What information are you ethically obligated to disclose?

4. You are a nurse in a busy emergency department. You frequently observe another nurse take repeated breaks outside and in the lounge in addition to taking long lunch breaks. Subsequently you find out that this nurse always writes "no lunch" and "no breaks" on her time sheet.

   a. Are employee time cards considered confidential?
   b. How does this nurse's actions affect resource allocation?
   c. What should be done to correct this situation?

SECTION 2: *Professional Nursing Issues: Staffing*

Safe and effective patient care depends on adequate, competent nursing staff. Specific staffing issues may have a profound effect on the nursing unit, as well as on the nursing profession as a whole. This section reviews specific staffing issues and their effects on resource allocation.

There are several facets of resource allocation. Currently, the most crucial allocation issue is maintaining an adequate number of nurses in the workforce to safely care for patients. This and many other countries are facing a serious nursing shortage, which is predicted to reach a crisis stage by the year 2020. In the past, increasing nurses' pay and benefits relieved shortages. However, the current shortage is not totally economically rooted. Rather, it is the result of declining enrollment in nursing schools, an aging workforce that will begin to retire in large numbers at the same time, and decreased retention of nurses in hospitals (Berliner & Ginzberg, 2002). Nurses are leaving hospital-nursing positions for other opportunities in nursing, such as outpatient and community-nursing positions. In addition, nurses with families or those who have been practicing for a number of years are choosing to spend fewer hours at work and have more free time. When these factors are combined with the increase in acutely ill patients that have shorter lengths of stay in the hospital, the responsibilities for hospital nurses increase and occasionally can become overwhelming.

STAFFING ISSUES

The American Nurses Association (ANA) (2001) Code of Ethics for Nurses states that nurses are responsible for the safety and well-being of their patients and that their primary commitment is to their patients. Nurses assume and incorporate this responsibility into their daily work environment. Increasingly, however, nurses are finding it difficult to maintain patient safety when they are assigned a large patient load. Many nurses are dissatisfied with the frequency of such unsafe assignments and want to be involved in decision-making regarding staffing ratios. Old staffing models used to determine nurse-to-patient ratios are now ineffective due to increased patient acuity and decreased lengths of hospital stays. Therefore, staff nurses now believe that they are the best judges of how many patients they can safely care for. Some members of the profession expect to have input into *all* levels of decisions, not just staff ratios (Bradford & Raines, 1992). Patients enter hospitals primarily to receive nursing care, yet nurses have limited input into health care decisions (Homsted & Nilsson, 2003). As a result of nurses' frustrations regarding safe staffing and competent patient care, they have begun to organize and present legislation for safe staffing levels. In 1999, California Assembly Bill 394 was passed to regulate minimum nurse-to-patient ratios in acute care hospitals (Kuehl, 1999). Many other states and nursing organizations are following this move to regulate the safe level of their nurse-to-patient ratios.

Another issue related to staffing levels is the staff mix. Research has shown that having a higher proportion of registered nurses leads to a higher quality of patient care and to lower patient mortality rates (Aiken, Smith, & Lake 1994; Kovner & Gergen, 1998). Many institutions also employ "supplemental staff" to assist registered nurses with patient care. "Supplemental staff" includes, among others, licensed practical nurses, nurse's aides, care technicians, secretarial support, environmental services, and transport staff. The staff mix may also include new graduates or orienting nurses.

An institution's staffing mix directly affects the quality of patient care delivered there. For example, one nurse and one care technician assigned to a group of five patients will probably, depending on the patients' acuity, result in the delivery of safe patient care. The nurse can delegate nonnursing responsibilities to the technician and spend more time performing nursing duties. On the other hand, if one nurse and two care technicians are assigned to a group of 10 patients, the nurse may not be able to provide safe nursing care to all of them, even with the additional technician support.

Another example that illustrates the effect of a staff's mix arises when two nurses are assigned 5 patients each and but share only one care technician. The technician is then responsible for 10 patients. If secretarial support is subtracted from this mix (so that either the nurses or the technician must also perform that role), the workload for each individual will be significantly different. This kind of situation increases the technician's workload and decreases his or her availability to assist both nurses. In addition, the absence of secretarial support means that the nurses will need to perform additional clerical responsibilities that will take time away from their provision of direct patient care. Just as an inadequate supply of nurses can lead to patient harm, so can an inappropriate staff mix. Although creative staff mixes can ease some of the nurses' workload, this lack of necessary resources may lead to ineffective patient care, or worse, unsafe patient care and preventable errors.

Solutions that many hospitals employ to deal with staffing shortages are to use nurses who float from units that have a low census to units that have a high census, in-house registry nurses who can work on any unit, and outside agency nurses (or traveling nurses).

Float nurses are reassigned from their primary nursing unit to other units that have greater staffing needs. The problem with reassignment is that the float nurses are often unfamiliar with the type of patient or the nursing focus of the reassigned unit. For example, a medical nurse is floated to the orthopedic-surgical unit. A patient who underwent a hip replacement asks, "Will you help me get up to go to the toilet?" A patient care technician enters the room and sees that the float nurse and the patient are not implementing the correct procedure for using crutches when transferring from the bed to a standing position, and shouts, "Stop, let me help you!" To prevent patient harm, it is essential for the reassigned nurse to explicitly state what functions he or she can or cannot perform. To ensure safe and organized patient care, it is also essential that the reassigned nurse receive a proper unit orientation. Even after all those requirements are met, the reassigned nurse may not be able to provide care for certain patients, so even though the new unit now has "enough nurses," the unit's regular nurses will still have increased responsibilities.

Registry nurses are typically hospital employees who work primarily on the nursing units in the hospital that need supplemental staff. These nurses are familiar with the institution's policies and procedures, and they are expected to be versatile in most types of patient care. Using registry nurses should provide for safe patient care, but there is still a potential for patients to be harmed because these nurses often work part-time, and so may not be proficient in every type of patient situation to which they are exposed. Furthermore, registry nurses are often evaluated by one nursing supervisor instead of by the unit leaders. This form of evaluation may limit the hospital's ability to act on the nurses' performance difficulties, and it may inhibit goal-setting and the delivery of additional education to the registry nurses.

Hospitals also utilize agency nurses as supplemental staff. Agency nurses typically work at several hospitals, and thus they may not be familiar with the policies of each institution. In addition, agency nurses work on a variety of nursing units, and they might not spend an extended period of time on any one unit. This can lead to fragmented and inconsistent patient care. Due to agency nurses' unfamiliarity with the hospitals at which they work, there is also an increased risk for them to make errors. Because the agency nurses do not know the other staff members, communication may be hampered. Maldistribution of nurses and the increased presence of temporary or part-time nurses may decrease the interaction and cohesiveness of the nurses on the unit. This fractured interaction may inhibit the communication of important or essential information (Anthony & Preuss, 2002).

Finally, *traveling nurses* contract with a particular hospital for 3 to 6 months at a time. Unlike agency nurses, traveling nurses are guaranteed employment for the terms of the contract. Although traveling nurses remain in the same institution for an extended period, they are initially unfamiliar with the environment, policies, and staff. This initial unfamiliarity can induce the same problems that are seen with agency nurses. In addition, because traveling nurses are temporary employees, they may not have a vested interest in the institution.

As illustrated in these examples, all methods of providing supplemental staffing may affect patient care and safety as a result of supplemental staffs' unfamiliarity, decreased communication, lack of organizational skills, lack of experience, and lack of competency in specialized nursing areas. Some hospitals avoid the use of supplemental staff by expecting/requiring their staff nurses to work overtime.

MANDATORY OVERTIME

Mandatory overtime, a common practice, has received increasing public attention as a safety issue in patient care. Mandatory overtime is the expectation that staff nurses will commit to work over their budgeted hours to provide adequate staffing levels on their nursing units. Although this practice may decrease the use of supplemental staff, it may also contribute to unsafe nursing practices, increased errors, and decreased patient safety. Working excess hours and forced overtime can be dangerous, and nurses who work long and tiring hours are at risk for making mistakes (Mee, 2001). Mandatory overtime can also be a major factor contributing to nurses' job dissatisfaction and to nurses leaving hospital nursing. As a result of the increased potential for errors and decreased patient safety and satisfaction, some nursing associations oppose the practice of mandatory overtime. The Arizona Nurses Association issued statements to be used as staffing tools that oppose mandatory overtime (Anonymous, 2002). Other professional organizations are also preparing statements that prohibit mandatory overtime. In addition, the Safe Nursing and Patient Care Act (H.R.791/S.351) is a legislative proposal that limits the use of mandatory overtime except in cases of local, state, or national emergencies. Whenever supplemental staffing or mandatory overtime becomes a part of staffing decisions, compensation also becomes an issue.

Compensation

Compensation takes on many forms. All nurses expect compensation for the jobs they perform. Compensation is typically rendered in the form of hourly wages (or a salary) and various kinds of benefits, which are considered a "just form of compensation." The most common problems that relate to compensation are disparate pay, bonuses, and "job hopping" from institution to institution for higher wages.

Just as the methods of health care delivery are matters of justice, so are the methods of reimbursement for nurses. Although the health care system has been restructuring and downsizing for years, the fact that nurses are essential to the existence of the agencies has not changed. Because the compensation of nurses is the predominant expenditure for hospitals, controlling nurses' wages is often a priority for institutions. In addition, hospitals are competing for the scarce resource of nurses and are changing their forms of compensation to remain competitive.

As stated earlier, this competition often takes the form of higher wages for new nurses or bonuses to attract new nurses to the institution. This becomes a problem, however, for the nurses currently working at the institution, who can feel devalued and unimportant to the institution and that they are being treated unfairly for remaining loyal to it. For example, Steve Theil has been employed for 5 years at the same hospital where he began as a new graduate. Nina Abbed, who also has 5 years of experience, has just been hired by the same hospital for a higher hourly wage than Steve receives. Although an experienced nurse has been added to the staff, a wage disparity has been created between nurses with equal nursing experience. The free market system in this country allows for institutions to compete for a scarce resource. The principle of distributive justice allows for fair and equitable distribution of resources (Beauchamp & Childress, 2001). This allows hospitals to fairly compete for nurses to ensure adequate staffing, maintain patient safety, and control their expenditures. However, this competition can also contribute to wage disparity and dissatisfaction for currently employed nurses, who might view this hiring practice as unjust and unfair.

Finally, as mentioned earlier, the use of supplemental staff can contribute to the perception of wage disparity. Supplemental staff such as agency nurses, traveling nurses, and hospital-registry nurses are paid higher hourly wages than regular staff nurses. Institutions justify the higher wages by saying they compensate for the benefits the staff nurses receive, who receive benefit packages, guaranteed hours, paid time off, and malpractice insurance through the hospital, whereas supplemental staff do not. In addition, supplemental personnel's absences are regulated by the agency, not by the hospital. Finally, as a trade-off for their higher wages and their increased control over their work hours, supplemental staff also must accept more variable assignments than staff nurses.

Lack of Equipment

Another resource issue that contributes to nurses' discontent is the lack of available (or properly functioning) equipment needed to safely provide patient care. Equipment purchases are often capital expenses that must be approved by the institutional governing board. If money was not allocated for the equipment in the fiscal budget, then the purchase of new equipment may have to be postponed until the next budget session. If nurses lack the appropriate equipment, patient safety and patient care can be compromised. Nurses' equipment needs can vary from properly functioning beds to adequate supplies of blood pressure cuffs and glucometers. For example, if a nursing unit has 20 patients who need blood-glucose checks four times a day but the unit only has one functioning glucometer, patients' treatment for altered glucose levels could be delayed. Another example of how a lack of equipment can compromise patient safety is a nursing unit that has a large population of patients at high risk for falling but does not have enough beds with fall alarms or enough light in the patients' rooms. If there is a considerable need for equipment and a limited supply of that equipment, patient care will be compromised. In addition, not only is borrowing equipment from one patient to treat another patient unsafe, but also it does not solve the equipment shortage. Borrowing equipment is a short-term solution to a resource issue.

There are several issues surrounding resource allocation that can adversely impact the nurses' role and patient care. Nurses need to be cognizant of the issues so they can advocate for themselves and for their patients. If nurses believe that they are being treated or compensated unjustly or that patient care and safety are being compromised, they need to seek support from the managers and advocates within their institutions. They can also seek guidance from the Code of Ethics for Nurses (ANA, 2001) (although the Code cannot be used as legal defense) or from their local or national nursing organizations. Finally, the National Labor Relations Board (NLRB) can offer answers to questions about compensation and fair labor practices.

SUMMARY

It now appears that the nursing shortage is far-reaching. Hospital restructuring has contributed to the shortage by driving the most experienced nurses, frustrated and disheartened, out of the profession (Weinberg, 2003). In a survey conducted by Aiken et al. (2001, p. 46), 22% of the surveyed U.S. nurses planned to leave the profession within the next year, and 33% of nurses younger than the age of 30 planned to leave. Canadian figures for nurses planning to leave the profession were 16.6% and 29.4%, respectively.

Because the shortage is multifactorial in nature, the resolution will need to be carefully planned. Nursing schools are currently unable to admit and graduate nurses at a faster rate than they are already. Because there is insufficient nursing faculty, nursing programs are turning away qualified candidates. With the profession's inability to replenish the supply of nurses as rapidly as they are leaving the workforce, the workload and responsibility of the remaining nurses becomes greater. With a diminishing workforce, staffing issues are already arising. It is essential for practicing nurses to be aware of the ethical issues created by decreased staffing and decreased resources.

Nurses' ethical responsibility continues to be that they safeguard patient care, despite staffing issues. Nursing leadership in institutions, professional associations, and nursing administration has an ethical responsibility to current and future patients and nurses to fight for the integrity and acceptable working conditions of their profession.

CLINICAL EXERCISES

1. Identify the mechanisms your agency uses to determine patient acuity and staffing ratios on different nursing units. What ethical principles are used to guide the nurses' workload?
2. Investigate whether the agency has a policy regarding overtime and/or mandatory overtime.

   - What criteria are used to determine the need for overtime? Do these criteria reflect any ethical commitments?
   - How is overtime allocated among employees?

3. Determine whether the state board of regulation for your state has a position statement regarding mandatory overtime.
4. Review nursing job advertisements and perform an online job search. Determine how often salary and bonuses (resources) are discussed in these sources. Identify which advertisements were the most attractive and why. Identify any disparity in resources within these advertisements and discuss the ethical justifications.

Discussion Questions

1. Review the Nurse Reinvestment Act (U.S. Department of Health and Human Services, HRSA, Bureau of Health Professions, 2002).

   a. What actions does this act take to relieve the nursing shortage?
   b. Are there actions that you believe are needed, but not addressed in this act? Explain.
   b. Is the Act sufficient to provide relief to the current and future nursing shortage? Defend your answer.

2. Discuss the current trend to have legislation mandate minimum nurse-to-patient staffing ratios.

   a. How are mandatory ratios ethical?
   b. Do you believe mandatory ratios improve patient care? Defend your answer.
   c. How does patient acuity still impact safe care even if ratios are upheld?
   d. What are the ethical consequences if the ratios cannot be maintained?
   e. Should mandatory ratios affect nurses leaving the unit for a coffee break?

3. Identify reasons nurses might give for or against mandatory overtime.

   a. Discuss the ethical justifications for mandatory overtime.
   b. Discuss alternatives to mandatory overtime.
   c. Describe ethical rationales for accepting/refusing to participate in mandatory overtime.

4. Review the ANA Code of Ethics for Nurses (2001) regarding nurses' accountability and responsibility.

   a. Discuss how the nursing shortage may affect responsibility and accountability.
   b. Discuss how staffing mix may affect the nurses' accountability.
   c. Discuss any ethical justifications for nurses' failure to be accountable and responsible for patient care and safety.

5. Review the agency's policy for nurse reassignment (floating) and the use of registry or agency nurses.

   a. Discuss the ethical implications of nurses floating to unfamiliar nursing units.
   b. Discuss nursing accountability for accepting/refusing patient assignments.
   c. Should a nurse be disciplined for refusing a patient assignment in an unfamiliar nursing environment?

SECTION 3: *Professional Nursing Issue: Management Issues*

The previous two sections discussed professional issues related to nurses' responsibilities in relation to confidentiality, truth-telling, and advocacy. They also discussed resource issues that are particularly related to staffing. This section ventures into broader issues related to *management's* role in health care organizations and how management decisions can affect nurses and patient care.

Within most institutions, there are several levels of management. Many hospitals have management layers comprising upper management, consisting of a president or chief executive officer (CEO) and a senior management team that includes vice presidents/department heads; middle management, consisting of supervisors/unit managers; and lower management, consisting of direct-line supervisors such as clinical leaders/charge nurses. Within all these layers, there are dual responsibilities toward the organizational mission and toward the employees. Each layer of management is accountable to the employees under their charge as well as to the next level of managers to whom they report. As a result of the dual nature of these positions, the possibility of ethical conflict is ever-present.

MANAGEMENT RESPONSIBILITIES

Top/Upper Management

Organizational management decisions traditionally begin in the upper levels and filter down through the layers to the employees. Top managers, such as the CEO or president, are ultimately accountable for the agency. The vice presidents are also accountable for major agency decisions. Decisions regarding the budget, such as capital expenditures and salaries, are decided at this level. Upper-level managers are also accountable to governing and accreditation agencies, their board of directors (and stockholders, if it is a for-profit organization), and patients, physicians, and the community.

Often, major organizational decisions are made at this level, and other managers and employees are simply informed of the decisions, a "top-down" approach. Decisions made unilaterally at this level that affect employees' salaries, benefits, or working conditions may elicit negative reactions from employees. Employees may perceive that these decisions were made autocratically and without input from those individuals who are most affected by them. For instance, the CEO of a hospital makes a unilateral decision, for budgetary reasons, to cut nursing staff by 20%. The CEO does not consider the effect this decision could have on patient care. The consequences of this decision could include medication errors, patient dissatisfaction, and even an increase in patient mortality. Ethically, this decision is not in the best interests of the patients, and by making this decision, the hospital is not acting as an advocate for patient safety and good care. Once the CEO makes this decision, other members of the senior management team are responsible for making sure the CEO really had the correct information regarding the effect that decreasing the nursing staff would have on patient care. This is why the agencies that monitor health care organizations try to ensure that major policies and decisions are not authoritarian and paternalistic in nature.

Middle Management

Members of middle management have more contact with employees and therefore are usually part of decisions that directly affect employees and patients. Middle management has an important, but often precarious, responsibility to advocate for the institution's employees while also maintaining the agency's values and mission.

Middle managers are accountable to upper management and are responsible for the line managers and the employees. Middle managers often are more visible to employees than are members of upper management. However, being in the middle often places these managers in the position of balancing the goals of the institution with the needs of the employees.

Middle managers represent different departments in a hospital such as Hospitality Services, Communications, and Patient Care. The most common scenario is that a hospital will have a director of nursing to oversee all aspects of nursing within the organization. The director of nursing is accountable for staffing decisions, unit budgets, nursing policies, patient care and safety, and even physician relationships. He or she is ultimately responsible for ensuring that staffing is adequate to meet patient needs, and is also accountable to upper management for maintaining a budget that can sustain safe staffing.

In addition, the director of nursing is responsible for working with ancillary services to ensure that nurses have the proper level of support needed to perform their jobs. For example, to admit new patients, a busy nursing unit that has rapid patient turnover requires that rooms be cleaned quickly. If housekeeping personnel are unable to clean the rooms in a timely fashion, patients will be backlogged in the emergency room or surgical areas. Because the problem now involves numerous areas in the hospital, the director of nursing needs to confer with the director of housekeeping to resolve the issue. The director of nursing has to serve as an advocate for the patients to uphold the agency's mission. He or she needs to use the unit managers to coordinate the organization's goals with those of the staff.

Unit (Lower) Management

Line supervisors or unit managers oversee the daily operations of specific nursing units and comprise the next level of management. Managers at this level are responsible for the day-to-day functioning of the nursing units, and they have 24-hour accountability for the units. They are responsible for the unit's budget, patient care, staffing ratios, and enforcing the policies of the hospital and the unit. They are also responsible for multiple levels of staff, such as nurses, patient-care technicians, and secretarial support. Unit managers address concerns from staff, physicians, and patients and/or their families. For example, a nephrologist is making rounds on the nursing unit and complains that the patients are not being weighed daily. The nurse–manager not only discusses the issue with the physician, but also needs to investigate the problem and, with staff input, resolve it so that patients are weighed daily. The manager then informs the physician again, of the resolution to the problem. This advocacy role not only improves patient care, but also relays to the physician that his or her concerns are important and need to be resolved.

Another example of the unit manager's role is disciplining staff, according to hospital policy, for excessive absence. For instance, a staff nurse has called off once a week for the last 2 months. She has a very ill child and needs to be available for him. She has been at the hospital for 11 years and is usually very reliable. The manager's responsibility lies in not only addressing the nurse's behavior, but also in covering the nurse's absence.

Patient care is compromised when nurses call off for their assigned shifts. In covering for the absent nurse, other nurses may have to exceed their normal patient load, which can severely jeopardize patient safety. If the covering nurses refuse to accept the additional patient assignments for safety reasons, care can be even further jeopardized.

If the nurse–manager authorizes the use of supplemental staff, this becomes a resource issue due to the extra expense of agency nurses. It also continues to be a safety issue if the float nurses are unfamiliar with the unit and/or the types of patients on the unit. The nurse–manager must make the decision that is in the best interest of patient safety, but must also consider the staff nurses' concerns. In addition, the nurse–manager must proceed, according to hospital policy, with disciplining the nurse with the frequent absences. In a case like this, the nurse–manager and the unit staff usually will support the nurse with the ill child so that the situation does not deteriorate into one requiring disciplinary action. The Family Medical Leave Act permits the nurse to take time off without pay, and the nurse's colleagues decide to share the extra shifts to cover the unit without using supplemental staff. The nurse–manager who cares about his or her staff will provide mechanisms jointly to solve problems with them and support them in their time of need while also finding ways to assure upper management that patient needs are being met within the unit's budget.

Nurse–managers are accountable for the orientation and education of the unit's nurses (Yoder-Wise, 2003). For example, a critical care manager accepts the transfer of a nurse from a medical unit to an intensive care unit. This nurse has been employed by the hospital for a few years. In the ICU, the nurse began to make serious medication errors. The manager initiates disciplinary action against the nurse. In addition to the disciplinary action, the nurse is also continuously assigned a preceptor. However, the nurse continues to make medication errors. Just as the manager is about to terminate the nurse, it is discovered that the nurse never completed the medication portion of the orientation program and has not taken the required medication test. The nurse is placed in the orientation class and given the required education on critical care medications. After completing the medication course, the nurse is again closely supervised and continues to make medication errors. Ultimately, the nurse is dismissed for failure to meet the job requirements. The nurse–manager ensured that the nurse was given the opportunity to improve his or her skills, but the nurse failed to demonstrate competency and therefore was not retained on the critical care unit. The principle of non-maleficence applied; the potential for harm was greater with that nurse practicing in the ICU, so that nurse needed to be placed in a position that reduced the possibility of patient harm due to medication errors.

Charge Nurses

Finally, each unit usually has designated *charge nurses* who assume management responsibilities during afternoon, night, and weekend shifts in the absence of the unit manager. Because they are staff nurses who assume management responsibilities for a limited time, charge nurses are placed in a difficult position. They also have limited authority and are frequently prevented from making major decisions without consulting with the unit manager/supervisor. Different charge nurses may use their authority in different fashions, and how they use it will affect the daily milieu of the nursing unit.

Charge nurses may or not be compensated for their additional responsibilities; if they are not compensated, some nurses may refuse to take on the role. In some instances, nurses decrease the number of hours they work so that they are ineligible for charge nurse responsibilities. Another issue that arises concerning charge nurses is that collective bargaining units are attempting to delineate whether charge nurses are "management" or "employees." This distinction is important because nurses in management are not protected by union contracts (Schraeder & Friedman, 2002) and are ineligible for overtime pay.

Different institutions and units handle the charge nurse role differently. In some instances, charge nurses do not provide direct care while in charge. This makes the role a little more manageable and desirable. In other cases, the charge nurses take on either a decreased patient load or a full patient assignment. Such scenarios make the role of charge nurse more difficult.

Charge nurses are responsible for enforcing hospital policies in the absence of the unit managers. They make decisions regarding staffing for their assigned shifts. These decisions may include deciding to reassign staff, accept reassigned staff, or use agency staff. Charge nurses delegate responsibilities and patient assignments to other nurses. They are responsible for the provision of safe and effective patient care during their shift. They may also have to solve problems and deal with physician, patient, or family issues.

Because the role of charge nurse is so variable, ethical issues may present on a regular basis. For example, a nurse who is a friend of the charge nurse may receive a more desirable patient assignment. This favoritism may not be in patients' best interests; it is not a just or fair method of patient assignment, and other nurses may interpret it unfavorably.

Because the role of charge nurse is temporary (for the shift or for the weekend), charge nurses often do not wish to be involved in problem-solving or confrontations. For example, a family member requests to talk to the charge nurse about patient care. The family member is concerned that a patient technician is rough and impatient with the patient. The charge nurse listens to the concern but takes no action and does not relay the information to the unit manager. The following day, the same technician is assigned to the patient, and the family member questions whether the issue had been addressed with the technician. There is a different charge nurse on duty that day, though, and he or she has no knowledge of the family member's concern. The family member is upset and requests to speak with a higher-level manager. Now a situation of mistrust has developed, and the family may believe that the unit staff is not concerned about and not advocating for the patient. As this example shows, regardless of what level a manager is on, his or her management will affect many aspects of patient care and the unit's milieu.

Management Styles

Although there are "management theories" and "management styles," many institutions use the term "leadership" in place of "management." Leaders still perform management duties, but the term "leadership" more broadly describes the responsibilities of the role (Yoder-Wise, 2003). Management styles include authoritarianism, democracy, and laissez-faire.

An *authoritarian style* of management describes leaders who have sole decision-making authority and tend to impose rules, expect obedience, and oppose individual freedom. Within a health care setting, this management style would preclude nurses from autonomous decision-making and individual choice. Ethically, authoritarian leaders act autocratically. When autocracy is present, the rights and wishes of others are often overlooked at the desire of the manager. This authoritarian style of leadership may diminish nurses' beneficence (ability to do good) by infringing on their autonomy.

Nurses who are not free to make professional choices that are consistent with their clinical judgment may eventually leave the unit or institution, leading to compromised patient care, or may choose to stay and take a stand against the manager. For example, nurses working on a particular oncology unit are not allowed to make schedule changes or trade shifts with other nurses without the manager's permission. It is Saturday, and Hector wishes to switch his Sunday shift with Adrienne. The manager is unavailable, and the nurses' fear that there will be repercussions if they make the change without notifying the manager. Subsequently, Hector calls in sick for the shift, leaving the unit one nurse short and compromising patient care because of the resulting understaffed shift. Although Hector did not make the best choice in this case, the unit nurses' lack of autonomy and fear of repercussions from the manager may have encouraged this action. This kind of severe authoritarianism is not common because leaders have learned that it can cause staff to feel unsupported and lead to compromised patient care and unit functioning.

A style of leadership that is less restrictive than authoritarianism is the *democratic style*. Democratic management implies that everyone will have a voice in all decisions. In a democracy, the leader should represent the ideas of the group. A democratic leadership style may contribute to achieving the goal of utilitarianism, the maximum benefit for the most individuals. If a democratic leader is constantly attempting to please most of the staff, patient care may be compromised and the institutional goals or mission may be violated. For example, hospital policy designates that each unit choose a uniform color and one pattern for the entire unit's staff to wear. This policy was instituted so that patients could recognize more easily which employees were staffed on specific units. The staff on a particular medical unit complain to their manager that the dress code is too restrictive. To please all of the nurses, and, she hopes, retain them, their democratic nurse–manager allows them to wear whatever they want. The hospital CEO receives complaints from patients on that unit that it is difficult for them to tell who the nurses are because all the nurses dress differently. The nurse–manager violated a silly, but nevertheless required, hospital policy in an attempt to please the staff. Now, when the manager enforces the hospital dress code, the staff may rebel and accuse the manager of not being democratic.

As another example of democratic leadership, nurses working on an oncology unit have been permitting patients that are terminally ill to smoke in their rooms. The nurses reason that these patients should not have to experience nicotine withdrawal in addition to the other discomforts associated with dying. It is against hospital policy for patients to smoke on hospital grounds, but these patients are not able to go off the hospital grounds. In this case, the oncology nurse–manager supports the nurses' violation of the policy but is reprimanded by her supervisor, who believes there is no justification for allowing anyone to smoke on hospital property. This manager may have been advocating for the nurses' concerns, but in doing so, she violated the institution's policy.

A primary source of dissatisfaction for nurses is their lack of input into important decisions. Newer management trends are less restrictive, but they may still pose ethical issues. One of the more recent leadership theories in practice is *transformational leadership*. This style of leadership requires role modeling. Transformed leaders create an environment that is responsive to staff as well as to patient needs. Under transformational leadership, nurses can become *empowered* and can promote ethical, research-based practice (Yoder-Wise, 2003). Therefore, this style of leadership raises employee motivation levels.

Even with transformational leadership, ethical issues may still develop. If employees' motives are not congruent with those of the institution, the results of this style of leadership can be obstructive instead of constructive. For example, a manager encourages his nurses to address and resolve issues as they arise. One of the unit's nurses consistently complains about pharmacy and their failure to deliver medications on time. When the issue is not resolved through the staff nurse's efforts, the manager addresses the issue with the pharmacy, only to discover that the nurse's allegations are unfounded. In going back to readdress the issue with the unit nurse, the manager discovers that the nurse actually had a specific issue only with a particular pharmacy employee. This situation has not only altered the manager's perception of that nurse's motives, but it may also have damaged the nursing/pharmacy relationship for that particular nursing unit. In transformational leadership, the nurse–manager needs to educate the staff, encourage them to discuss their intradepartmental problems, and strategize with them to develop plans to resolve their problem without abdicating the leadership role to the staff nurses.

SUMMARY

All institutions use some type of management philosophy. In addition, each nursing unit within the institution will have a leadership style that is developed by the unit manager. Although different leadership styles will create different environments, there may be drawbacks to each of the styles. Nurses need to be cognizant of the possible ethical situations that can develop in relation to each of the leadership models.

CLINICAL EXERCISES

1. Identify the management style of the unit manager and the charge nurse on your unit.

   - Observe how the staff responds to the manager or charge nurse.
   - Observe the unit milieu for cooperation and team work.

2. Review the job descriptions for the unit manager and charge nurse and identify any ethical conflicts that could result from these descriptions.
3. Discuss with the charge nurse how he or she would handle a patient complaint about care.

Discussion Questions

1. You are a staff nurse on an oncology unit. As a staff nurse, you are required to attend mandatory in-services prior to chemotherapy administration. You observe that one of your peers never attends the in-services but continues to administer the medications.

   a. Discuss the manager's ethical responsibility for staff education.
   b. Discuss the ethical implications for the patients receiving medications from the untrained nurse.

    c. Discuss the nurse's ethical responsibility to deal with the peer who administers the medications without the training.

2. You are a staff nurse working on a unit with an authoritarian leader. The nurse leader mandates that every nurse work equal amounts of every shift (days, evenings, and nights) and that the nurses rotate shifts each week.

    a. Discuss the ethical consequences of this policy for the nurses.
    b. Discuss the ethical duty of the manager to adequately staff the unit.
    c. Discuss the options for a nurse who cannot rotate shifts.
    d. Discuss the ethical consequences for the patients.

3. You are staff nurse on a pulmonary unit in which many of the patients are on ventilators. When Sally is the charge nurse you constantly receive at least three patients on ventilators in your patient assignment while the other nurses receive only one or no ventilator patients and Sally does not have a patient assignment.

    a. Discuss the ethical issues that are present in this situation.
    b. Discuss how to approach this situation with Sally.
    c. Discuss the next step to take if Sally ignores your concerns.

SECTION 4: *Professional Nursing Issue: Nursing's Voice and Power*

Ideally, nurses have many opportunities to partake in decision-making at the nursing-unit, the institutional, and, often, the societal level. Of course, not many nurses become elected officials, but that should not lessen the affect that nurses can have on legislative issues. Nurses may participate in decision-making at the unit level by being part of a shared governance model. Nurses may also choose to increase their decision-making power by being represented in a collective group through a bargaining unit (a nursing union). It is important to consider the ethical implications and responsibilities of having a voice and power.

    Nurses undertake the role of advocate for patients, but at times they must become self-advocates as well as advocates for the profession. Shared governance and collective bargaining are two mechanisms that allow nurses to participate in decision making and advocate for patient care and the nursing profession. It is essential that nurses maintain an awareness of the ethical problems that may arise when they exercise their voices and become empowered. This section discusses shared governance, collective bargaining, and the political activity of nurses and the problems that might be encountered in each situation.

SHARED GOVERNANCE

Shared governance is shared decision-making. The governance is shared by professional-practice groups such as governing boards, managers, nurses, and physicians. Nurses become responsible and accountable for nursing practice within the institution (Marquis & Huston, 2000). Shared governance is a mechanism for nurses to participate in not only nursing-unit decisions, but also institutional decisions and, eventually, policy-making. Shared governance gives nurses a degree of power and a voice in nursing-related decisions and allows them to be advocates for themselves and for their patients. Nurses who participate in shared decision-making are more likely to be satisfied with their nursing roles and to remain with the institution. A study of Magnet hospitals (hospitals that have applied and received recognition through the ANA for nursing excellence) revealed that nurses are likely to experience less stress and be more satisfied with their jobs if they receive support as professionals, participate in decision-making and shared governance, and are positively recognized for their accomplishments (Upenieks, 2003).

Shared governance has been shown to improve job perceptions and the practice environment, but it may also have problems. It might affect unit-based decisions, such as flexible staffing, or hospital-based decisions regarding patient complaints. An example of a unit-based decision might be one regarding how adequate staff coverage is provided on holidays. A common practice is to place all staff into a fixed holiday rotation, which means that staff are assigned to work certain holidays one year and then are off on those holidays the next year. This rotation is designed to provide adequate staffing for the holidays for years to come. A problem arises when staff do not approve of the rotation in which they are placed and call in sick on their designated holiday. Another problem with a fixed rotation is that attrition from the nursing unit can leave the remaining staff working most of the holidays from year to year, which causes discontent among the nurses. In a shared governance situation, the staff can develop a task force of unit nurses to review the problems that occur with holiday staff coverage. The task force could poll the current staff about their opinions of holiday rotation. The task force could also suggest and implement creative staffing methods for the hardest-to-staff holidays, such as splitting shifts into smaller increments so that all staff members can enjoy some holiday time off.

Shared governance can also contribute to more effective problem-solving for larger issues, for example, how other issues affecting nursing time are handled. For example, a physician asks nurses on a busy unit to record detailed information about patients on a form that the physician provides. The information is already documented in various areas in the medical record, but the physician wants to save time and have all the information recorded on this new form. This doubles the amount of time it takes for nurses to document this information for each of the physician's patients. The nurses refer the physician to the documentation committee, a multidisciplinary committee that is part of their shared governance organization, to have this request and form reviewed. Through established processes, the nurses' views and the physician's needs are examined. One resolution to this problem may be that the existing form is revised to accommodate the physician's needs without doubling nurses' documentation time. As illustrated in this example, the existence of a shared governance process to review physician requests prevents one physician from making a unilateral mandate that would significantly affect nursing time on a particular unit.

When the mechanisms of shared governance work, they can lead to increased patient satisfaction and decreased stress for nurses by involving the nurses in decision-making and, in turn, advocating for the patients and the nurses. Although shared governance should increase decision-making and empowerment among the nurses, if the concept is not fully supported, it will be ineffective for facilitating change. Some of the problems with the shared governance model include reluctant managers, the increased time needed to make decisions, the complexity of the decision-making process, the absence of nurse accountability, and the absence of commitment by either the nurses or the organization. In these cases, shared governance may exist in name only or may not be taken seriously. The institution may use the shared governance committee structure just to fulfill accreditation requirements for which they would otherwise have needed to employ additional nurses. In these cases, staff nurses who devote uncompensated time to committee work fulfill the institution's accreditation requirements but have no real say in the institution's governance. When nurses perceive that their opinion is not valued or when they are alienated from making important decisions and become dissatisfied, they may look for collective bargaining representation.

Collective Bargaining

Traditionally, and in most institutions, nurses have not organized into a union. However, nurses are discovering that by joining forces they create a more powerful voice for the profession. Nurses are increasingly seeking *collective bargaining* as a solution to their quality-of-care issues, their high patient-to-nurse ratios with large numbers of acutely ill patients, and their lack of decision-making opportunities (Schraeder & Friedman, 2002). "When nurses show signs of job dissatisfaction—feeling frustrated, stressed, and powerless—they're sending nurse-leaders a wake-up call" (Steltzer, 2001, p. 35). Fitzpatrick (2001) cited a survey of nurses who were asked about unionizing. Sixty-six percent of 598 nurses agreed that nurses should unionize. The factors most often noted that increased interest in unions included inadequate staffing, mandatory overtime, reassignment, humiliation, unfair wages, lack of recognition, intimidation by managers, feeling unsupported, and being undervalued. In areas where nurses are more dissatisfied, union activity is higher (Steltzer, 2001). Just as increased involvement in decision-making equates to nurse satisfaction, devaluation by supervisors can contribute to union organization.

One factor that is often closely linked to unionization is the opportunity unions provide for nurses to strike. Administrators have long warned nurses that a strike would be considered "patient abandonment." However, if nurses remain cognizant of their responsibilities to patients, as well as of their rights to organize, they can initiate strike activity without incurring charges of patient abandonment. If nurses follow the appropriate guidelines for a strike, there is sufficient time for the institution to ensure safe patient care. In 2000, the Massachusetts Nurses Association supported a nurses' strike against mandatory overtime (Miller, 2000). Nurses most often organize to improve working conditions or decrease practices that adversely affect patient care.

One consequence of nurses belonging to a collective bargaining unit (or union) is the potential for adverse relationships to develop between nurses and managers. Managers are exempt from joining a collective bargaining unit, and they must abide by the union contract that covers the nurses that work under their supervision. When managers attempt to enforce stringent policies that are not negotiated by the union, their decisions will likely be challenged. In the prior example of working holidays, the union contract may specify the mechanism of wages for the holiday, but not the holiday hours. A manager could then schedule the nurses for long shifts, such as 12-hour shifts, or for shifts that they generally do not work, such as a day nurse working a night shift. Managers will usually work cooperatively with unions to avoid having employees file grievances for unfair labor practices, though.

Another consequence of nurses joining unions is that union contracts specifying "progressive discipline" processes can make it difficult for managers to dismiss poorly performing employees or employees who break certain rules. The spirit behind progressive discipline is to inform nurses of unacceptable actions and teach and retrain them. With each disciplinary step, the nurse is made aware of corrective actions and of the risk of dismissal. If all efforts to change the unacceptable action fail, then the manager can dismiss the nurse. If the fellow nurses are eager for the problem employee to be dismissed, their morale may be affected during this lengthy process, but they all have the same protections under the union. Most union rules and activities are aimed toward productive goals and enhanced working conditions that will improve patient care and nurse satisfaction.

A positive factor in nurses' unionizing is the benefit gained from having the shared voice of a large group of professionals. Large groups of organized professionals are more likely to be heard than individuals. In addition, nurses who are unionizing are doing so for safe workplace environments, fair treatment and wages, respect, and patient safety. Therefore, these nurses are advocating for themselves and for their patients. For example, unionized nurses may have a greater effect on adverse patient-care conditions than nonunionized nurses. Organized nurses have had a positive effect on mandatory overtime and nurse-to-patient ratios in recent years. Finally, organized groups of nurses may elicit changes on a broader horizon than just at local hospitals. Organization allows for mass support of political candidates, candidates who can then take forward the messages of nurses.

Political Activity

There are several ways in which nurses can become involved in *political activity*. First, they can collectively support candidates for local, state, or federal offices who support the advancement of patient care and of the nursing profession. State and national nursing associations are powerful political voices that can support candidates and can lobby for improved health care provisions and conditions.

In California, organized nurses who collaborated with state legislators were able to pass a bill that mandated safe nurse-to-patient ratios (Kuehl, 1999). Other states are also seeking legislative support for safe nurse-to-patient ratios and for eliminating mandatory overtime. The Nurse Reinvestment Act (U.S. Department of Health and Human Services, HRSA, Bureau of Health Professions, 2002) was enacted in response to the national nursing shortage. It provides grants and funds for the retention of nurses and various other funds to assist with addressing the nursing shortage.

Nurses can also become politically involved through various specialty-nursing organizations. Nurses who become members or officers in national nursing organizations may be in positions to exert political influence. In addition, nurses who are politically active may seek local, state, or even federal office to promote and advance nursing. It is increasingly more common to see health care professionals become political figures and work to advance health care and protect public welfare. Political activity among nurses can enhance the profession's advocacy for its members as well as for its patients; therefore political activity may become an integral piece of the nursing role.

SUMMARY

There are several mechanisms for nurses to have voices and power in their practice arenas. It is essential for nurses to become involved, whether on the unit level in shared governance models or on the legislative level, with regard to areas that affect nursing practice. Regardless of their level of involvement, nurses must be aware of the ethical implications of organizing for change, and they must work within those ethical boundaries.

CLINICAL EXERCISES

1. Observe the nurses unit at the clinical agency for examples of cooperative decision-making. Ask the nurses to give you examples of how they have input into unit decisions or institutional decisions
2. Observe the practices for making patient assignments or scheduling. What are the ethical consequences of such practices?
3. Access the ANA website (www.nursingworld.org) and review any legislative updates in your region that affect nursing practice.

Discussion Questions

1. You are a staff nurse who is working at an institution with unionized nurses. One of your peers frequently calls in but does so in a pattern outside of disciplinary parameters

   a. Discuss how this practice affects other nurses.
   b. Discuss the principle of justice as it applies to this situation.
   c. Debate the ethical implications for the union contract that permits this employee's behavior.

2. You are a staff nurse at a small community hospital. One of your peers is unhappy with the schedule, benefits, and salary and has begun to contact union representatives.

   a. Discuss the ethical implications of this nurse contacting a union.
   b. Develop an argument supporting and refuting the idea for unionization.

3. You are a staff nurse working at a small rural hospital with a collective bargaining unit for the nurses. Some of the nurses are unhappy about recent cutbacks in ancillary help (patient-care technicians and secretaries). One of the nurses announces, "Let's go out on strike."

   a. Discuss the ethical consequences of a strike (both positive and negative) for the nurses, present patients, future patients, and the institution.
   b. Discuss plans that should be in place or are needed to protect patients during a strike.
   c. Discuss the positive and negative aspects of crossing a picket line during a strike.

Resources

American Nurses Association. (2001). Commission on workplace advocacy. Retrieved May 1, 2003, from www.nursingworld.org/wpa/infolinks.htm

National Labor Relations Board. Retrieved May 1, 2003, from www.nlrb.gov/

Phoenix Health Systems. (2002). HIPAA advisory: HIPAA primer. Retrieved September 10, 2003, from www.hipaadvisory.com/regs/HIPAAprimer1.htm

U.S. Department of Health and Human Services, HRSA, Bureau of Health Professions (2002). Nurse Reinvestment Act of 2002. Retrieved October 13, 2005, from http://bhpr.hrsa.gov/nursing/reinvesttext.htm

References

Aiken, L., Clarke, S. P., Sloane, D. M., Sochalski, J. A., Busse, R., Clarke, H., et al. (2001). Nurses' reports on hospital care in five countries. *Health Affairs, 20*(3), 43–53.

Aiken, L. H., Smith, H. L., & Lake, E. T. (1994). Lower Medicare mortality among a set of hospitals known for good care. *Med Care, 32*, 771–787.

American Nurses Association. (2001). *The code of ethics for nurses with interpretive statements.* Washington, DC: Author.

Anonymous. (2002). Arizona Nurses' Association position statement. *Arizona Nurse, 56*(1), 6.

Anthony, M. K., & Preuss, G. (2002). Models of care: The influence of nurse communication on patient safety. *Nursing Economics, 20*(5), 209–215.

Beauchamp, T. L., & Childress, J. F. (2001). *Principles of biomedical ethics* (5th ed.). New York: Oxford University Press.

Berliner, H. S., & Ginzberg, E. (2002). Why the nursing shortage is different. *JAMA, 288*(21), 2742–2744.

Bradford, L., & Raines, C. (1992). *Twentysomething.* New York: Master Media.

Fitzpatrick, M. (2001). Collective bargaining: Vulnerability assessment. *Nursing Management, 32*(2), 40–42.

Homsted, T., & Nilsson, M. (2003). Safe staffing: A serious concern. *The Florida Nurse, 51*(1), 1–3.

Kovner, C., & Gergen, P. J. (1998). Nurse staffing levels and adverse events following surgery in US hospitals. *Image Journal of Nursing Scholarship, 30*, 315–321.

Kuehl, S. (1999). Health facilities. Nursing staff assembly bill No. 394. California Business and Professional Code, 2725.3. Sacramento, CA.

Marquis, B. L., & Huston, C. J. (2000). *Leadership roles and management functions in nursing.* Philadelphia: Lippincott.

Mee, C. L. (2001). Mandatory madness. *Nursing, 31*(9), 6.

Miller, N. (2001). Strikes and strife causing rifts. *Nursing Economics, 18*(4), 212–213.

Safe Nursing and Patient Care Act of 2005. (H.R.791/S.351). Retrieved on December 7, 2005, from http://www.house.gov/stark/news/109th/legislation/nursing%20summary%20109.htm

Schraeder, M., & Friedman, L. H. (2002). Collective bargaining in the nursing profession: Salient issues and recent developments in healthcare reform. *Hospital Topics, 80*(3), 21–24.

Steltzer, T. M. (2001). Collective bargaining: A wake up call. *Nursing Management, 32*(4), 35–37.

Trossman, S. (1998). Striking reflections: Why nurses are willing to walk the line. *The American Nurse, 30*(4, July/August). Retrieved October 14, 2005, from http://nursingworld.org/tan/98julaug/strike.htm

Upenieks, V. (2003). Recruitment and retention strategies: A magnet hospital prevention model. *Nursing Economics, 21*(1), 7–12.

U.S. Department of Health and Human Services, HRSA, Bureau of Health Professions (2002). Nurse Reinvestment Act of 2002. Retrieved October 13, 2005, from http://bhpr.hrsa.gov/nursing/reinvesttext.htm

Weinberg, D. B. (2003). *Code green: Money-driven hospitals and the dismantling of nursing.* Ithaca, NY: Cornell University Press.

Yoder-Wise, P. S. (2003). *Leading and managing in nursing.* St. Louis, MO: Mosby.

Appendix: Reports of Presidential Commissions

National Commission for the Protection of Human Subjects of Biomedical and Behavioral Research (appointed by Secretary of Health, Education and Welfare Caspar Weinberger, 1974)

1975
Research on the fetus.

1976
Report and recommendations: Research involving prisoners.

1977
Psychosurgery: Report and recommendations.
Research involving children: Report and recommendations.

1978
Research involving those institutionalized as mentally infirm: Report and recommendations.
Report and recommendations: Institutional review boards.
Ethical guidelines for the delivery of health services by DHEW.
The Belmont report: Ethical principles and guidelines for the protection of human subjects of
    research.

President's Commission for the Study of Ethical Problems in Medicine and Biomedical and Behavioral Research (appointed by President Jimmy Carter in 1978)

1981
Defining death: A report on the medical, legal, and ethical issues in the determination of death.
Protecting human subjects: First biennial report on the adequacy and uniformity of federal
    rules and policies, and their implementation, for the protection of human subjects in bio-
    medical and behavioral research.

1982

Whistle blowing in biomedical research: Proceedings of a workshop held September 21–22, 1981.

Compensating for research injuries: A report on the ethical and legal implications of programs to redress injuries caused by biomedical and behavioral research.

Making health care decisions: The ethical and legal implications of informed consent in the patient–practitioner relationship. Vol. I: Report.

Making health care decisions: The ethical and legal implications of informed consent in the patient–practitioner relationship. Vol. II: Appendices. Empirical studies of informed consent.

Making health care decisions. The ethical and legal implications of informed consent in the patient–practitioner relationship. Vol. III: Appendices. Studies on the foundations of informed consent.

Splicing life: A report on the social and ethical issues of genetic engineering with human beings.

1983

Screening and counseling for genetic conditions: A report on the ethical, social, and legal implications of genetic screening, counseling, and education programs.

Deciding to forego life-sustaining treatment: A report on the ethical, medical, and legal issues in treatment decisions.

Securing access to health care: The ethical implications of differences in the availability of health services.

Implementing human research regulations: A second biennial report on the adequacy and uniformity of federal rules and policies, and of their implementation, for the protection of human subjects.

Summing up: A final report on studies of the ethical and legal problems in medicine and biomedical and behavioral research.

National Bioethics Advisory Commission (appointed by President Bill Clinton, 1995)

1997

Cloning human beings: Report and recommendations of the National Bioethics Advisory Commission.

Cloning human beings: Views of scientific societies and professional associations on human nuclear transfer cloning research.

Cloning human beings: Religious perspectives on human cloning.

1998

National Bioethics Advisory Commission: 1996–1997 Annual Report.

Research involving persons with mental disorders that may affect decision-making capacity. Volume 1: Report and recommendations of the National Bioethics Advisory Commission.

Report 1998: Annual Report.

1999

Research involving persons with mental disorders that may affect decision-making capacity. Volume 2: Commissioned papers by the National Bioethics Advisory Commission.

Research involving human biological materials: Ethical issues and policy guidance. Volume 1: Report and Recommendations of the National Bioethics Advisory Commission.

National Bioethics Advisory Commission: 1998–1999 Biennial Report

2000

Research involving human biological materials: Ethical issues and policy guidance. Executive summary; Volume 1: Report and recommendations of the National Bioethics Advisory Commission; Volume 2: Commissioned papers.

2001
Ethical and policy issues in research involving human participants. Executive summary, Volume 1 and Volume 2.
Ethical and policy issues in international research: Clinical trials in developing countries. Executive summary, Volume 1 and Volume 2.

President's Council on Bioethics (appointed by President George W. Bush, 2002)

2002
Human cloning and human dignity: An ethical inquiry.

2003
Beyond therapy: Biotechnology and the pursuit of happiness.
Being human: Readings from the President's Council on Bioethics.

2004
Monitoring stem cell research.
Reproduction and responsibility: The regulation of new biotechnologies.

2005
White paper: Alternative sources to human pluripotent stem cells.
Taking care: Ethical caregiving in our aging society.

Glossary

Abandonment: "occurs when the provider ends the relationship with the client without proper notification." (Ladd, Pasquerella, & Smith, 2002)

Abortion, induced: termination of a pregnancy before week 20 of gestation through evacuation of uterine contents by surgery, vacuum extraction, prostaglandin infusion, or other chemical means of expelling the fetus from the uterus

Abortion, natural: loss of pregnancy before week 20 of gestation not due to induced means

Academic dishonesty: "dishonesty in connection with any University activity. Cheating, plagiarism or knowingly furnishing false information to the University. . . . Moreover, knowingly to aid and abet, directly or indirectly, other parties in committing dishonest acts is in itself dishonest" (Purdue, 2003, p. 1)

Adult-onset genetic disease: a medical condition that has a genetic cause but the symptoms of which do not present until adulthood

Advance directive: a legal document that allows a legally competent adult to identify his or her wishes about aggressiveness of treatment and end-of-life care

Advocacy: an ethical principle that requires health care providers to ensure that the needs, concerns, and wishes of patients or profession are heard and respected

Age of majority: the age, usually eighteen, at which time the person is considered to be an adult

Altruism: "an unselfish concern for the welfare of others" (Steinberg, 2003, p. 21)

Anonymity: the state of being nameless, unknown, and/or unidentified

Appeal to conscience: refusal to act based on the belief that acting would cause harm to one's self

Artificial nutrition and hydration: administration of food and water through a tube either into the gastrointestinal system or intravenously

Assent: affirmative agreement, for example, a child's agreement to participate in research

Assisted reproduction: medical techniques for achieving a successful pregnancy, such as in vitro fertilization, oocyte donation, preimplantation diagnosis

Assisted suicide: "makes the means of death available, but does not act as the direct agent of death" (American Nurses Association [ANA], 1994b)

Autonomy: a fundamental ethical principle based on respect for persons that requires one to accept the free and informed choices of competent patients or their designated decision-makers

Baby Doe regulations: based on the Baby Doe case in Bloomington, Indiana, in 1982, federally mandated changes in child abuse and neglect laws in every state to prevent discrimination by the withholding of medical treatment from newborns based on a handicapping condition

Beneficence: a fundamental ethical principle that requires that one first do no harm, and then seek to do or produce good for others

Best interests: an evaluation of whether an action/option will promote a person's ability to achieve his or her goals and/or be free from harm

Best interests standard: criterion by which a decision by a surrogate is such as to "promote the patient's good" (President's Commission for the Study of Ethical Problems in Medicine and Biomedical and Behavioral Research, 1983, p. 179)

Bioethics: the ethical issues in health and the delivery of health care; may broadly encompass the ethics of medical, nursing, and other health care professionals

Boundary violations: intentional or unintentional actions that disrespect the typical social behavioral convention between two persons

Brain death: the irreversible cessation of whole-brain function based on repeated clinical assessments and tests such as an electroencephalogram to yield a clinical diagnosis (American Academy of Pediatrics, 1987)

Cadaver organ donation: retrieving an organ, such as heart, lung, or kidney, from a dead body

Cardiopulmonary resuscitation (CPR): use of chest percussions and/or ventilation (e.g., mouth-to-mouth or an endotracheal tube connected to a ventilator) to reestablish a person's pulse and respirations

Caregiver burden: physical, financial, psychological, and emotional toll from providing care to another, usually one family member caring for another ill or disabled family member

Challenging patient: a patient who denies "both the authority and therapeutic value of the nursing staff" (Breeze & Repper, 1998, p. 1301)

Charge nurse: a nurse who assumes management responsibilities for a nursing unit for a given period of time, such as a specific shift

Chemical restraint: "the use of chemicals to control behavior" (Parker, 1995, p. 26)

Circumcision: in the male, removal of the foreskin of the penis; in the female, the procedure may vary from the removal of the clitoral hood to the removal of the clitoral hood, clitoris, labia minora and majora and the suturing of the remaining tissue, leaving a small opening for urination and menstrual flow

Clinical equipoise: the state of not knowing which treatment is better

Clinical trial: procedure in which a new intervention is compared to the standard intervention; subjects agree to be randomized to a control group (standard treatment) or an experimental group (experimental treatment)

COBRA: Consolidated Omnibus Budget Reconciliation Act of 1986, provides for health care coverage when an employee leaves employment; the employee must pay the entire insurance premium to remain covered for up to 18 months

Codes of ethics: a profession's ideal ethical standards and expectations as endorsed by its professional associations

Collective bargaining: negotiation of wages or other conditions of employment by an organized body of employees

Comfort care: care focused on maintaining a person's comfort level and not on cure

Communitarianism: a type of moral theory that considers the community as the primary moral unit, with individuals being constituted and supported by the community

Compassion: an ethical principle that requires one to approach others with consideration for and sensitivity to the pain and suffering that they may be experiencing

Competence: the condition of being adequately qualified or capable

Competency: legal term referring to the ability of a person to make his or her own decisions

Confidentiality: an ethical principle that requires one to protect and secure the personal information of others and to see that it is only shared with those who have a need and right to know

Conscience: the mental faculty used to determine the rightness or moral appropriateness of a person's actions

Conscientious objection: refusal to participate based on a religious belief or the equivalent moral conviction

Consequentialism: a moral theory that claims that the right act in any given situation is the one that will produce the best overall consequences

Contraception: prevention of pregnancy through abstinence, use of a barrier method, spermicides, hormones, an intrauterine device, or timing of intercourse during infertile periods (rhythm method)

Controlled-drug misuse: "the improper use, unlawful misapplication, or incorrect use of one or more controlled drugs that were illegally diverted from patient use for the purpose of self-administration" (Bell, McDonough, Ellison, & Fitzhugh, 1999, p. 136) or sale to other

Culture: a "collection of beliefs, values, and behaviors that permit a group of people to interact effectively with their environment" (Jones, 1992, p. 282)

Culture of silence: the unspoken expectation that an individual will not report an act of violence or abuse

Cupping and bleeding: procedure performed on the skin over certain points on the body as part of Chinese medicine (Ergil, 2001)

Dangerous to self: the perceived likelihood that a person might act in a manner that would cause physical or emotional harm to himself or herself

Deception: any verbal or nonverbal communication done with "the intention of misleading others . . . [to] believe what we ourselves do not believe" to be true (Bok, 1999, pp. xxiii)

Decision-maker: the identified person responsible for choosing an action to resolve an ethical situation

Decision-making capacity: the ability of a person to make his or her own decisions; the person must be able to understand the information relevant to the decision, be able to reason and manipulate the information, appreciate the implications of the decision, and make a choice (Grisso & Appelbaum, 1998)

Deinstitutionalization: "The massive discharge of clients from state hospitals that began in the 1950s, accelerated in the 1960s and 1970s, and continues today as psychiatric treatment continues to move from inpatient to outpatient settings" (Conn, 2003, p. 169)

Delegation: a procedure by which the professional nurse assigns tasks to and supervises employees who report to him or her, such as unlicensed assistive personnel

Deontology: a moral theory that claims that right action is determined by whether an act is consistent with a person's moral duties and obligations

Discriminate: to make an unjust distinction based on race, gender, sexual orientation, or ethnicity

Distributive justice: the fair allocation of the benefits and burdens of society

Double effect: the doctrine that provides grounds for determining the moral justifiability of acts that produce both benefit and harm

Due diligence: an ethical principle that requires that reasonable care be exercised in a given situation to ensure that one does not harm another person

Durable power of attorney for health care: an advance directive that allows a legally competent adult to (1) identify a surrogate decision-maker to make decisions on his or her behalf if he or she becomes unable to participate in decision-making and (2) state his or her wishes about aggressiveness of treatment and end-of-life care

Elder abuse: "any knowing, intentional, or negligent act by a caregiver or any other person that causes harm or serious risk of harm to a vulnerable adult" older than age 65 (National Center on Elder Abuse, 2003, p. 1)

Emancipated minor: a person younger than 18 years of age who has the same rights as an adult

Empowerment: the ability to enable or give authority to another; can also be a feeling of control over one's life and/or environment

EMTALA: Emergency Medical Treatment and Active Labor Act, commonly referred to as the "antidumping" law, "a statute which governs when and how a patient may be (1) refused treatment or (2) transferred from one hospital to another when he is in an unstable medical condition" (Garan Lucow Miller, P.C., n.d.).

End-of-life choices: decisions about preferences for how a person chooses to die

Errors: "the failure of a planned action to be completed as intended or the use of a wrong plan to achieve an aim" (Institute of Medicine, 2000, p. 28); an error is not an intentional act, but rather a deviation from the standard accepted way of acting

Ethical analysis: a way of thinking and a way of breaking down concepts and examining them in a context and from various perspectives

Ethical decision-making: the process of determining what ought to be done to resolve an ethical question, issue, or quandary

Ethical situation: a situation that involves an ethical question, issue, or quandary

Ethics committees: an interdisciplinary committee responsible for reviewing and providing ethical analysis and recommendations about a clinical ethics situation or a question on request

Ethics of care: a corrective emphasis to moral theory with origins in feminist thought that stresses the importance of paying attention to relationships and emotional commitments when trying to understand ethical duties

Eugenics: manipulation of the gene pool through laws regarding marriage and sterilization in an effort to eliminate "undesirable" hereditary traits

Euthanasia: "often called 'mercy killing' and has been taken to mean the act of putting to death someone suffering from a painful and prolonged illness or injury" (ANA, 1994a, p. 1)

Excuses: reasons proposed in an attempt to eliminate or escape the blame from someone or some action (Bok, 1999)

Fabrication: the presentation of data or information that has no factual basis

Fee-for-service: situation in which patients see the health care provider of their choice and authorize their insurance to pay the physician bill, hospital bill, tests, equipment, and so on

Female genital mutilation: ranges from removal of the clitoral hood to infibulation; female circumcision

Fidelity: an ethical principle that requires one to honor matters of trust and other expectations in a clinician–patient relationship

Futile treatment: an intervention judged as not achieving an ultimate goal, such as cure, and therefore as being of no benefit to a patient; for example, CPR in a dying patient may postpone death temporarily, and so is not futile in restoring vital signs, but will not ultimately prevent death; futility is a negotiated concept between the patient or surrogate and the health care provider

Gene: a sequence of DNA that specifies the sequence of amino acids in a particular polypeptide (Lewis, 1994, p. 369)

Genetic marker: "a detectable piece of DNA that is closely linked to a gene of interest whose precise location is not known" (Lewis, 1994, p. 369)

Genetic testing: molecular techniques for examining DNA for specific genes and/or gene sequences

Grievance: a real or imagined cause for a complaint

Harassment: continuous trouble or annoyance

Health care rationing: in the case that not enough resources are available to meet all health care needs, decisions made as to which health care services are provided and which needs will go unmet

Health disparities: differences in incidence, prevalence, morbidity, and/or mortality based on race, ethnicity, and socioeconomic level

Health Insurance Portability and Accountability Act of 1996 (HIPAA): federal legislation that mandates that certain employers continue health care coverage for employees who leave their employment; also requires health care providers to adopt national standards for electronic health care transactions and adopt security and privacy standards to protect personal health information

Health maintenance organization (HMO): a form of managed care; patients pay a monthly premium to the HMO and are required to go to providers within the HMO network and obtain prior authorization for utilization of health care resources

Hill-Burton Act: also known as the Hospital Survey and Construction Act of 1946; federal law mandating that hospitals receiving these funds cannot turn away patients based on ability to pay

Human Genome Project: a collaborative scientific project created with the goal of creating a map of all the human genes

Human subjects research: scientific experimentation conducted on humans

Illegal practice: actions taken that violate a local, state, or federal law

Impaired practice: a condition caused by drugs, alcohol, or mental illness that result, in "the inability to carry out professional duties and responsibilities in a reasonable manner consistent with nursing standards" (Smith, Taylor, & Hughes, 1998, p. 106)

Incompetent: lacking the ability to make one's own decisions, as adjudicated in a court of law

Incompetent practice: practice that occurs when a person does not possess or does not apply the necessary knowledge or abilities to meet the established standard of care

Index patient: a person with a suspected or confirmed disease who is the initial case reported to the health department; the index case may or may not be the source case

Infibulation: a form of female circumcision in which the labia minora and majora are removed and the remaining tissue is sewn together, almost completely covering the perineum

Informed consent: an ethical principle that requires that patients receive all pertinent information about their health condition and the options with risks, benefits, and alternatives for treatment and that they explicitly choose their own treatments

Institutional review board (IRB): an oversight committee that reviews a detailed proposal in which the investigators describe the purpose of the study, previous research, all procedures that will be done with human subjects, the potential risks and benefits, measures that will be taken to minimize risks, any alternatives to participation, copies of the consent form, all instruments, recruitment scripts, and advertisements, and the sponsor's project booklet, if applicable; approval by the IRB is required before the investigator can conduct the research

Integrity: demonstrated actions over time that consistently reflect a commitment to the person's or society's moral standards

Intersex: infants born with genitalia that do not clearly indicate the infant's gender (ambiguous genitalia)

Interstate compact: "the legal agreement between two or more states that enables nurses licensed in those states to practice in the other states agreeing to the compact" (Kulig, 2001, p. 51)

Justice: a fundamental ethical principle that requires that all people be treated fairly

Life-sustaining treatment: "Any medical treatment that is used to keep a person from dying. A breathing machine, CPR, and artificial nutrition and hydration are examples of life-sustaining

treatments" (American Academy of Family Physicians, 1999, p. 2)

Linkage analysis: testing that identifies the "location of genes on the same chromosome" (Lewis, 1994, p. 371)

Living organ donation: retrieving an organ, such as a kidney or liver segment, from a living person who has decisional capacity

Living will: an advance directive that allows a legally competent adult to reject death-delaying procedures in the event that the patient is imminently dying of a terminal illness

Lying: "a statement (a) that the speaker knows is false or believes to be false and (b) that is intended to mislead the listener" (Lo, 2000, p. 52)

Managed care: a form of health insurance in which the person pays a premium to a company or physician group practice in return for health care; intended to contain health care costs

Mandatory overtime: mandated work hours that exceed the nurse's budgeted hours; mandatory hours may be prescheduled or placed on an on-call list

Mandatory reporting: the legal requirement to notify the agency or person about a specific incident, usually suspicion or actual abuse and/or neglect

Maternal–fetal conflict: situations in which maternal conditions may jeopardize fetal welfare and health care providers cannot satisfactorily meet both maternal and fetal needs; a typical situation is maternal substance use or maternal refusal for Caesarean section when it is medically indicated

Mature minor: a child who has been declared mature by a court proceeding for the purposes of giving or refusing consent for medical treatment

Medical ethics: the ethical rules by which how physicians practice medicine and address the ethical issues they encounter in their practice; the terms "ethics in medicine" and "medical ethics" are interchangeable

Medical neglect: the denial of medically indicated care

Medicaid: health care insurance programs managed by each state to provide coverage for the poor and/or disabled

Medicare: the federal government program that pays for health care for people who are 65 years of age or older, on hemodialysis, blind, or otherwise disabled

Menopause: cessation of menses due to hormonal changes associated with aging, surgical removal of ovaries, or chemotherapy and/or radiation treatment

Mental health disorder (MHD): "a clinically significant behavioral or psychological syndrome experienced by a person and marked by distress, disability, or the risk of suffering, disability, or loss of freedom" (Johnson & Mohr, 2003, p. 3)

Moderate paternalism: limiting people's freedom from harming themselves, for example, via seatbelt and helmet laws

Moral courage: willingness to take a risk to advocate for a patient or correct a wrong or an injustice

Moral distress: emotional discomfort people (e.g., nurses) experience when they know the right action to take but are constrained from taking it (Jameton, 1984)

Morally neutral: when providing genetic counseling, not communicating a moral stance about the available options or judge the decisions made by the patient

Moxibustion: the heating of the skin at acupuncture points through the burning of dried leaves

Mutual recognition model: "the plan proposed by National Council of State Boards of Nursing that allows a nurse who holds a license in one state to practice in others without additional licenses (Kulig, 2001, p. 51)

Noncompliance: patient behavior when his or her goals are different from those identified by the health care professional

Nondirective: when providing genetic counseling, not giving an opinion about what action should or ought to be taken

Nonmaleficence: a fundamental ethical principle that requires that one not inflict harm on others

Nontherapeutic research: research that will not provide any direct benefit to the subject

Nursing ethics: the ethical rules governing how nurses practice nursing and how they address the ethical issues they encounter in their practice; the terms "ethics in nursing" and "nursing ethics" are interchangeable

Nursing process: a five-step process used to plan, implement, and evaluate nursing care; the steps are assessment, diagnosis, goals, interventions with rationale, and evaluation

Paternalism: an ethical principle derived from beneficence that obliges one to act for the good of another without consulting or heeding the expressed wishes of the other, which results in overriding another's preferences or freedom

Physical restraint: "any manual method or physical or mechanical device, material or equipment attached or adjacent to the client's body that he or she cannot easily remove that restricts freedom of movement or normal access to one's body" (Health Care Financing Administration; Medicare and Medicaid Programs; Hospital Conditions of Participation: Patient's Rights; Interim Final Rule; effective August 2, 1999; as cited in American Psychiatric Nurses Association, 2000)

Pedigree: "a chart showing the relationships of relatives and indicating which ones have a particular trait" (Lewis, 1994, p. 373)

Persistent vegetative state: a condition in which "a person is unconscious with no hope of regaining consciousness even with medical treatment. The body may move and the eyes may be open, but as far as anyone can tell, the person can't think or respond" (American Academy of Family Physicians, 1999, p. 2)

Peyote: a hallucinogen used in some Native American medicoreligious rituals (Shultes & Hoffman, 1992)

Placebo: an inert substance, such as a sugar pill or saline intravenous flush, that is presented as if it were an active medication

Preferred provider organization (PPO): a panel of providers who negotiate discounted prices for their services with companies; the companies in turn ask their employees to select a provider from the panel; less restrictive than an HMO

Presymptomatic diagnosis: testing to determine whether an individual has inherited the genetic mutation responsible for a specific disease before he or she manifests symptoms of the disease

Privacy: "That which is not open to or controlled by the public; of or concerning a particular person; that which is secret and not shared" (ANA, 1995, p. 6)

Promises: "a commitment to act in a certain way in the future, either to do something or to refrain from doing it. Promises generate expectations in other people" (Lo, 2000, p. 62)

Proportionality: an ethical principle that requires one to choose the action or option that produces greater good than harm or has the highest ratio of benefit to burden

Randomization: the procedure by which, in a clinical trial, all participants are given an equal opportunity for being selected or assigned to the control or experimental group, with the objective of minimizing bias in findings by having comparable groups

Reciprocity: in the nursing context, the situation in which "two states have a reciprocal agreement to honor one another's licensure" (Hall, 1996, p. 1999)

Recruitment: the process of identifying and, after informed consent is obtained, enrolling subjects into a research study

Research ethics committee (REC): the Canadian equivalent of an institution review board (IRB)

Resource allocation: the distribution of resources and services

Respect: an ethical principle that requires that one act in considerate ways and in such a way as to preserve the dignity of others

Right: a justifiable claim a person can make regardless of time or location; a right creates related obligations on the part of its holder as well as others to support and protect it

Scope of practice: "describes the *who, what, where, when, why,* and *how* of nursing practice" (ANA, 2004, p. 1)

Seclusion: "the involuntary confinement of a person in a room or an area where the person is physically prevented from leaving" (Health Care Financing Administration; Medicare and Medicaid Programs; Hospital Conditions of Participation: Patient's Rights; Interim Final Rule; effective August 2, 1999; as cited in APNA, 2000)

Sexually transmitted infection (STI): a communicable infection, which may lead to disease, contracted through sexually intimate contact, such as vaginal or anal intercourse or oral sex; some infections, such as hepatitis B, are considered sexually transmitted diseases even though they can be acquired through exchange of bodily fluids such as blood

Shared governance: a management model that empowers nurses and allows them to participate in decisions regarding issues that affect patient care

Single-payer program: a proposed health care insurance program managed by a single payer, such as the U.S. government, to cover the entire U.S. population

Staffing mix: the mixture of staff assigned to provide direct patient care; may include registered nurses, licensed practical nurses, and care technicians

Staffing ratio: the ratio of number of patients to each individual nurse or care team

Standard treatment: the usual and customary treatment

Standards: "authoritative statements by which the nursing profession describes the responsibilities for which its practitioners are accountable" (ANA, 2004 p. 1)

Sterilization: a procedure to render a person infertile, typically tubal ligation in women or vasectomy in men; with microsurgery, it is sometimes possible to reverse, but should be considered permanent

Substance abuse: "using alcohol or drugs to become intoxicated or using prescription drugs beyond their stated purpose" (Griffith, 1999, p. 20)

Substituted judgment standard: situation in which a surrogate makes the decision that the incapacitated adult would make using the adult's values and beliefs

Suicide: the act of taking one's own life

Supererogation: the act of seeking or producing good for others that goes beyond the moral obligation of the agent; such acts are known as supererogatory acts

Supplemental staff: additional staff assigned to a nursing unit to provide direct or indirect patient care; may include nurses (in-house registry, agency, or traveling nurses), care technicians, housekeeping or secretarial staff, or transport personnel

Terminal condition: "An ongoing condition caused by injury or illness that has no cure and from which doctors expect the person to die even with medical treatment." (American Academy of Family Physicians, 1999, p. 2)

Therapeutic misconception: the mistaken belief of a patient that although he or she is told that there may be no direct benefit to participating in research, his or her physician would not ask him or her to participate if the physician did not believe it would benefit the patient

Therapeutic relationships: ongoing relationships between patients and health care providers to achieve the patient's health goals

Therapeutic research: research that has potential to provide a direct benefit to subjects

Trust: the unrestricted certainty that another (person, agency, or even inanimate object) will always perform as expected

Truth: a statement or belief that corresponds to the reality

Truth-telling: verbal or nonverbal communication of factual information

Unethical practice: actions that violate accepted professional standards, such as the American Nurses Association's (2001) Code of Ethics for Nurses with Interpretive Statements

United Network for Organ Sharing (UNOS): the national system for coordinating the matching of organs for donation to individuals waiting for transplantation

Unsafe practice: "is more than a mistake: it consists of a pattern of practice that is dangerous to patients. It involves more than a single event or a single event of such magnitude that this incident shows incompetence" (Tranbarger, 1997, p. 33)

Universal coverage: a health care insurance program that could cover the entire U.S. population

Utilitarianism: a consequentialist moral theory that claims that the right act in any given situation is the one that produces the greatest amount of pleasure or freedom from pain for the greatest number of people judged from an impersonal standpoint and giving equal weight to the interests of each person

Veracity: an ethical principle that requires a "comprehensive, accurate, and objective transmission of information, as well as the way the professional fosters the patient's or subject's understanding" (Beauchamp & Childress, 2001, p. 284)

Whistle-blowing: an extraordinary action by which an individual goes outside of an organization's hierarchy to disclose illegal, incompetent, or unethical practices within the organization

Withdrawing treatment: stopping a treatment after it is started

Withholding treatment: not providing or initiating a specific intervention

Workplace violence: "incidents where staff are abused, threatened or assaulted in circumstances related to their work, including commuting to and from work, involving an explicit or implicit challenge to their safety, well-being or health" (International Labour Office, International Council of Nurses, World Health Organization, & Public Service International, 2002, p. 3)

References

American Academy of Family Physicians. (1999). Sample Advance Directive Form. Retrieved September 2, 2003, from http://www.aafp.org/afp/990201ap/617.html

American Academy of Pediatrics Task Force on Brain Death in Children. (1987). Report of the special task force: Guidelines for determination of brain death in children. *Pediatrics, 80(2)*, 278.

American Nurses Association. (1994a). Position statements: Active euthanasia. Retrieved September 3, 2003, from http://nursingworld.org/readroom/position/ethics/eteuth.htm

American Nurses Association. (1994b). Position statements: Assisted suicide. Retrieved September 3, 2003, from http://nursingworld.org/readroom/position/ethics/etsuic.htm

American Nurses Association. (1995). The right to accept or reject an assignment. Retrieved October 12, 2005, from www.nursingworld.org/readroom/position/workplac/wkassign.htm

American Nurses Association. (2004). *Nursing: Scope & standards of practice*. Washington, D.C.: nursingbooks.org

American Nurses Association. (2001). *The code of ethics for nurses with interpretive statements*. Washington, D.C.: Author.

American Psychiatric Nurses Association. (2000). Position statement on the use of seclusion and restraint. Retrieved April 16, 2005, from www.apna.org/resources/positionpapers.html

Beauchamp, T. L., & Childress, J. F. (2001). *Principles of biomedical ethics* (5th ed.). New York: Oxford University Press.

Bell, D. M., McDonough, J. P., Ellison, J. S., & Fitzhugh, E. C. (1999). Controlled drug misuse by certified registered nurse anesthetists. *AANA Journal, 67(2),* 133–140.

Bok, S. (1999). *Lying: Moral choice in public and private life.* New York: Vintage Books.

Breeze, J. A., & Repper, J. (1998). Struggling for control: The care experiences of "difficult" patients in mental health services. *Journal of Advanced Nursing, 28(6),* 1301–1311.

Conn, V. (2001). Working with individuals. In W. K. Mohr (Ed.). *Johnson's psychiatric-mental health* nursing (5th ed., pp. 135–150). Philadelphia: Lippincott Williams & Wilkins.

Ergil, K. V. (2001). Chinese medicine. In M. S. Micozzi (Ed.). *Fundamentals of complimentary and alternative medicine* (2nd ed., pp. 303–344). New York: Churchill Livingstone.

Garan Lowcow Miller, P. C. (n.d.). News about EMTALA. Retrieved February 24, 2003, from www.emtala.com

Griffith, J. (1999). Substance abuse disorders in nurses. *Nursing Forum, 34(4),* 19–28.

Grisso, T. & Appelbaum, P. S. (1998). *Assessing competence in consent for treatment: A guide for physicians and other health professionals.* New York: Oxford University Press.

Hall, J. K. (1996). *Nursing ethics and law.* Philadelphia: WB Saunders.

Institute of Medicine. (2000). *To err is human: Building a safer health system.* Washington, D.C.: National Academy Press.

International Labour Office, International Council of Nurses, World Health Organization, & Public Service International. (2002). *Framework guidelines for addressing workplace violence in the health sector.* Geneva: Authors. Retrieved May 14, 2005, from http://icn.ch/guide_violence.pdf

Jameton, A. (1984). *Nursing practice: The ethical issues.* Englewood Cliffs, NJ: Prentice Hall.

Johnson, B. S., & Mohr, W. K. (2003). Introduction to psychiatric mental health nursing. In W. K. Mohr (Ed.). *Johnson's psychiatric-mental health* nursing (5th ed., pp. 135–150). Philadelphia: Lippincott Williams & Wilkins.

Jones M. J. (1992). Cultural influences on community health. In. M. J. Clark (Ed.). *Nursing in the community* (pp. 280–341). Norwalk, CT: Appleton & Lange.

Kulig, N. (2001). Interstate licensure: Nursing beyond your state's borders. *Nursing, 31(2),* 51.

Ladd, R. E., Pasquerella, L., & Smith, S. (2002). Ethical issues in home health care. *Newsletter on Philosophy & Medicine, 291,* 196–197.

Lewis, R. (1994). *Human genetics: Concepts and applications.* Dubuque, IA: Wm. C. Brown Communications, Inc.

Lo, B. (2000). *Resolving ethical dilemmas: A guide for clinicians* (2nd ed.). Philadelphia: Lippincott Williams & Wilkins.

National Center on Elder Abuse. (2003). Frequently asked questions. Retrieved December 12, 2003, from http://www.elderabusecenter.org/default.cfm?p=faqs.cfm

Parker, J. G. (1995). Chemical restraints and children: Autonomy or veracity? *Perspectives in Psychiatric Care, 31(2),* 25–29.

President's Commission for the Study of Ethical Problems in Medicine and Biomedical and Behavioral Research. (1983). *Deciding to forego life-sustaining treatment.* Washington, D.C.: U.S. Government Printing Office.

Purdue University, Office of the Dean. (2003). Academic integrity: A guide for students. Retrieved September 29, 2005, from http://purduekelley.iupui.edu/academic/integrity.aspx

Shultes, R. D., & Hoffman, A. (1992). Plants of the gods: Their sacred, healing, and hallucinogenic powers. Retrieved September 21, 2004, from www.peyote.org

Smith, L. L., Taylor, B. B., & Hughes, T. L. (1998). Effective peer responses to impaired nursing practice. *Nursing Clinics of North America, 33(1),* 105–118.

Steinberg, D. (2003). The antemortem use of heparin in non-heartbeating organ transplantation. A justification based on the paradigm of altruism. *Journal of Clinical Ethics, 14(1/2),* 18–25.

Tranbarger, R. E. (1997). A nurse executive's nightmare: The rogue nurse. *Nursing Management, 28(2),* 33–36.

Index